LEADERSHIP
AND NURSING CARE MANAGEMENT

SEVENTH EDITION

LEADERSHIP
AND NURSING CARE MANAGEMENT

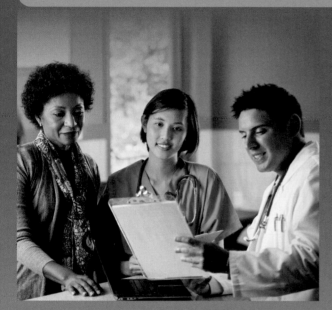

DIANE L. HUBER
PHD, RN, NEA-BC, FAAN
Professor Emeritus
College of Nursing and College of Public Health
The University of Iowa
Iowa City, Iowa

M. LINDELL JOSEPH
PHD, RN, FAONL, FAAN
Clinical Professor,
Director, Health Systems/Administration Program
College of Nursing
University of Iowa
Iowa City, Iowa

ELSEVIER

ELSEVIER

3251 Riverport Lane
St. Louis, Missouri 63043

LEADERSHIP AND NURSING CARE MANAGEMENT, SEVENTH EDITION   ISBN: 978-0-323-69711-8

Notices

Practitioners and researchers must always rely on their own experience and knowledge in evaluating and using any information, methods, compounds or experiments described herein. Because of rapid advances in the medical sciences, in particular, independent verification of diagnoses and drug dosages should be made. To the fullest extent of the law, no responsibility is assumed by Elsevier, authors, editors or contributors for any injury and/ or damage to persons or property as a matter of products liability, negligence or otherwise, or from any use or operation of any methods, products, instructions, or ideas contained in the material herein.

Library of Congress Number: 2020952283

Senior Content Strategist: Yvonne Alexopoulos
Senior Content Development Manager: Lisa Newton
Publishing Services Manager: Shereen Jameel
Senior Project Manager: Umarani Natarajan
Designer: Amy L. Buxton

Printed in India

Last digit is the print number: 9   8   7   6   5   4   3   2

CONTRIBUTORS

Kupiri "Piri" Ackerman-Barger, PhD, RN, CNE, FAAN
Associate Dean for Health Equity, Diversity, and Inclusion
University of California Davis
Betty Irene Moore School of Nursing
Sacramento, California

Mary Jo Assi, DNP, RN, NEA-BC, FAAN
Senior Vice President, Clinical Excellence Solutions
    and Associate Chief Nursing Officer
Press Ganey,
Dallas, Texas

Jennifer Bellot, PhD, RN, MHSA, CNE
Associate Dean of Academic Practice Integration
Jefferson College of Nursing
Thomas Jefferson University
Philadelphia, Pennsylvania

Michele A. Berg, MSHI, RN-NIC
Nursing Informaticist
Rush University Medical Center
Chicago, Illinois

Richard J. Bogue, PhD, FACHE
Associate Clinical Professor, University of Iowa College
    of Nursing,
Iowa City, Iowa
President, Courageous Healthcare, Inc.
Bryan, Texas

Debra V. Craighead, PhD, RN, CNL
Associate Professor, CNL Track Leader
Kitty DeGree School of Nursing
University of Louisiana at Monroe
Monroe, Louisiana

Laura Cullen, DNP, RN, FAAN
Evidence-Based Practice Scientist
Office of Nursing Research and EBP
University of Iowa Health Care
Iowa City, Iowa

Cindy J. Dawson, MSN, BSN
Chief Nurse Executive and Associate Director,
University of Iowa Health Care
Iowa City, Iowa

Bob Dent, DNP, MBA, RN, NEA-BC, CENP, FACHE, FAAN, FAONL
Vice President, Chief Nursing Officer
Emory Decatur Hospital, Decatur, Georgia
Emory Hillandale Hospital
Lithonia, Georgia
Emory Long-Term Acute Care Hospital
Lithonia, Georgia

Christina Dempsey, DNP, MBA, MSN, RN, CNOR, CENP, FAAN
Chief Nursing Officer, President for Clinical Excellence
    Solutions
Springfield, Missouri

Karen Dunn-Lopez, PhD, MPH, RN
Associate Professor and Director of the Center for
    Nursing Classification & Clinical Effectiveness
College of Nursing
University of Iowa
Iowa City, Iowa

Cole Edmonson, DNP, RN, NEA-BC, FACHE, FAONL, FNAP, FAAN
Chief Experience and Clinical Officer,
AMN Healthcare
Dallas, Texas

Michele Farrington, BSN, RN-BC
Program Manager
University of Iowa Health Care
Iowa City, Iowa

Ellen Fink-Samnick, MSW, ACSW, LCSW, CCM, CRP, DBH(s)
Principal/Owner, EFS Supervision Strategies, LLC
Burke Virginia
Adjunct Faculty: George Mason University
College of Health and Human Services Social Work
    Department
Part-time Faculty: University of Buffalo, School of
    Social Work
EFS Supervision Strategies, LLC
Burke, Virginia

Therese A. Fitzpatrick, PhD, RN, FAAN
Senior Vice President, Kaufman Hall and Associates
Assistant Professor, University of Illinois–Chicago
Chicago, Illinois

Betsy Frank, PhD, RN, ANEF
Professor Emerita
School of Nursing
Indiana State University
Terre Haute, Indiana

Mary Louanne Friend, PhD, MN, RN
Assistant Professor, Community Medicine and
    Population Health
The University of Alabama
College of Community Health Science/Rural Health
    Research
Tuscaloosa, Alabama

Kirsten Hanrahan, DNP, ARNP, CPNP-PC, FAAN
Director, Nursing Research and Evidence-Based
    Practice
Department of Nursing and Patient Care Services
University of Iowa Health Care
Iowa City, Iowa

Kimberly K. Hatchel, DNP, MHA, MSN, RN, CENP
Chief Nursing Officer
Blake Medical Center
Bradenton, Florida

Melinda Hirshouer, DNP, RN, MBA, MHSM
Director of Nursing, Cardiovascular and Neurosciences,
Texas Health Dallas
Dallas, Texas

Diane L. Huber, PhD, RN, NEA-BC, FAAN
Professor Emeritus
College of Nursing and College of Public Health
The University of Iowa
Iowa City, Iowa

Palma D. Iacovitti, DNP, MBA, RN
Program Director Surgical Oncology Clinics
Baptist MD Anderson Cancer Center
Jacksonville, Florida

Lisa Janeway, DNP, MSN, RN-BC, CPHIMS
Nursing Informaticist
Northwestern Memorial Healthcare
Resurrection University (Adjunct Faculty)
Chicago, Illinois

(Carol) Susan Johnson, PhD, RN, NPD-BC, NE-BC, FAAN
Founder & Principal
RN Innovations, LLC
Fort Wayne, Indiana

M. Lindell Joseph, PhD, RN, FAONL, FAAN
Clinical Professor,
Director, Health Systems/Administration Program
College of Nursing
University of Iowa
Iowa City, Iowa

Susan R. Lacey, PhD, RN, FAAN
Kitty DeGree Eminent Scholars
Professor and Endowed Chair for Nursing
Kitty DeGree School of Nursing
University of Louisiana Monroe
Monroe, Louisiana

Lyn Stankiewicz Losty, PhD, MBA, MS, RN
Contributing Faculty
Walden University
Minneapolis, Minnesota

Christopher J. Louis, PhD, MHA
Clinical Associate Professor of Health Law, Policy and
    Management
Boston University School of Public Health
Boston, Massachusetts

Joy Parchment, PhD, RN, NEA-BC
System Director, Nursing Strategy Implementation &
    Magnet® Program
Orlando Health
Orlando, Florida

Luc R. Pelletier, MSN, APRN, PMHCNS-BC, FAAN, CPHQ, FNAHQ
Clinical Nurse Specialist
Sharp Caster Institute for Nursing Excellence
San Diego, California

Beverly Quaye, EdD, RN, NEA-BC, FACHE
Assistant Professor
California State University
Fullerton, California

Veronica Rankin, DNP, RN-BC, NP-C, CNL
Director of Nursing Excellence—Magnet Program
    Director
Clinical Nurse Leader Program Administrator
Atrium Health
Charlotte, North Carolina

Barbara Seifert, PhD, LCSW, CPC
President/Owner, Committed to Your Success
    Coaching & Consulting
President, Elite Leadership Success Institute
Associate Adjunct Professor – Webster University
Adjunct Professor – Florida Institute of Technology
Orlando, Florida

Erin M. Steffen, MSN, RN
Assistant Nurse Manager, Procedure and Imaging Suite,
    Pediatric APEC
University of Iowa Stead Family Children's Hospital
University of Iowa Health Care
Iowa City, Iowa

Sandra Lynne Swearingen, PhD, RN, MSN, MHA
Director Leadership Development
Courageous Healthcare, Inc.
Bryan, Texas

Linda B. Talley, MS, RN, NE-BC, FAAN
Vice President and Chief Nursing Officer
Children's National Hospital,
Washington, DC

Diane H. Thorgrimson, MHSA, BS
Advisor to the CNO
Children's National Hospital
Washington, DC

Teresa M. Treiger, RN-BC, MA, CCM, CHCQM, FABQAURP
Principal
Ascent Care Management
Quincy, Massachusetts

ANCILLARY WRITERS

Stephanie C. Evans, PhD, APRN, CPNP-PC
Assistant Professor
The Houston J. and Florence A. Doswell College of
    Nursing
T. Boone Pickens Institute of Health Sciences
Texas Woman's University
Dallas Texas
Test Bank; NCLEX® Review Questions

Charla K. Hollin, RN, BSN
Allied Health Division Chair
University of Arkansas Rich Mountain
Mena Arkansas
TEACH for Nurses, PowerPoint Slides

REVIEWERS

Rebecca Davidson, PhD, MSN, RN
Assistant Professor of Nursing
Caylor School of Nursing
Lincoln Memorial University
Harrogate Tennessee

Kari Lynn Koenig, MS, RN
Associate Degree Nursing Program Director
Nursing
Northland Community and Technical College
East Grand Forks MN

Judy Kay Ogans, DNP, RN, CNE
BSN Program Director and Assistant Professor of
    Nursing
Nursing
The University of Oklahoma Health Sciences Center
    College of Nursing
Oklahoma City Oklahoma

Judith T. Pfriemer, RN, MSN
Assistant Professor of Nursing
School of Nursing
Arkansas State University
Jonesboro Arkansas

With the publication of the seventh edition of *Leadership and Nursing Care Management*, we start a new and exciting phase of incorporating Dr. M. Lindell Joseph as coeditor of the book. The history of this book began with the publication of the first edition in 1996, when Dr. Diane Huber wrote the whole first edition. She rewrote the whole second edition but invited chapter authors for the third edition in 2006, making it an edited book. The new phase means that a broader range of chapter authors were solicited, and there is double the editorial expertise. Welcome Lindell!

The development of the seventh edition occurred at a time of change and uncertainty in health care. This has reverberated within health care organizations and systems, in nursing professional organizations, and in the work life of nurses in leadership and administration. Hospitals and health care organizations are struggling with financial and workforce pressures. Nursing professional organizations, such as the American Organization of Nurse Executives (AONE) [now: American Organization for Nursing Leadership (AONL)] and the Council on Graduate Education for Administration in Nursing (CGEAN) [now: Association for Leadership Science in Nursing (ALSN)], have changed their names, as did the Institute of Medicine [now: the National Academies of Sciences, Engineering, Medicine, Health and Medicine Division] in 2016.

It is clear that nurses matter to health care delivery systems. Yet the United States is in the midst of a continuing and projected nurse shortage. Strong nurse leaders and managers are important for clients (and their safety), delivery systems (and their viability), and payers (and their solvency). Pressures remain to balance cost and quality considerations in a complex, chaotic, and turbulent health care environment.

Although society's need for excellent nursing care remains the nurse's constant underlying reason for existence, nursing is much more than that. Because nurses offer cost-effective expertise in solving problems related to the coordination and delivery of health care to individuals and populations in society, they have become a crucial linchpin in health care delivery and are highly valued for their clinical judgment. Nurses are well prepared to lead clinical change strategies and effectively manage the coordination and integration of interdisciplinary teams, population needs, and systems of care across the continuum. This has been increasingly important following implementation of the 2010 Patient Protection and Affordable Care Act (ACA), and nurses are needed to address care coordination and integration across the health care delivery system.

It can be argued that nursing is a unique profession in which the primary focus is caring—giving and managing the care that clients need. Thus, nurses are both health care providers and health care coordinators; that is, they have both clinical and managerial role components. Beginning with the first edition of *Leadership and Nursing Care Management*, it has been this text's philosophy that these two components can be discussed separately but in fact overlap. Because all nurses are involved in coordinating client care, leadership and management principles are a part of the core competencies they need to function in a complex health care environment.

Nurses need a strong background in nursing leadership and care management to be prepared for contemporary and future nursing practice. As nurses mature in advanced practice roles and as the health care delivery system restructures, nurses will become increasingly pivotal to cost-effective health care delivery, and research is bearing this out. This also is seen in the national trend to determine the most optimal organizational structure to effectively use and deploy large numbers of advanced practice providers such as nurse practitioners. Leadership and management are crucial skills and abilities for complex and integrated community and regional networks that employ and deploy nurses to provide health care services to clients and communities.

Today's nurses are expected to be able to lead and manage care across the health care continuum—a radically different approach to nursing from what has been the norm for hospital staff nurses. The COVID-19 pandemic in 2020 showed how critical it is to have nurses' expertise in care management. In all settings, including both nurse-run and interdisciplinary clinics, nursing leadership and management are complementary skills that add value to solid clinical care and patient- and client-oriented practice. Thus there is an urgent need to advance nurses' knowledge and skills in leadership and management. In addition, nurses who are expected to make and implement day-to-day management decisions need to know how these precepts can be practically applied to the organization and delivery of nursing care in a way that conserves scarce resources, reduces costs, and maintains or improves quality of care. This is the emphasis on adding value, innovation, and prevention interventions.

The primary modality for health care in the United States has moved away from acute care hospitalization. As prevention, wellness, and alternative sites for care delivery become more important, nursing's already rich experiential tradition of practice in these settings is emerging. This text reflects this contemporary trend by blending the hospital and non-hospital perspectives with an eye toward systems leadership and management.

PURPOSE AND AUDIENCE

The intent of this text is to provide both a broad introduction to the field and a synthesis of the knowledge base and skills related to both nursing leadership and nursing care management. It is an evidence-based blend of practice and theory that breaks new ground by explaining the intersection of nursing care with leading people and managing organizations and systems. It highlights the evidence base for care management. It combines traditional management perspectives and theory with contemporary health care trends and issues and consistently integrates leadership and management concepts. These concepts are illustrated and made relevant by practice-based examples.

The impetus for writing this text comes from teaching both undergraduate and graduate students in nursing leadership and management and from perceiving the need for a comprehensive, evidence- and practice-based textbook that blends and integrates leadership and management into an understandable and applicable whole.

Therefore the main goal of *Leadership and Nursing Care Management* is twofold: (1) to clearly differentiate traditional leadership and management perspectives and (2) to relate them in an integrated way with the evidence base, contemporary nursing trends, and practice applications. This textbook is designed to serve the needs of nurses and nursing students who seek a

foundation in the principles of leading and coordinating nursing services in relation to patient care, peers, superiors, and subordinates.

ORGANIZATION AND COVERAGE

This seventh edition continues the format first used with the third edition. The first two editions were Dr. Huber's single-authored texts. The edited book approach draws together the best thinking of experts in the field—both nurses and non-nurses—to enrich and deepen the presentation of core essential knowledge and skills. Beginning with the first edition, a hallmark of *Leadership and Nursing Care Management* has been its depth of coverage, its comprehensiveness, and its strong evidence-based foundation. This seventh edition continues the emphasis on explaining theory in an easily understandable way to enhance comprehension and is an easy-to-understand bridge to the evidence-based management practices from AONL.

The content of this seventh edition integrates leadership and care management topics with the nurse executive leadership competencies of the 2015 American Organization of Nurse Executives (AONE)/American Organization for Nursing Leadership (AONL). AONL has identified the evidence-based core competencies in the field, and this book has been aligned accordingly to reflect the knowledge underlying quality management of nursing services, thereby synthesizing theory, evidence-based management principles, and application exercises. This will help the reader develop the crucial skills and knowledge needed for core competencies.

The organizational framework of this book groups the 26 chapters into the following five parts:

Part I: Leadership aligns with the AONL competency category of the same name and provides an orientation to the basic principles of both leadership and management. Part I contains chapters on Leadership and Management Principles, Change and Innovation, and Organizational Climate and Culture, and Managerial Decision-Making.

Part II: Professionalism aligns with the AONL competency category of the same name and addresses the nurse's role and management of professional nursing practice. The reader is prompted to examine the role of the nurse leader and manager. Part II discusses the content areas of Managing Time and Stress, Role Management, and Legal and Ethical Issues.

Part III: Communication and Relationship Building aligns with the AONL competency category of the same name. Part III focuses on Communication Leadership, Team Building and Working with Effective Groups, Power and Conflict, and Workplace Diversity. These are essential knowledge and skill areas for nurse leaders and managers as they work with and through others in care delivery.

Part IV: Knowledge of the Health Care Environment covers the AONL competency category of the same name and features a broad array of chapters. Part IV encompasses Organizational Structure, Decentralization and Shared Governance, Strategic Management, Professional Practice Models, Case and Population Management, Evidence-Based Practice: Strategies for Nursing Leaders, Quality and Safety, and Measuring and Managing Outcomes. This discussion highlights the importance of understanding the health care organizational structures within which nursing care delivery must operate. This section includes information on traditional organizational theory, professional practice models, and the dynamics of decentralized and shared governance.

Part V: Business Skills aligns with the AONL competency category on business skills and principles and contains an extensive grouping of chapters related to Prevention of Workplace Violence; Nursing Workforce Staffing and Management; Budgeting, Productivity, and Costing Out Nursing; Performance Appraisal; Emergency Management and Preparedness; Data Management and Clinical Informatics; and Marketing. These chapters discuss the opportunities and challenges for the nurse leader-manager when dealing with the health care workforce. The wide range of human resource responsibilities of nurse managers is reviewed, and resources for further study are provided. The significant share of scarce organization budgets consumed by the human resources of an institution makes this area of management a key challenge that requires intricate skills in leadership and management. This section examines some of the important factors that nurse leader-managers must consider in the nursing and health care environment. Also in this section are chapters that build on organizational theory and demonstrate the importance of integrating organizations and systems with the current technology and theory applications, including data management and informatics, strategic management, and marketing.

The 26 chapters in this text are organized in a consistent format that highlights the following features:

- Concept definitions
- Theoretical and research background
- Leadership and management implications
- Current issues and trends
- Case Studies and Critical Thinking Exercises
- Research Notes

This format is designed to bridge the gap between theory and practice and to increase the relevance of nursing leadership and management by demonstrating the way in which theory translates into behaviors appropriate to contemporary leadership and nursing care management. Case Studies and Critical Thinking Exercises offer opportunities for synthesis, application, and active learning.

TEXT FEATURES

This book contains several interesting and effective aids to readers' comprehension, critical thinking, and application.

CRITICAL THINKING EXERCISES

Found at the end of each chapter, this feature challenges readers to inquire and reflect, analyze critically the knowledge presented, and apply it to the situation.

RESEARCH NOTES

These summaries of current research studies are highlighted in every chapter and introduce the reader to the liveliness and applicability of the available literature in nursing leadership and management.

CASE STUDIES

Found at the end of each chapter, these vignettes introduce the reader to the "real world" of nursing leadership and management and demonstrate the ways in which the chapter concepts operate in specific situations. These vignettes show the creativity and energy that characterize expert nurse administrators as they tackle issues in practice.

NEXT-GENERATION NCLEX® (NGN) EXAMINATION CONTENT

The National Council of State Boards of Nursing (NCSBN) administers the national licensure exam for registered nurses (RNs), called NCLEX®. In 2013–2014 the NCSBN conducted a Strategic Practice Analysis that highlighted the complexity of decisions new nurses make while doing patient care. That prompted the question: Is the NCLEX® measuring the right things? To answer this question, the NCSBN launched the Next Generation NCLEX® (NGN), a research project to determine whether clinical judgment and decision making in nursing practice can reliably be assessed (https://www.ncsbn.org/next-generation-nclex.htm). They have developed a Clinical Judgment Measurement Model and analyzed the current NCLEX® item bank for clinical judgment domain distribution. The conclusion was a need for more research and the use of new item types on the NCLEX®. The research and development continue. As this text goes to press, it is projected that a revised NCLEX® exam will be rolled out in 2023.

The imperative for nursing students preparing to take the licensure exam and for nurse educators is to move into high gear with preparations for NCLEX®'s assessment of clinical decision-making testing even as the new test is in the development phase. New item types include enhanced multiple response, extended drag and drop, cloze items, enhanced hot spots, and matrix/grid. Layer 3 of the NCSBN's Clinical Judgment Measurement Model is focused on patient care and how the nurse recognizes cues, analyzes cues, prioritizes hypotheses, generates solutions, takes actions, and evaluates outcomes.

Leadership and Nursing Care Management, seventh edition, is not primarily focused on individual patient care (one nurse with one patient), but rather on the leadership and management of patient care delivery and the work of nurses. The content is most directly aligned with Layer 4 of the NCSBN's Clinical Judgment Measurement Model (https://www.ncsbn.org/14798.htm): Environmental Factor Examples. There are eight Environmental Factor Examples: (1) environment, (2) client observation, (3) resources, (4) medical records, (5) consequences and risks, (6) time pressure, (7) task complexity, and (8) cultural considerations. Layer 4 is concerned with the context within which a nurse is making clinical judgments and taking action. This is the realm of leadership and management of patient care. For example, the environment,

situation, time pressures, resources, and cultural factors all have an influence on the nurse's clinical judgment and subsequent choice of action. The NGN focus is on what the nurse should do. This also applies to leadership and management in clinical practice.

Although NGN is still in development, and we are not informed as to how contextual/environmental content will be tested, we have addressed the NGN initiative in three ways: (1) ever since the first edition of *Leadership and Nursing Care Management*, each chapter has had a case study and a critical thinking exercise feature that promotes the analysis and integration of the application of the content and provides practice in managerial decision-making; (2) there is a dedicated chapter (Chapter 4) on managerial decision-making; and (3) as a new feature in this seventh edition, we have composed an NGN-type single episode case study for five selected chapters. Following the American Organization for Nursing Leadership's (AONL, 2015) Nurse Executive Competencies, which forms the broad structure of five parts of the content, the chapters chosen highlight the core of the five competencies: (1) leadership (Chapter 1), (2) professionalism/managing time and stress (Chapter 5), (3) communication (Chapter 8), (4) knowledge of the health care environment/decentralization and governance (Chapter 13), and (5) business skills/nursing workforce staffing and management (Chapter 21).

Students using this book may begin to prepare for NCLEX® (NGN) by using the NGN case studies. In addition, practice leaders or colleagues of future nurses can use these new case studies to foster their clinical imagination and model high-level thinking to help new graduate nurses prepare for NCLEX® (NGN).

LEARNING AND TEACHING AIDS

For Students

The Evolve Student Resources for this book include the following:

NCLEX® Review Questions, including rationales and page references

For Instructors

The Evolve Instructor Resources for this book include the following:

- *TEACH for Nurses* lesson plans, based on textbook chapter Learning Objectives, serve as ready-made, modifiable lesson plans and a complete road map to link all parts of the educational package. These concise and straightforward lesson plans can be modified or combined to meet your particular scheduling and teaching needs.

- *Test Bank* in ExamView format, featuring over 650 test items, complete with correct answer, rationale, cognitive level, nursing process step, appropriate NCLEX label, and corresponding textbook page references. The ExamView program allows instructors to create new tests; edit, add, and delete test questions; sort questions by NCLEX® category, cognitive level, and nursing process step; and administer and grade tests online.

- *Next-Generation NCLEX® (NGN)-Style Case Studies for Leadership and Nursing Care Management*: Four NGN-style case studies focused on Leadership and Management.

- *PowerPoint Presentations* with more than 650 customizable lecture slides.

- *Audience Response Questions* for i-clicker and other systems with two to three multiple-answer questions per chapter to stimulate class discussion and assess student understanding of key concepts.

ACKNOWLEDGMENTS

This book is dedicated to my children, Brad Gardner and Lisa Witte, and their spouses, Nonalee Gardner and John Witte, for their enthusiasm, caring support, and love. I am forever privileged that they are in my life. I thank them for the gifts of Kathryn Anne Gardner, Anthony James Gardner (A.J.), Logan Thomas Witte, and Olivia Morgan Witte. I love being Grandma to these wonderful people.

To my professional colleagues who inspired me and served as examples of excellence in nursing, I am grateful that you came alongside me and engaged in my life. I also am most grateful for my interdisciplinary health care colleagues who have taught me, role-modeled caring behaviors, and offered invaluable opportunities to learn and grow. To my nursing students, my thanks for being a source of continual intellectual stimulation and challenge. To all of you who have read and used this book, thank you. It is so very humbling and heartwarming when you mention this to me as we intersect on professional pathways. I am glad it is of use to you.

This book's first two editions evolved under the tender care of Thomas Eoyang, former editorial manager at W.B. Saunders Company, whose guidance, support, and caring were invaluable. To the editors in the Elsevier Nursing Division who worked so hard to facilitate everything related to the seventh edition, and to the excellent staff at Elsevier, a sincere thank you.

No acknowledgement is complete without an expression of sincere appreciation to Lindell Joseph for taking on the coeditor role. This textbook is truly enriched by your special talents. Together, all is better.

Diane L. Huber

My contributions in this book are dedicated to Dr. Diane L. Huber, an unbelievable mentor, colleague, and friend. I will always be thankful for her belief and support in my abilities. I am grateful to God, my mother Mary Madelina Joseph, husband Hector Guadalupe, daughter Geneva Guadalupe, cousin Caroline Norbal, aunts Albertha Corneille, Christine Corneille, Tenose Corneille, and Nicholina Felix, extended family members, friends, and Drs. Rose Sherman (Chief Editor of *Nurse Leader*) and Robyn Begley (CEO of AONL) for their ongoing support.

Recently, I had the privilege of observing the care management of my deceased nephew Kimani Joseph. During his battle with lupus, I observed many opportunities where the content in this book would have been useful. I hope that aspiring and current leaders could use this book as a resource to develop or improve care management practices.

I am truly honored and grateful to be the coeditor of the seventh edition of *Leadership and Nursing Care Management*. I am thankful to my colleagues who were invited to provide their expertise on specific content areas. Diane and I are hopeful that readers will find new insights for future leadership and care management practices. Once again, I am thankful to the selfless acts that Dr. Huber has demonstrated toward my personal and professional development.

M. Lindell Joseph

CONTENTS

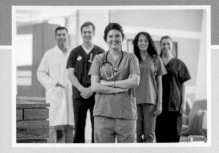

Leadership and Management Principles

Diane L. Huber

ⓔ http://evolve.elsevier.com/Huber/leadership

Health care is a challenging sector to lead and manage. Both the practice of health care professionals and the effectiveness of health care organizations are affected by change, complexity, and environmental turbulence. The twin skills of leadership and management are crucial to nurses' effectiveness and organizational survival. Fortunately there is an evidence base of knowledge about leadership and management, and both can be learned.

Issues of cost, access, methods, and structures of care delivery, human capital management, and quality surround the broader context of health care. The effect on nursing is an urgent need for leadership and management at all levels and places where nurses work. With approximately 3 million licensed registered nurses (RNs) in the United States (US Bureau of Labor Statistics, 2019), RNs are the largest segment of the health care workforce. Strong and prepared leaders are needed to guide their practice. Leading and managing are essential skills, made more acutely urgent given health care system characteristics of rapid change, complexity, and chaos.

Ongoing health care reform, integration of new technologies, and patient-centered care influence the health care delivery system by redefining both how care is delivered and the role of the nursing workforce (The National Academies of Sciences, Engineering, Medicine; Health and Medicine Division, 2020). Emerging care delivery models, with a focus on managing health status and preventing acute health issues, will likely contribute to new growth in demand for nurses as they assume new and/or expanded roles in preventive care and care coordination. An example is the explosion in the growth of roles for Advanced Practice Providers, including nurse practitioners. Supply and demand for nurses will continue to be affected by numerous factors, including population growth, increases in chronic conditions, the aging of the nation's population, overall economic conditions, aging of the nursing workforce, and changes in health care reimbursement.

Leaders guide and motivate nurses to achieve their care provision goals as they practice nursing. Managers organize and guide nurses' work in organizations where they practice. Together the result is structures and processes that deliver desired outcomes. For the health care system, there are two predominant sets of desired outcomes. The first is the six aims for the health care system (Agency for Healthcare Research and Quality, 2018): health care needs to be safe, effective, patient centered, timely, efficient, and equitable. The second is the Institute for Healthcare Improvement's (IHI) (2020) Triple Aim: health care needs to simultaneously improve the health of the population, enhance the experience and the outcomes of the patient, and reduce per capita cost of care to benefit communities. The Triple Aim has been extended to a fourth element ("Quadruple Aim") that focuses on the workforce and is aimed at improving the experience of providing care (Sikka et al., 2015).

The major national leadership initiatives in nursing are the Institute of Medicine's (IOM, now called The National Academies of Sciences, Engineering, Medicine; Health and Medicine Division) (IOM, 2011) report *The Future of nursing: Leading change, advancing health* and the Magnet Recognition Program® (American Nurses

Photo used with permission from FatCamera/Getty Images.

Credentialing Center [ANCC], n.d.). As nurses seek to embed themselves and grow in jobs and careers within health care services, leadership and management knowledge, skills, and abilities are important to overall effectiveness.

In nursing, leadership is studied to increase the knowledge, skills, and abilities that nurses need to facilitate clinical and administrative outcomes while working with people across a variety of situations, settings, and sites. Effective leadership can also increase understanding and control of nurses' professional work settings. *Effective* leadership is important in nursing, specifically because of its impact on the quality of nurses' work lives, because it functions as a stabilizing influence during constant change, and because it underpins nurses' productivity and quality of care delivery.

Nurse leaders and managers are responsible for designing, developing, implementing, and sustaining the organizational infrastructure and environment that enable both large- and small-scale interventions for quality and safety. Research has shown that there are organizational and cultural factors that mediate hospital or system-wide interventions. These include the prevailing culture, such as being patient-centered and having available effort and resources; human relationships, including leadership styles and teamwork; and an approach used for routine monitoring of systems and services (Clay-Williams et al., 2014; Stetler et al., 2014).

This chapter presents definitions and a detailed overview of both leadership and management. Theories are reviewed and important elements are discussed. There is a long history, rich literature, and evidence base regarding leadership theories, much of it from outside of nursing. Nursing has drawn from both classic and contemporary thinkers, especially from business management.

DEFINITIONS

There are a variety of definitions of **leadership**, one of which is the process of influencing people to accomplish goals. It has been described as "the art of motivating a group of people to act toward achieving a common goal" (Ward, 2020). Key concepts related to leadership are influence, vision, communication, group process, goal attainment, and motivation. Hersey et al. (2013) defined leadership as a process of influencing the behavior of either an individual or a group, regardless of the reason,

to achieve goals in a given situation. Leaders mobilize others so that they want to make extraordinary things happen (Kouzes & Posner, 2017).

Most leadership definitions incorporate the two components of an interaction among people and the process of influencing. Thus leadership is a social exchange phenomenon. At its core, leadership is about influencing people. In contrast, management involves influencing employees to meet an organization's goals and is focused primarily on organizational goals and objectives. Thus the leader focuses on people, whereas the manager focuses on systems, processes, and structures. A leader innovates; a manager administers.

Management is defined as the coordination and integration of resources through planning, organizing, coordinating, directing, and controlling to accomplish specific institutional goals and objectives. Hersey et al. (2013) defined management as a process of working with and through individuals and groups, using resources (such as equipment, capital, and technology) to accomplish organizational goals. They identified management as a special kind of leadership that concentrates on the achievement of organizational goals.

Followership is defined as "a process whereby an individual or individuals accept the influence of others to accomplish a common goal" (Northouse, 2019, p. 295).

LEADERSHIP AND CARE MANAGEMENT DIFFERENTIATED

Leadership theory is often discussed separately from management theory. Some say leadership and management are two very different things. Yet clearly there is overlap in that an individual can be *both* leading and managing simultaneously in some cases. The area of overlap may not be clear or explained. The premise of this book is that leadership and management are not identical ideas. This can be seen in their distinct definitions, yet sometimes they occur together or via multitasking. Northouse (2019) differentiated leadership and management on elements of activities and outcomes: management produces order and consistency; leadership produces change and movement.

If the delivery of nursing services involves the organization and coordination of complex activities in the human services realm, then both leadership and management are important elements. Both are used to accomplish goals; each has a different focus. Management is focused on task accomplishment, and leadership is focused on human relationship aspects. They may be sequential, and they are interrelated. Clearly, a balance of the two is necessary. Leadership and management have some shared characteristics. There is a "gray area" in which the focus of their outcomes overlaps. In this area of overlap, the processes and strategies look similar and may be employed for a similar outcome or blended together to accomplish goals. This overlap occurs where the two processes are integrated or synthesized to accomplish goals and where the same strategies are employed even though the goals may differ. For example, a nurse may use leadership strategies or management strategies to motivate others, but the desired outcome of the motivation is likely to be different. For example, leadership may be used to empower nurses and management to reduce costs.

Leadership and management are equally important processes. Because they each have a different focus, their importance varies according to what is needed in a specific situation. Hersey et al. (2013) thought that leadership was a broader concept than management. They described management as a special kind of leadership. This view would position management as a part of leadership, not as a distinct concept. However, according to the definitions, characteristics, and processes, the concepts of leadership and management are different; but at the area of overlap they look similar. For example, directing occurs in both leadership and management activities (the area of overlap), whereas inspiring a vision is clearly a leadership function. Both leadership and management are necessary. Leadership occurs in an interactive mode rather than through a stepwise linear process. The interactive nature makes relationships and relationship building fundamental elements. "Transformational change happens one relationship at a time" (Koloroutis, 2004).

Jennings et al. (2007) took an evidence-based approach to differentiating nursing leadership from management to identify discrete competencies through an integrative content analysis of the literature base. In 140 articles reviewed, they found 894 competencies, of which 862 (96%) were common to both leadership and management. Thus the overlap area appeared to be larger than previously thought. However, leadership and management do serve distinct purposes. Perhaps it is time to apply leadership and management

concepts and competencies by setting, level of role responsibility, career stage, and social context to more fully apply the evidence base to practice. For example, the American Organization for Nursing Leadership (AONL, formerly AONE) (2015) promulgated two levels of administrative competencies: nurse manager and nurse executive.

LEADERSHIP OVERVIEW

Leadership is an activity of human engagement and a relationship experience founded in trust, communication, inspiration, action, and "servanthood". The four essential dimensions of leadership are process, influence, group setting (context), and vision (Miles & Scott, 2019). Leadership has elements of process, personalities, power relationships, actions, transformation, and skills, all of which are designed to influence. Ideally, for effectiveness, styles are matched. Northouse (2019, p. 5) found five core leadership components: (1) leadership is a process, (2) leadership involves influence, (3) leadership occurs in groups, and (4) leadership involves common goals. The leadership role is so important because it embodies commitment and forward-reaching action. Arising from a drive to make things better, leaders use their power to bring teams together, spark innovation, create positive communication, and drive forward toward group goals.

Leadership is important to study, learn, and practice in today's complex, rapidly changing, turbulent, and chaotic health care work environment. Such an environment generates challenges to the nurse's identity, coping skills, and ability to work with others in harmony. It also presents the opportunity to lead, challenge assumptions, consolidate a purpose, and move a vision forward. Leadership is important for nurses because they need to possess knowledge and skills in the art and science of solving problems in work groups, systems of care, and the environment of care delivery. The effectiveness of an individual nurse depends partly on that individual's competence and partly on the creation of a facilitating environment that contains sufficient resources to accomplish goals. This is an underappreciated reality when it is assumed that results occur from only individual competence and effort. However, health care delivery is a team effort.

The nurse leader combines clinical, administrative, financial, and operational skills to solve problems in the care environment so that nurses can provide cost-effective care in a way that is satisfying and health promoting for patients and clients. Such an environment does not simply happen; it requires special skills and the courage and motivation to move a vision into action. For example, it may be easier to continue on the way things have always been done, but this strategy would not capture the advantages of new innovations. Thus the study of nursing leadership and care management directs critical thinking toward what it takes to be a nursing "environment architect," transition leader, and administrator of care delivery services.

Strong evidence for the nurse leader's critical role both in the business of a health care organization and in the quality and safety of service delivery can be found in influential documents by the IOM (2004), the ANCC's Magnet Recognition Program® (ANCC, n.d.a), and the AONL (2015). The IOM emphasized evidence-based management practice and focused on the following five areas of management practice:

- Implementing evidence-based management
- Balancing tensions between efficiency and reliability
- Creating and sustaining trust
- Actively managing the change process through communication, feedback, training, sustained effort and attention, and worker involvement
- Creating a learning environment

The ANCC's Magnet program acknowledges excellence in nursing services and leadership based on five components: transformational leadership, structural empowerment, new knowledge, exemplary professional practice, and empirical outcomes (ANCC, n.d.a). The Magnet Recognition Program® focuses specifically on nursing, is considered the "gold standard" in nursing, and is addressed in several chapters in this book because of its centrality to the evidence-based management

practice called for by the IOM (2004). AONL's (2015) nurse executive competencies are described as falling within the following five domains of skill: communication and relationship management, leadership, business skills and principles, knowledge of the health care environment, and professionalism. Taken together, these source documents overlap and converge on the primary attributes, knowledge domains, abilities, and skills that nurse leaders need to lead people and manage organizations in health care.

The Two Roles of a Nurse

Nursing is a service profession, the core mission of which is the care, restoration of health, and nurturing of human beings in their experiences of health and illness. This is the role of the nurse as a direct care provider. The nurse's care provider or "doing" role is sometimes seen as the most important and valued aspect of nursing. The nurse's second role, the coordinator/integrator role, is a complementary function that arises from nursing's central positioning in the day-to-day coordination of service delivery and central location at the hub of information flow regarding care and service delivery. This linkage relationship is shown visually in Fig. 1.1.

With the shift to primary care and care coordination, the nurse's care management role has become more prominent, needed, and valued. The delivery of nursing services involves the organization and coordination of complex activities. Nurses use managerial and leadership skills to facilitate delivery of quality nursing care. A current example is the shift to population health management (PHM), which is in concert with the Quadruple Aim. Nurses have emerged as well-prepared practitioners, especially at the clinical nurse leader (CNL) and nurse practitioner levels of preparation (Joseph & Huber, 2015).

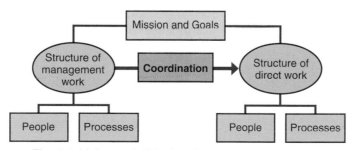

Fig. 1.1 Linkage of clinical and management domains.

The Leadership Role

Leadership is a unique role and function. It can be part of a formal organizational managerial position, or it can arise spontaneously in any group. Certain characteristics, such as being motivated by challenge, commitment, and autonomy, are thought to be associated with leadership. Effectiveness is a key outcome of leadership efforts in health care. It has been suggested that there is a scarcity of leaders and a crisis in leadership in nursing. In times of chaos, complexity, and change, leadership is essential to provide the guidance, direction, and sense of stability needed to ensure followers' effectiveness and satisfaction. Nurses are challenged to respond with leadership and can best respond by demonstrating vision, using innovativeness (Joseph, 2015; Joseph et al., 2016), adapting to changes, seeking new tools for dealing with the new health care environment, and leading the way with client-centered strategies. Effective leaders are change agents and promote innovation. Innovation is seen as a viable mechanism to address care delivery complexity and is further discussed in Chapter 2.

Leadership Skills

Leadership is a natural element of nursing practice because the majority of nurses practice in work groups or units. Possessing the license of an RN implies certain leadership skills and requires the ability to delegate and supervise the work of others. Leadership can be understood as the ability to inspire confidence and support among followers, especially in organizations in which competence and commitment produce performance.

Leadership is an important issue related to how nurses integrate the various elements of nursing practice to ensure the highest quality of care for clients. Every nurse needs two critical skills to enhance professional practice. One is a skill with interpersonal relationships. This is fundamental to leadership and the work of nursing. The second is skill in applying the problem-solving process. This involves the ability to think critically, identify problems, and develop objectivity and a degree of maturity or judgment. Leadership skills build on professional and clinical skills. Hersey et al. (2013) identified the following three skills needed for leading or influencing:

1. *Diagnosing:* Diagnosing involves being able to understand the situation and the problem to be solved or resolved. This is a cognitive competency.

2. *Adapting:* Adapting involves being able to adapt behaviors and other resources to match the situation. This is a behavioral competency.
3. *Communicating:* Communicating is used to advance the process in a way that individuals can understand and accept. This is a process competency.

Emotional Intelligence

Relational and emotional integrity are hallmarks of good leaders. Among the important personal leadership skills for nurses is **emotional** intelligence (EI). EI traits are emotional factors consisting of five defining attributes: self-awareness, self-regulation or discipline, motivation, social awareness, and relationship management. EI can be understood as a constellation of self-perceptions of the person's empathy, impulsivity, and assertiveness, also including elements of social and personal intelligence. EI is seen as an intellectual skill helping to understand and assess the meaning of emotions, to reason, and to problem solve. EI has a strong and positive impact on organizational climate. A positive organizational climate is less likely to contain counterproductive work behaviors or unethical dysfunctional organizational behavior (Al Ghazo et al., 2019). EI has been studied in nursing and shown to be related to transformational leadership (Spano-Szekely et al., 2016), nursing team performance and cohesiveness (Quoidbach & Hansenne, 2009), quality of care (Adams & Iseler, 2014), and as a moderator of **stress** and **burnout** (Görgens-Ekermans & Brand, 2010). Spano-Szekely and colleagues recommended that EI characteristics be considered during the hiring of nurse managers.

Adaptive thinking abilities are needed for leadership in the complex, volatile, and unpredictable environment of health care (Spano-Szekely et al., 2016). This is because the leader operates in a crucial cultural and contextual influencing mode within the organizational environment. The leader's behavior, patterns of actions, attitude, and performance have a special impact on the team's attitude and behaviors and on the context and character of work life. Followers observe and respond to all aspects of what leaders say and do (or do not do). Followers need to be able to depend on role consistency, balance, and behavioral integrity from the leader. The four EI skill sets needed by good leaders are as follows:

1. *Self-awareness:* Ability to read one's own emotional state and be aware of one's own mood and how this affects staff relationships

2. *Self-management:* Ability to take corrective action so as not to transfer negative affect to staff relationships
3. *Social awareness:* An intuitive skill of empathy and expressiveness in being sensitive and aware of the emotions and moods of others
4. *Relationship management:* Use of effective communication with others to disarm conflict and the ability to develop the emotional maturity of team members

Relationship Management and Relational Coordination

High performance, organizational health, and effectiveness are organizational goals. Relationship-based care has been proposed as a model for nursing care that promotes organizational health, thus resulting in positive outcomes (Koloroutis, 2004). Relationship-based care focuses on the care provider's three crucial relationships: relationship with patients and families, with self (nurtured by self-knowing and self-care), and with colleagues (commitment to healthy interpersonal relationships) (Creative Health Care Management, 2020).

Gittell (2016) emphasized the centrality of relationship management because patient care is a coordination challenge. She noted that relational coordination drives quality and efficiency outcomes and health care performance. Relational coordination is defined as "… coordinating work through relationships of shared goals, shared knowledge, and mutual respect" (p. 13). Relational coordination focuses on *relationships among roles* rather than between individuals.

Interpersonal relationship skills are crucial to the work of leadership. Leaders are pivotal for connecting the efforts of followers to organizational goals in order to produce outcomes. However, good leaders manage relationships and are anchors to the vision and the larger mission, guides to coping and being productive, and champions of energy and enthusiasm for the work.

BACKGROUND RELATED TO LEADERSHIP

Terms related to leadership are *leadership styles, followership,* and *empowerment.* **Leadership** styles are defined as different combinations of task and relationship behaviors used to influence others to accomplish goals. **Followership** is defined as an interpersonal process of participation: "a process whereby an individual or individuals accept the influence of others to accomplish a common goal" (Northouse, 2019, p. 295). **Empowerment**

means giving people the authority, responsibility, and freedom to act on their expert knowledge and skills.

Self-awareness is an important aspect of both leadership and followership. This means that nurses can assess themselves to better understand their own style and leadership characteristics. Self assessment tools are available to assist nurses in awareness of both leadership and followership behaviors. Examples are the LEAD instruments developed by Hersey et al. (2013), the Multifactor Leadership Questionnaire (MLQ) (Bass & Avolio, 2019), and multiple training instruments. Leadership related research instruments were identified, compared, and evaluated by Huber and colleagues (2000). Some instruments are useful for research and others for leadership training or self-diagnosis. A wide variety of tools are available to help individuals increase their effectiveness through greater awareness and subsequent honing of both their leadership and followership skills.

Leadership can be best understood as a process. Much attention has been focused on leadership as a group and organizational process because organizational change is heavily influenced by the context or environment. Nurses need to have a solid foundation of knowledge in leadership and care management at all levels, although the depth and focus of care management roles and skills may vary by level. For example, the clinical nurse care provider or direct care ("bedside") nurse concentrates on the coordination of nursing care to individuals or groups and is a leader and manager within his or her scope of practice. This may include such activities as arranging access to services, providing direct care, doing referrals, and supporting a patient's family.

Nurses without formal positional authority are **informal leaders**. They influence peers and administrators and function in an influence sphere within interdisciplinary teams. They have varying forms of power, but they are a part of the shadow organization that operates behind the scenes of the formal chain of command in informal networks of people and influence. They serve as advocates for the work being done and heighten the contributions of themselves and others through influence, relationship building, knowledge, and expertise. These nurses can be developed and empowered to affect unit performance and culture.

At the next level, the nurse manager concentrates on the day-to-day administration and coordination of services provided by a group of nurses. The nurse executive's role and functions concentrate on long-term administration of an institution or program that delivers nursing services, focusing on integrating the system and building a culture. CNLs and advanced practice registered nurses (APRNs) provide leadership in the care and care transitions of individuals and populations while providing expertise to the organization in specialty areas.

LEADERSHIP: FIVE INTERWOVEN ASPECTS

Hersey et al. (2013) noted that the leadership process is a function of the leader, the followers, and other situational variables. The leadership process includes five interwoven, connected but distinct, aspects: (1) the leader, (2) the follower, (3) the situation, (4) the communication process, and (5) the goals. Fig. 1.2 shows how these components relate to one another. All five elements interact within any given leadership circumstance.

Process Part 1: The Leader

The values, skills, and style of the leader are important. His or her internalized pattern of basic behaviors influences actions and the ability to lead. Leaders' perceptions of themselves, their roles, and their expectations also have an impact on their followers. Self-awareness is crucial to leadership effectiveness and is an EI skill. Among the internal forces in leaders that impinge on leadership style are values, energy level, confidence in employees, leadership inclinations, motivation for leadership, and sense of security in uncertainty. Interpersonal, emotional, and social intelligence skills also contribute to effective leadership.

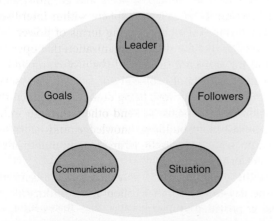

Fig. 1.2 Components of a leadership moment.

Self-awareness is an important aspect of both leadership and followership. This means that nurses can assess themselves to better understand their own style and leadership characteristics. Self-assessment tools are available to assist nurses in awareness of both leadership and followership behaviors. Examples are the LEAD instruments developed by Hersey et al. (2013), the Multifactor Leadership Questionnaire (MLQ) (Bass & Avolio, 2019), and multiple training instruments. A wide variety of tools are available to help individuals increase their effectiveness through greater awareness and subsequent honing of both their leadership and followership skills.

Process Part 2: The Follower and Followership

Followership is the flip side of leadership. It is likely that without followers there is no leadership. Followers are vital because they accept or reject the leader and determine the leader's personal power (Hersey et al., 2013). Followership skill is underappreciated. Grossman and Valiga (2017) suggested that leaders are only leaders if they have followers. Followership can be learned and consciously developed. Northouse (2019) differentiated followership based on roles or positions within an organizational structure versus based on relationships in an interpersonal context.

Types of Followers

There are several typologies that distinguish types of followers. Styles can be plotted along the two axes of passive to active and dependent to independent. Grossman and Valiga (2017) identified types of followers on dimensions of activity and independence: effective or exemplary, alienated, yes people, and sheep.

Understanding types of followers is as important as understanding types of leaders: it creates the ability to match leadership style to effectiveness in care delivery. Effective followers are an asset to be nurtured, developed, and valued. Effective followers contribute to success in organizations because they contribute motivation, enthusiasm, expertise, energy, innovation, and goal-orientation. Nurses can and should examine their own behavior and ask themselves the question, "In this situation, what kind of follower am I?"

There are types of followers, ranging from being vital to the success of the group to being passive and unthinking. Using the variables of performance initiative (high to low) and relationship initiative (high to low), Grossman and Valiga (2017) developed a grid of four followership styles: subordinate, contributor, partner, and politician. Effective followers show characteristics of assertiveness, determination, willingness to challenge ideas, an ability to act, and openness to new ideas. Followers also need self-awareness to know themselves and their expectations. Situations in which members of a group are not accustomed to working together or do not hold shared expectations frequently lead to conflict. Followership is based on trust. Groups have personalities that include a discernible level of trust. The wise leader assesses the trust and readiness to change levels of the group. Northouse (2019) discussed four typologies of followership. For example, Kelley's Typology plots active/passive and independent/dependent critical thinking into five types: passive, conformist, alienated, pragmatic, and exemplary. Other typologies plot dominance versus passivity, support versus challenge, and followers' levels of engagement.

Followership is not as simple as it seems. Followership can be assessed similar to leadership style and becomes a part of self-awareness (e.g., Followership Questionnaire in Northouse, 2019).

Leaders do not operate in isolation. Instead, leadership involves cooperation and collaboration. The basic nature of leadership is interactive; it revolves around the interpersonal relationships among leaders and followers. Therefore cooperation and collaboration between the leader and followers enhance the group's effectiveness. Although it may seem obvious, followership quality is important. There is a dynamic relationship between leaders and followers, and both are important.

Followership is an interpersonal process of participation. It implies an engagement of the follower with the leader, and possibly a group, by which the follower takes guidance and direction from the leader to accomplish group goals. The importance of followership is emphasized because leadership requires the presence of followers. The relationship between the leader and the followers defines leadership. The corollary to leadership is followership, which is helping to get the job done. A good leader clearly needs good followers, and this relationship is based on giving direction, trust, and hope. Kouzes and Posner (2017) noted that for people to follow willingly, they need to believe the leader is honest, forward looking, competent, and inspiring. With these three elements in place, followers are empowered in their participation efforts. Any situation can be analyzed to determine whether the desired leader attributes are present and to what extent.

Process Part 3: The Situation

The specific circumstances surrounding any given leadership situation will vary. Elements such as work demands, control systems, amount of task structure, degree of interaction, amount of time available for decision-making, and external environment shape the differences among situations (Hersey et al., 2013). For example, in acute care hospitals, staffing levels and policies strongly influence many aspects of a nurse's work life. Organizational culture and ethos are also important factors in the situation. For example, in one setting the culture may resemble one big happy family, with an emphasis on teamwork and morale boosting. The cultural aspects of that leadership situation are different from those of an organization where there is a fast-paced tempo and people seem too busy and/or in a bullying environment. Environmental or cultural differences also cause the leadership situation to vary. The leadership situation in a group that is knowledgeable and experienced in solving problems is very different from the leadership situation in a group that is not experienced at the task or at working together. The personality styles of both superiors and subordinates have an influence on the situation, the work demands, and the amount of time and resources available.

Process Part 4: Communication

Communication processes vary among groups regarding the patterns and channels used and the degree to which the communication flow is open or closed. Communicating is basic to the process of influencing and thus to leadership (see Chapter 8). Almost every issue or problem contains a communication aspect. Through communication, the leader's vision and message are received by the followers. After choosing a channel, the sender transmits a message, but the message is filtered through the receiver's perception. Communication is transmitted through both verbal and nonverbal modes. Organizations include a variety of communication structures and flows. These may be downward, upward, horizontal, grapevines, or networks. Communication may be formal or informal (Hersey et al., 2013). Certain acts performed by leaders have positive effects and make people feel more respected; listening and informal chatting are prime examples because they foster interpersonal and relational trust and social cohesion.

Process Part 5: Goals

Organizations have goals, and individuals working in organizations also have goals. These goals may or may not be congruent. For example, the goal of the organization may be to decrease costs or increase revenue. In contrast, the goal of the individual nurse may be to spend time counseling and teaching clients because that is what is seen by the nurse as the most important activity. Goals may thus be in conflict, in which case there is tension and a need for leadership.

Clearly, leadership is a complex and multidimensional process. Nurses need to be aware of the interacting elements in any leadership situation. Critical thinking can be applied to diagnosing and analyzing the five elements, adapting to the situation, and communicating for effectiveness. For example, if a nurse works in a situation in which there is a high level of frustration, it may be time to step back and analyze the basic five elements. Doing so sets the stage for better decision-making about change strategies and strategic management.

LEADERSHIP THEORIES

Leadership is so critical that it has been studied for a very long time, especially in the business literature. There are numerous theories and extensive research. The condensation here will highlight core concepts and common theories.

Leadership is fundamentally about the two basic elements of tasks and relationships. **Tasks** are the job aspects that must be done to produce the product (e.g., nursing care). Human **relationships** are the "people element": the interpersonal workings of humans in a job environment.

Hersey et al. (2013) have done a thorough overview of leadership and organizational theory up through the situational leadership school of thought. From an early awareness of the leader's need to be concerned about both tasks and human relationships (output and people) sprang a long history of leadership theories that can be grouped as *trait, attitudinal*, and *situational* (Hersey et al., 2013). The trait approach focuses on identifying specific characteristics of leaders. The attitudinal approach measures attitudes toward leader behavior. The situational approach focuses on observed behaviors of leaders and how leadership styles can be matched to situations.

Trait Theories: Characteristics of Leadership

Leadership theories have evolved away from an early focus on the traits or characteristics of the leader as a person because it was found that it is not possible to predict leadership from clusters of traits, yet interest remains in the characteristics to look for in good leaders. In the trait approach, theorists have sought to understand leadership by examining the characteristics of leaders, leading to multiple lists of traits proposed to be essential to leadership. One result was the awareness that leadership skills can be both taught and learned. It is important for nurses to recognize that they can learn, practice, and improve their personal leadership competencies.

Leaders are active, not passive. Leaders engage their environment with behaviors of doing, influencing, and moving. These are action terms that need to be melded with expertise and empathy. Leaders are those who talk about adventures into new territory and take the risks inherent in innovation (Kouzes & Posner, 2017). Leadership means giving guidance and using a focused vision.

Characteristics such as knowledge, motivating people to work harder, trust, communication, enthusiasm, vision, courage, ability to see the big picture, and ability to take risks are associated with important leadership qualities in research findings. Kouzes and Posner (2017) found that for people to be willing followers, the leader needs to be honest, forward-looking, competent, and inspiring. They identified the Five Practices of Exemplary Leadership that correlate with leadership excellence:

1. *Model the way*: Leaders set an example and structure events so that incremental progress is celebrated as small wins.
2. *Inspire a shared vision*: Leaders envision the future and enlist others in sharing the dream.
3. *Challenge the process*: Leaders go beyond the status quo to search for opportunities, experiment, and take risks to achieve lofty goals.
4. *Enable others to act*: Leaders foster collaboration and develop and strengthen others so that the whole team performs well.
5. *Encourage the heart*: Leaders appreciate and recognize individual contributions and formally celebrate accomplishments.

This model of leadership has been used in nursing research looking at staff nurse clinical leadership (Patrick et al., 2011).

Vision and Trust

Although the lists of leadership characteristics and competencies vary somewhat, the functions of visioning, setting the direction, inspiration, motivation, and enabling systems and followers are at the core of leadership activity. The one specific defining quality of leaders is vision: the ability to create a vision and put it into operation.

Leadership is founded on trust: "Trust is the emotional glue that binds leaders and employees together and is a measure of the legitimacy of leadership" (Malloch, 2002, p. 14). Organizations that focus on sustaining a healing culture rebuild organizational trust by focusing on trust in relationships with employees. Behaviors that build trust include sharing relevant information, reducing controls, and meeting expectations. Trust-destroying behaviors include being insensitive to beliefs and values, avoiding discussion of sensitive issues, and encouraging competition via winners and losers. Trust goes both ways and needs to be nurtured. Nurses can start by examining their own behaviors and then taking deliberative actions to strengthen trust in the environment.

Leadership Styles Theories

As leadership theories evolved, leadership came to be viewed as a dynamic process and an interaction among the leader, the followers, and the situation. Leadership theory began to move beyond a focus on traits to explore the concept of leadership styles. Styles of leadership range from authoritarian to permissive to democratic and from transactional to transformational. The individual nurse's task is to determine in which environments he or she functions best and is most comfortable

or where he or she most likely will succeed. This facilitates placement for success and a better match between leader and follower.

Leadership styles are defined as different combinations of task and relationship behaviors used to influence others to accomplish goals. They are sets or clusters of behaviors used in the process of effecting leadership. Hersey et al. (2013) defined these terms as follows:

- *Task behavior*: The extent to which leaders organize and define roles; explain activities; determine when, where, and how tasks are to be accomplished; and endeavor to get work accomplished
- *Relationship behavior*: The extent to which leaders maintain personal relationships by opening communication and providing psycho-emotional support and facilitating behaviors

Hersey et al. (2013) said that leadership styles are the consistent behavior patterns exhibited in influencing the activities of others by working with and through them, as perceived by those others. Different styles evoke variable responses in different situations. A leader's leadership style is some combination of task and relationship behavior. A style may range from democratic to authoritarian (or subordinate centered to leader centered) (Fig. 1.3). Schooley (2019) identified nine different leadership styles:

1. **Autocratic leadership:** The leader primarily uses directive behaviors. Decisions of policy are made solely by the leader, who tends to dictate tasks and techniques to followers. Leaders tell the followers what to do and how to do it. This style emphasizes a high concern for task. Authoritarian leaders are

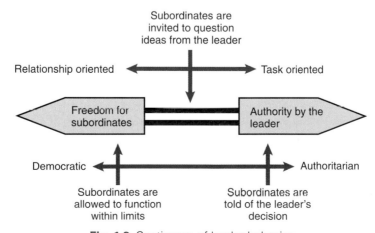

Fig. 1.3 Continuum of leader behavior.

characterized by giving orders. Their style can create hostility and dependency among followers; this may also stifle creativity and innovation. On the other hand, this style can be very efficient, especially in a crisis or during a code situation.

2. **Bureaucratic leadership:** Although not as strict as autocratic leaders, bureaucratic leaders tend to strictly enforce regulations and statuses in the hierarchy. They strive to maintain the status quo. They carry out policies and procedures. This leadership style can be effective in complex healthcare and safety environments or where there is high risk and stability is desired.

3. **Charismatic leadership:** Charismatic leaders have an infectious presence that attracts followers and motivates their team to follow their lead. Their likability helps achieve success. This leadership style can be effective in high-energy work environments that need a lot of positive motivation and team morale. The danger arises in following the "cult of personality" instead of using critical thinking.

4. **Democratic leadership:** A democratic leader often welcomes subordinate participation in decision-making. This approach implies a relationship and person orientation. Policies are a matter of group discussion and decision. The leader encourages and assists discussion and group decision-making. Human relations and teamwork are the focus. The leader shares responsibility with the followers by involving them in decision-making. In nursing, interdisciplinary teamwork is a major element in effectiveness. The democratic style may appear to move more slowly and is thought to take longer than using an authoritarian style. This is because group consensus needs time and facilitation to be fostered. Furthermore, the needs of disenfranchised minority groups must be balanced. Intergroup cohesion is a focus with this style. The challenge of the democratic style is to get people with different professional backgrounds, personal biases, and psychological needs together to focus on the problem and next action steps. Motivating participation is a constant challenge. This leadership style is often admired and can be effective in creative work environments that do not require quick decisions.

5. **Laissez-faire leadership:** Laissez-faire leaders have a hands-off approach and let their employees assume responsibility in the decision-making process, although they must still set expectations and monitor performance. This style promotes complete freedom for group or individual decisions. There is a minimum of leader participation. A leader using this style may seem to be apathetic. Because the style is based on noninterference, a clear decision may never be formulated. The laissez-faire style results in a decision, conscious or otherwise, to avoid interference and let events take their own course. The leader is either permissive and fosters freedom or is inept at guiding a group. Followers may need greater structure than the leader gives them. Despite its potential drawbacks, this style has advantages when used with some circumstances involving groups of fully independent care providers or professionals working together. This leadership style is seen as effective when working with highly experienced and confident employees.

6. **Servant leadership:** Servant leaders are those who share power and decision-making with their subordinates and direct the organization based on the interests of the team. Servant leaders put others first. They choose to make sure that other people's highest-priority needs are being served in a way that promotes personal growth and helps others become freer and more autonomous. This leadership style can be effective for humanitarian organizations, nonprofits, and teams that need to create diversity, inclusion, and morale.

7. **Situational leadership:** Situational leaders see the use of leadership style as situational or contingent based on what produces effectiveness. They first do a specific assessment of all aspects of the situation and then modify their style to match the situation based on the needs of their employees and the environment. Because of its versatility, this type of leadership can be effective in most organizations.

8. **Transactional leadership:** A transactional leader is focused on day-to-day operations and uses a reward/consequence system to motivate employees to achieve success or discourage them from failure. Transactional leadership is a social exchange (this for that). This leadership style can be effective for teams or individuals who are motivated by rewards or immediate needs.

9. **Transformational leadership:** Similar to charismatic leaders, transformational leaders use their inspiring energy and personality to create a magnetic workplace. They engage with others so that leaders and

followers raise each other to higher levels of motivation. The transformational type is often more effective than charismatic leadership, because it also is centered on the followers', not the leader's, needs and goals and motivates teams to build confidence, skills, achievement, and accountability. Transformational leadership can be effective in organizations with intellectual team members who thrive in interactive environments.

There is no one "right" style. Each has its strengths. Effectiveness comes from pairing leadership styles with organizational fit, timing, and needs. There are situational and contextual factors to consider when choosing a style. Styles should vary according to the appropriateness of the situation with reference to an evaluation of effectiveness. Flexibility is important. For example, if a nurse prefers to operate in a democratic style yet suddenly a code situation occurs, then the nurse must rapidly switch from a democratic to an authoritarian style. Some democratic leaders cannot vary their style sufficiently to handle crises. On the other hand, in a staff meeting, an authoritarian leader may be ineffective with a group of professionals and would need to be flexible enough to switch to a democratic or laissez-faire style, depending on the circumstances. The basic needs are for leader self-awareness and knowledge of the group's ability and willingness levels before examining the situational elements and choosing a leadership style. Self-awareness is key to strategically using leadership styles.

Feminist Leadership Perspective

Leadership styles appear to have a gender component. The feminist perspective on leadership was presented originally by Helgeson (1995a, 1995b). She identified female leadership as a web-like structure that is dynamic and continuously expanding and contracting. It is characterized by a concern for family, community, and culture. The inclination is for a democratic power style, and the emphasis is on the importance of establishing relationships, maintaining connections with others, and deriving strength from empowering others. By contrast, leadership approaches described by men, as a generalization, tend to be influenced by the military and participating in team sports. Men tend to spend their time on meetings and tasks requiring immediate attention, focusing on completion of tasks and achievement of goals. Women tend to focus on process; men tend to focus on achievement and closure. Women tend to be

more flexible and value cooperation, connectedness, and relationships. Exploring the feminist perspective on leadership is valuable in that it provides food for thought as health care organizations and the predominantly female nurses working in them struggle with not wanting to let go of the familiar hierarchical management style yet needing to reconfigure to the circular or web structure to be effective. It is not known whether gender differences are permanent characteristics or are culturally mediated artifacts that blur with time.

Reynolds (2011) explored the thesis that servant leadership is a gender-integrative, partnership-oriented approach to leadership, using the feminist ethic of care. Leadership is a system for organizing activity, and gender is a system for organizing meaning. Yet mainstream leadership theory has ignored gender-related aspects of power. Scholars of communication and leadership have identified the management of meaning as one of the significant acts of leadership.

Situational Leadership Theories

A group of leadership contingency theories posit that organizational behavior is contingent on the situation or environment. This means that which theory or style is the best all depends on the situation at hand. What is needed by the leader is diagnostic ability. The leader observes and analyzes which abilities and motives are present in the followers. With sensitivity, cues in the environment can be identified and used to make choices regarding leadership style. One choice a leader has is to alter his or her own behavior and the leadership style used. Personal flexibility and leadership skills are needed to vary one's style when the followers' needs and motives change or vary. The ability to diagnose, choose, and alter behavior to implement a leadership style best matched to the situation is a critical skill needed for effective leadership (Hersey et al., 2013).

In situational leadership theories, leadership in groups is never a static circumstance. The situation is dynamic and subject to change. In a very difficult situation, relationships may be the leader's preferred emphasis. However, if interpersonal relationships are not an immediate problem or if the group is on the verge of collapse, then strong authoritative direction is needed to get the group moving and accomplishing. For this situation, the task-oriented leader is a more effective match between leader and job. However, groups do not remain static; they move back and forth through stages. When the problem is no longer just the need to get the group moving but also includes solving numerous interpersonal conflicts, a relationship-oriented leader is better matched to the situation. Eventually, as the situation progresses, a relationship-oriented leader can become less effective. This occurs because once the group has less conflict, individuals may begin to coast along, and positive motivation may be lost as individuals become apathetic. Once again, a task-oriented style is called for to challenge individuals by using the motivation they need to continue to produce. Because of the factor of constant change, maintaining good leadership is complicated for any group.

The Situational Leadership® Model

The Situational Leadership® Model of Hersey et al. (2013; The Center for Leadership Studies, 2020) focuses on the interplay among three elements: the amount of guidance and direction (task behavior) a leader gives; the amount of socioemotional support (relationship behavior) a leader provides; and the Performance Readiness® Level that individuals or teams (followers) exhibit in performing specific activity, task, or job. Using a grid that results from task and relationship axes ranging from high to low, task behavior is plotted on the horizontal axis, and relationship behavior is plotted on the vertical axis. See the grid on The Center for Leadership Studies' (2020) website: https://situational.com/situational-leadership/. This makes it possible to describe leader behavior in four quadrants: (1) high task, low relationship (S1, telling); (2) high task, high relationship (S2, selling); (3) high relationship, low task (S3, participating); and (4) low task, low relationship (S4, delegating). As applied to the continuum of authoritarian versus democratic styles, telling would be authoritarian and participating would be democratic.

To choose an appropriate style, the leader needs to be knowledgeable about the Performance Readiness® level of the followers. This leads to the third dimension of effectiveness: the situation, or environment, which determines the effectiveness of a leader's behavior style (Hersey et al., 2013). Thus the difference between effective and ineffective styles often will not be the actual behavior of the leader but rather the appropriateness of the leader's behavior as matched to the environment in which it is used.

Found below the basic grid is a continuum of Performance Readiness® ranging from low to high.

The Performance Readiness® level of an individual or group is determined by both ability and willingness. The first consideration regarding readiness is the followers' ability. *Ability* is the demonstrated knowledge, experience, and skill that a follower brings to a task or activity. *Knowledge* is demonstrated understanding of the task. *Skill* is the demonstrated proficiency in the task. *Experience* is the demonstrated ability gained from performing a task (Hersey et al., 2013).

The other part of readiness is *willingness*. Willingness is the extent to which a follower has demonstrated confidence, commitment, and motivation to accomplish a specific task. *Confidence* is demonstrated self-assurance in the ability to perform a task. *Commitment* is demonstrated dedication to perform a task. *Motivation* is demonstrated desire to perform a task (Hersey et al., 2013). Both ability and willingness need to be assessed; then they can be plotted on the grid to determine readiness.

Hersey et al. (2013) combined the aspects of ability and willingness and showed them displayed on the grid in four levels of readiness: (1) R1: both unable and unwilling or insecure; (2) R2: unable but willing or confident; (3) R3: able but unwilling or insecure; and (4) R4: both able and willing or confident. The Situational Leadership® Model correlates the four different levels of Performance Readiness® to the four basic leadership styles. The result is a visual display and model that provides the opportunity for the leader to assess a follower's behavior and identifies a way to understand and select the leadership style that has the highest probability of effectively influencing a specific person for a specific task.

Thus at the Situational Leadership® Model's core, Hersey et al. (2013) emphasized the importance of the readiness of followers. Any leader behavior is predicted to be more or less effective depending on the Performance Readiness® of the followers that the leader is attempting to influence. The leader's chosen leadership style would have to consider where the followers are in terms of their Performance Readiness® level. The principles of the Situational Leadership® Model can be applied to a work group. The leader begins with assessment and analysis. Have the members worked together for a long time in the job, or are they new employees? The culture is more solidified in a work group that has worked together for many years on a unit. Using the Situational Leadership® Model, leaders (1) identify the specific job, task or activity, (2) assess current Performance Readiness®, and (3) match and communicate by selecting and exhibiting the appropriate leadership style: S1, S2, S3, or S4 (Hersey et al., 2013). For example, telling is an appropriate leadership style to use with followers who are at the novice level and with followers who are unable, unwilling, or insecure. An example is when a nurse is appointed as chair of a committee. The nurse needs to assess and then adapt his or her leadership style to match the Performance Readiness® level of the followers in order to be most effective.

Thus in this view of leadership, it is situational or contingent and concerned with what produces effectiveness. Hersey et al. (2013) noted that the common themes include the following: the leader needs to be flexible in behavior, able to diagnose the leadership style appropriate to the situation, and able to apply the appropriate style given the Performance Readiness® of followers.

Transactional and Transformational Leadership

Another way of looking at leadership is how leaders produce quantum results. The concept of leadership styles

broadened over time to include two types of leaders: the transactional leader and the transformational leader.

A *transactional leader* is defined as a leader or manager who functions in a caretaker role and is focused on day-to-day operations. Such leaders survey their followers' needs and set goals for them based on what can be expected from the followers. A transactional leader is focused on the maintenance and management of ongoing and routine work. Transactional leadership is a social exchange: one thing is exchanged for another, generally to accomplish daily work (Steaban, 2016).

A *transformational leader* is defined as a leader who motivates followers to perform to their full potential over time by influencing a change in perceptions and by providing a sense of direction. Transformational leaders use charisma, individualized consideration, and intellectual stimulation to produce greater effort, effectiveness, and satisfaction in followers. Transformational leaders grow and develop others by empowering them (Steaban, 2016). Fig. 1.4 distinguishes between transactional and transformational leadership.

The transactional leader is more common. This type of leader approaches followers in an exchange posture, with the purpose of exchanging one thing for another,

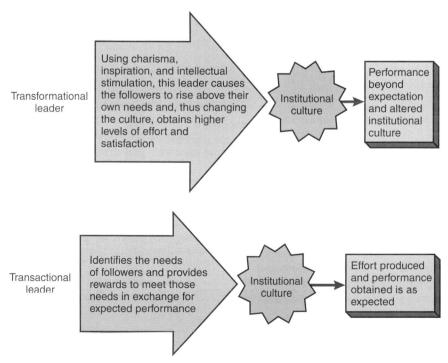

Fig. 1.4 Transactional and transformational leadership.

such as a politician who promises jobs for votes. Transactional leadership is about the exchange of valued things. Therefore transactional leadership is comparable to a bargain or contract for mutual benefits that aids both the leader and the follower. The transactional leader works within the existing organizational culture and is an essential component of effective leadership at the level of task accomplishment. Examples would be the exchange of a salary for the services of a nurse to provide care or when a leader offers release time or paid time to entice staff members to do project or committee work. Continuous or incremental change, the first order of change, can be handled well at the transactional level.

Transformational leadership occurs when persons engage with others so that leaders and followers raise each other to higher levels of motivation. Instead of emphasizing differences between the leader and the followers, transformational leadership focuses on collective purpose and mutual growth and development. Transformational leadership augments transactional leadership by being committed, having a vision, and empowering others to heighten motivation in a way that attains extra effort beyond performance expectations. Transformational leadership is used for higher-order change and to change the organization's culture. Circumstances of growth, change, and crisis call forth transformational leaders, and transformational leadership has been studied regarding successful change management (Deschamps et al., 2016).

There is nursing research to demonstrate the positive outcomes of transformational leadership. The American Nurses Credentialing Center's (ANCC, n.d.a) Magnet Recognition Program® has emphasized transformational leadership approaches. For example, the chief nursing officer of Magnet-designated organizations' transformational leadership style has been shown to have a positive impact on the work environment (Buck & Doucette, 2015). Transformational leadership was the type of leadership most often reported in early Magnet research studies (Upenieks, 2003a; 2003b). A transformational leadership style has been shown to generate greater follower commitment, follower satisfaction, and overall effectiveness (Kleinman, 2004). In nursing homes, the most transformative style of top managers (consensus managers) was found to be associated with better quality outcomes (Castle & Decker, 2011). Deschamps et al. (2016) found that leadership is an important factor in implementing changes, but justice is also a crucial factor. The positive impact of transformational leadership is mediated by organizational justice.

Transformational leaders have been shown to have an impact on both organizations and individuals. Organizational impacts include increased organizational citizenship, stronger organizational culture, and clearer organizational vision (Thomson et al., 2016). Improvements in outcomes for individuals, including empowerment, job satisfaction, commitment, trust, self-efficiency, beliefs, and motivation, have also been linked to transformational leadership (Givens, 2008). Transformational leadership is also associated with a decrease in staff turnover (Weberg, 2010). Overall, transformational leadership qualities appear to be better suited to the work of professionals and important for leadership in nursing.

CONTEMPORARY LEADERSHIP: INTERACTIONAL AND RELATIONSHIP-BASED

In this information age there has been a metamorphosis in health care organizations as they transform into knowledge or learning organizations. Nurses are knowledge workers who use expertise and specialized knowledge in the care of patients. They need matching organizational structures that will value, nurture, and foster the acquisition of the data, information, and knowledge needed for effectiveness. Today's health care environments demand that frontline workers such as nurses have and maintain the expertise and have the information necessary (e.g., evidence-based practice) to take action to solve problems. They need leadership that is interactional, relational, and transformational at all levels.

Arising in conjunction with the application of complexity theory and chaos theory (as discussed under Contemporary Management Theories), leadership was described by Wheatley (2006) as having important elements of connectedness and relationships within self-organizing systems. Nursing has a natural niche within interactional and relationship leadership theories. Optimal health care delivery is truly interdisciplinary, holistic, and highly team based. When connections and relationships are strong, patients benefit. Contemporary definitions of leadership describe leadership as being the result of a relationship between leaders and followers where a distinct set of competencies is used to allow the relationship to achieve shared goals. This is complex and requires nurses to be creative and flexible. It is proposed that "quantum" leadership is needed to produce results in today's health care environment. Quantum leadership is about discovering using an ongoing process of exploration, curiosity, and asking questions. Driven by organizational stress and the feeling that something more and different in work life is needed, quantum leadership is one type of leadership strategy that helps nurses focus on the future, stretch and break boundaries, and encourage breakthrough thinking to solve problems in a complex and fluid care environment. Quantum approaches build on feminist and transformational leadership perspectives and dive more deeply into the behavioral, relational, and interactional elements that form the activities and functions of a leader. Innovation is desired and encouraged.

Complexity Leadership

Traditional leadership theories were developed during the industrial era and describe traits, situations, and a role with power concentrated in a position in the organization. The focus is on maximizing production and reducing variance. Linear models assume input will yield a proportional output (linear processes). Weberg (2012) argued that a focus on linear systems requires management, not leadership, because it removes the capacity for the system to change and innovate. Using complexity science principles and systems thinking, Weberg advocated for complexity leadership because it gives a context for organizational operations whereby the behaviors of leadership foster interaction, increase network strength, and generate stability in order to create the energy for constant change, growth, and adaptation. Interconnectedness and change become normal operating conditions. Complexity leadership is a type of leadership "based on adaptive capacity, understanding the external environment and connecting with the internal organizational culture and thriving in situations where groups need to learn their way out of unpredictable problems" (Weberg, 2012, p. 271). In health care, this will require a shift toward complexity behaviors that embrace complex systems and continually search for value-added innovations. Leaders need to develop innovation competence.

Servant Leadership

Another popular contemporary leadership concept is called *servant leadership*. Greenleaf (2002) originally used the term to describe leaders who choose first to serve others and then to be a leader, as opposed to those who are leaders first (often because of a power drive or need to acquire material possessions) and later choose to serve. When applied to health care, servant leadership is an attractive alternative to the traditional bureaucratic environment experienced by nurses. The servant leadership model draws attention to the necessity for leaders to be attentive to the needs of others and is a model that enhances the personal growth of nurses, improves the quality of care, values teamwork, and promotes personal involvement and caring behavior. Reynolds (2011) melded the feminist and servant leadership perspectives, calling servant leadership gender-integrative leadership that values equally the masculine and feminine dualities, qualities, activities, and behaviors. Hanse et al. (2016) studied the impact of servant leadership dimensions on leader–member exchange among health care professionals and found that servant leadership dimensions are likely to help develop stronger exchange relationships between nurse managers and individual subordinates. A servant leader culture involves interpersonal interaction and promotes strong relationships and trust between leaders and followers.

Authentic Leadership

Following from the IHI's Triple Aim and moving to the Quadruple Aim, focus has now turned to the importance of employees thriving in organizations for organizational performance. Thriving at work is defined as a state where individuals at work experience both a sense of vitality and a sense of learning (Mortier et al., 2016) and is an aspect of work life and nurse vitality. Mortier and colleagues found that nurse managers' authentic leadership enhances nurse thriving.

Authentic leadership was described by Avolio and Gardner (2005) as a leadership style rooted in the concept of authenticity ("to thine own self be true"), where the leader is a fully functioning person in tune with themselves and their basic nature, self-actualizing, and having strong ethical convictions. Authentic leaders are "those who are deeply aware of how they think and behave and are perceived by others as being aware of their own and others' values/moral perspectives, knowledge, and strengths; aware of the context in which they operate; and who are confident, hopeful, optimistic, resilient, and of high moral character" (Avolio & Gardner, 2005, p. 321).

There are four aspects of authentic leadership:

- Self-awareness: how the leaders perceive themselves in comparison with the world and with their understanding of their own strengths and weaknesses
- An internal moral perspective: leaders align their beliefs with their actions and are not often persuaded by external pressures
- Balanced processing: their decision-making is based on analyses of all relevant data, being positive or confirming information or negative clues
- Relational transparency: how openly the leader presents him- or herself to others

The authentic leadership style is seen as fair and supportive and one that provides a healthier and more ethical work environment (Avolio & Gardner 2005; Mortier et al., 2016). This style has been studied in nursing and shown to have a positive effect on nurse job satisfaction and performance (Wong & Laschinger, 2013).

Clinical Leadership

All nurses in all positions exhibit leadership. For example, the "bedside" nurse uses informal leadership to influence high quality care delivery. Mannix et al. (2013) used an integrative review of literature on clinical leadership to elicit defining attributes of contemporary clinical leadership in nursing. The technical and practical skills necessary for competent clinical practice and leading a team emerged. The data were grouped into three categories of clinical leadership with either a clinical, follower/team, or personal qualities focus. "Clinical leaders who demonstrate clinical competence, possess effective communication and are supportive of colleagues have been linked to building healthy workplaces" (Mannix et al., 2013, p. 19). For example, one staff nurse who worked on a surgical and neuroscience intensive care unit recognized that there was incomplete and incorrect spinal cord injury/surgical patient assessment and documentation, which is critical when a patient's condition declines so that the degree of change is known. She took the initiative and contacted the nurse manager, invited other staff nurses to join her, set up a small committee, updated and simplified the assessment tool, and led the education of the staff on the revised tool with positive outcomes. This is clinical leadership.

There is a renewed focus on clinical leadership models at the point of care. Typically aimed at a hospital unit where care is delivered, the crucial role played by nurses in quality, safety, care coordination, and related aims of the IOM and IHI are the centerpiece. Nursing roles of care coordinator, CNL, and APRN have emerged and show continued growth. Joseph and Huber (2015, p. 56) defined clinical leadership as "the process of influencing point-of-care innovation and improvement in both organizational processes and individual care practices to achieve quality and safety of care outcomes." Patrick et al. (2011) viewed every registered staff nurse as a clinical leader and used Kouzes and Posner (2017) model of transformational leadership as a framework to describe and measure clinical leadership practices. Their review of literature identified five key aspects of clinical leadership: clinical expertise, effective communication, collaboration, coordination, and interpersonal understanding. Empowering work environments create a supportive structure for staff nurses as clinical leaders to achieve the best outcomes of care. "Clinical leadership uses the skills of the RN and adds components of general leadership skills, skills in management of care delivery at the point of care, and focused skills in using evidence-based practice for problem solving and outcomes management. There is clearly a need for clinical leadership in nursing because of the many and varied point-of-care implementation problems that arise" (Joseph & Huber, 2015, p. 56).

EFFECTIVE LEADERSHIP

Effective leadership is an integrated blend of leadership principles and characteristics with management principles and techniques. Nurses can grow such skills by knowledge and awareness (e.g., through assessment tools) and then may put knowledge and skills to work through guided exercises and mentored experiences. This is especially true for succession planning and the development of nurse managers (Mackoff et al., 2013).

Leadership effectiveness is based on the ability to adapt in a complex and chaotic environment. Adaptive problems arise from change and chaos and are often systems problems that affect people, planning, institutional operations, or work processes. Effective leaders first have strong self-awareness of their leadership strengths and weaknesses as well as preferred or most comfortable leadership styles and flexibility. Then they expand this to a grasp of themselves, their team, their goals, nursing and health care, and important evaluative data for "dashboards." They use their personal style, vision, and energy to focus on goal attainment and group satisfaction. Starting with whatever natural talent a nurse possesses, essential leadership skills can be practiced over time for greater effectiveness. Effective leadership uses empowerment. For nurses, empowering means that the power over clinical practice decisions is invested in staff nurses, enabling them to do what they do best and make decisions related to their practice. This process is similar to nurses empowering clients. Leadership involves elements of vigor and vision and can be understood as a dynamic combination of competence, willingness to take responsibility, and strength of character to do what is right because it is the right thing to do. See Chapter 10 for further discussion of sources of power.

MANAGEMENT OVERVIEW

Along with an array of opportunities such as instantaneous communication across vast distances, health care organizations and the people in them struggle with an ever-accelerating rate of change, knowledge explosion, technology, and information flow. The recruitment, development, deployment, motivation, and leveraging of human capital (nurses) as scarce resources and prime assets are critical management issues for service industries in general and specifically for nursing and health care. At the core, managers manage people and organizations. People's time and effort—as well as organizations' money, facilities, and supplies—need to be directed in a coordinated effort to achieve best results and meet objectives. Managers focus on the needs of the organization and on getting the work done.

Because nurses are the central hub of care delivery and information flow, it is helpful to think of the work of nurses as having both care delivery and care coordination aspects. Although the coordination of care has always been a key nursing function, it is becoming more visible and valued in health care and as nurses assume care coordination roles that focus on integrating clinical care. However, the relative proportion of the nurse's role that is devoted to management and coordination functions varies within nursing according to the job category. Nurse managers balance two competing needs: the needs of the staff related to growth, efficiency, motivation, morale, and accomplishment with the outcome of staff satisfaction and the needs of the employer for productivity, quality, and cost effectiveness with the outcome of productivity.

DEFINITIONS

Management is defined as the process of coordination and integration of resources through activities of planning, organizing, coordinating, directing, and controlling to accomplish specific institutional goals and objectives. Management has been viewed as an art and a science related to planning and directing both human effort and scarce resources to attain established organizational goals and objectives.

Management, then, applies to organizations. The definition of leadership emphasizes actions that influence toward group goals; the definition of management focuses on organizational goals. The achievement of organizational goals through leadership and manipulation of the environment is management. In a systems approach to management, the inputs would be represented by human resources and physical and technical resources. The outputs would be the realization of goals through task accomplishment, culture development, removal of barriers, and efficiency optimization.

Thus management is a separate function with a specific purpose and related roles but one that is focused on organizations and operations. It is associated with important day-to-day functions geared toward maintenance and stability and associated with transactional leadership or "doing things right" via task accomplishment. To achieve organizational goals, managers are involved in activities such as analyzing issues, establishing goals and objectives, mapping out work plans, organizing assets and supplies, developing and motivating people, communicating, managing technology, handling change and conflict, measurement, analysis, and evaluation. Without talent and attention to these functions, effectiveness and morale drop. This affects quality. In addition, it is important to do the background work needed to keep the organization functioning ("making the trains run on time") so that services are delivered seamlessly. Effective managers are thought to be those who can weave strategy, execution, discipline, inspiration, and leadership together as they unite an organization toward achieving its goals.

BACKGROUND: THE MANAGEMENT PROCESS

Drucker (2004) suggested that effective executives do not need to be leaders. "Great managers may be charismatic or dull, generous or tightfisted, visionary or numbers oriented. But every effective executive follows eight simple practices" (Drucker, 2004, p. 59). These eight practices are divided into the following three categories:

A. Practices That Give Executives the Knowledge They Need
  1. They asked: "What needs to be done?"
  2. They asked: "What is right for the enterprise?"
B. Practices That Help Executives Convert Knowledge to Action
  3. They developed action plans.
  4. They took responsibility for decisions.
  5. They took responsibility for communicating.
  6. They were focused on opportunities, not problems.
C. Practices That Ensure That the Whole Organization Feels Responsible and Accountable
  7. They ran productive meetings.
  8. They thought and said "we" not "I."

Effective management also appears to be a result of artful balancing, because managers need to function at the point at which reflective thinking combines with practical doing. This is described as managerial mind-sets within the bounds of management practice. Managers interpret and deal with their world from the following five perspectives (Gosling & Mintzberg, 2003):

1. *Reflective mind-set*: Managing self
2. *Analytic mind-set*: Managing organizations
3. *Worldly mind-set*: Managing context
4. *Collaborative mind-set*: Managing relationships
5. *Action mind-set*: Managing change

These five mind-sets were described as being like threads for the manager to weave. The process is as follows: analyze, act, reflect, act, collaborate, reanalyze, articulate new insights, and act again.

Management is central to the work of nursing. **Nursing management** is defined as the coordination and integration of nursing resources by applying the management process to accomplish nursing care and service goals and objectives.

It is important to recognize that managers perform unique and discrete functions: they plan, organize, coordinate, and control. Nurses work to deliver care (produce the product); managers manage organizations toward goal achievement. Someone needs to monitor financial indicators; hire, train, and evaluate personnel; improve quality; coordinate work and effort; fix systems problems; and ensure that goals are met. In nursing, this means that nurses do the work of providing nursing care while nurse managers coordinate and integrate the work of individual nurses with the larger system and solve problems for them so they can deliver high quality care. These are distinctly different activities.

The four steps of the management process are planning, organizing, directing/leading, and controlling. These functions make up the scope of a manager's major effort. Planning involves determining the long-term and short-term objectives and the corresponding actions that must be taken. Organizing means mobilizing human and material resources to accomplish what is needed. Directing/leading relates to methods of motivating, guiding, and leading people through work processes. Controlling has a specific meaning closer to the monitoring and evaluating actions that are familiar to nurses. The management process can be compared with an orchestra performing a concert or a team playing a football game. There is a plan and an organized group of players. A director manages the performance and controls the outcome by making corrections and adjustments along the way but does not play an instrument or a position. The management process is a rational, logical process based on problem-solving principles.

Planning

Planning is the managerial function of selecting priorities, results, and methods to achieve results; setting the direction for a system; and then guiding the system. It is decision-making and determining courses of action. **Planning** is defined as "[a] basic management function involving formulation of one or more detailed plans to achieve optimum balance of needs or demands with the available resources. The planning process (1) identifies the goals or objectives to be achieved, (2) formulates strategies to achieve them, (3) arranges or creates the means required, and (4) implements, directs, and monitors all steps in their proper sequence" (BusinessDictionary.com, 2020a). Planning can be detailed, specific, and rigid, or it can be broad, general, and flexible. Planning is deciding in advance what is to be done and when, by whom, and how it is to be done. It is traditionally thought of as a linear process. Hersey et al. (2013) described planning as involving the setting of goals and objectives and developing "work maps" to show how they are to be accomplished. Planning activities include identifying goals, objectives, methods, resources, responsible parties, and due dates. There are two types of planning: strategic and tactical.

Strategic planning: More broad-ranged, this approach means determining the overall purposes and directions of the organization. This is often focused on mission, vision, and major goal identification (see Chapter 14).

Tactical planning: More short-ranged, this type means determining the specific details of implementing broader goals. Examples are project planning, staffing planning, and marketing plans.

Planning heavily depends on the decision-making process. Part of planning is choosing among a number of alternatives. Thus in nursing, the manager often must balance the needs of patients, staff, administrators, and physicians under conditions of limited resources.

Planning involves considering systems inputs, processes, outputs, and outcomes. The process of planning in its larger context means that planners work backward through the system. Starting with the results, outcomes, or outputs desired, they then identify the processes needed to produce the results and the inputs or resources needed to carry out the processes. Typical planning phases include the following:

- Identify the mission.
- Conduct an environmental scan.
- Analyze the situation (e.g., SWOT analysis of strengths, weaknesses, opportunities, and threats).
- Establish goals.
- Identify strategies to reach goals.
- Set objectives to achieve goals.
- Assign responsibilities and timelines.
- Write a planning document.
- Celebrate success and completion.

The nurse is engaged in a constant mental planning operation when deciding what specific things are to be accomplished for the patient. The same is true for the nurse manager who is deciding how to devise, implement, and maintain a positive and productive work environment for nurses. Planning is a function that assumes stability and the ability to predict and project into the future. A turbulent environment makes planning difficult. Learning and adapting are important abilities in a changeable environment.

Organizing

Organizing is a management function related to allocating and configuring resources to accomplish preferred goals and objectives. It is the activities done to collect and configure resources to implement plans effectively and efficiently and involves coordination. **Organizing** can be defined as "assembling required resources to attain organizational objectives" (BusinessDictionary.com, 2020b). It is the mobilizing of the human and material resources of the institution to achieve organizational objectives. The organizing function is focused on building up material and human structures into a working infrastructure. Authority, power, and structure are used for influence. The goal is to get the human, equipment, and material resources mobilized, organized, and working effectively. Organizing so that the goals and objectives can be accomplished includes forging and strengthening relationships between workers and the environment. The first step is to organize the work, then the people are organized, and finally the environment is organized. The essence of organizing is the integration and coordination of resources (Hersey et al., 2013).

There are a wide variety of topics related to organizing, which is considered to be one of the major functions of management. For example, organizing can be thought of as a process of identifying roles in relationship to one another. Thus organizing involves activities related to establishing a structure and hierarchy of jobs and positions within a unit or department. Responsibilities are assigned to each job. The complexity of this aspect of organizing is related to the size of the organization and the number of employees and jobs. Organizing in nursing also relates to the activities of budget management, staffing, and scheduling and to other human resources and personnel functions such as developing committees and bylaws, orientation, and staff in-service. Institutions organize by establishing a structure, such as a hierarchy with divisions or departments, and by developing some method for division of labor and subsequent coordination among subunits.

Directing/Leading

Directing/leading is the managerial function of establishing direction and then influencing people to follow that direction. This involves managing, motivating, and directing people/teams to carry out desired actions. Directing is defined as "a basic management function that includes building an effective work climate and creating opportunity for motivation, supervising, scheduling, and disciplining" (BusinessDictionary.com, 2020c).

Along with communicating and leading, motivation is often included with the description of the activities of directing others. Motivating is a major strategy related to determining the followers' level of performance and thereby to influencing how effectively the goals of the organization will be met. The amount of employee effort that can be influenced by motivation is thought to be from 20% to 30% at the low end and as high as 80% to 90% for highly motivated people (Hersey et al., 2013). A wide range of effort can be affected through motivation.

On a day-to-day basis, coaching is used as a technique to direct and motivate followers. The manager delegates activities and responsibilities when making assignments. The function of directing involves actions of supervising and guiding others within their assigned duties. The use of interpersonal skills is required to delicately balance the need to direct and supervise for task accomplishment with the need to create and maintain a motivational climate with high participation and positive outcomes.

Within nursing there is a legal aspect to the managerial directing function. Under some state licensing laws, supervision is a defined and regulated legal element of nursing practice. Because delegation and supervision are viewed legally as a part of the practice of nursing, nurses have a specific need to know and understand this area of nursing responsibility within their scope of practice. Nurses carry responsibility and accountability for the quality and quantity of their supervision, as well as for the quality and quantity of their own actions regarding care provision. Nurse managers carry the added responsibility and accountability for the coordination of groups of nurse providers and assistive or ancillary personnel, sometimes across settings and sites of care. Nurse managers also have an overall responsibility to monitor and provide surveillance or vigilance regarding situations that can lead to failure to rescue, patient safety errors, or negligence. Too many hours worked, nurse fatigue from stress, too heavy a patient workload, and other systems problems are situations to monitor regarding legal accountability.

Controlling

Controlling is the management function of monitoring and adjusting the plan, processes, and resources to effectively and efficiently achieve goals. It is a way of coordinating activities within organizations by systematically figuring out whether what is occurring is what is wanted. It is the activities focused on monitoring and evaluating what is occurring. The controlling aspect of the managerial process may seem at first to carry a negative connotation. However, when used in reference to management, the word *control* does not mean being negatively manipulative or punitive toward others. Managerial controlling means ensuring that the proper processes are followed. In nursing, the term *evaluation* is used to refer to similar actions and activities. Control or evaluation means ensuring that the flow and processes of work, as well as goal accomplishment, proceed as planned. **Controlling** is defined as "the basic management function of (1) establishing benchmarks or standards, (2) comparing actual performance against them, and (3) taking corrective action, if required" (BusinessDictionary.com, 2020d). Thus it is concerned with comparing the results of work with predetermined standards of performance and taking corrective action when needed by taking some action to modify, remediate, or reverse variances.

The coordination of activities of a system is one aspect of managerial control, along with financial management, compliance, quality and risk management, feedback mechanisms, performance management, policies and procedures, and research and trend analysis. Ongoing, careful review using standardized documents, informatics systems, and standardized measures prevents drift and the waste of time and resources that occur when direction is vague. Well-exercised, managerial control is flexible enough to allow innovation yet present enough to effectively structure groups and organizations toward goal attainment. This is an artful balance.

The management function of controlling involves feeding back information about the results and outcomes of work activities, combined with activities to follow up and compare outcomes with plans. Appropriate adjustments need to be made wherever outcomes vary or deviate from expectations (Hersey et al., 2013). For example, when a standardized clinical practice protocol is used in nursing to track client care, the variances are analyzed and corrected as a function of managerial control. The controlling function of management is a constant process of internal reevaluation.

CONTEMPORARY MANAGEMENT THEORIES

Human organizations are complex in nature. It is tricky to provide overall direction for an organization in times of rapid environmental change. The recent focus of leadership theory has been on interactional, relational, and transformational leadership to guide organizations through successful change and chaos. However, less attention has been focused on how to advise managers who are working toward the organization's goals and trying to use resources effectively and efficiently under conditions of change, scarcity, and complexity. Forces such as technology, the Internet, social media, increasing diversity, and a global marketplace create pressure to be more sensitive, flexible, and adaptable to stakeholders' expectations and demands. This is like a fine dance on a balance beam.

The result has been a push toward reconfiguration or restructuring of many organizations from the classic hierarchical, top-down, rigid form to a more fluid, organic, team-based, collaborative structure. Health care is evolving toward multidisciplinary team-based care. This has had an impact on how managers manage. Managers cannot control continued rapid change. Old familiar plans and behaviors no longer provide clear direction for the future. Managers now need to focus on two major aspects of management: managing change through constant assessment, guidance, and adaptation and managing employees through worker-centered teams and other self-organizing and self-designing group structures. Bureaucratic management is out; organic and virtual management is in.

A variety of contemporary theories of management have arisen to help organize management thought. Four major management theories now predominate: contingency theory, systems theory, complexity theory, and chaos theory. Each one contributes principles useful for nursing management and administration and for nurse managers working to coordinate and integrate health care delivery.

Contingency Theory

Contingency theory is considered a leadership theory, but it also applies to management. The basic principle is that managers need to consider the situation and all its elements when making a decision. Managers need to act on the key situational aspects with which they are confronted. Sometimes described as "it all depends" decision-making, contingency theory is most often used for choosing a leadership or management style. The "best" style depends on the situation. This relates to concepts of situational leadership theory.

Systems Theory

Systems theory has helped managers to recognize their work as being embedded within a system and better understand what a system is. Managers have learned that changing one part of a system inevitably affects the whole system. General systems theory is a way of thinking about studying organizational wholes. A system is a set of interrelated and interdependent parts that are designed to achieve common goals. Systems contain a collection of elements that interact with each other in some environment. The elements of an open system and related examples in health care are shown in Table 1.1.

A key principle of systems theory is that changes in one part of the system affect other parts, creating a ripple effect within the whole. Using systems theory implies a rational approach to common goals, a global view of the whole, and an emphasis on order rather than chaos. The input–throughput–output model exemplifies this linear thinking aspect of general systems theory.

Systems theory is easy to understand but difficult to apply in bureaucratic systems or organizations with strong departmental "silos." This is because coordinators and integrators with sufficient organizational power to cross the system are needed but often not deployed. Without integrators, systems parts tend to make changes

TABLE 1.1 Open System Elements and Health Care Examples	
Open System Elements	**Health Care Examples**
Inputs to the system (resources)	Money, people, technology
Transforming processes and interactions (throughputs)	Nursing services, management
Outputs of the system	Clinical outcomes, better quality of life
Feedback	Customer and nurse satisfaction, government regulation, accreditation, lawsuits

without consideration of the whole system. Shifting to systems theory thinking helps managers view, analyze, and interpret patterns and events through the lens of interrelationships of the parts and coordination of the whole.

In health care, concepts such as interrelatedness and interdependence fit well with multidisciplinary teamwork and shared governance professional models (see Chapter 13). However, concepts of attaining a steady state and equilibrium are difficult to reconcile with the reality of uncertainty, risk, change, and ambiguity that characterize the turbulence of the change occurring in the health care delivery environment. An example of the use of systems theory is basing an analysis of a planned change, such as implementing a new program, on systems concepts by identifying inputs, throughputs, outputs, and feedback loops to more effectively plan how the new program fits into the existing system. Sometimes this process is used for short time frame or rapid response team projects.

Complexity Theory

Complexity theory is a more general umbrella theory that encompasses chaos theory. Arising in scientific fields such as astronomy, chemistry, biology, geology, and meteorology and involving disciplines such as engineering, mathematics, physics, psychology, and economics, the body of literature on the behavior of complex adaptive systems has been growing since the late 1980s. Complexity theory explains the behavior of the whole system. Complex systems are networks of people exchanging information and are self-organizing. Complexity theory core concepts are self-organization, interaction, emergence, system history, and temporality (Chandler et al., 2015). The focus of complexity theory is the behavior over time of certain complex and dynamically changing systems. The concern is about the predictability of the behavior of systems that perform in regular and predictable ways under certain conditions but in other conditions change in irregular and unpredictable ways, are unstable, and move further away from starting conditions unless stopped by an overriding constraint. What is most intriguing is that almost undetectable differences in initial conditions will lead to diverging reactions in these systems until the evolution of their behavior is highly dissimilar?

Stable and unstable behavior can be thought of as two zones. In the stable zone, a disturbed system returns to its initial state. In the unstable zone, any small disturbance leads to movement away from the starting point and further divergence. Which subsequent type of behavior will occur depends on environmental conditions? The area between starting and divergence is called *chaotic behavior*. This refers to systems that have behavior with certain regularity yet defy prediction based on that regularity. This unpredictability was puzzling.

Complexity theory has informed classical management theories. Previous management theories heavily emphasized rationality, predictability, stability, setting a mission, determining strategy, and eliminating deviation. Discoveries from complexity and chaos theories include the fact that the natural world does not operate like clockwork machinery.

Managers need to alter their reflexive behaviors, put an emphasis on "double-loop learning" that also examines the appropriateness of operating assumptions, foster diversity, be open to strategy based on serendipity, welcome disorder as a partner, use instability positively, provoke a controlled ferment of ideas, release creativity, and seek the edge of chaos in the complex interactions that occur among people. Change management takes on a noticeably different form when complexity theory is used. Complexity theory is being used in health care to explain the complexity of the social context in order to better explain the organization of health care and patterns of professional behavior (Chandler et al., 2015). "A new style of leadership is required in complex adapting organizations. This style is one in which the leader serves their people with vision and guidance to see the interconnectedness of the whole system. The leaders must first gain and communicate a shared identity and then be able to allow the organization ownership of that identity" (Berry, 2006, p. 2).

Chaos Theory

Most would agree that one characteristic of nursing is its unpredictability and its chaos and complexity. To use a theory about chaos and complexity is intuitively attractive. Sometimes no matter how hard nursing leaders try to maintain consistency and control, things do become chaotic. Projects seem to take off on their own and defy direction. Chaos is commonly known as disorganization and disorderliness, but the meaning for this concept in chaos theory is quite different. It refers to behavior that is unpredictable despite certain regularities.

Randomness and complexity are two principal characteristics of chaos. There is a paradox in the fact that even in the simplest of systems, it is extraordinarily difficult to accurately predict the course of events, yet some order arises spontaneously even in these simple systems. Patterns form in nature. Some are orderly, and some are not. Concepts of nonlinearity and feedback help explain situations of complexity without randomness (with order). Chaos theory suggests that simple systems may give rise to complex behavior, and complex systems may exhibit simple behavior. At the essence of chaos is a fine balance between forces of stability and those of instability. Two examples are snowflake formation and the behavior of the weather.

Chaos has become one concept of complexity theory. Over the past three or four decades, complexity theory has been the focus of scientific disciplines such as astronomy, chemistry, physics, evolutionary biology, geology, and meteorology. Systems studied in these disciplines have phenomena in common, which seem to pass from an organized state through a chaotic phase and then emerge or evolve into a higher level of organization. There are examples from sciences such as pharmacology, where chaos theory and complexity theory seemed relevant to some patients' unpredictable responses to drugs. The field of research called pharmacogenomics has emerged as a part of precision medicine to address this chaos by studying how a patients' genes affect how they respond to medications.

In management, the traditional focus for leaders is to identify organizational goals and to make decisions facilitating goal achievement. Control is central to logical management processes, but in complexity theory, the idea of control is considered a delusion because uncertainty and deviations would be denied and disregarded. The natural world, according to this theory, does not operate this way and is continually evolving to a higher level of complexity. In complexity theory, the future is so unpredictable that long-term planning is not helpful. Rather, it is suggested that managers need to look for instability and complex interactions among people so that learning occurs and the best result "emerges." The idea of the interconnectedness of the parts (people) of the whole suggests that communication among the parts (people) is a key feature of complexity theory.

Chaos, as used in complexity theory, is not utter confusion and disorder but rather a system that defies prediction despite certain regularities. Chaos is the boundary zone between stability and instability, and systems in chaos exhibit bounded instability and unpredictability of specific behavior within a predictable general structure of behavior. At first, this seems to make no sense. However, chaos theory principles can be applied in health care. For example, managerial planning for an evidence-based practice change such as bedside reporting can produce chaos and unpredictable results. An example of chaos theory in action is when a seemingly small change, such as using assistive personnel instead of professionals, in effect creates ripples and larger impacts on the system than preplanning would seem to indicate. This is why organizations use small tests of change.

As many health care organizations move away from bureaucratic models and recognize organizations as whole systems, more organic and fluid structures are replacing the older ones. Sometimes referred to as "learning organizations," these structures are tapping into the inherent capacity for individuals to exhibit self-organization. In the transition, experiences of change, information overload, entrenched behaviors, and chaos reflect human reactions to organizations as living systems that are adapting and growing (Wheatley, 2006). Complexity and a sense of things being beyond one's control create a search for a simpler way of understanding and leading organizations.

The manager's job is to reveal and handle the mostly hidden dynamics of the system and forge a direction for the organization as a complex adaptive system. The goal is for a self-managed system with people capable of engaging in cooperative behavior, using feedback to learn and adapt, self-organizing, and operating with flexibility.

LEADERSHIP AND MANAGEMENT IMPLICATIONS

It can be argued that all nurses are managers. Staff nurses are the employees at the most critical point in fulfilling the purpose of health care organizations: They are in close and frequent contact with the patient at the point of care, and they coordinate the delivery of health care services.

As nurses work in a rapidly changing practice environment, leadership is important because it affects the climate and work environment of the organization. It affects how nurses feel about themselves at work and about their jobs. By extension, leadership affects organizational and individual productivity. For example, if nurses feel goal-directed and think that their contributions are important, they are more motivated to do the work. Important for the professional practice of nurses is how they feel about themselves and how satisfied they are with their jobs. Both aspects have implications for how well nurses are retained and recruited. Leadership cannot be overlooked because leaders' function as problem finders and problem solvers. They are people who help everyone else overcome obstacles. The leadership role is one of bridging, integrating, motivating, and creating organizational "glue."

Leadership in nursing is crucial. *First*, it is important to nurses because of the size of the profession. Nurses make up the largest single health care occupation and one that is experiencing critical shortages. Pressures in the health care environment, including costs, thrust nurses into leadership roles in highly complex and stressful work situations.

Given the challenges of cost containment, increased chronic conditions, an aging population needing more health care services, and issues of access and quality of care, nurse leaders are experiencing greater pressure to perform and produce more effective alignment of key processes, functions, and resources. Organizations have underinvested in nursing leadership skill development. Thus there is a call for structured transition management and leadership development programs for nurses assuming leadership and management responsibilities in organizations (Campbell, 2016).

Second, nursing's work is complex, often conducted in complex and chaotic settings. Tremendous changes in nursing have occurred. Leadership is needed to guide and motivate nurses and health care delivery systems toward positive achievements for better patient care. Leadership in nursing is needed to influence the organizational context of care for greater effectiveness and productivity because leaders establish norms and values, define expectations, reward behaviors, and reinforce culture. Authenticity and caring are valued in nurse leaders as are people who are genuine, trustworthy, reliable, and believable and who create a positive environment.

Third, nurses are knowledge workers in an information and high-tech age. Knowledge workers respond to inspiration, not supervision. Nurses as functioning professionals in complex systems need protection and support from leaders and managers in order to be creative and innovative followers and deliver care in complex environments. Leaders need to model what they want. Nurses can read, learn, and practice effective leadership and followership.

CURRENT ISSUES AND TRENDS

Current issues and trends that have significance for leadership in nursing include the dramatic US demographic data related to both the aging of the baby boom generation and the demographic profile of nursing in the United States. A major societal and public policy issue related to the aging of a large demographic bulge of baby boomers is beginning to reach a critical point. Called the "2030 problem" (Bahrampour, 2013), this socioeconomic and demographic phenomenon is real, looming, urgent, and fraught with health care challenges. Statistics show that there are approximately 49.2 million Americans ages 65 years and older, representing 15.2% of the population, or one in seven Americans (Administration on Aging, 2018). The percentage of Americans 65 years of age and older has tripled since 1900. Issues related to health burdens and chronic illness are characteristic of older adults. In fact, persons 85 years of age and older may spend up to half of their remaining lives inactive or dependent.

US population and health trends are assessed and monitored by governmental agencies such as the US Census Bureau, Administration on Aging, Centers for Disease Control and Prevention, Bureau of Labor Statistics, and Health Resources and Services Administration. The statistics related to the baby boom generation are impressive. Born between 1946 and 1964, baby boomers in 2030 will be between the ages of 66 and 84 years, are projected to include 60 million people, thus one in five (20%) Americans will be 65 or older. In addition to baby boomers, the US population in 2030 is projected to also include 9 million people born before 1946. By 2029, all of the baby boomers will be 65 years or older, making more than 20% of the population over the age of 65 years. The projected population of people 65 years and older in 2050 is 88.5 million (US Census Bureau, 2014). This predictable tidal wave will make chronic illness and long-term care a huge economic burden. Medical costs and the costs of long-term care loom large. An overwhelming economic burden could occur if tax rates need to be raised dramatically, economic growth is retarded because of high service costs, or future generations of workers have worse general well-being because of service costs or income transfers. Nurses and the health care system will be challenged to find evidence-based care delivery and service systems models and strategies that address the projected growth industry in chronic illness care. One response has been the emphasis on prevention and wellness, targeting behavior change upstream from the development of chronic illness.

Leadership is considered key to the success of health care organizations. Nurses are pressed to demonstrate the outcomes of their care and provide evidence of the effectiveness of their service delivery. The link between leadership style and staff satisfaction highlights the importance of leadership in times of chaos. A nurse leader needs to be dynamic, show interpersonal skills, and be a visionary for the organization and the profession. The ability to inspire and motivate followers to carry out the vision is crucial. Effective leadership has a profound impact on nurse recruitment and retention.

The classic notions of management and managerial work were developed in a sociopolitical era of industrialization and bureaucratization. Competitive pressures and economic forces now are compelling organizations to adopt new flexible strategies and structures. Organizations are being urged to become leaner, more entrepreneurial, and less bureaucratic. This trend has created levels of complexity and interdependency that challenge nurse leaders and managers.

Current and emerging issues in health care are complex and ethically challenging for managers. The "big three" issues of access, cost, and quality continue to be persistent themes that affect any organization's internal operations. Medical insurance coverage is an issue of access, as is the geographical location of facilities, providers, and services. Increased complexity and technology prompt provider specialization and affect cost. Consumer preferences and increased health care awareness affect both cost and quality. Critical medical errors and patient safety issues create pressure related to the need for quality. Complexity, randomness, and chaos created by change call for new management and leadership strategies.

As health care reconfigures, health care delivery settings will likely be knowledge-based organizations composed primarily of specialists whose performance is directed by organized feedback from colleagues, patients, and data analytics. Nurses are positioned at the care coordination intersection and have needed skills for facilitating flow and integrating care delivery. Nurses' roles may change, but their need for leadership inspiration and managerial competence will remain. Nurses are well prepared to serve as leaders, care providers, integrators, and facilitators of patient care. This is the age of the nurse as leader and manager.

RESEARCH NOTE

Source

Shaughnessy, M.K., Quinn Griffin, M.T., Bhattacharya, A., & Fitzpatrick, J.J. (2018). Transformational leadership practices and work engagement among nurse leaders. *Journal of Nursing Administration*, 48(11), 574–579.

Purpose

Transforming the work environment is important to support the work of nurses and meet the challenges of a complex health care system. The purpose of this study was to identify and describe transformational leadership (TL) characteristics and work engagement (WE) by clinical nurse leaders in the United States. The research question asked about the relationship between TL and WE among nurse leaders.

Discussion

Transformational leadership has been shown to inspire followers and create an environment that enhances nurse satisfaction, recruitment, and retention. Work engagement has been shown to be connected to organizational outcomes such as lower levels of burnout and sustaining a culture of professional nursing practice. To explore the relationship between TL and WE, a descriptive correlational study was done with a convenience sample of clinical nursing leaders such as Chief Nurse Officers (CNOs), nurse managers, and educators, who attended the American Nurses Credentialing Center's National Magnet Conference in October 2016. The Leadership Practices Inventory (LPI) by Posner and Kouzes, the Utrecht WE Scale (UWES), and a demographic questionnaire were administered to 218 RNs. Of note, half of the sample was master's prepared, and about 75% were certified. Descriptive statistics were computed, including correlation analyses. A statistically significant positive relationship of moderate strength was shown between LPI and UWES total scores.

RESEARCH NOTE—cont'd

Application to Practice

This study sample was different regarding the level of education and job titles (higher than comparison studies). Nurse leaders' lowest scores were on future vision, taking risks, and supporting innovation, with "inspiring a shared vision" being the weakest leadership behavior. In the literature, an adapted clinical leadership program on leadership competencies was found to create significant improvement. TL can be learned. Leaders play a crucial role in infusing followers with a shared vision and by taking risks and supporting innovation. Nursing practice benefits from greater WE that fosters autonomy and professional growth.

NEXT-GENERATION NCLEX® EXAMINATION-STYLE CASE STUDY

The medical/surgical units at St. Helens Community Hospital are busy with a complex mix of patient diagnoses and conditions and have a staff of 88 employees, with a few nurses of long tenure, but mostly new graduates and nurses with less than 2 years of experience. They have 4 very different leaders:

1. Nurse Manager Dan has 3 years of experience as a nurse manager. He prefers to tell the followers what to do and how to do it in order to get tasks done.
2. Nurse Manager Maria has 3 years of experience as a nurse manager. She prefers to use her outgoing personality and likability to achieve success, using positive motivation and team morale.
3. Nurse Manager Jorge has 3 years of experience as a nurse manager. He prefers to have a hands-off approach and let his employees assume responsibility in the decision-making process.
4. Nurse Manager Olivia has 3 years of experience as a nurse manager. Her unit is busy with a complex mix of patient diagnoses and conditions. She prefers to use her inspiring energy and personality to create a magnetic workplace by engaging with others, centering on followers' needs and goals, and thus raising each other to higher levels of motivation.

Use the numbered scenarios above, to indicate the best approach and priority area to lead the unit.

Nursing Situation	Best Approach
The entire facility has a power outage in a storm. Backup generators do not come on in the ICU.	
Nurses complain about being understaffed for Christmas vacation.	
Nurses have organized a shared governance committee.	
The bariatric unit does not have an adequate number of Hoyer lifts, and the NM is concerned about future back injuries.	

CRITICAL THINKING EXERCISE

Nurse manager Mike Catney has a problem. He has detected angry venting and counterproductive work behavior affecting the morale of the clinic. He goes to observe and assess. It was the end of another long, hectic, and frustrating day in Ambulatory Clinic A for Nurse John Folkrod. There were daily issues with sluggish patient flow and long wait times for patients in the waiting room. John's usual reaction was to bottle up the frustration, causing personal health issues, or to vent it by complaining to colleagues. Neither method influenced a positive change in the situation. Fortunately, the nurse manager is a visionary, authentic leader. However, John has not approached him, assuming that the situation was obvious to the manager and not desiring to "make waves" or be seen as a troublemaker. In the meantime, Nurse Catney evaluates the organizational climate (how the surroundings are perceived by the staff) and reviews principles of EI. He consults the literature (Al Ghazo et al., 2019).

1. What is the problem?
2. Whose problem is it?

3. What are John's followership role and options for followership strategies to resolve the situation?
4. What leadership behaviors and styles might be effective? What should nurse manager Catney do?
5. How might the situation be analyzed using relationship-based care and EI principles?

REFERENCES

Adams, K. L., & Iseler, J. I. (2014). The relationship of bedside nurses' emotional intelligence with quality of care. *Journal of Nursing Care Quality, 29*(2), 174–181.

Administration on Aging (AoA), Administration for Community Living, US Department of Health and Human Services. (2018). *2017 Profile of older Americans.* Washington, DC: Author. Retrieved from https://acl.gov/sites/default/files/Aging%20and%20Disability%20in%20America/2017OlderAmericansProfile.pdf.

Agency for Healthcare Research and Quality. (2018). *Six domains of healthcare quality.* Retrieved from https://www.ahrq.gov/talkingquality/measures/six-domains.html.

Al Ghazo, R. H., Suifan, T. S., & Alnuaimi, M. (2019). Emotional intelligence and counterproductive work behavior: The mediating role of organizational climate. *Journal of Human Behavior in the Social Environment, 29*(3), 333–345. https://doi.org/10.1080/10911359.2018.1533504.

American Nurses Credentialing Center (ANCC). (n.d.). *ANCC Magnet Recognition Program.* https://www.nursingworld.org/organizational-programs/magnet/.

American Organization for Nursing Leadership (formerly AONE). (2015). Nurse executive competencies. Chicago, IL. https://www.aonl.org/resources/nurse-leader-competencies.

Avolio, B. J., & Gardner, W. L. (2005). Authentic leadership development: Getting to the root of positive forms of leadership. *The Leadership Quarterly, 16*(3), 315–338.

Bahrampour, T. (2013). Huge shortage of caregivers looms for baby boomers, report says. https://www.washingtonpost.com/national/health-science/huge-shortage-of-caregivers-looms-for-baby-boomers-report-says/2013/08/25/665fb2aa-0ab1-11e3-b87c-476db8ac34cd_story.html.

Bass, B. M., & Avolio, B. J. (2019). *Multifactor Leadership Questionnaire™. Mind Garden.* https://www.mindgarden.com/16-multifactor-leadership-questionnaire.

Berry, B. L. (2006). There is a relationship between systems thinking and W. Edwards Deming's theory of profound knowledge. The Berrywood Group. https://pdfs.semanticscholar.org/a090/48ae9c5cd2efbe90f3feb8a2b9ca57a9f6e9.pdf?_ga=2.49216102.1570324709.1578433890-316060041.1578433890.

Buck, S., & Doucette, J. N. (2015). Transformational leadership practices of CNOs. *Nursing Management, 46*(9), 42–48.

BusinessDictionary.com. (2020a). Planning. http://www.businessdictionary.com/definition/planning.html.

BusinessDictionary.com. (2020b). Organizing. http://www.businessdictionary.com/definition/organizing.html.

BusinessDictionary.com. (2020c). Directing. http://www.businessdictionary.com/definition/directing.html.

BusinessDictionary.com. (2020d). Controlling. http://www.businessdictionary.com/definition/controlling.html.

Campbell, G. (2016). Growing and developing our future nurse leaders. *Voice of Nursing Leadership, 14*(4), 4–6.

Castle, N. G., & Decker, F. H. (2011). Top management leadership style and quality of care in nursing homes. *The Gerontologist, 51*(5), 630–642.

Chandler, J., Rycroft-Malone, J., Hawkes, C., & Noyes, J. (2015). Application of simplified complexity theory concepts for healthcare social systems to explain the implementation of evidence into practice. *Journal of Advanced Nursing, 72*(2), 461–480.

Clay-Williams, R., Nosrati, H., Cunningham, F. C., Hillman, K., & Braithwaite, J. (2014). Do large-scale hospital- and system-wide interventions improve patient outcomes: A systematic review. *BMC Health Services Research, 14*, 369. https://doi.org/10.1186/1472-6963-14-36.

Creative Health Care Management. (2020). Relationship-based care. https://chcm.com/solutions/relationship-based-care/.

Deschamps, C., Rinfret, N., Lagace, M. C., & Prive, C. (2016). Transformational leadership and change: How leaders influence their followers' motivation through organizational justice. *Journal of Healthcare Management, 61*(3), 194–22.

Drucker, P. F. (2004). What makes an effective executive. *Harvard Business Review, 82*(6), 58–63.

Feather, J., McGillis Hall, L., Trbovich, P., & Baker, G. R. (2018). An integrative review of nurses' prosocial behaviours contributing to work environment optimization, organizational performance and quality of care. *Journal of Nursing Management, 26*(7), 769–781.

Gittell, J. H. (2016). *Transforming relationships for high performance: The power of relational coordination.* Stanford, CA: Stanford University Press.

Givens, R. J. (2008). Transformational leadership: The impact on organizational and personal outcomes. *Emerging Leadership Journeys, 1*(1), 4–24.

Görgens-Ekermans, G., & Brand, T. (2010). Emotional intelligence as a moderator of the stress-burnout relationship: A questionnaire study on nurses. *Journal of Clinical Nursing, 21*(15–16), 2275–2285.

Gosling, J., & Mintzberg, H. (2003). The five minds of a manager. *Harvard Business Review, 81*(11), 54–63.

Greenleaf, R. K. (2002). *Servant leadership: A journey into the nature of legitimate power and greatness* (25th anniversary ed). Mahwah, NJ: Paulist Press.

Grossman, S. C., & Valiga, T. M. (2017). *The new leadership challenge: Creating the future of nursing* (5th ed.). Philadelphia, PA: F.A. Davis Company.

Hanse, J. J., Harlin, U., Jarebrant, C., Ulin, K., & Winkel, J. (2016). The impact of servant leadership dimensions on leader-member exchange among health care professionals. *Journal of Nursing Management, 24*, 228–234.

Helgeson, S. (1995a). *The web of inclusion: A new architecture for building organizations.* New York, NY: Doubleday.

Helgeson, S. (1995b). *The female advantage: Women's ways of leadership* (2nd ed.). New York, NY: Doubleday.

Hersey, P. H., Blanchard, K. H., & Johnson, D. E. (2013). *Management of organizational behavior: Leading human resources* (10th ed.). Upper Saddle River, NJ: Pearson Education.

Institute for Healthcare Improvement (IHI). (2020). Triple aim for populations. http://www.ihi.org/Topics/TripleAim/Pages/default.aspx.

Institute of Medicine (IOM). (2004). *Keeping patients safe: Transforming the work environment of nurses.* Washington, DC: National Academies Press.

Institute of Medicine (IOM). (2011). *The future of nursing: Leading change, advancing health.* Washington, DC: National Academies Press.

Jennings, B. M., Scalzi, C. C., Rodgers, J. D. III., & Keane, A. (2007). Differentiating nursing leadership and management competencies. *Nursing Outlook, 55*, 169–175.

Joseph, M. L. (2015). Organizational culture and climate for promoting innovativeness. *Journal of Nursing Administration, 45*(3), 172–178.

Joseph, M. L., & Huber, D. L. (2015). Clinical leadership development and education for nurses: Prospects and opportunities. *Journal of Healthcare Leadership, 2015*(7), 55–64.

Joseph, M. L., Rhodes, A., & Watson, C. A. (2016). Preparing nurse leaders to innovate: Iowa's innovation seminar. *Journal of Nursing Education, 55*(2), 113–117.

Kleinman, C. (2004). The relationship between managerial leadership behaviors and staff nurse retention. *Hospital Topics, 82*(4), 2–9.

Koloroutis, M. (2004). *Relationship-based care: A model for transforming practice.* Minneapolis, MN: Creative Health Care Management.

Kouzes, J. M., & Posner, B. Z. (2017). *The leadership challenge: How to make extraordinary things happen in organizations* (6th ed.). Hoboken, NJ: John Wiley & Sons, Inc.

Mackoff, B. L., Glassman, K., & Budin, W. (2013). Developing a leadership laboratory for nurse managers based on lived experiences: A participatory action research model for leadership development. *Journal of Nursing Administration, 43*(9), 447–454.

Malloch, K. (2002). Trusting organizations: Describing and measuring employee-to-employee relationships. *Nursing Administration Quarterly, 26*(3), 12–19.

Mannix, J., Wilkes, L., & Daly, J. (2013). Attributes of clinical leadership in contemporary nursing: An integrative review. *Contemporary Nurse, 45*(1), 10–21.

Miles, J. M., & Scott, E. S. (2019). A new leadership development model for nursing education. *Journal of Professional Nursing, 35*(1), 5–11.

Mortier, A. V., Vlerick, P., & Clays, E. (2016). Authentic leadership and thriving among nurses: The mediating role of empathy. *Journal of Nursing Management, 24*, 357–365.

Northouse, P. G. (2019). *Leadership: Theory and practice* (8th ed.). Thousand Oaks, CA: Sage.

Patrick, A., Laschinger, H. K. S., Wong, C., & Finegan, J. (2011). Developing and testing a new measure of staff nurse clinical leadership: The clinical leadership survey. *Journal of Nursing Management, 19*, 499–460.

Quoidbach, J., & Hansenne, M. (2009). The impact of trait emotional intelligence on nursing team performance and cohesiveness. *Journal of Professional Nursing, 25*(1), 23–29.

Reynolds, K. (2011). Servant-leadership as gender-integrative leadership: Paving a path for more gender-integrative organizations through leadership education. *Journal of Leadership Education, 10*(2), 155–171.

Schooley, S. (2019). What kind of leader are you? 9 leadership types and their strengths. Business News Daily. https://www.businessnewsdaily.com/9789-leadership-types.html.

Shaughnessy, M. K., Quinn Griffin, M. T., Bhattacharya, A., & Fitzpatrick, J. J. (2018). Transformational leadership practices and work engagement among nurse leaders. *Journal of Nursing Administration, 48*(11), 574–579.

Sikka, R., Morath, J. M., & Leape, L. (2015). The Quadruple Aim: Care, health, cost and meaning in work. *BMJ Quality & Safety, 24*(10), 608–610.

Spano-Szekely, L., Quinn Griffin, M. T., Clavelle, J., & Fitzpatrick, J. J. (2016). Emotional intelligence and transformational leadership in nurse managers. *Journal of Nursing Administration, 46*(2), 101–108.

Steaban, R. L. (2016). Health care reform, care coordination, and transformational leadership. *Nursing Administration Quarterly, 40*(2), 153–163.

Stetler, C. B., Ritchie, J. A., Rycroft-Malone, J., & Charns, M. P. (2014). Leadership for evidence-based practice: Strategic and functional behaviors for institutionalizing EBP. *Worldviews on Evidence-Based Nursing, 11*(4), 219–226. https://doi.org/10.1111/wvn.12044.

The Center for Leadership Studies. (2020). Situational leadership. https://situational.com/situational-leadership/.

The National Academies of Sciences, Engineering, Medicine; Health and Medicine Division. (2020). The future of nursing 2020–2030. http://www.nationalacademies.org/hmd/Activities/Workforce/futureofnursing2030.aspx.

Thomson, N. B., Rawson, J. V., Slade, C. P., & Bledsoe, M. (2016). Transformation and transformational leadership: A review of the current and relevant literature for academic radiologists. *Academic Radiology, 23*(5), 592–599.

Upenieks, V. (2003a). Nurse leaders' perceptions of what compromises successful leadership in today's acute inpatient environment. *Nursing Administration Quarterly, 27*(2), 140–152.

Upenieks, V. (2003b). What constitutes effective leadership? *Journal of Nursing Administration, 33*(9), 456–467.

US Bureau of Labor Statistics. (2019). Occupational employment statistics: Occupational employment and wages, May 2018, 29-1141 Registered Nurses. https://www.bls.gov/oes/current/oes291141.htm.

US Census Bureau. (2014). The baby boom cohort in the United States: 2012 to 2060: Population estimates and projections. https://www.census.gov/prod/2014pubs/p25-1141.pdf.

Ward, S. (2020). The definition of leadership. https://www.thebalancesmb.com/leadership-definition-2948275.

Weberg, D. (2010). Transformational leadership and staff retention: An evidence review with implications for healthcare systems. *Nursing Administration Quarterly, 34*(3), 246–258.

Weberg, D. (2012). Complexity leadership: A healthcare imperative. *Nursing Forum, 47*(4), 268–277.

Wheatley, M. J. (2006). *Leadership and the new science: Discovering order in a chaotic world* (3rd ed.). San Francisco, CA: Berrett-Koehler.

Wong, C. A., & Laschinger, H. K. S. (2013). Authentic leadership, performance, and job satisfaction: The mediating role of empowerment. *Journal of Advanced Nursing, 69*(4), 947–959.

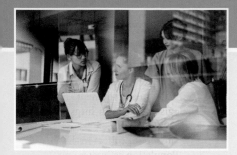

2

Change and Innovation

Beverly Quaye

 http://evolve.elsevier.com/Huber/leadership

As we enter our third decade of the 21st century, we reflect on significant health care changes in the United States since 2000. These include national health care reform with provider incentives for Medicare and Medicaid, and an option for purchasing insurance on state exchanges as a result of the Patient Protection and Affordable Care Act (ACA, 2010). ACA incorporates individual mandates, accompanying subsidies, tax credits, health benefits, and discrimination protections, such as preexisting conditions (Department of Health and Human Services [DHHS], 2018, p. 19432). There is more emphasis on coordination across the full care delivery continuum, and an increase in evidence about health promotion, disease prevention, and early detection of disease. Other achievements are more emphasis on increasing alternatives to traditional medicine, significant growth in retail and urgent care clinics (Heath, 2017), and rapid expansion in telemedicine. ACA has driven reform and innovation needs by health care leaders due to economic, quality, access to care, and service implications as a result of this new direction.

Care delivery has shifted from health care institutions that were individualized to collaboration across organizations and expanding and strengthening networks (Raus et al., 2018). There is also a shift from a business to a person-centered model that may also be due to changing demographics, that is, senior and diverse population growth, an information-driven society, social media in real-time, and global communication. Additionally, the use of personal health devices in telemedicine for monitoring and sharing data such as blood sugar, cardiac rhythms, blood pressure, and weight with providers (Centers for Medicare & Medicaid Services [CMS],

2019) is proliferating. Lastly, physician networks' use of health care professional extenders, telemedicine, and hospitalists is on the rise and is resulting in economic efficiencies, better access to care, evidence-based and quality services, improved patient safety and enhanced experiences, and maximization of technology (Raus et al., 2018).

It is imperative that mastering change and innovation calls for preparing our future nurse administrative *and* clinical leaders to (1) comprehend an idealized future state, and (2) acquire skills that will positively impact nursing practice, care delivery, patient outcomes, and health care policy. Changes in 21st century health care have been described as "revolutionary" (Longenecker & Longenecker, 2014). Today's frontline nurses are accustomed to changing processes, systems, roles, and responsibilities. Those at the point of care are often charged with leading, implementing, and evaluating the effects of change. As professionals, nurses frequently desire to maintain their emphasis on humanism and healing in the face of ongoing and perpetual change (Perregrini, 2019). This may be stressful for nurses, often leading to change fatigue resulting in lowered job performance and satisfaction, as well as health issues (Sherman, 2018).

Change is complex and disruptive. Initiating, following through, and sustaining change is challenging, whether on a personal or organizational level. Even planned personal "healthy" changes, such as smoking cessation, weight loss, a new exercise program, or continuing education, can be challenging and contribute to stress. In the work setting, when change is directive, not understood, or threatens nurse autonomy and security, it can result in conflict and resistance. To facilitate the change process, nursing management and leadership need to follow evidence-based practice grounded in change theory, research, and successful process and systematic outcomes to support nurses in accepting and adapting to change and creating a culture of innovation.

DEFINITIONS

Consistency in language via definitions will contribute to better understanding in acquiring new knowledge, skills, and the ability to translate this information into practice.

Change—an alteration to make something become different (Cambridge Dictionary, 2020a). Change is a complex process that occurs over time and is influenced by any number of unpredictable variables.

Planned change—"any kind of alternation or modification which is done in advance and differently for the improvement of present position into brighter one is called planned change" (Bank of Information, 2014, p. 1).

Emergent change assumes that change is a continuous, open-ended, and unpredictable process of aligning and realigning an organization to its changing environment (Burnes, 2009).

Transformation—"a complete change in the appearance or character of something or someone, especially so that thing or person is improved" (Cambridge Dictionary, 2020b).

Resistance—to refuse to accept or be changed by something, a force that acts to stop the progress of something or make it slower (Clarke, 2013).

Change agent—a person who encourages people to change their behavior or opinions and who may function as a change facilitator (Cambridge Dictionary, 2020c).

THEORETICAL FRAMEWORK

There are multiple change theories and models in the literature that impact how change in organizations is accomplished. Shanley's (2007) seminal work on planned or emergent change was selected as framework throughout this chapter because it addresses planned and emergent change and remains highly relevant today. Although planned change is critical in operationalizing organizational goals and strategies, modifications of Shanley's original work to meet the needs of our current

health care environment often are needed. Critics of Shanley's traditional approach object to sequential and linear methods employed in his planned change work in most current situations. Due to the complexity of health care operations requiring multidimensional perspectives and flexibility, there is more demand for emergent change methods.

Shanley's classic model was characteristic of a top-down leadership approach and a strong role of managers that needs adaptation in most contemporary scenarios. The dominant role of management has shifted to a more participatory and collaborative one in planning, managing, and executing change projects, with benefits from diverse views and skills from other professional and support staff, affiliated partners, and external suppliers. Principles and processes of change become central especially when there has been limited or no time for planning, strategizing, and supporting what is needed to be effective (Longenecker & Longenecker, 2014; Shanley, 2007) in emerging change. Shanley's model will be demonstrative in the understanding of both planned and emerging change needs as well as the associated roles and responsibilities, including change agents and recipients, in creating and sustaining change.

BACKGROUND

For the past three decades, a 70% failure rate in organizational change outcomes (Hammer, 1990; Kotter, 1995) frequently has been reported and has produced negative attitudes and beliefs about change by both change experts and the lay public. It can be said this has become a self-fulfilling prophecy in organizational change and remains commonplace today. Curious about how to break some of these long-standing assumptions, Hughes (2011) critically reviewed five separate publications that identified a 70% failure rate and concluded there was no valid and reliable empirical evidence to support this claim. Participants who experience emergent problems in the change process often revert to this negative and toxic bias, resulting in disengagement and eventual failure in their change process. Klein and O'Brien (2017) found that people assume failure as a more likely expected result of a change process compared with success, and attribute positive outcomes as luck and negative results as undeniable proof that change is difficult and often escapes us. Despite the effort required to ward off this issue, their research also discovered that most people who commit to change initiatives do eventually succeed. Studies have found that people do successfully improve with minimal effort and are quicker to notice improved changes versus setbacks. Based on this evidence, Tasler (2017) believed that it is timely to change our thinking, and an opportunity exists to write a new story by reminding us that "adaptation is the rule of human existence, not the exception."

Structurally, too often organizational change initiatives are initiated and based on top-down planned change tactics. Too frequently the focus is on the role of administrators and top managers in the change process. The reasons for this are generally pressure from decision makers desiring fast change, noncompliance from regulatory and accrediting bodies requiring immediate corrective action, health system directives, an overall lack of infrastructure to support change management and sustainability, and a lack of leadership acumen in evidence-based proven results. Table 2.1 displays contrasting views of change.

Research supports that not only is top-down change undesirable, but it does not result in successful outcomes and sustainability (Balogun, 2006; Longenecker & Longenecker, 2014). Porter-O'Grady and Malloch (2015) conceptualized this as "moving from the center, or the point of service (POS), outward." Staff and other "recipients" of change at the POS must be viewed as assets rather than barriers who are integral to the process. Representatives from all levels and parts of the system need to participate in all steps of the process: readiness, justification of need, assessment, planning, implementation, measurement, evaluation, and sustaining goals.

In addition, when considering the processes of change, issues of power and how individuals make sense of the change are essential.

Little evidence is available in the literature on the success of specific approaches to planned change (Hallencreutz & Turner, 2011). Current evidence supports an emergent view of change (Shanley, 2007) that is more likely to produce positive outcomes (Balogun, 2006; Packard & Shih, 2014). The literature points to a shift in the roles and responsibilities of executives to those affected at the frontline when change needs have been identified and needs to be executed. The traditional planned approach has often been too simplistic, made too many assumptions, and has not allowed for the analysis of the increased complexity of the aspects of change over time. Leadership needs to acknowledge that improved technology, fast-paced information technology, and increased use of personal mobile devices have accelerated access to real-time information and communication, resulting in a consumer-driven society. Today, change efforts need to be localized and incorporate a variety of approaches (Hallencreutz & Turner, 2011), since organizations have become more complex, need to keep pace with competition in services and care delivery, and accommodate consumer needs and choices.

Organizational Change

A current definition of organizational change is "a change in organizational structure, its system/subsystems, employees and relationships between them in a planned or non-planned way" (Bejinariu et al., 2017, p. 322). Management efforts are employed to transition

TABLE 2.1 Contrasting Views of Change		
	Planned Change (Traditional View)	**Emergent View**
Direction	Top-down, linear	Multidirectional, multidimensional
Initiator	Leader initiated	Diffuse
Process	Planned, step-by-step process	Principles to guide process
Organizational culture	May be considered	Essential to consider
Power issues	Not considered or not spoken	Essential to consider
Role of staff/recipients of change	Resisters	Participants in change process
View of the change recipients	May be assessed so they can be changed or manipulated	Essential to process

an organization from a current state to a desired future state to increase organizational functioning when there is an identified need for this type of change. Suddaby and Foster (2017) theorized that organizational change was positively influenced by the capacity of leadership to develop a historical consciousness. He suggested that leaders should aim for a heightened self-awareness of feelings, reactions, and appreciation of how their assumptions about the past may influence their understanding of the organization's current state and an envisioned future state. By reframing attitudes and preconceived notions about the past, successful change can occur (Suddaby, 2016). Organizational change is recognized in today's context as a complex process that is not necessarily linear (Jansson, 2013), and innovative approaches to organizational change that are consistent with emergent views are common in the evidence.

Nursing's Contribution

The role of nurses in change management is a critical leadership competency for nurses and is congruent with the human side of change. Nurses take part in most patient/client health care needs in a multitude of settings, and also have the most direct contact with them. Nurses' education is comprehensive, their scope of practice and span of control is broad, their practice ranges from general to highly specialized, and roles, functions, and responsibilities are immense. Because of this variety and scope, registered nurses have outstanding knowledge and expertise in working within organizations and fully engaging in change management.

The *Nurse Executive Competencies* of the American Organization of Nurse Executives (AONE), now the American Organization for Nursing Leadership (AONL) (2015), emphasized the need for change management knowledge, skills, and abilities. The ground-breaking report *The future of nursing: Leading change, advancing health* of the Institute of Medicine (IOM), now the National Academies of Sciences, Engineering, and Medicine, Health and Medicine Division (HMD 2010), called on nurses to use their expertise and influence to act in leading roles that support and promote health care change and innovation.

CHANGE THEORIES/MODELS

Nurse leaders, from the frontline to the executive suite, need to understand and be able to apply a variety of change theories, individualizing them to their organization and situation. Theories of change that focus on the human side of change are person-centered, align with consumer demand, and support leader–collaborator relationships that are desirable. Nurse leaders who assess and respect participants' responses to change, are mindful of political and power issues, and are sensitive to departmental and organizational values and culture will be more successful at facilitating and sustaining change (Longenecker & Longenecker, 2014). Nurse leaders are called upon to focus on the importance of human relationships in the change process.

Anderson and Anderson's (2009) work examined traditional hierarchical mind-sets of relying on power and control and top-down, manager-driven approaches, determining these were unsuccessful. They learned that when leaders focused on the process of change and human relationship aspects, better outcomes in change projects were achieved. The researchers identified the emerging mind-set, like other complexity views, as one grounded in wholeness and relationship, embracing co-creation and participation. By utilizing relationship-based change methods, an industrial mind-set used by organizational leaders shifted to an emerging mind-set. The industrial mind-set had a mechanistic worldview that relied on power and control, certainty, and predictability. A component of the emerging mind-set is that leaders need to move to what they call *conscious change leadership.*

Conscious change leaders are aware of the dynamics of change (Carson, 2016) and are more apt to lead from the principles of an emerging mind-set. Conscious change leaders need to be willing to look internally to transform their own mind-set (Carder, 2015) by expanding their thinking about process and systems and evolve their own unique leadership style.

Other models or worldviews that influence organizational change, that is, systems theory, complexity theory, and chaos theory, are also consistent with the foundations of the emerging mind-set (see Chapter 1). The focus of these theories is on interrelationships, processes, and systemic behavior. These models are congruent with the behaviors of complex systems characterized by nonlinearity, spontaneity, and self-organization. Small changes can often lead to larger dynamic changes and effects that are often unintentional. Systems, complexity, and chaos theories help

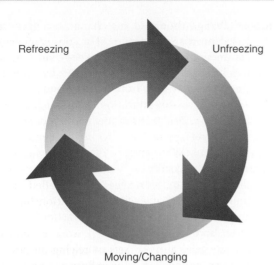

Refreezing   Unfreezing

Moving/Changing

Fig. 2.1 Elements of a successful change. Data from Lewin, K. (1947). Frontiers in group dynamics: Concept, method, and reality in social science; social equilibrium and social change. *Human Relations, 1*(1), 5–41; Lewin, K. (1951). *Field theory in social science: Selected theoretical papers*. New York, NY: Harper & Row.

navigate changes in complex systems and understand how to enable systems to adapt to change (Porter-O'Grady & Malloch, 2015).

The majority of change theories originated or were influenced by Kurt Lewin (1947; 1951) and his seminal work on the three elements for successful change processes: (1) unfreezing, (2) moving, and (3) refreezing (Fig. 2.1). Some view his ideas as more consistent with traditional views of planned change (Burnes, 2004); however, his model is currently and frequently used to frame how groups and organizations change and also serves as the basis for many newer theories.

Lewin's Change Process

Lewin coined the term *planned change* to distinguish the process from accidental or imposed change (Burnes, 2004). Lewin's (1947, 1951) theory of change used ideas of equilibrium within systems. *Unfreezing*, the first stage of change, is characterized as a process of "thawing out" the system. Unfreezing creates an awareness of the need for change and defines motivation and readiness for change. This first stage solicits a cognitive exposure to the change idea, diagnosis of the problem, and work to generate alternative solutions. When those

involved in the change process understand and generally accept the necessity of change the unfreezing stage is complete.

Moving, the second stage of change, demonstrates proceeding to a new level of behavior, evidenced by the occurrence of the actual visible change. After the individuals involved collect adequate information that clarifies and identifies the problem, the change itself can be planned and initiated. Lewin (1951) observed that a process of "cognitive redefinition"—or looking at the problem from a new perspective—happens. As a first step to launch a change, a pilot test may be performed so that the change can be pretested, and a transition period launched.

Refreezing, the final change stage, is when new changes are integrated and stabilized. Behavioral reinforcement is crucial as individuals integrate the change into their own value system and organizational culture. Leadership strategies to recognize and reward new behaviors and change, such as *positive feedback, encouragement*, and *constructive criticism* are effective means of reinforcement. Refreezing is a significant step in the sustainability plan for lasting change.

Lewin's (1947, 1951) planned change process stages can be compared with the nursing process and the generic problem-solving process (Table 2.2). *Unfreezing* is like assessing in the nursing process and like problem identification and definition in the problem-solving process. *Moving* is similar to planning and implementing in the nursing process and similar to problem analysis and seeking alternative solutions in the problem-solving process. *Refreezing* is like evaluation in the nursing

TABLE 2.2   Similarities of Change, Nursing Process, and Problem Solving

Change	Nursing Process	Problem Solving
Unfreezing	Assessing	Problem identification and definition
Moving	Planning and implementing	Problem analysis and seeking alternatives
Refreezing	Evaluation	Implementation and evaluation

Data from Workman, R., & Kenney, M. (1988). The change experience. In S. Pinkerton, & P. Schroeder (Eds.), *Commitment to excellence: Developing a professional nursing staff* (pp. 17–25). Rockville, MD: Aspen.

process and like implementation and evaluation in the problem-solving process.

Individuals and systems are like organisms in that they naturally strive for equilibrium. Lewin (1951) saw this as a balance between driving forces that promote change and restraining forces that inhibit change. Both driving and restraining forces exist within any change situation. To create change, the equilibrium is broken by altering the relative strengths of driving and restraining forces. The relative strengths of these forces may be analyzed. A force field analysis facilitates the identification and analysis of driving and restraining forces in any situation. *Unfreezing* occurs when disequilibrium is introduced into the system to disrupt the status quo. *Moving* is the change to a new status quo. *Refreezing* occurs when the change becomes the new status quo and new behaviors are frozen. The process of change may flow back and forth among stages. It is not a simple linear process in which one step follows the preceding one. The process may move rapidly or may stall in any of its stages. The goal of planned change is to manage the planning, and control and evaluate the change. Lewin's theory (1947, 1951) depicted a classic foundation for other change theories. Successive theorists were inspired and created new change theories based on further understanding and application of Lewin's theory.

Lippitt (1973) refined and expanded Lewin's (1947, 1951) work to identify seven phases of change that more fully supported planned change in dynamic and complex situations. The first three steps correlate to Lewin's unfreezing, steps 4 and 5 to moving, and steps 6 and 7 to refreezing Lewin's (1947, 1951). Lippitt's model consists of the following seven steps:

Kotter (1995) introduced his change management model based on his experiences as a consultant with businesses undergoing change. Like other change models, Kotter's has not been empirically tested, but its popularity seems to derive both from its direct and practical format and its successful utilization in multiple settings (Appelbaum et al., 2012). His model consists of the following eight steps:

1. Establish a sense of urgency.
2. Create a guiding coalition.
3. Develop a vision and strategy.
4. Communicate the change vision.
5. Empower employees for broad-based action.
6. Generate short-term wins.
7. Consolidate gains and produce more change.
8. Anchor new approaches in the culture.

Kotter's model is inclusive of employees and focuses on both engaging them in the change process and empowering them to be involved. Its emphasis is on helping others to see the need for the change and to embrace it. One potential shortcoming is that Kotter (2012) insisted that the eight steps be implemented in order, without substantial overlap. Because studies have suggested that organizations prefer to use change strategies that best fit their culture, such strict adherence to the plan may be harder to adapt. After reviewing the work of Lewin, Lippitt, and Kotter, it is evident that the various conceptualizations of the stages of the process of change bear similarity to one another but vary in emphasis (Table 2.3).

Lippitt's model consists of the following seven steps:

1. Diagnosis of the problem
2. Assessment of motivation and capacity to change
3. Assessment of the change agent's motivation and resources
} Unfreezing

4. Selecting progressive change objectives
5. Choosing an appropriate role for the change agent
} Moving

6. Maintaining the change once it is started
7. Termination of the helping relationship with the change agent
} Refreezing

TABLE 2.3 Comparisons of the Process of Change Theories

Lewin	Rogers	Lippitt	Kotter
Unfreezing	Awareness, interest, evaluation	Steps 1, 2, 3	Stages 1–6
Moving	Trial	Steps 4, 5	Stage 9
Refreezing	Adoption	Steps 6, 7	Stage 10

THE PROCESS OF CHANGE

Change in health care has been continuous, rapid, and accelerating. It may appear to be like a continuum from haphazard drift at one end to a structured, planned change at the other. Van Woerkum et al. (2011) acknowledged that "change happens" and that there are three ways by which it happens: (1) the emergence of events—essentially change by chance; by the use of language—how we arrive at new interpretations and ideas, (2) talking with one another about them, and (3) the development of practices—the result of a chain of activities, purposeful and planned.

Within nursing and health care, change is often circumstantial, whether it be updating policies and procedures because of lessons learned from a natural disaster, or changes in practice needed for new regulatory, accreditation, or licensing requirements. Through language, which may include information from meetings, investigations, reports, other documents, and records, nurses make conscious efforts to change and meet the latest requirements for quality improvements or safety standards. The development of modified and/or new practices in response to new evidence or best practices (evidence-based practice [EBP]) occurs regularly and falls under planned change. One example is the broad adoption of evidence-based protocols and practices as a way of making sure that desirable outcomes are achieved.

Readiness Assessment

Assessment of organizational readiness for change (ORC) may be helpful when preplanning the management of change and can empower leaders with a greater understanding of how increased levels of readiness may positively affect change outcomes. The ORC definition

most widely accepted today is "the extent to which organizational members are psychologically and behaviorally prepared to implement change" (Weiner et al., 2008, p. 381). However, readiness for change assessments has been mostly measured on individuals and less on organizations. Several tools are available in publications, from consultants, and on the Internet that purport to capture employees' opinions on readiness for change. However, like so many other areas in the study of organizational change, there continues to be limited evidence of reliability and validity of most of the published tools for assessing readiness for change (Weiner et al., 2008; Weiner, 2009).

Collecting data on organizational readiness includes how employees consume, process, and interpret information related to change within their work setting (Petrou et al., 2016). There are many methods that have been tried for data collection utilizing different approaches: manual or electronic surveys, focus groups, open forums, mailers, and interviews, yet reliability and validity have been problematic. According to Shea et al. (2014), as a result of their testing, psychometric evidence supports a newly created theory-based tool of ORC named "Organizational Readiness for Implementing Change" (ORIC). Phillips (2017) compared the laboratory-tested results of ORIC to a field-proven scenario using the same tool. His study found change valence and informational assessment were positive and significantly associated with increased ORC scores ($\beta = 1.778$, $P < .001$, and $\beta = 1.392$, $P < .001$, respectively). In a principal components analysis of the ORC score, change commitment and efficacy were both favorable.

Another valid and reliable tool available is the "Organizational Readiness for Knowledge Translation" (OR4KT) (Puchalski Ritchie & Straus, 2019), based on the framework of Holt et al. (2010). The OR4KT includes individual and organizational psychological and structural factors and levels of analysis. There are some limitations to the OR4KT tool, such as its length, average time for completion of 15–20 minutes, and limited use in high-income country settings based on its testing (Gagnon et al., 2018). Therefore, the change agent/leader needs to proceed with caution in selecting and using a tool, selecting one that is consistent with organizational culture and using judgment in the application of the findings. Open communication within the change process, early involvement of staff, listening to their input and concerns, and engaging them in the change may continue to be the most effective means to assess readiness for change.

Change Fatigue

To ensure that the process of change is effective, it is important to understand how unintended consequences can result in change fatigue from ineffective communication and top-down planning. The focus needs to change from one of top-down control to one of participation and communication. Five strategies to help staff manage change fatigue are to (1) utilize effective communication using common language to frame people, situations, and events that staff will find logical and believable, (2) show support and meet staff where they are in the acceptance of the change process by listening and not being indifferent, (3) forfeit control and involve staff in the change process by empowering them on how to implement the change in their department, (4) identify where and how staff can fit into the change process to alleviate anxiety and build staff optimism, and (5) give them hope by modeling a positive outlook and energy that will mobilize and energize staff (Sherman, 2018).

Emergent Process Methods

With the emphasis on patient safety and quality goals in today's health care environment, there is a need to make small rapid changes to improve care. Two related models can be used: (1) rapid cycle change, and (2) Transforming Care at the Bedside (TCAB) (Robert Wood Johnson Foundation [RWJF], 2018). Both use the plan-do-study-act (PDSA) model (Agency for Healthcare Research and Quality [AHRQ], 2015), originated by W. Edwards Deming, as a foundation (Leis & Shojana, 2016). Rapid cycle change is based on the idea that changes should first be piloted on a small scale to see how they work. TCAB was a program created by RWJF that ran from 2003 through 2008. Its goal was to improve quality and safety on medical–surgical acute care units by engaging in changes to improve practice. The idea was to create a small test, evolve the idea, get feedback, make modifications based on feedback, and proceed with the next cycle of change, until the best outcome was achieved. Once the process reached that level, it was approved, and the process continued its use by replication based on the evidence of achievement of positive outcomes and sustainability. RWJF has a downloadable toolkit on its website (RWJF, 2018) to help organizations use the process. Numerous projects were implemented and carried out between 2003 and 2008. They included the creation of rapid response teams, the initiation of multidisciplinary rounds at the bedside, and planned interventions to prevent or decrease patient falls. One of the key features of TCAB is that it was not a top-down approach, but engaged clinicians at the bedside in the design and implementation of new work practices and systems (RWJF, 2018). TCAB also emphasized that the improvement process was continuous, not a one-time occurrence.

Rapid cycle change, a methodology adapted from Toyota Production System principles, uses a small, focused, rapid process to make process improvements (AHRQ, 2015). Rather than initiating long research studies, in rapid cycle change staff are encouraged to brainstorm new ideas, try a potential change, and test its effectiveness. This can be done with one nurse, one shift, and one patient. Demonstrating the effectiveness of small change encourages nurses to try others. Rapid cycle change is often discussed and used in conjunction with TCAB but has broad application for most process changes (Valente, 2011).

Resistance

Where there is change, there is *resistance*. Resistance is inevitable, and of concern because it impacts the change process. If resistance is anticipated as a naturally occurring phenomenon in the process of change, and treated as such, the results of working through it collaboratively can be a growth experience for individuals, groups and the organization at large. Historically in some change situations, nurses have been characterized as the targets or victims of change, irrational resisters, and problems to overcome rather than as co-creators of change. Nurses are the largest group of health care providers and are central to change within health care and are influential in success, failure, and sustenance of change depends on the commitment to the change by those on the frontline. Their resistance is typically rooted in fear, anxiety, anger, and egos. Reducing and/or eliminating resistance in the work setting is not just a management and leadership function, but a disruption that needs to be identified, opened, and embraced by those involved in the change process.

According to Caruth and Caruth "change produces uncertainty, threatens stability, elicits defensive reactions, triggers feelings of angst and prompts thoughts of failure" (Caruth & Caruth, 2018, p. 21). The authors' definition of resistance is three-fold: (1) observable behavior in response to the challenge or disagreement as a result of the introduction of new ideas, methods, or devices, (2) the degree to which those within the department or organization oppose the idea of anything new, and (3) the external orientation toward an implemented change.

Interpreting change and resistance as two opposing forces may also result in *stereotyping* one group as irrational resisters rather than as partners in and co-creators of change. Strategies for disseminating information about the change and intervening when resistance is identified so that individuals and groups can achieve adoption of the change process should be integrated into the plan.

The repercussions of not identifying or taking action on employees' overt and covert resistant actions intended to prevent, interrupt, or damage the change process is problematic for the organization. It is disruptive to operations, fosters a lack of commitment, erodes loyalty, contributes to turnover, is costly, and may be irreparable if not detected or addressed. From an individual point of view, some may have a vested interest in the status quo, others may believe that change diminishes their informal/formal power and negatively affects their personal network of interpersonal relationships. Change can threaten employees' sense of control, income/benefits, and employment. Delayed, inaccurate, or absent communication regarding change fuels resistance efforts. When resistance is perceived as a warning to management or the change agent(s), it can be a wake-up call. It creates an opportunity to understand their perspective, and to reevaluate the change, clarify the purpose, and improve messaging. It is a time for leadership to take pause and reconceptualize their approach to the change. Using a strategy to reconceptualize frontline nurses as assets and problem solvers is critical. Vos and Rupert (2018) found that when change agents created space to enable employees to think and act differently by employing creative behavior, this actually resulted in higher levels of resistance. However, when the change agents used positive framing to facilitate an emotional connection between the employees and the change, resistance significantly improved.

Leaders also need to understand that resistance is an adaptive response to power (Thomas & Hardy, 2011). When those affected by change have played a part in negotiating the process of change, there is more likelihood they will buy into the change. In addition, when it is understood that power and resistance act together, the focus can change. It shifts the question to: how do relations of power and resistance operate together in producing change? (Thomas & Hardy, 2011). Leaders who understand the power–resistance relationship will be more equipped to guide change in their settings.

Nurses live with change daily. The common belief that nurses resist change is just not accurate. One way to reframe perceptions of resistance is to consider the positive effect that resisters and resistance have played in history and in US development. Examples include rebels in the Boston Tea Party, antislavery abolitionists, passive Civil Rights protestors, and me-too protestors. These resisters led and inspired others to work for change. Just as the resisters reconceptualized a future state for others as the co-creators of change by providing an alternative view, so can health care leaders reconceptualize a new vision that they share with staff and create new strategies collaboratively for moving organizations toward change.

Managing Responses to Change

Dealing with change evokes emotional responses for all involved. Although individuals must devote personal resources and energy to accomplish change, organizations may also consider creative options. Krügel and Traub (2018) did an experimental study to determine if employees would increase change approval if the employees engaged in reciprocity towards the employer. The intervention was for the employees to play a combination of a gift exchange and a threshold contribution game. Employees were grouped, and in each group of five, one employer chooses a wage and then each group decides on their effort. If the employees exert at least a minimum threshold of effort, it is conceived as an increase in change approval. The authors found that uncertainty over payoffs does not necessarily lead to resistance, and if the employer is able to trigger reciprocal behavior in employees by offering a fair wage, employee resistance was significantly reduced. The likelihood of reform approval is especially high if the employer is able to trigger reciprocal behavior in employees by offering a fair wage, which confirms the authors' hypothesis.

Mid-level managers can provide emotional support to staff in periods of stress and change. Some effective strategies to consider are active listening, promoting action steps and solutions, keeping staff informed of decisions, soliciting input and encouraging participation, and reframing difficult messages. The meaning that a change has for the individual and/or department is important and influences how the staff view the change. The meaning that the initiator of change intends is not always what the recipient of change perceives. For example, a hospital implementing professional shared governance saw this as an opportunity for increased empowerment for the staff, yet many of those on the receiving end saw it as an increase in workload. Any perceived positive gain was negated by the personal feelings of added work. Additional factors influencing this implementation were the role of emotional contagion and staff perception of inadequate, infrequent, and poorly timed education. Emotions can play a strong role in change effort, and the associated emotional contagion was due to the staff influencing one another. Although most people inherently distrust change, change can be viewed either positively or negatively. To facilitate the change process, leaders or change agents need to actively involve the recipients of change, work to understand their view, and plan adequate, timely education on the change. An additional intervention might be to monitor unit-level reactions and understanding, because individuals who understand change better tend to view it more positively. It is helpful for leaders of change and change agents to identify early adopters of the change processes and other participants who can contribute to enthusiastically spread the work.

Transtheoretical Stages of Change Model (TTM)

This classic biopsychosocial model introduced by Prochaska and DiClemente (1983) defined self-change stages for individuals in need of behavioral change, specifically smoking cessation. Since the original work there has been widespread application inclusive of behavioral health, physical rehabilitation, weight loss, and alcoholism and other substance disorders. This model was ground-breaking in that it took an integrative process approach to intentional behavior change. Individuals could be successful at deciding on and incrementally changing personal behavior by working through a series of stages to modify behavior. The time an individual spends in each stage is variable; the tasks in each stage are not. The five stages are (1) precontemplation, (2) contemplation,

(3) preparation, (4) action, and (5) maintenance. Patient stages have correlated to specific health care provider actions (stage-matched interventions) and facilitated desired behavior change. Although TTM has been used extensively to guide health promotion changes in care delivery since the advent of the ACA's goal of improving population health, its stages may also be used to positively impact individual, team, and organizational behavior during periods of significant change and innovation.

LEADERSHIP AND CHANGE

Never doubt that a small group of thoughtful, committed citizens can change the world.
Indeed, it is the only thing that ever has.

Margaret Mead

Nurse leaders are an essential part of the change process, and their values, approaches, and skills brought to change efforts are integral to success outcomes. Change is so critical to this systematic process that Burns (1978) introduced a novel model he termed *transformational leadership* (TL), emphasizing a central concept that embodied change over 40 years ago. Hindsight is 20/20, but we can all appreciate how TL has evolved into the most popular model used in nursing leadership today. In 1994, Rost conceived leadership as no longer positional but as an active process that inspired people to work collaboratively within organizational structures (Rost, 1994). The value of Rost's definition is that there was no longer a need to depend on positional structure but to re-define the leader's role and responsibilities as adaptable and driven by the needs of the organizational entity and its desired change. As these classic theories and leadership methods evolved, they were consistent with the external changes in the US healthcare arena engendering a paradigm shift to managing from an emergent change perspective. As leaders tailored their roles during these transitional times, they often struggled with their own intense emotions and likened them to feelings associated with disasters, catastrophes, and even abuse (Shanley, 2007). Managing stress for self-care as well as supporting direct reports in the work environment posed risk for negative morale, disengagement, motivational issues, and low self-esteem to grow if the management of change and human reactions was not effective.

Nurse executives and administrators are responsible for providing and sharing the vision of a preferred future, initiating change, and helping guide the direction of change that is aligned with the organization's mission, vision, values, and philosophy. As a member of the executive team, they are the colleague and liaison to effectively communicate, influence, and collaborate, garnering support for high-value patient care needs for change. Members of the change team are inclusive of middle-level and first-level managers, educators, clinical specialists, nurse practitioners, case managers, navigators, frontline staff, and other non-clinical nursing support roles, as well as other health care providers; and recipients of change take on roles as change agents, opinion leaders, and early adopters of innovations. Change agents can follow several steps in the process of change:

- Articulate a clear need and justification for change.
- Group participation in details at the point-of-service changes.
- Provide reliable information and details to the implementers of the change.
- Motivate through rewards and benefits to maintain engagement and progress.
- Do not promise anything that cannot be delivered.

For example, when implementing a planned change to a new care delivery system, the change agent's clarity and consistent messaging regarding the benefits of the change is critical throughout its inception and the entire change process. Benefits might include greater nurse autonomy, patient/staff safety, higher quality outcomes, improved patient experience, staff satisfaction, improved process effectiveness, and an overall healthy work environment with joy in the work setting. After reliable and detailed evidence is presented to the change team, the details of implementation should be arrived at by consensus of group members. Specific, realistic, and achievable goals should be the foundation for the motivation for change, reinforced by rewards and benefits— not demands or threats about performance scrutiny. High performing teamwork itself may be motivating, provide a high degree of internal satisfaction, and contribute to career development within the organization.

POWER AND POLITICS

When planning for change, power issues and politics are often overlooked and need to be incorporated into change management plans. Shanley (2007) suggested

that change initiators ask, "Whose needs are being met by the change, and whose interests are being served by the change?" If hierarchical managerial practices and top-down directives are unavoidable, understanding power may assist the leadership in this scenario to reframe their views of resistors and engage them as co-creators of change. For example, powerful change can occur through professional shared governance mechanisms that bolster empowerment and sustainability, such as developing a unit-based council or integrating this project into one that already exists. Also, creating incentives for meeting criteria for career ladder advancement, or acquiring other skills related to change projects, that is, Six Sigma, STEPPS, or nursing informatics, can build competencies and proficiencies in areas that may prepare nurses for other organizational opportunities.

The business aspects of health care, running the gamut from organizational ownership changes, physician practice changes, contractual loses, shifting demographics, and reimbursement reductions, to a whole host of other non-controllable issues and often unpredictable events, can have downstream negative effects on employees, services, and the community at large.

These types of changes are usually externally imposed and require cost reductions and/or containment to survive. Top-down decisions and actions often result in negative consequences for those affected based on increased demands, fewer resources, bigger workloads, reductions in force, less benefits, changes in positions, and reporting relationships. The impact can be demoralizing and instill feelings of loss, anger, depression, disloyalty, and increased turnover contributing to lowered performance, increased sick time, reduced quality, higher risk and safety issues, shortages in labor, and more. These economic or political forces may pressure nurse leaders to make organizational changes or enact restructuring to alleviate immediate or short-term problems. Unfortunately, the long-term effects of these changes may be difficult to foresee or to quantify. There are unintended consequences. Nurses at all levels must learn to speak up, articulate, and support the value of their role and evaluate change for the long term. As nurses assume more leadership responsibilities in the health care system, as suggested in the *Future of nursing* report (IOM, 2011), they can use their own positional power and influence to chart nursing's own destiny and, hopefully, prevent further destructive practices that do not necessarily serve the better good.

INNOVATION THEORY

Change and *innovation* are companion terms, but many authors differentiate innovation from change. An *innovation* is defined as something new, the introduction of a new process or new way of doing something. Innovation implies creativity and doing things differently. According to Hernandez et al. (2013, p. 167), innovation is "a process involving several steps from the creation of a novel idea to its adoption, implementation, and spread (diffusion) within and/or across organizations." Research has determined that leaders in practice and academia experience significant gaps in innovation competencies in formal and continuing education (White et al., 2016). Leaders need to develop skill proficiency that promotes innovation and contributes to a culture that incorporates the most effective evidence-based practices. This will help to meet needs of patients and for providers to gain or maintain a competitive advantage in health care service delivery.

Research on innovation in nursing began to emerge (Joseph, 2015) to solve complex problems by adopting behaviors, processes, and systems that foster innovation. A good example is how Kaiser Permanente created their Innovation Model to develop, test, improve, transform, and spread new ideas, equipment, products, care procedures, and services. The Innovations Unit was designed as an inpatient unit where operational and process innovations are trialed.

The Deloitte Center for Healthcare Solutions (DCHS) has developed a framework based on expected fundamental changes to the health care industry, driven by consumerism, data availability and use, and scientific innovation (Batra & Shukla, 2020). DCHS is tracking progress on innovations made by several public and private entities. The Centers for Medicare & Medicaid Services (CMS) has Blue Button 2.0 application (Verdict Medical Devices, 2018) that allows 53 million Medicare beneficiaries to access health information on their mobile devices. Access to their personal data (i.e., prescriptions, coverage, and costs) can also be shared with other health care providers to support decision-making. Apple Health Records® has an application that allows over 100 million Apple iPhone® consumers to link personal health data from several different sources on conditions, medications, claims and utilization, genomics, and wellness, and can also share it with other health care providers to support decision-making (Muoio, 2019; Terry, 2019).

The first step to innovation for leaders is to realize forces of innovation and change have mobilized. In order to change mindsets, learned ways of thinking, communication, and decision-making, leaders must be open to increase knowledge of what is happening apart from the current setting and comfort level. Considerations to include in a personal development plan for innovation are (1) share data, (2) review analyses and transformative work in data architecture, (3) continue to improve access to health care, (4) empower the consumer with convenience and transparency, and (5) support care and services that integrate digital tools, such as artificial intelligence, remote devices, and sensors, and (6) stay abreast of the scientific communities' innovative work (Batra & Shukla, 2020).

Rogers' Innovation Theory

First published in 1962 by the late Everett M. Rogers, Innovation Theory is the best-known theory on innovation (Kapoor et al., 2014). Known as the "inventor" of innovation, Rogers produced multiple editions of his book, with the 5th edition published in 2003. Rogers (2003) described a cognitive innovation-decision process that individuals and groups go through. He delineated five stages of the innovation-decision process: (1) first knowledge of an innovation's existence and functions, (2) persuasion to form an attitude toward the innovation, (3) decision to adopt or reject, (4) implementation of the new idea, and (5) confirmation to reinforce or reverse the innovation decision (Rogers, 2003). The innovation-decision process is a sequence of actions, behaviors, and choices beginning with the evaluation of a new idea and ending with a decision to accept or reject the incorporation of the innovation into practice. The perceived newness and associated uncertainty are distinctive aspects of the innovation.

Individuals need to be interested in the innovation and committed to making change occur. Hersey et al. (2013) suggested that effective change must involve people in four levels of change: (1) knowledge, (2) attitude, (3) individual behavior, and (4) group or organizational behavior. Typically to test out an innovation, the change agent would begin to work on awareness-knowledge, then address attitudes and emotions, but a focus on the development of how-to skills is the driver of creating sustainable behavioral change. Most change agents concentrate on creating knowledge and raising awareness, but Rogers (2003) believed that concentrating on practical how-to information was more critical when adopters needed to change individual, group, and organizational behaviors. Once the innovation has been tested, a knowledge-attitude-practice gap (KAP-gap) emerges. This is when individuals have gained awareness knowledge and how-to knowledge about an innovation, have formed a favorable attitude towards it, but have not acted upon it. The KAP-gap informs and influences a reevaluation of the new idea, product, or practice (Singer, 2019), and, based on the level(s) of change the individuals/group members are falling out at, will determine what modifications to make to fill the gap.

Individual members of a group or social system will adopt an innovation at different rates. This time element of the adoption of an innovation usually follows a normal, bell-shaped curve when plotted over time on a frequency basis. However, if the cumulative number of adopters is plotted, an S-shaped curve appears (Rogers, 2003). The normal adopter frequency distribution was segmented into the following five categories of innovators, early adopters, early majority, late majority, and laggards (Rogers, 2003).

Change agents can anticipate these five categories as an expected phenomenon, identify followers as to early adopter category, and target interventions accordingly. This means that for effective change, nurse leaders can recognize that there will be individual variance in acceptance of an innovation, plan for this with targeted strategies to decrease resistance, and capitalize on the power of innovations and early adopters.

Individuals need to be interested in the innovation and committed to making change occur. The outcomes of change are that the change is either accepted, adopted, or rejected. If the change is accepted, it can be either continued or eventually dropped. If the change is rejected, it can remain rejected or be adopted later in some other form. Rogers' theory (Rogers, 2003) described change as more complex than Lewin's (1947, 1951) three stages. Rogers (2003) identified the following five factors as determinants of successful planned change:

1. *Relative advantage*: The degree to which change is thought to be better than the status quo.
2. *Compatibility*: The degree to which change is compatible with values of the individuals/group.
3. *Complexity*: The degree to which a change is perceived as difficult to use and understand.

4. *Trialability*: The degree to which a change can be tested out on a limited basis.
5. *Observability*: The degree to which the results of a change are visible to others.

Kapoor et al. (2014) conducted an extensive meta-analysis of research on innovation. They found that of the five factors that Rogers (2003) identified, only *relativity* and *compatibility* could be positively correlated with successful change and that complexity was *negatively* correlated. None of the other factors were found significant in those studies. Simply stated, if members of an organization perceive a change to be better than the status quo, consistent with their values and relatively easy to understand, there will be a much better chance of adoption.

Rogers (2003) did the initial research on how acceptance of a new idea spread and was the original creator of the *Diffusion of Innovations* model. Innovators need tools to test whether their new ideas, products, or practices will be used.

Singer (2019, p. 1) defined diffusion as "the process by which an innovation is communicated through certain channels over time among the members of a social system." When leaders determine what level of change the people are in, they must communicate with the members of the social system with enthusiasm, new information, and authority about the likelihood of adoption. It also raises questions for ongoing steps toward dissemination of the innovation, such as should we conduct user research to make sure we solve actual problem(s)? What metrics are the most important ones to track? What advertising strategies should we use so we attract people who will be interested in our offering?

Innovation in Health Care

For nurses to be equipped to participate and/or lead in viable improvements in health care, they need to be open and mindful of new methods to try out via innovation. Innovation in health care requires creativity and ownership of practice solutions. Two government agencies, CMS (n.d.) and Agency for Healthcare Research and Quality (AHRQ)(n.d.), and private organizations such as the Center for Creative Leadership (CCL, 2014) have developed resources useful to nurses and health care providers wishing to innovate. In CCL's white paper, *Innovation leadership: How to use innovation to lead effectively, work collaboratively, and drive results*, they noted that underlying the pressure on individuals and organizations to adapt is the need to innovate. Their six innovative thinking skills are paying attention, personalizing, imaging, serious play, collaborative inquiry, and crafting. To begin experimenting with innovation they recommend reframing the challenge, focusing on the customer experience, and rapid prototyping. Nurses can use these resources to apply innovative thinking to the solution of problems.

AHRQ (n.d.) has a Health Care Innovations Exchange (https://innovations.ahrq.gov/) that offers Innovation Profiles and quality tools, articles and collections, and sponsored learning communities on high-priority patient care delivery topic areas.

CMS (n.d.) has an Innovation Center (https://innovation.cms.gov/) that supports development and testing of innovative health care payment and service delivery models. The website offers webinars, forums, reports, and datasets to the community of health care innovators, data researchers, and policy analysts.

Recognizing innovations created by nurses promotes a better understanding of the nurse role in innovation. Johnson & Johnson Nursing (2019) shared the stories of five nurse innovators at https://nursing.jnj.com/nursing-news-events/nurses-leading-innovation/5-nurses-making-waves-in-healthcare-innovation.

How might leaders best identify, support, and promote innovators? First, they need to seek out people who are not afraid to take risks (Cullen, 2015). Cullen characterized innovators as having the following assets: questions common beliefs and practices, comfort level with uncertainty and failures, expert knowledge, identifies innovations that may apply in their organization, and connects with other innovators through their professional network.

Nurse leaders need to create plans to add or develop existing innovation groups within their organization. Producing environments that support innovation empowers nurses to generate creative ideas and design the way of our future. Providing opportunities for frontline nurses to share ideas with colleagues both within and outside the organization and health care environment, can inspire clinical and administrative solutions that embrace ambiguity and reinforce the art of possibilities (Cullen, 2015). Innovation-promoting behaviors are relatively new considering other professions have been studying and developing evidence for a long time. To keep pace with the rapid and changing demands in health care, the value to the organization of having frontline caregivers contribute to meaningful innovation is immeasurable.

Disruptive Innovation

In contrast to system-related views of innovation, it is important to understand the history behind another type, *disruptive innovation*. Christensen and colleagues from Harvard Business School described disruptive innovation as a process wherein a simplifying technology takes root and displaces more established technologies or business practices that are slower to change, rooted in tradition, or constrained by regulation and the status quo (Christensen et al., 2000). Disruptive innovations were defined by Christensen et al. (2000, p. 104) as: "*disruptive innovations—*cheaper, simpler, more convenient products or services that start by meeting the needs of less-demanding customers."

As an example, Christensen et al. identified a portable low-intensity x-ray machine designed to be used in clinics, doctors' offices, and in the field. The technology was estimated to cost 10% of traditional x-rays, but it did not gain acceptance in the market at that time. The assumption was that this was because it threatened current business models. Further analysis suggested that regulators were encouraged not to approve the technology; insurance companies would not approve the reimbursement because they could charge more in other radiology settings; and hospitals were driven to reap a return on investment in newly purchased equipment, radiologists in their medical staff, and radiology centers. Christensen et al. (2000) also identified other disruptive innovations that held promise to improve health care in the United States, that is, increasing use of nurse practitioners in primary care, and further expanding the care continuum by increasing ambulatory services and home care. An example of a disruptive innovation is shown in Box 2.1. Christensen et al. (2000) had evidence and vision for health care reform, creative leaders, and flexible organizations to incorporate new ideas and innovations, yet the business and economics of health care appears to have thwarted progress in some areas.

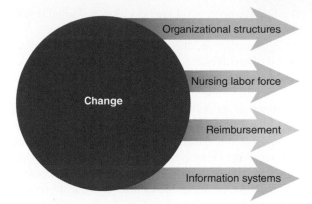

Fig. 2.2 Areas of major change in health care and nursing.

BOX 2.1 Example of Disruptive Innovation in Health Care

Disruptive innovations were described by Christensen et al. (2000) as simplifying "technology" that takes root. One such innovation that fits his definition was a barber-based blood pressure control program for African American men (AHRQ, n.d.). In this innovation, "trained barbers in African American owned shops provided ongoing monitoring of blood pressure to African American male patrons during each haircut, along with printed educational materials and feedback designed to encourage those with elevated blood pressure to visit the doctor." African American men suffer higher rates of hypertension than the rest of the population and often have higher rates of disability because of it. By providing this screening and educational materials at every haircut, the program significantly improved treatment rates and blood pressure control in hypertensive patrons. This outside-the-box innovation was a low-cost approach that was successful in meeting a community health need.

LEADERSHIP AND MANAGEMENT IMPLICATIONS

Change is a current expectation of leadership by envisioning future states as a necessity and mastering skills to develop achievable processes that are mutually agreeable to the frontline. The essentials of leadership are the ability to communicate and share the vision, collaborate on issues inherent in the change, support inclusivity from all key stakeholders in the change process, and incorporate into the organization's culture. Role modeling leader access, visibility at all levels, and support of creative and innovative ideas that translate into change initiatives will inspire and gain commitment from the change team.

Emblematic of transformational leaders, strategic change work includes being able to ignite a vision and have the ability to support changes in structure, mindsets, and power structures, and empowers others to fully participate in change initiatives (Robbins & Davidhizar, 2007). When trust and cooperation are achieved between the frontline and administration, a high performance is the norm.

Because of a current state of continuous change, the nursing perspective has also adapted to include four key areas signifying major change areas in nursing practice: (1) organizational structure, (2) nursing labor force, (3) reimbursement, and (4) information systems (Fig. 2.2). First, organizational structures have been modified and reconfigured in response to changes in health care reimbursement and other external and internal environmental factors. Population-based care, insurance and contractual reform, patient- and family-centered care, and patient safety initiatives are examples of redesigns in patient care systems to accommodate the aforementioned environmental factors.

After a decade, the ACA has resulted in more integrated networks, advancements of technological support across care settings, increased remote care improving patient access to care, a rise in digital personal devices providing real-time clinical information to providers, and consumer ownership of health care information, options, and care decisions. The complexion of the nurse workforce has experienced exponential change, and a new wave of leaders from all generations and at all career levels is emerging and rising to the challenges in health care.

Learning Organizations

An organization committed to keeping pace with health care needs and demands needs to embrace continuous life-long learning principles from a systems perspective. Porter-O'Grady and Malloch (2015) endorsed four practices for current workplaces that foster learning organizations:

(1) empowerment, (2) shared decision-making, (3) self-direction, and (4) shared governance.

Senge popularized the concept of a learning organization based on his belief that "every organization is a product of how its members think and interact" (Senge et al., 1994, p. 48). A learning organization requires an infrastructure that supports ongoing learning and knowledge acquisition by using systems thinking, mental models, personal mastery, team learning, and shared vision. Its aim is to transform behaviors within an organization resulting in a learning culture that is adaptable and responsive. Essentially the creation, acquisition, and transference of knowledge are used to adapt behavior to establish new evidence, new knowledge, and new insights at all levels.

CURRENT ISSUES AND TRENDS

At the end of the last century, multiple authors identified future trends in health care. They predicted that these amounted to major paradigm shifts. In 1996, Issel and Anderson identified the following six interconnected transformations that are major areas of change still influencing health care today:

1. From person-as-customer to the population-as-customer
2. From illness care to wellness care and prevention
3. From revenue management to cost management
4. From autonomy of professionals to their interdependence
5. From client as non-consumer to consumer of cost and quality information
6. From continuity of provider to continuity of information.

There have been continual shifts toward those changes. For example, the ACA (2010) is not just a payment or insurance program; its aims are to guide the United States to shift health care priorities from a disease and illness mindset to wellness and prevention.

Another area of important change in health care is reimbursement. For example, reimbursement (payment) for physicians has changed, driven previously by the federal government's relative value units' determinations, pay for performance, pay based on outcomes, and now value-based purchasing and population health management. Reimbursement for nurse practitioners is allowed now under Medicare/Medicaid. Payment reforms are likely to continue and change. The cost areas include physician payment, already being ratcheted down; pharmaceutical costs; and equipment and technology costs. The government will continue to review and analyze health care expenditures to reduce a huge national budget deficit fueled partly by health care costs.

A massive transformation in computerized information systems occurred with the upgrade from manual medical records to electronic health records (EHR) and meaningful use initiatives. Powerful computers and sophisticated software programs have a pattern of frequently undergoing updates and generational changes, which creates challenges of compatibility, archival retrieval, maintaining currency, and staff training. Compatibility among systems, such as relational databases, remains challenging.

These changes have and will continue to alter the health care delivery system. They present both opportunities and challenges, and nurses need to be able to anticipate and monitor trends for their immediate and long-term effects on practice. Nurses can participate in and even lead some of these trends, as they create new environments or establish new organizational documents to shape the direction of health care. It is a question of which courses of action are the best and what is the best way to direct the transformations.

The health care environment has been described as turbulent because of the rapid rate of change and the perceived constancy of change. However, change can be growth producing, renewing, and invigorating for individuals and organizations. This occurs as individuals and organizations enlist creativity to derive an innovation that improves the environment or client care delivery. Believe in the impossible.

> "There is no use trying," said Alice. "One can't believe impossible things." "I daresay you haven't had much practice," said the Queen. "When I was your age, I always did it for half an hour a day. Why, sometimes I've believed as many as six impossible things before breakfast."
>
> **Lewis Carroll**

BEST PRACTICE SUGGESTIONS FOR NURSE LEADERS

There are multiple models and approaches to change, but little evidence on what works or what will work for a particular setting. This is understandable, as organizational change is decidedly difficult to research. There are multiple confounding variables and differences in settings (from systems to specific units to individual nurses). Here are a few "take-aways" for best practice in considering the information presented in this chapter:

- Assess your particular setting and the type of change proposed.
- There is no ONE best theory or model to follow; find a model or process (or combination) suited to your specific setting.
- Communicate the vision for the change.
- Avoid top-down implementation.
- Involve the frontline and those who are at the point of care.

- Engage the "early adopters"; have them help you to influence others.
- Remember that power and resistance go hand-in-hand.
- Reassess and reevaluate frequently, and modify the strategy when needed.
- Maintain the change by making it part of the new culture.
- Communicate, communicate, communicate.
- Listen, listen, listen.

Change and innovation is a complex process with multiple approaches and models. The transfer of this knowledge coupled with applying new skills and managing the change process will determine the "best way" for a nurse to proceed in implementing and mastering change as a leader.

RESEARCH NOTE

Source

"Nursing innovation is a fundamental source of progress for healthcare systems around the world."

Joseph, M.L. (2015). Organizational culture and climate for promoting innovativeness. *Journal of Nursing Administration*, 45, 172–178. https://doi.org/10.1097/NNA.0000000000000178.

Purpose

This qualitative study had dual purposes: (1) to find out more about the experiences of nurses and nurse leaders in a hospital with a mission to support innovation, and (2) to generate a thematic map of the experience.

Discussion

Because nurses are critical in developing innovations that impact patient care, it is important to understand how you, as leader, can best create a healthy work environment that supports innovation. This study consisted of two phases: the first phase was based on semi structured interviews of six staff nurses and six nurse leaders, and the second phase involved focus groups to validate the model. The qualitative data were analyzed using content analysis methods, which entails reviewing and analyzing the data, immersion in the data to gain a sense of the

whole, identifying commonalities that led to coding and labeling, and sorting into categories. A model demonstrating innovativeness in nursing was developed from newly acquired evidence from the analysis (see Fig. 2.3).

Results

Joseph identified:

Five concepts as preconditions for innovativeness:
  (1) organizational values, (2) workplace relationships, (3) organizational identification, (4) organizational support, and (5) relational leadership.

Six additional concepts emerged that revealed a social process for innovativeness:
  (1) trust, (2) inquiry, (3) idea generation, (4) support, (5) trialing, and (6) learning.

Three key concepts related to innovativeness in nursing:
  (1) relationships, (2) leadership style, and (3) context.

Application to Practice

Study results support the need for the leader to build a strong relationship with staff aligned with organizational values and to create an innovative climate that positively affects the organization's culture. Leaders need to have an impact at all staff and organizational levels that fosters consistency across departments and sustainability.

continued

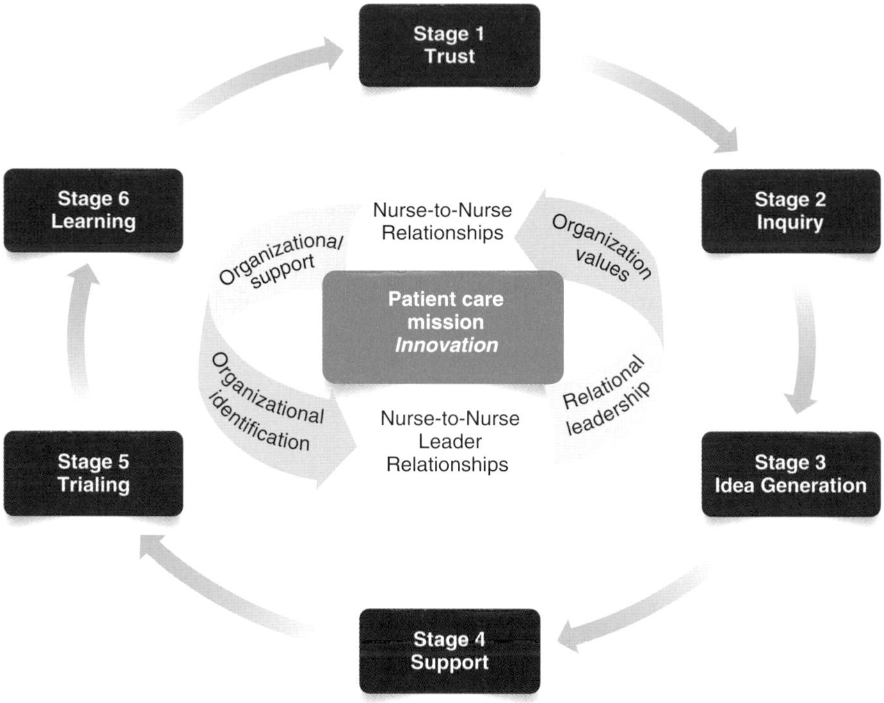

Fig. 2.3 Innovativeness in nursing. (Reprinted with permission from Joseph, M.L. [2015].)

CASE STUDY

Amanda Gonzalez, RN and Gus Lopez, RN work as diabetic case managers (DCMs) who support the family practice and internal medicine areas in a large community health care system. The case management and education departments are charged with restructuring some of the processes to improve efficiency and comply with the National Committee for Quality Assurance.

In the midst of these changes, researchers from the local university approached departmental administrators to seek assistance in recruiting qualified patients for a blood pressure research study. The administrators decided that the DCMs should be the ones to take on the recruitment responsibilities, but Amanda and Gus were not consulted about the change, nor was their workload discussed. This responsibility to recruit participants for the research study was presented to the DCMs in addition to their current responsibilities, which include contacting patients post hospital discharge, monitoring an assigned case load, educating diabetic patients, and monitoring their diet, activity, blood sugars, and medications.

The DCMs believe the additional responsibility has a negative impact on the quality of their patient education. They are concerned that because of the increased workload, they may increase risk for omissions or errors in care and jeopardize patient safety. Since this change was initiated, the DCMs are not able to meet all patient care needs due to these unrealistic additions to their workload.

CASE STUDY—cont'd

They are stressed and confused about the expectations they were not consulted on prior to this decision. There was a lack of discussion and collaboration within the work unit regarding this new responsibility. The DCMs are receiving more patient applications for the study than they can accommodate. The result so far has been slow recruitment to the research protocol, potential patient safety issues, and poor patient and staff satisfaction.

1. What type of change would you call this? How was it initiated?
2. Has this been a successful change so far?
3. Where do you think the leaders went wrong in approaching this change?
4. List three strategies that the administrators might have used to increase the possibility of a positive change.

■ CRITICAL THINKING EXERCISE

Carol Butterworth, RN, is a staff nurse in a 22-bed critical care unit within a large health care organization for over 10 years. She returned to school for a master's degree in nursing last year and would like to do her graduate project in her clinical area. Carol identified the rate for hospital-acquired ventilator associated pneumonia (VAP) was higher than local, state, and national benchmarks. She gathered information about sedation and intubation in her intensive care unit (ICU) and decided that an evidence-based nurse-directed sedation protocol could improve patient outcomes. She plans to enlist the support of the VAP committee that includes members of the interdisciplinary team and frontline health care workers. She first seeks consultation from the Advanced Practice Provider, who is a nurse practitioner.

Carol wants to develop and implement policies, procedures, physician order sets, and establish a sedation protocol based on national clinical guidelines. She has identified key stakeholders, that is, physicians, frontline nurses, clinical nurse specialists (CNS), ICU mid-level managers, pulmonary technicians, and directors of intensivists, critical care, and pharmacy. She is contemplating how to gain support for this project that will be piloted on this one unit. Critical care nurses as well as the intensivists will receive sufficient education on this evidence-based guideline and its protocol.

1. Analyze some of the issues that Carol must anticipate.
2. Explain what theory or model might be useful and why?
3. Who should be recruited for the committee and why?
4. Describe Carol's first step in the innovation process and why it is a priority?
5. How might Carol and the committee problem-solve staff resistance?

REFERENCES

Agency for Healthcare Research and Quality (AHRQ). (n.d.). *AHRQ health care innovations exchange*. https://innovations.ahrq.gov/.

Agency for Healthcare Research and Quality (AHRQ). (2015). *Plan-Do-Study-Act (PDSA): Directions and examples*. https://www.ahrq.gov/health-literacy/quality-resources/tools/literacy-toolkit/healthlittoolkit2-tool2b.html.

American Organization for Nursing Leadership (AONL). (2015). AONE nurse executive competencies. *Nurse Leader, 3*(1), 15–21.

Anderson, L. A., & Anderson, D. (2009). *Awake at the wheel: Moving beyond change management to conscious change leadership*. http://www.beingfirst.com/.

Appelbaum, S. H., Habashy, S., Malo, J., & Shafiq, H. (2012). Back to the future: Revisiting Kotter's 1996 change model. *Journal of Management Development, 31*(8), 764–782. https://doi.org/10.1108/02621711211253231.

Balogun, J. (2006). Managing change: Steering a course between intended strategies and unanticipated outcomes. *Long Range Planning, 39*, 29–49.

Bank of Information. (2014). *Planned change*. http://bankofinfo.com/definition-of-planned-change/.

Batra, N., & Shukla, M. (2020). *Six assumptions for measuring health disruption: The future of health is further along than some might think*. The Deloitte Center for Health Solutions. https://www2.deloitte.com/content/dam/Deloitte/ec/Documents/life-sciences-health-care/DI_Six-assumptions-for-measuring-health-disruption.pdf.

Bejinariu, A. C., Jitarel, A., Sarca, I., & Mocan, A. (2017). Organizational change management: Concepts definitions and approaches inventory, 321–331. Paper presented at the "Management Challenges in a Network Economy" conference, *Management, Knowledge and Learning International Conference Technology, Innovation and Industrial Management*. Lublin, Poland. http://www.toknowpress.net/ISBN/978-961-6914-21-5/papers/ML17061.pdf.

Burnes, B. (2004). Kurt Lewin and complexity theories: Back to the future? *Journal of Change Management, 4*(4), 309–325.

Burnes, B. (2009). Reflections: Ethics and organizational change—time for a return to Lewinian values. *Journal of Change Management, 9*(4), 359–381. https://doi.org/10.1080/14697010903360558.

Burns, J. (1978). *Leadership*. New York, NY: Harper & Row.

Cambridge Dictionary. (2020a). *Change*. https://dictionary.cambridge.org/us/dictionary/english/change.

Cambridge Dictionary. (2020b). *Transformation*. https://dictionary.cambridge.org/us/dictionary/english/transformation.

Cambridge Dictionary. (2020c). *Change agent*. https://dictionary.cambridge.org/us/dictionary/english/change-agent.

Carder, B. (2015). A psychological theory of culture: Balancing the conscious and unconscious mind to improve leadership. *The Journal for Quality & Participation, 38*(3), 18–22.

Carson, F. (2016). Why personal change is important for a conscious leader. *Industrial and Commercial Training, 48*(6), 300–302 https://doi.org/10.1108/ICT-12-2015-0085.

Caruth, D. L., & Caruth, G. D. (2018). Managing workplace resistance to change. *Industrial Management, 60*(4), 21.

Center for Creative Leadership (CCL). (2014). *Innovation leadership: How to use innovation to lead effectively, work collaboratively, and drive results*. https://www.ccl.org/openenrollmentprograms/?keyword=center%20for%20creative%20leadership&matchtype=e&gclid=CjwKCAiA7t3yBRADEiwA4GFlI57-kAETFU6yLk0Ht4ozCG6eJUYHkqgYyP-eMrdEPUVlP4sqUe6hU8hoCI0EQAvD_BwE.

Centers for Medicare & Medicaid Services (CMS). (2019). *Telemedicine*. https://www.medicaid.gov/medicaid/benefits/telemedicine/index.html.

Centers for Medicare & Medicaid Services (CMS). (n.d.). *CMS Innovation Center*. https://innovation.cms.gov/.

Christensen, C. M., Bohmer, R., & Kenagy, J. (2000). Will disruptive innovations cure health care? *Harvard Business Review, 78*(5), 102–112.

Clarke, C. S. (2013). Resistance to change in the nursing profession: Creative transdisciplinary solutions. *Creative Nursing, 19*, 70–76 https://doi.org/10.1891/1078-4535.19.2.70.

Cullen, L. (2015). Evidence into practice: Awakening the innovator in every nurse. *Journal of PeriAnesthesia Nursing, 30*, 430–435.

Department of Health and Human Services. (2018). Clarification of final rules for grandfathered plans, preexisting condition exclusions, lifetime and annual limits, rescissions, dependent coverage, appeals, and patient protections under the Affordable Care Act. *Federal Register, 83*(86), 19431–19436.

Gagnon, M. P., Attieh, R., Dunn, S., Grandes, G., Bully, P., Estabrooks, C. A., et al. (2018). Development and content validation of a transcultural instrument to assess organizational readiness for knowledge translation in healthcare organizations: The OR4KT. *International Journal of Health Policy Management, 7*(9), 791–797.

Hallencreutz, S. S., & Turner, D. (2011). Exploring organizational change best practice: Are there any clear-cut models and definitions? *International Journal of Quality and Service Sciences, 3*, 60–68.

Hammer, M. (1990). Reengineering work: Don't automate—obliterate. *Harvard Business Review, 68*(4), 104–112.

Heath, S. (2017). *What is the difference between urgent care, retail health clinics?* https://patientengagementhit.com/news/what-is-the-difference-between-urgent-care-retail-health-clinics.

Hernandez, S. E., Conrad, D. A., Marcus-Smith, M. S., Reed, P., & Watts, C. (2013). Patient-centered innovation in health care organizations: A conceptual framework and case study application. *Health Care Management Review, 38*(2), 166–175. https://doi.org/10.1097/HMR.0b013e31825e718a.

Hersey, P., Blanchard, K. H., & Johnson, D. E. (2013). *Management of organizational behavior: Leading human resources* (10th ed.). Upper Saddle River, NJ: Pearson Education.

Holt, D. T., Helfrich, C. D., Hall, C. G., & Weiner, B. J. (2010). Are you ready? How health professionals can comprehensively conceptualize readiness for change. *Journal General Internal Medicine, 25*(Supplement 1), 50–55. https://doi.org/10.1007/s11606-009-1112-8.

Hughes, M. (2011). Do 70 per cent of all organizational change initiatives really fail? *Journal of Change Management, 11*(4), 451–465. https://doi.org/10.1080/14697017.2011.630506.

Institute of Medicine (IOM). (2011). *The future of nursing: Leading change, advancing health.* Washington, DC: National Academies Press.

Issel, L. M., & Anderson, R. A. (1996). Take charge: Managing six transformations in healthcare delivery. *Nursing Economic$, 14*(2), 78–85.

Jansson, N. (2013). Organizational change as practice: A critical analysis. *Journal of Organizational Change Management, 26,* 1003–1019. https://doi.org/10.1108/JOCM-09-2012-0152.

Johnson & Johnson Nursing. (2019). *Five nurses making waves in healthcare innovation.* https://nursing.jnj.com/nursing-news-events/nurses-leading-innovation/5-nurses-making-waves-in-healthcare-innovation.

Joseph, M. L. (2015). Organizational culture and climate for promoting innovativeness. *Journal of Nursing Administration, 45,* 172–178. https://doi.org/10.1097/NNA.0000000000000178.

Kapoor, K. K., Dwivedi, Y. K., & Williams, M. D. (2014). Rogers' innovation adoption attributes: A systematic review and synthesis of existing research. *Information Systems Management, 31,* 74–91. https://doi.org/10.1080/10580530.2014.854103.

Klein, N., & O'Brien, E. (2017). The power and limits of personal change: When a bad past does (and does not) inspire in the present. *Journal of Personality and Social Psychology, 113*(2), 210–229. https://doi.org/10.1037/pspa0000088.

Kotter, J. P. (1995). Leading change: Why transformation efforts fail. *Harvard Business Review, 73*(2), 59–67.

Kotter, J. P. (2012). *Leading change.* Boston, MA: Harvard Business Review Press.

Krügel, J. P., & Traub, S. (2018). Reciprocity and resistance to change: An experimental study. *Journal of Economic Behavior & Organization, 147,* 95–114. https://doi.org/10.1016/j.jebo.2017.12.017.

Leis, J. A., & Shojania, K. G. (2016). A primer on PDSA: executing plan-do-study-act cycles in practice, not just in name. *BMJ Quality & Safety, 26*(7), 572–577. https://doi.org/10.1136/bmjqs-2016-006245.

Lewin, K. (1947). Frontiers in group dynamics: Concept, method, and reality in social science; social equilibrium and social change. *Human Relations, 1*(1), 5–41.

Lewin, K. (1951). *Field theory in social science: Selected theoretical papers.* New York, NY: Harper & Row.

Lippitt, G. (1973). *Visualizing change: Model building and the change process.* La Jolla, CA: University Associates.

Longenecker, C. O., & Longenecker, P. D. (2014). Why hospital improvement efforts fail: A view from the front line. *Journal of Healthcare Management, 59,* 147–157.

Muoio, D. (2019, June 28). Apple Health Records now available to all US providers with compatible EHRs. *Mobihealthnews.* https://www.mobihealthnews.com/news/north-america/apple-health-records-now-available-all-us-providers-compatible-ehrs.

National Academies of Sciences, Engineering, and Medicine, Health and Medicine Division (HMD). (2010). *The future of nursing: Leading change, advancing health.* http://www.nationalacademies.org/hmd/Reports/2010/The-Future-of-Nursing-LeadingChange-Advancing-Health.aspx.

Packard, T., & Shih, A. (2014). Organizational change tactics: The evidence base in the literature. *Journal of Evidence-Based Social Work, 11,* 498–510. https://doi.org/10.1080/15433714.2013.831006.

Patient Protection and Affordable Care Act [ACA]. (2010). https://www.dpc.senate.gov/healthreformbill/healthbill04.pdf.

Perregrini, M. (2019). Mitigating resistance to change in the workplace. *Creative Nursing, 25*(2), 154–156. https://doi.org/10.1891/1078-4535.25.2.154.

Petrou, P., Demerouti, E., & Schaufeli, W. B. (2016). Crafting the change: The role of employee job crafting behaviors for successful organizational change. *Journal of Occupational Health Psychology.* https://doi.org/10.1177/0149206315624961.

Phillips, J. E. (2017). *Effects of change valence and informational assessment on organizational readiness for change.* Minneapolis, MN: Walden University. https://scholarworks.waldenu.edu/cgi/viewcontent.cgi?article=5119&context=dissertations.

Porter-O'Grady, T., & Malloch, K. (2015). *Quantum leadership: Building better partnerships for sustainable health* (4th ed.). Sudbury, MA: Jones and Bartlett.

Prochaska, J. O., & DiClemente, C. C. (1983). Stages and processes of self-change of smoking: Toward an integrative model of change. *Journal of Consulting and Clinical Psychology, 51*(3), 390–395.

Puchalski Ritchie, L. M., & Straus, S. E. (2019). Assessing organizational readiness for change. *International Journal of Health Policy Management, 8*(1), 55–57. https://doi.org/10.15171/ijhpm.2018.101.

Raus, K., Mortier, E., & Eeckloo, K. (2018). The patient perspective in health care networks. *BMC Medical Ethics, 19*–52. https://doi.org/10.1186%2Fs12910-018-0298-x.

Robert Wood Johnson Foundation (RWJF). (2018). *The transforming care at the bedside (TCAB) toolkit.* Princeton, NJ: Robert Wood Johnson Foundation. https://www.rwjf.org/en/library/research/2008/06/the-transforming-care-at-the-bedside-tcab-toolkit.html.

Robbins, B., & Davidhizar, R. (2007). Transformational leadership in healthcare today. *The Healthcare Manager, 26,* 234–239.

Rogers, E. M. (2003). *Diffusion of innovations* (5th ed.). New York, NY: Free Press.

Rost, J. C. (1994). Leadership: A new conception. *Holistic Nursing Practice, 9*(2), 1–8.

Senge, P., Kleiner, A., Roberts, C., Ross, R., & Smith, B. (1994). *The fifth discipline fieldbook*. New York, NY: Doubleday.

Shanley, C. (2007). Management of change for nurses: Lessons from the discipline of organizational studies. *Journal of Nursing Management, 15*, 538–546. https://doi.org/10.1111/j.1365-2834.2007.00722.x.

Shea, C. M., Jacobs, S. R., Esserman, D. A., Bruce, K., & Weiner, B. J. (2014). Organizational readiness for implementing change: A psychometric assessment of a new measure. *Implementation Science, 9*(7), 1–15. https://doi.org/10.1186/1748-5908-9-7.

Sherman, R. (2018). Managing change fatigue. *Emerging Nurse Leader*. https://www.emergingrnleader.com/managing-change-fatigue/.

Singer, L. (2019). *Thoughts on human behavior and making software (blog). On the diffusion*. https://leif.me/2016/12/on-the-diffusion-of-innovations-how-new-ideas-spread/.

Suddaby, R. (2016). Toward a historical consciousness: Following the historic turn in management thought. *M@n@gement, 19*(1), 46–60.

Suddaby, R., & Foster, W. M. (2017). History and organizational change. *Journal of Management, 43*(1), 1–20. https://doi.org/10.1177/0149206316675031.

Tasler, N. (2017). *Stop using the excuse "Organizational change is hard"*. https://hbr.org/2017/07/stop-using-the-excuse-organizational-change-is-hard.

Terry, K. (2019, July 3). *Apple opens iPhone EHR feature to all healthcare organizations. Medscape*. https://www.medscape.com/viewarticle/915208.

Thomas, R., & Hardy, C. (2011). Reframing resistance to organizational change. *Scandinavian Journal of Management, 27*, 332–331.

Valente, S. (2011). Rapid cycle change projects improve quality of care. *Journal of Nursing Care Quality, 26*(1), 54–60.

Van Woerkum, C., Aarts, N., & Van Herzele, A. (2011). Changed planning for planned and unplanned change. *Planning Theory, 10*, 144–161. https://doi.org/10.1177/1473095210389651.

Verdict Medical Devices. (2018, December 19). Heavily promoted Medicare Blue Button 2.0 will speed up machine learning in healthcare. *eClinicalWorks*. https://www.medicaldevice-network.com/comment/heavily-promoted-medicare-blue-button-2-0-will-speed-up-machine-learning-in-healthcare/.

Vos, J. F. J, & Rupert, J. (2018). Change agent's contribution to recipients' resistance to change: A two-sided story. *European Management Journal, 36*(4), 453–462. https://doi.org/10.1016/j.emj.2017.11.004.

Weiner, B. J., Amick, H., & Lee, S. Y. (2008). Conceptualization and measurement of organizational readiness for change: A review of the literature in health services research and other fields. *Medical Care Research Review, 65*(4), 379–436. https://doi.org/10.1177/1077558708317802.

Weiner, B. J. (2009). A theory of organizational readiness for change. *Implementation Science, 4*(1), 67–76. https://doi.org/10.1186/1748-5908-4-67.

White, K. R., Pillay, R., & Huang, X. (2016). Nurse leaders and the innovation competence gap. *Nursing Outlook, 64*(3), 255–261. https://doi.org/10.1016/j.outlook.2015.12.007.

Workman, R., & Kenney, M. (1988). The change experience. In S. Pinkerton, & P. Schroeder (Eds.), *Commitment to excellence: Developing a professional nursing staff* (pp. 17–25). Rockville, MD: Aspen.

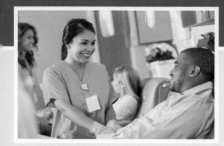

3

Organizational Climate and Culture

Jennifer Bellot

 http://evolve.elsevier.com/Huber/leadership

Since the 1960s, health care organizations have systematically responded to economic, social, and financial challenges that have ultimately caused a transformation in health care delivery. Health care organizations now compete in a marketplace based on their ability to demonstrate lean performance, increased efficiency, and quality health outcomes. Particularly since the implementation of the Affordable Care Act (ACA) in the United States, the payment structure for health care has largely shifted from fee-for-service to prospective payment to pay-for-performance and outcomes.

Crossing the quality chasm (IOM, 2001), a landmark report of the Institute of Medicine (IOM, now called the National Academies of Sciences, Engineering, and Medicine, Health and Medicine Division), described the challenge of care provision in the 21st century and was one of the first publications to detail the shift from provider-centered care to patient-centered care. Inclusion of patient and family values, norms, customs, and family/caregiver participation are now dominant factors in treatment decisions. Furthermore, recent inquiry regarding patient safety has emphasized patient outcomes as well as the processes and behaviors that lead to safe care. An explosion in information technology capacity is altering the speed and transparency of communication and information delivery. Interprofessional care is gaining prominence, showing mixed to positive evidence that teamwork leads to better patient outcomes (Reeves et al., 2013). The impact of a nurse shortage, the increasing demand for nursing care, and the drive to incorporate evidence-based practice are changing the face of nursing care. Taken together, these issues have transformed health care structures and delivery,

creating a fast-paced and ever-changing practice environment for nurses to negotiate. There is an inevitable impact on organizational climate and culture.

An appreciation for workplace culture is critical for today's nurse leader. In the perfect storm, nurses may wonder how the issues detailed here link with organizational culture, the professional role of the nurse, and nurse leaders. Nurses' insight into organizational culture enables them to understand staff behaviors and relationships, norms, change processes, expectations, and communications. This holds true for all levels of nurses—from novice to expert practitioner and from direct care provider to administrator. This chapter provides an overview of culture, focusing on the factors that affect the culture within an organization. This chapter also discusses organizational culture and climate and their relationship to the nursing work environment, workforce, and practice.

DEFINITIONS

Culture

Organizational culture is rooted in anthropology, psychology, sociology, and management theory. It first appeared in the academic literature in 1952. **Culture** is the set of values, beliefs, and assumptions that are shared by members of an organization. An organization's culture provides a common belief system among its members. Culture provides a common bond so that members know how to relate to one another and how to show others who are outside of the organization what is valued. For example, organizational culture can encompass things like the mission statement, policies, procedures, organizational positions, the way people dress, and the language they use. Additionally, culture encompasses what is implicit in the organization, such as the unwritten rules and customs that pervade the work environment. Collectively, these variables define the character and norms of the organization.

Culture is represented in several ways. One example is that the care delivery model that guides nursing practice helps interpret the culture. For instance, when a relationship-based nursing care model is used, it represents an underlying belief in patient-centered care. Open visiting hours in the intensive care unit convey the importance of family as partners in care delivery. How new nurses are oriented expresses values about the socialization of new nurses. Many visible aspects of culture reflect the underlying values of the organization.

Culture is a multifaceted phenomenon, difficult to comprehend and unravel. The health care system is incredibly complex. High-quality health care delivery is dependent on good communication and collaboration between providers, patients, and their families. One way to better understand such relationships is to appreciate how the hospital culture affects nursing units, nursing practice, and patient outcomes. For a nurse to function effectively in an organization, a solid grasp of organizational culture, characteristics, and operations is essential.

Culture has been measured both quantitatively and qualitatively. Initially it was thought that something as diffuse and intangible as culture could only be measured using qualitative techniques. Bellot (2011, p. 33) stated that "early culture researchers believed that standardized, quantitative instruments were inappropriate for cultural assessment because they would be unable to capture the subjective and unique aspects of each culture." A strictly qualitative approach to cultural assessment can be time consuming, expensive, less generalizable, and difficult to interpret. Thus, various quantitative tools have been developed to more quickly assess culture and allow for comparison across different work environments. In reality, it is likely that a combination of qualitative and quantitative measures are best for capturing organizational culture (Bellot, 2011). As with any selection of a measurement tool, the choice of a measurement instrument should be directed by definition, purpose, and context for cultural assessment.

Because of the confusion around the tendency to use organizational culture and climate interchangeably and definitional confusion, measuring these two can be difficult. Gershon et al. (2004) searched the literature and identified and described 12 organizational climate and culture instruments. They described the dimensions and subconstructs of each instrument and then displayed five major dimensions of leadership, group behaviors and relationships, communications, quality of work life, and health care worker outcomes by instrument. Recommendations for use were presented. A rigorous assessment of the organizational culture and climate sets the stage for planned change. Choosing the right instrument is important.

Climate

Organizational climate is a concept that is closely linked to the organization's culture and is often confused with it. Although many people use *culture* and *climate* interchangeably, the terms are not the same. **Climate** is an *individual* perception of what it feels like to work in an environment (Snow, 2002). It is how nurses perceive and feel about practices, procedures, and rewards (Sleutel, 2000). People form perceptions of the work environment because they focus on what is individually important and meaningful to them. This explains why some aspects of culture may be interpreted differently. A key feature of culture is its *group* orientation.

Climate can be easier to identify than culture. Researchers who study climate describe various components of the work environment that influence behaviors (Sleutel, 2000). Some characteristics that are used to study climate are decision making, leadership, supervisor support, peer cohesion, autonomy, conflict, work pressure, rewards, feeling of warmth, and risk (Stone et al., 2005). Within organizations, it is common to identify sub-climates that focus on specific aspects of the organizations (e.g., climates related to patient safety, ethics, and learning). For example, some organizations have adopted principles of a learning organization to establish an organizational culture change using knowledge and learning.

Culture–Climate Link

Climate research has formed the basis for the definition and research surrounding organizational culture, and the two are closely linked (Bellot, 2011). Regardless of the practice setting, a link exists between culture and climate. That link is what is important to understanding attitudes, motivations, and behavior among nurses (Stone et al., 2005). Culture and climate can be described as the interaction of shared values about what things are important, beliefs about how things work, and behaviors about how things get done.

Nurse Practice Environment

Although organizations usually have a single, overarching culture, many climates can exist within that culture—from unit to unit, for instance. Groups and organizations exist within society and develop a culture that has a significant effect on how members think, feel, and act. Culture becomes a learned product of the group experience. In general, nurses work together in a group such as on a nursing unit, in home care, in long-term care, or in communities. The nursing unit is a small geographical area within the larger organization where nurses work interdependently to care for patients. Nursing work groups naturally spend time together and set up their own norms, values, and ways to communicate with each other. These factors contribute to that work group having its own climate, or perception of what it feels like to work within a geographical area, contributing to the **nurse practice environment**. The nurse practice environment is also often referred to as the "professional practice environment."

Climate is evident in staff perceptions of policies, practices, and goal achievement. Some authors have described this as an organizational subculture (Hatch & Cunliffe, 2013). Understanding organizational culture from the perspective of individual nurse practice environments can offer an unprecedented view of nurses' work. Creating an environment with a culture and climate that empowers nurses to practice in ways that support a positive professional practice environment can maximize both nurse and patient outcomes.

Using strict social science definitions, the predominance of nursing organizational research focuses on *organizational culture*—or employs the more general term *work environment*—rather than climate. For the purposes of the everyday nurse leader, the terms are interchangeable, although "organizational culture" or "work environment" are typically distinguished more precisely in the research literature.

BACKGROUND

The business focus on culture is as the means to achieve organizational success and competitive advantage. Industry leaders in the corporate world quickly realized that the philosophy and values of an organization could determine success and secure market advantage (Wooten & Crane, 2003). The health care industry has been slower than the corporate world to embrace culture as a means to optimize organizational performance.

Organizational culture is defined as "the set of shared assumptions that relate to the core values of the organization" (Levine et al., 2020, p. 131). These shared assumptions guide members on how to problem solve, adapt to the external environment, and manage relationships. The mission statement for an organization offers a snapshot of strategic priorities and is an important way to get a sense of organizational values.

Organizational culture affects the quality of nursing care and patient outcomes. Shared meanings—the taken-for-granted practice and assumptions of a work group—can exert a significant effect on performance and outcomes. Basic underlying assumptions are those that are never questioned and make up an integral part of the fabric of an organization that extends to the unit work level, such as a commitment to excellence and to the surrounding community. Each organizational unit and work group has cultural norms and values that blend the social realities and features that shape interactions among staff, patients, and families. The manner in which the staff perceives organizational culture, manages boundaries, and translates implied values to the unit level has a direct effect on patient care (Carthon et al., 2015).

RESEARCH

Since the mid-1990s a growing body of research has confirmed that the relationship between nurse staffing and patient outcomes is influenced by culture or climate and the organizational characteristics of the structure in which nurses practice (Wong et al., 2013). More recently, studying the impact of culture has shifted from the organizational level to the unit level, where caregiver relationships, communication, and autonomy intersect to inform care decisions that affect individual outcomes. To understand how the culture of the organization and climate of a unit are related to professional practice, five contemporary trends in achieving a culture/climate of quality are discussed here: the Magnet Recognition Program®, the professional practice environment, patient safety culture, healthy work environments, and just culture.

Magnet Recognition Program®

In 1983, the American Academy of Nursing's Task Force on Nursing Practice in Hospitals studied nursing service best practices by surveying 163 hospitals. The goal was to identify and describe those factors that, when present, created an environment that attracted and retained qualified RNs who delivered quality care. The 41 best hospitals were called "Magnet hospitals" because of their clear ability to attract professional nurses. The 14 original characteristics they displayed were identified and called "Forces of Magnetism." Now administered by the American Nurses Credentialing Center (ANCC, n.d.), the Magnet Recognition Program® has become the gold standard for excellence in nursing.

Magnet hospitals are an example of a positive culture that affects nurse and patient outcomes. Today, hospitals and long-term care facilities wanting to achieve Magnet Recognition Program® status must meet five key components identified by the ANCC (n.d.): transformational leadership; structural empowerment; exemplary professional practice; new knowledge, innovations, and improvements; and empirical outcomes. In 1998 Magnet recognition was expanded to include long-term care facilities, although Magnet designation still largely applies to the acute care, hospital environment.

In Magnet-designated organizations, a strong visionary nurse leader nurtures a professional nursing environment and advocates for, and is supportive of, excellence in nursing practice. Magnet-designated hospitals have been recognized over the years for excellence in patient care, strong nursing practice environments, and the ability to attract and retain nurses. The advancement of professionalism, autonomy, and nursing's knowledge base are hallmarks. Periodically, the ANCC queries Magnet-designated facilities to establish an official national research agenda that is current and germane to ongoing professional development.

Aiken and colleagues have transformed the initial Magnet hospital work into a program of research congruent with quality of care and organizational effectiveness through study of the links between hospital organizational culture and care outcomes. Magnet hospitals were conceptualized as those institutions that have a specific organizational culture with characteristics of autonomy, practice control, and collaboration. In a seminal work, Aiken et al. (1994) examined mortality rates in 39 Magnet hospitals and 195 control hospitals using multivariate matched control sampling. Magnet hospitals had a significantly lower mortality rate (4.6% lower) for Medicare patients than did control hospitals. The Magnet-designated hospitals' cultures provided higher levels of autonomy and control of practice for nurses and fostered stronger professional relationships among nurses and physicians than did non–Magnet-designated hospitals. In one study RNs had significantly lower work engagement after the loss of Magnet designation (Wonder et al., 2017).

Magnet research and an organizational framework developed by Aiken et al. (1997) provide the means to better understand the link between unit culture characteristics and adverse events. A nursing unit culture that supports and values nurse autonomy and the provision of adequate resources and effective communication among providers most likely constitutes an environment where practice excellence is the norm. Examples of research regarding Magnet-designated hospitals show associations with lower central-line-associated bloodstream infections (Barnes et al., 2016), lower selected-cause readmissions (McHugh & Ma, 2013), lower rates of hospital-acquired pressure ulcers (Ma & Park, 2015), more positive patient experiences (McCaughey et al., 2020), and multiple other nurse and patient outcomes (Kutney-Lee et al., 2015). A repository of research references on Magnet research can be found at https://www.nursingworld.org/organizational-programs/magnet/program-resources/research-materials/

Professional Practice Environment

In the journey toward Magnet designation, research and evidence-based practice become important in meeting the core criteria and representing a culture and climate of learning that is supportive of a professional practice environment that involves continuous learning and professional nursing development. A **professional practice environment** is characterized by a shared and positive perception of the value of learning to enhance practice, quality, and outcomes. This may be reflected in principles of a learning organization.

Cultures in which continuous learning is valued are less likely to become outdated and stale. In the past, it was not unusual to hear nurses say in relation to their practice, "We have always done it this way." Today, a professional practice environment encourages nurses to propose new ideas and adopt and implement evidence-based practices to promote clinical excellence. Moving new research findings into practice has historically taken many years. In a culture that supports professional practice, nurses are challenged to ask, "How can this be done better?" Nurses interact with many patients on a daily basis. Patients are experts about themselves, and nurses are experts about nursing practice. Blending these areas of expertise puts nurses in the best position to ask the question, "How can practice and the environment in which practice occurs be improved?" Nursing practice then becomes a vehicle for generating questions that are important to practice. This idea, along with creating a culture of lifelong learning, is one cornerstone of the IOM report *The future of nursing: Leading change, advancing health* (IOM, 2011). Progress in nursing recognition and positive workforce culture has led to the Robert Wood Johnson Foundation commissioning a second Future of Nursing study (2020–2030), currently in production, and focusing on the nurses' role in addressing social determinants of health and health equity.

The formation of the team at the unit level creates a collective vision for continuous learning and professional practice. In turn, the norm for learning intersects with the desire for good practice and forms a cohesive unit that shares a value for learning that generates excitement for moving beyond traditional practice. Cultures in which knowledge is freely shared can have a groundswell effect. Examples of outward and visible signs that support nurses' shared values for professional practice include activities such as journal clubs, unit presentations, poster displays, and participation in evidence-based practice teams.

Patient Safety Culture and Climate

An emphasis on an organization's patient safety culture and climate has driven an avalanche of research and change in hospital practices since the publication of the IOM's (1999) report *To err is human: Building a safer health system*, which suggested that 98,000 persons die annually in hospitals because of errors. A safety culture is an outgrowth of the larger organizational culture and emphasizes the deeper assumptions and values of the organization toward safety, whereas the safety climate is the shared perception of employees about the importance of safety within the organization (DeJoy et al., 2004). Like organizational climate, the safety climate has a number of different components, including leadership, involvement, blameless

culture, communication, teamwork, commitment to safety, beliefs about errors and their cause, and others (Blegen et al., 2005).

Safety climate refers to keeping both patients and nurses safe. Strong surveillance skills regarding patients are at the heart of safety. Because they are on the front line of patient care, nurses are in an optimal position to monitor patients to prevent adverse events or near misses of adverse events. The ability of nurses to understand a patient's baseline status and recognize early, critical warning signs or changes in health status is a skill derived from having a strong nursing knowledge base. It is not simply task application. Astute recognition of deviations from normal and timely interventions signify that nurses understand the patient's baseline status and are capable of intervening to prevent or remediate an adverse event. Knowledge of the patient and the patient's baseline status is derived through subjective, objective, and intuitive observations that are honed as nurses develop a level of expertise in working with specific patient populations. Factors that influence a nurse's ability to watch over patients to avoid errors and adverse events include managerial leadership, communication style and clarity, staffing levels, excess fatigue, and lack of education and experience (Higgins, 2015; McHugh et al., 2016; Van Bogaert et al., 2014). Other aspects of a safety climate and culture, such as Six Sigma and lean health care organizations, are techniques related to creating quality.

Healthy Work Environments

Included in the concept of a safety culture/climate is a focus on nurses' health and safety. Nurses working in hospitals have one of the highest rates of work-related injuries, including back injury, needle sticks, and chemical exposures (Stokowski, 2014). When fewer nurses are working, less help is available to provide care to patients. This results in more work needing to be done in a shorter time and can lead to taking shortcuts, also known as workarounds, which can result in injury to the nurse and/or poor patient outcomes. To address these issues, the American Nurses Association (2016) has created a variety of resources, position papers, and compiled research on a healthy work environment (HWE) (https://www.nursingworld.org/practice-policy/work-environment/). The ANA has defined an HWE as one that is safe, empowering, and satisfying. Paramount is a culture of safety for both patients and health care workers. General workplace improvements such as in decision making, communication, and collaboration, along with provision of authentic leadership and meaningful recognition are needed. In addition, an HWE would have programs in place to address specific workplace issues such as fatigue management, safe handling of patients, bullying and violence, infection control and prevention, sharps injury, environmental health, and disaster preparedness to demonstrate the organization's commitment to partnership with nurses.

Regardless of whether the focus of safety is on the patient or the nurse, the likelihood of injury can be lessened where there is a cohesive team. When there is a shared perception among a group of care providers about the value and importance of safety, they are more likely to work together effectively toward common goals. Espousing the values of a safety climate and endeavoring to prevent, detect, and mitigate the effect of errors and injuries increases the likelihood of improved outcomes. As nurses work together as a team, they share information, can anticipate events, and are more likely to respond appropriately to unanticipated events.

Just Culture

One major shift in an organization's safety culture/climate is the move from a punitive and reactive culture to a fair and just culture. The concept of a **just culture** was first developed by John Reason in 1997. A just culture represents the middle ground between patient safety and a culture that supports error reduction (Reason, 1997). In a fair and just culture, expectations for system and individual learning and accountability are transparent. Underlying these beliefs, the overall organizational strategy must effectively implement a fair and just culture. When an organization can freely discuss mistakes with the intention of learning from them, and when it takes the time and resources needed to understand the mistakes using root cause analysis, the organizational culture changes from punitive to respectful and open to learning. For example, within a systems-oriented approach, learning from adverse events can encourage error reporting, rather than concealment, and lead to new wisdom and improved ways of doing things. This is called a just culture. In 2010 the American Nurses Association published a position statement, formally endorsing the creation of a just culture for nurses across the health care work environment (American Nurses Association, 2010).

LEADERSHIP AND MANAGEMENT IMPLICATIONS

Nurses work in a wide variety of health care organizations, such as clinics, educational organizations, health insurance organizations, health care associations, home health care, hospitals, long-term care facilities, physician practices, mental health organizations, public health departments, rehabilitation centers, and research institutions. These organizations vary as to their business configuration, ownership, and mission, such as for-profit, not-for-profit, or governmental. The type of organization in which the nurse works has an impact on the differences seen in organizational culture and climate.

Culture is characterized by complexity and is relatively enduring, making it hard to change. Climate, on the other hand, can be easier to change. Regardless, the basic elements that constitute culture and climate must be understood before any change. Change that begins at the unit level may be most influenced by nursing leadership. Nurses have the ability to create or change a work culture, climate, or environment to accomplish a change that may affect productivity and satisfaction and promote safe, high-quality, patient-centered care. For example, units experiencing high turnover can make strategic and evidence-based decisions about processes and relationships in order to convert to a more satisfying work environment that attracts and retains nurses.

A key role of a nursing leader is to influence the culture and the climate. A primary task of the leader is to create a convincing vision that inspires and engages the entire team to move it forward. Values drive behaviors. The leader communicates this vision by influencing norms and values and creating a shared perception through role modeling and ensuring role clarity, accountability, and a nurse practice environment that promotes safe patient- and family-centered care.

Unit-based nurse managers serve as bridges between the senior nursing leadership and direct care nursing staff. Nurse Managers are instrumental in shaping and managing the core values of their staff. There are a multitude of tools available to document the relationship between nursing management behavior and registered nurse (RN) job satisfaction (Feather et al., 2015). Professional organizations such as the American Organization for Nursing Leadership and the American Nurses Association have long campaigned for healthy work environments that reflect positive nurse management. Increasingly, studies are showing that the nurse manager is important in retention (Al-Hamdan et al., 2016), stress management (Parry et al., 2014), and work environments (D'Ambra & Andrews, 2014).

Key areas within the leader's scope of control are recruiting and retaining staff, welcoming new staff, providing orientation, celebrating and recognizing staff accomplishments, facilitating change, and promoting a just culture and professional practice environment. Climate is evident in how policies are enacted, unit norms, dress code and appearance, environment, communication, and teamwork. The nurse manager can articulate the vision, mission, and goals of the organization and work with staff to translate them into unit-level values for performance, thus linking the context of the organization to clinical practice.

Values drive the way resources are distributed. They contribute to a general attitude and sense about the quality of work life and reflect the organization's core goals. Clues can be gleaned from organizational documents such as philosophy statements and meeting minutes. Caring values of the organization are reflected in the way the organization treats its staff. Organizational values may not mirror professional values. The leader's role is to bridge such values with the values of individual team members to shape the individual unit climate. Values support the mission and the related vision, which, in turn, support strategies and action plans. The key platform is shared values. Given the complexity and diversity of the nursing workforce, developing and sustaining a set of shared values is no easy task and requires leadership skill.

Leaders are expected to chart a clear course for change and mobilize staff to accomplish organizational goals. This means implementing change effectively. Effective cultural change requires communication, passion, and clear understanding of the existing culture. The nurse manager can create such opportunities by using focus groups, holding team meetings, coaching and mentoring, posting minutes from staff meetings, using clear and directive communication, and empowering staff by soliciting their input. The value of communication cannot be overstated.

In their landmark organizational behavior research, Peters and Waterman (1982) stressed that the greatest professional need people have is to find meaning in their work life. Finding meaning at work is a fundamental motivational strategy related to job satisfaction. The job of managers is to help create meaning through the use of stories, slogans, symbols, rituals, legends, and myths that convey the values, beliefs, and meanings shared among the staff. Managers should function as passionate leaders to motivate staff.

The challenges of leadership belong to every nurse, not just those in formal administrative or management roles. Leadership at the staff level may be informal and simply take a different form. For example, a staff nurse adapting to a challenging patient assignment, taking initiative to change practice through performance improvement, or challenging the status quo is participating in unit culture construction. Informal clinical leadership is manifested among peers, for example, when a staff nurse sees an area for improvement and mobilizes peers or the unit-based council to pursue a solution. This can create a positive unit climate with a "can do" attitude. Further, staff nurses are critical to founding and maintaining a Magnet-designated organization.

Nurse leaders with an accurate and comprehensive assessment of culture and climate can identify strategic areas for change. A thorough understanding of organizational culture and climate is a powerful diagnostic tool that may be used to identify both troubled and high-performance areas. An effective organizational culture empowers nurses to practice to the full extent of their education and training (IOM, 2011). The culture of a nursing unit practice environment may exert a significant and independent effect beyond that of staffing and skill mix by enhancing or impeding interventions once problems are detected. Nurses serve as the surveillance system for early detection of adverse events.

Culture and Strategy

"Culture eats strategy for breakfast."
—attributed to Peter Drucker

A principal responsibility for nursing leadership and management is short- and long-term planning, creating a strategy for the unit and organization as a whole. Organizational culture is a key component to consider when creating strategy. Having a thorough baseline assessment of organizational culture and current resources (workforce, technology, financial, etc.) will inform the nurse leader if the desired vision, goals, and outcomes included in a strategic plan are appropriate given the characteristics of the organization/unit.

Regardless of the organization's or leader's priorities for a strategic plan, they will be unsuccessful in realizing those goals unless there is cultural congruence, employee buy-in, and sufficient resources to support the strategic plan.

CURRENT ISSUES AND TRENDS

At the beginning of the chapter, a number of forces were identified that have had significant influence in changing the culture of health care delivery. Several of these forces have particular impact on nursing care, and a brief discussion of patient- and family-centered care, generational diversity, and the Quality and Safety Education for Nurses (QSEN, 2020) initiative follows to exemplify current issues and trends related to organizational climate and culture.

Patient-Centered Care and the Patient-Centered Medical Home

Beginning in 2001 with the IOM's landmark report *Crossing the quality chasm*, it has been widely promulgated that the culture of patient care must transition from care that is driven by providers to care that is patient centered and family centered, in which patient and family norms, values, and preferences are respected. Shortly thereafter, the Agency for Healthcare Research and Quality (AHRQ) agreed with these recommendations and discussed four other features of optimal primary care to create national recognition for the patient-centered medical home (PCMH) model of primary care delivery.

First introduced in the 1960s as a means to coordinate primary and specialty care for children, the PCMH model evolved to include other areas of primary care. In this model, nurses work as part of an interprofessional team to deliver care that helps to improve patient outcomes, the patient experience, and value. There is a large body of research that supports the success of the PCMH model, and it has since been advocated for as a best practice for primary care by the AHRQ and many major payers.

There are five core functions and attributes in the PCMH model: comprehensive care, patient-centered, coordinated care, accessible services, and quality and safety. Comprehensive care is providing care that is inclusive of both physical and mental health care, wellness, prevention, and illness care. Comprehensive care requires a team of providers, and this is where

the nurses' role is central. Patient-centered care is relationship-based, inclusive of the whole person, and respectful of the patient's values, culture, and preferences. Coordinated care coordinates information across all levels and sites of care. For example, this would include primary and specialty care, inpatient, outpatient, home, subacute, and long-term care. Accessible services refer to providing care that is easiest for patients to obtain such as offering telephonic access, shorter wait times, and hours conducive to the patients' needs. Finally, quality and safety refers to a provider employing evidence-based care and clinical decision support tools. For more information about the PCMH model, including the wide base of supportive research, see the AHRQ website at www.pcmh.ahrq.gov.

Beginning research on the PCMH model showed small to moderate effects on nurse outcomes and experiences (Jackson et al., 2013). It has been noted in some studies that the transition to this model inherently results in a conflict with how a nurse traditionally organizes and structures the workday (Bellot, 2012; Stewart et al., 2015). Although the PCMH model is an admirable way to encourage comprehensive, holistic patient care that is informed by interprofessional, team-based communication, it is also important to consider the practice and cultural transformation that must occur to facilitate its implementation.

Culture Change in Long-Term Care

After the passage of the Nursing Home Reform Act legislation (OBRA, 1987, https://www.congress.gov/bill/100th-congress/house-bill/3545) a series of quality improvement programs were implemented in nursing homes. By the mid-1990s the culture change movement had begun to gain popularity and continues to spread today. Culture change is distinguished from typical quality improvement activities in its attempt to simultaneously alter multiple aspects of care and caregiving in the nursing home. Culture change is so named because of its aim to adopt an entirely new philosophy in long-term elder care. There is no universal operational definition of what specific elements constitute culture change programming. Instead, culture change refers to the movement to reorganize nursing home care completely. Included under this umbrella are several different initiatives that address staff, resident, environmental, or behavioral outcomes or some combination of these factors. Most culture change initiatives are focused upon resident-directed (patient-centered) care, providing services that are directed by the strengths and preferences of the individual resident and/or family.

Research has been done to evaluate various culture change initiatives, but some models have been promulgated and replicated more than others. Early culture change initiatives, although generally dedicated to the same principles of resident-directed care and homelike social structures, were unique from organization to organization. Despite the wide range of programming, research has found that nursing homes that have engaged in culture change activities report declines in avoidable hospitalizations and 30-day hospital readmissions (Zimmerman et al., 2016), declines in bedfast residents (Afendulis et al., 2016), and decreased Medicare spending (Grabowski et al., 2016).

In 1995, at a meeting of the National Citizens' Coalition for Nursing Home Reform (NCCNHR), a panel of administrators whose nursing homes were engaged in culture change initiatives was convened. This group grew in size and strength and became known as the Pioneer Network. Today, the Pioneer Network is an organization of facilities engaged in many diverse culture change initiatives dedicated to a common set of values. These values include returning the locus of control to residents, enhancing the capacity of frontline staff to be responsive, and establishing a homelike environment that values choice, dignity, respect, self-determination, and purposeful living (https://www.pioneernetwork.net/). Some of the most prominent culture change models include the Eden Alternative, the Green House Project, and the Wellspring Program.

Development of a new model or culture change must be preceded by comprehensive assessment of the organization culture, an understanding of the patient population, what members of the staff need to care for them, and what roles are required to form the change team. There is no one right model, nor does one size fit all settings. The work entails a deliberative process to facilitate change that will improve outcomes. Culture development must be an essential component of any new culture change. Transparency and frequency of clear communication is critical for cultural transformation and buy-in from all staff (Bellot, 2012).

Engagement

Nurse engagement is a term of growing interest and emphasis in nursing leadership, quality and outcomes research. Nurse engagement is defined as "nurses'

commitment to and satisfaction with their jobs…nurses' level of commitment to the organization that employs them and their commitment to the nursing profession itself" (Dempsey & Reilly, 2016, p. 1). Some regard nurse engagement as the opposite of burnout. It is a burgeoning area of nursing research and a major area of focus for initiatives such as Press Ganey surveys, the National Database of Nursing Quality Indicators (NDNQI) and other sources of key data that drive the Magnet Recognition Program®. Nurse engagement has been found to correlate with safety, quality and patient experience outcomes (Day, 2014; Laschinger & Leiter, 2006; Nishioka et al., 2014; Press Ganey, 2013).

The nurse leader needs to consider culture as a key ingredient to stimulate employee engagement. The Advisory, Conciliation and Arbitration Service (ACAS) has identified four factors that lead to a more satisfied and productive workforce. These factors are:

- Leaders with a vision who value how individuals contribute
- Managers who empower, rather than control their staff
- Values that are lived, not just spoken, leading to a sense of trust and integrity
- Employees who have the chance to voice their views and concerns (ACAS, n.d.)

These four factors are important for the nurse leader to consider when creating a work environment that engages and rewards its employees.

There are a number of other ways the nurse leader can promote positive nurse engagement in the workplace. For example, Kutney-Lee et al. (2016) found increased nurse engagement when the professional practice environment incorporates higher levels of shared governance. As ACAS promotes, it is intuitive for a nurse leader to posit that employees who have the chance to voice their views and concerns (shared governance) will enjoy higher satisfaction and commitment to the workplace (engagement). Other strategies for nurse leaders to promote nurse engagement include recognition and empathy for the difficulty of work and talent required to do the job of a nurse, adequate resources in areas ranging from emotional support to safe staffing levels, trust and delegation so that the nurse feels valued and respected, and encouragement for and modeling of a work/life balance. When these values are promoted in the professional practice environment *and* modeled by nurse leaders, it sends a clear signal to nurses that they are valued contributors.

Predictive Analytics

The use of predictive analytics in nursing management and leadership is a new application of an old method. Predictive analytics, broadly, refers to using statistical or data-driven modeling to determine outcomes based on current or historical data. Predictive analytics have been applied in various aspects of the professional practice environment including determining if a potential nurse employee is a good cultural match for the unit, modeling safe staffing in uncertain conditions and determining risk for 30-day readmissions and undesirable patient outcomes given nursing workforce resources. As sources of big data such as the electronic medical record become more robust, it is expected that predictive analytics will be used increasingly to modulate the professional practice environment.

Generational Differences

The importance of a positive work climate on organizational, patient, and nurse outcomes is firmly established and evidence-based. However, creating a work environment for nurses that meets their personal and professional values can be a challenge. In 2008, for the first time since the inaugural National Sample Survey of RNs, the numbers of nurses working who were under age 30 years and over age 60 years were almost equal (US Department of Health and Human Services, 2010). Because nurses from each of these generations were raised with a different set of priorities and values, a work environment supportive to each generation is an important retention strategy. For example, baby boomer nurses value rewards. Recognition and pay may be motivators for them. In contrast, Generation X nurses are concerned with a better balance of work and life. Further, Generation Y (sometimes called Millennials) have shown indications of increased mobility and higher willingness to move to another job when dissatisfied with the work environment and culture (Tourangeau et al., 2013). Tailoring the work environment to meet generational and life-stage needs is a recurrent theme in being able to address successfully the impending nursing shortage.

As Generations X and Y become a larger proportion of the nursing workforce, a marked shift in values has been noted. Research from the Pew Research Center (2018) has indicated that younger workers place a higher emphasis on finding a professional practice environment that promotes work/life balance, flexible working arrangements, and values-driven work. Younger generations tend to place less value on material items like pay and more value on time and flexibility. A 2019 survey of 20,000 RNs discussed how care is becoming more complex, demand for services is increasing, and there is a wave of Baby Boomer retirements (Edmonson & Marshall, 2020). These forces generate rising consumer demand coupled with a limited nursing workforce supply. Issues from the 2019 survey highlighted that there is a growing burden on the nursing workforce as reflected in (Edmonson & Marshall, 2020, p. 131):

- The significant percentages of nurses working second jobs
- The reality that many nurses are unable to spend the time they need with patients
- Concerns that their jobs are affecting their health
- Plans to leave their current jobs within a year
- The need for greater work-life balance

Professional practice environments and policies that support well-being, making healthy choices, and clear communication and expectations are highly desired by new nurses. Nurse leaders may want to consider, although the physical work of the bedside nurse cannot be made remote, perhaps other things required of the job such as evaluations or professional development can be more flexible regarding where they occur. Perhaps a more meaningful recognition than a chair massage or tote bag during Nurses Week would be a demonstrated commitment from nursing leadership to creating a sustainable year-round professional practice environment and considering recognition and rewards in the form of a day off or preferred/discounted parking. Taking these generational preferences into account is important as nurse leaders consider recruitment strategies as well as retention. Younger generations have shown greater mobility and intent to leave when they are dissatisfied with the work environment. As evidenced by the #metoo movement, younger generations typically have a much lower tolerance for hostile work environments and will simply leave for a workplace more suitable to their needs.

Quality and Safety Education for Nurses

In 2005, Quality and Safety Education for Nurses (QSEN, 2020), a joint project of the Robert Wood

Johnson Foundation and the National League for Nursing, was announced. The purpose of QSEN is "to address the challenge of preparing future nurses with the knowledge, skills and attitudes (KSAs) necessary to continuously improve the quality and safety of the health care systems in which they work" (QSEN, 2020, Project Overview page). Widespread rollout of the QSEN program has resulted in extensive nursing faculty education that is designed to create nursing curriculum that emphasizes organizational culture attributes such as the implementation of patient-centered care, emphasis on teamwork and collaboration, integration of evidence-based practice, and creation of a culture that supports quality improvement, safety, and

informatics. To this end, QSEN's key tenets are geared toward teaching nursing students the competencies they will need to affect organizational culture and create an environment that maximizes patient safety and health outcomes.

By incorporating these elements into nursing education, it is believed that nurses will enter the workforce with the tools necessary to help create an organizational culture that fosters high-quality nursing care. QSEN has now expanded to target nurses both prelicensure and at the advanced practice level and is permeating into practice at the direct care level. This initiative is an example of how to make large-scale cultural change in nursing.

RESEARCH NOTE

Source
Levine, K.J., Carmody, M., & Silk, K.J. (2020). The influence of organizational culture, climate and commitment on speaking up about medical errors. *Journal of Nursing Management, 28*(1), 130–138.

Purpose
To make patient safety a priority, nurse managers have an important role in creating the communication culture that fosters speaking up. However, there is high variability with regard to whether medical errors are reported. The purpose of this study was to understand how a hospital's culture and climate impact nurses' active behavior of speaking up about medical errors.

Discussion
Using an online survey given to 162 medical professionals and support staff at one Midwestern hospital, data were collected about organizational commitment, importance of reporting medical errors, consequences for reporting medical errors, supervisory responsiveness, and ease of reporting medical errors to determine their impact on intentions to speak up about medical errors. Organizational commitment used an existing scale. Data gathered from focus groups and one-on-one interviews were used to develop the remaining scales.

Organizational commitment, culture, and climate to understand why medical errors go unreported. Organizational commitment is an established measure of the relative strength of a person's identification and involvement in an organization. Organizational responsiveness and the importance of reporting medical errors measure the

culture. Organizational climate is measured by ease of reporting medical errors and interpersonal consequences of reporting. The results of the study showed a strong culture in this hospital: if people feel that reporting is important, then they have a great likelihood of reporting. However, findings suggest that the culture reflects one value but the climate makes fulfilling that value difficult. The perception of reporting an error is that this is like writing up a co-worker or "tattling." The existing culture is one of fear, mistrust, and intimidation. By contrast, in a culture where near misses and errors are commonly reported, there is a greater focus on quality of care. The bottom line is a confusing set of messages coming from upper management about speaking up about medical errors.

Application to Practice
In this study employees reported high levels of organization and group/unit commitment. However, the organization's culture and climate worked against an overarching organizational goal of effective and proactive patient care. Thus the major organizational goal is over-shadowed by working environment realities. Nurse Managers need to be assertive in communications about the problem of speaking up to assure patient safety. The literature indicates that teaching strategies for assertive communication were linked to higher levels of reporting medical errors by residents and interns. Nurse Managers are crucial to affecting change; they can be a pivotal force in changing organizational culture and climate by realizing the connection between organizational culture and patient safety.

CASE STUDY

Several months ago, a sentinel event occurred on an acute rehabilitation unit in which the mother of a high-profile community member suffered severe anoxic brain injury by becoming trapped between her mattress and the bed rails. This event was heavily reported by the media and a competing rehabilitation hospital in the neighboring county decided to tout their image as the "safest, most alert rehab for your loved one." The competitor hospital then required its nurses to take five different measurements of the gap between the bed frame and mattress at the beginning of each shift. Nurses, already stretched tightly for staffing, were upset because obtaining these measurements was time-consuming when they felt they could be providing more important patient care. There were no tape measurements provided for this task; nurses had to take paper rulers from wound care kits. Further, nurses were not advised what was an acceptable versus dangerous gap, nor what to do if the gap was deemed "too big." Some nurses placed pillows between the mattress and bed frame to lessen the gap...which angered other nurses, who felt pillows should be reserved for therapeutic positioning. One nurse refused to take measurements at all, loudly stating that it was a useless activity since every time the bed was adjusted or sheets were changed, the measurements would change anyway. After a week of this new policy, most of the nurses simply copied over the measurements from the previous shift and did not perform any new measurements.

At the monthly management meeting, all staff were re-advised of the original policy and several nurses were informed that they were being placed on disciplinary probation for falsifying their charting by using previous measurements. Tension was high. Nurses claimed they were not consulted in the initial policy, that it was not evidence-based, and that they were given no direction on how to interpret measurements or rectify a gap that was "too big." Management thought that nurses were being lazy and inflexible, but they were sure that using the threat of disciplinary probation would convince the nurses that they were "serious about safety." Several people left the meeting in tears and two considered finding another job.

1. What are the problems?
2. Identify challenges faced by nurses and by management.
3. What steps would you take to define a culture of safety?
4. How would you define the culture of this facility? How would you change it?
5. What can the nurses do? What can management do?

CRITICAL THINKING EXERCISE

The Magnet Recognition Program's® website offers case studies about Magnet designation that showcase culture change. One example of multiple Magnet designations is the Carle Foundation Hospital/Carle Physician Group of Urbana, Illinois (https://www.nursingworld.org/organizational-programs/magnet/program-resources/case-studies/).

In presenting their case study, the Carle Foundation Hospital noted that it launched its first Magnet® journey as a strategy to improve nurse recruitment and retention. The process involved nursing leaders reviewing the Magnet standards. They realized that Magnet is focused on doing the right thing, including for nurses, the organization, and patients. They achieved their initial designation with great pride of accomplishment in 2009.

This pride drove their re-designation journey four years later. Because Magnet status put the hospital among the nation's elite, everyone was determined to maintain Magnet designation at the time of re-designation. However, there was a new environmental and cultural change to account for: the recent integration with Carle Physician Group. The integration of a hospital with a physician group posed some challenges. The climate and culture of the physician's group clinic differed from the hospital. For example, certification rates in the ambulatory clinic were low, and nurses showed little enthusiasm to pursue specialty credentials. To address this situation, nursing leaders developed and implemented a policy of paying the certification fee in advance for RNs. Rates for certification skyrocketed from 14% to 36% in just 8 weeks.

Other benefits to Carle from Magnet designation include a bolster to its mission to provide high-quality, world-class health care that garners national recognition. It is an important recruitment and retention tool. Physicians and nurses cite the hospital's Magnet status when choosing to work for Carle. Employees are proud to say they work for a Magnet organization.

Magnet appraisers named their New Nurse Residency Program an exemplar during their most recent site visit because the program boasted a 96% retention rate its first year.

Pursuit of Magnet standards improved outcomes. For example, implementation of Chlorhexidine gluconate (CHG) (basinless) bathing in the cardiovascular intensive care unit significantly reduced surgical site infection rates, with no deep/organ space infections for more than a year. This successful program has been expanded to other surgical areas.

Evidence of a culture of Magnet, with resources and programs to support nurses in enhanced competence, is seen in providing tuition assistance (rather than reimbursement) to nurses to pursue educational goals. This initiative produced a steady increase in Bachelor of Science in nursing (BSN) rates since the hospital's first designation in 2009. Now 46% of nurses have BSNs, and there is a clear plan to get to 80% by 2020 as recommended by the IOM (2011).

Carle's nursing leaders call Magnet an "indispensable roadmap" for success because it directs the organization to where they need to focus and pinpoints what they need to do to achieve desired outcomes. The Magnet journey is seen as a continuous, evolving process. Clearly, their pursuit of excellence is not a once-every-4-year goal, but rather it is an integral part of the organization's daily work.

1. What are three examples of a professional practice environment for nurses at Carle Foundation Hospital/Medical Group?
2. Based on the information provided in the case study, what are likely some prominent features of Carle's culture? Climate?
3. Based on the information provided in the case study, how might Carle continue to capitalize on their successes innovatively?
4. What steps would you take to implement one of Carle's programs in your own work environment?
5. What are some barriers you might anticipate to culture change in your work environment?
6. How might you think about planning proactively to address barriers to culture change in your work environment?

REFERENCES

Advisory, Conciliation and Arbitration Service (ACAS). (n.d.). *Employee engagement: Happy and productive people equals growth.* https://archive.acas.org.uk/engagement.

Afendulis, C. C., Caudry, D. J., O'Malley, A. J., Kemper, P., & Grabowski, D. C. for the THRIVE Research Collaborative. (2016). Green house adoption and nursing home quality. *Health Services Research, 51*(1 Pt 2), 454–474.

Aiken, L. H., Lake, E. T., Sochalski, J., & Sloane, D. M. (1997). Design of an outcomes study of the organization of hospital AIDS care. *Research in the Sociology of Health Care, 14*, 3–26.

Aiken, L. H., Smith, H. L., & Lake, E. T. (1994). Lower Medicare mortality among a set of hospitals known for good nursing care. *Medical Care, 32*, 771–785.

Al-Hamdan, Z., Nussera, H., & Masa'deh, R. (2016). Conflict management style of Jordanian nurse managers and its relationship to staff nurses' intent to stay. *Journal of Nursing Management, 24*(2), E137–E145.

American Nurses Association. (2010). *Position statement: Just culture.* https://www.nursingworld.org/practice-policy/nursing-excellence/official-position-statements/id/just-culture/.

American Nurses Association. (2016). *Healthy work environment.* https://www.nursingworld.org/practice-policy/work-environment/.

American Nurses Credentialing Center (ANCC). (n.d.). *ANCC Magnet Recognition Program®.* https://www.nursingworld.org/organizational-programs/magnet/.

Barnes, H., Rearden, J., & McHugh, M. D. (2016). Magnet® hospital recognition linked to lower central line-associated bloodstream infection rates. *Research in Nursing & Health, 39*(2), 96–104.

Bellot, J. (2011). Defining and assessing organizational culture. *Nursing Forum, 46*(1), 29–37.

Bellot, J. (2012). Nursing home culture change: What does it mean to nurses? *Research in Gerontological Nursing, 5*(4), 264–273.

Blegen, M. A., Pepper, G. A., & Rosse, J. (2005). *Safety climate on hospital units: A new measure.* http://www.ncbi.nlm.nih.gov/books/NBK20592/.

Carthon, J. M. B., Lasater, K. B., Sloane, D. M., & Kutney-Lee, A. (2015). The quality of hospital work environments and missed nursing care is linked to heart failure readmissions: A cross-sectional study of US hospitals. *BMJ Quality & Safety, 24*(4), 255–263.

D'Ambra, A. M., & Andrews, D. R. (2014). Incivility, retention and new graduate nurses: An integrated review of the literature. *Journal of Nursing Management, 22*(6), 735–742.

Day, H. (2014). Engaging staff to deliver compassionate care and reduce harm. *British Journal of Nursing, 23*(18), 974–980. https://doi.org/10.12968/bjon.2014.23.18.974.

DeJoy, D. M., Schaffer, B. S., Wilson, M. G., Vandenbert, R. J., & Butts, M. M. (2004). Creating safer workplaces: Assessing the determinants and role of safety climate. *Journal of Safety Research, 35*, 81–90.

Dempsey, C., & Reilly, B. A. (2016). Nurse engagement: What are the contributing factors for success? *OJIN, 21*(1), 2. https://doi.org/10.3912/OJIN.Vol21No01Man02.

Edmonson, C., & Marshall, J. (2020). Keeping the human in health care human capital: Challenges and solutions for RNs in the next decade. *Nurse Leader, 18*(2), 130–134.

Feather, R. A., Ebright, P., & Bakas, T. (2015). Nurse manager behaviors that RNs perceive to affect their job satisfaction. *Nursing Forum, 50*(2), 125–136.

Gershon, R. R. M., Stone, P. W., Baaken, S., & Larson, E. (2004). Measurement of organizational culture and climate in healthcare. *Journal of Nursing Administration, 34*(1), 33–40.

Grabowski, D. C., Afendulis, C. C., Caudry, D. J., O'Malley, A. J., & Kemper, P. for the THRIVE Research Collaborative. (2016). The impact of green house adoption on Medicare spending and utilization. *Health Services Research, 51*(1 Pt 2), 433–453.

Hatch, M. J., & Cunliffe, A. L. (2013). *Organization theory: Modern, symbolic and postmodern perspectives*. New York: Oxford University Press.

Higgins, E. A. (2015). The influence of nurse manager transformational leadership on nurse and patient outcomes: Mediating effects of supportive practice environments, organizational citizenship behaviours, patient safety culture and nurse job satisfaction. *Electronic Thesis and Dissertation Repository*. Paper 3184. vhttp://ir.lib.uwo.ca/cgi/viewcontent.cgi?article=4453&context=etd.

Institute of Medicine (IOM). (1999). *To err is human: Building a safer health system*. Washington, DC: National Academies Press.

Institute of Medicine (IOM). (2001). *Crossing the quality chasm*. Washington, DC: National Academies Press.

Institute of Medicine (IOM). (2011). *The future of nursing: Leading change, advancing health*. Washington, DC: National Academies Press.

Jackson, G. L., Powers, B. J., Chatterjee, R., Bettger, J. P., Kemper, A. R., Hasselblad, V., et al. (2013). The patient-centered medical home: A systematic review. *Annals of Internal Medicine, 158*(3), 169–178.

Kutney-Lee, A., Germack, H., Hatfield, L., Kelly, S., Maguire, P., Dierkes, A., Del Guidice, M., & Aiken, L. (2016). Nurse engagement in shared governance and patient and nurse outcomes. *Journal of Nursing Administration, 46*(11), 605–612. https://doi.org/10.1097/NNA.0000000000000412.

Kutney-Lee, A., Stimpfel, A. W., Sloane, D. M., Cimiotti, J. P., Quinn, L. W., & Aiken, L. H. (2015). Changes in patient and nurse outcomes associated with Magnet hospital recognition. *Medical Care, 53*(6), 550–557.

Laschinger, H. K., & Leiter, M. P. (2006). The impact of nursing work environments on patient safety outcomes. *The Journal of Nursing Administration, 36*(45), 259–267.

Levine, K. J., Carmody, M., & Silk, K. J. (2020). The influence of organizational culture, climate and commitment on speaking up about medical errors. *Journal of Nursing Management, 28*(1), 130–138. https://doi.org/10.1111/jonm.12906.

Ma, C., & Park, S. H. (2015). Hospital Magnet status, unit work environment, and pressure ulcers. *Journal of Nursing Scholarship, 47*(6), 565–573.

McCaughey, D., McGhan, G. E., Rathert, C., Williams, J. H., & Hearld, K. R. (2020). Magnetic work environments: Patient experience outcomes in Magnet versus non-Magnet hospitals. *Health Care Management Review, 45*(1), 21–31.

McHugh, M. D., & Ma, C. (2013). Hospital nursing and 30-day readmissions among Medicare patients with heart failure, acute myocardial infarction, and pneumonia. *Medical care, 51*(1), 52.

McHugh, M. D., Rochman, M. F., Sloane, D. M., Berg, R. A., Mancini, M. E., Nadkarni, V. M., et al. (2016). Better nurse staffing and nurse work environments associated with increased survival of in-hospital cardiac arrest patients. *Medical Care, 54*(1), 74–80.

Nishioka, V. M., Coe, M. T., Hanita, M., & Moscato, S. R. (2014). Dedicated education unit: Student perspectives. *Nursing Education Perspectives, 35*(5), 301–307. https://doi.org/10.5480/14-1380.

Parry, J. S., Calarco, M. M., & Hensinger, B. (2014). Unit-based interventions: De-stressing the distressed. *Nursing Management, 45*(8), 38–44.

Peters, T., & Waterman, R. H. (1982). *In search of excellence*. New York, NY: Warner Communications.

Pew Research Center. (2018). *Millennials are the largest generation in the U.S. labor force*. https://www.pewresearch.org/fact-tank/2018/04/11/millennials-largest-generation-us-labor-force/.

Press Ganey Associates, Inc. (2013). *Every voice matters: The bottom line on employee and physician engagement*. South Bend, IN. http://healthcare.pressganey.com/2013-PI-Every_Voice_Matters.

Quality and Safety Education for Nurses (QSEN). (2020). *QSEN Institute*. https://qsen.org/.

Reason, J. (1997). *Managing the risks of organisational accidents*. London, UK: Ashgate Publishing.

Reeves, S., Perrier, L., Goldman, J., Freeth, D., & Zwarenstein, M. (2013). Interprofessional education: Effects on professional practice and healthcare outcomes (update). *Cochrane Database of Systematic Reviews, (3)*, Article CD002213.

Sleutel, M. R. (2000). Climate, culture, context, or work environment? Organizational factors that influence nursing practice. *Journal of Nursing Administration, 30,* 53–58.

Snow, J. (2002). Enhancing work climate to improve performance and retain valued employees. *Journal of Nursing Administration, 33*(2), 111–117.

Stewart, K. R., Stewart, G. L., Lampman, M., Wakefield, B., Rosenthal, G., & Solimeo, S. L. (2015). Implications of the patient-centered medical home for nursing practice. *Journal of Nursing Administration, 45*(11), 569–574. https://doi.org/10.1097/NNA.0000000000000265.

Stokowski, L. A. (2014). The risky business of nursing. *Medscape.* January 14, 2014 http://www.medscape.com/viewarticle/818437.

Stone, P. W., Harrison, M. I., Feldman, P., Linzer, M., Peng, T., Roblin, D., et al. (2005). *Organizational climate of staff working conditions and safety: An integrative model.* http://www.ncbi.nlm.nih.gov/books/NBK20497/.

Tourangeau, A. E., Thomson, H., Cummings, G., & Cranley, L. A. (2013). Generation-specific incentives and disincentives for nurses to remain employed in acute care hospitals. *Journal of Nursing Management, 21*(3), 473–482.

US Department of Health and Human Services: Health Resources and Services Administration. (2010). *The registered nurse population: Findings from the 2008 National Sample Survey of Registered Nurses.* https://bhw.hrsa.gov/sites/default/files/bhw/nchwa/rnsurveyfinal.pdf.

Van Bogaert, P., Timmermans, O., Weeks, S. M., van Heusden, D., Wouters, K., & Franck, E. (2014). Nursing unit teams matter: Impact of unit-level nurse practice environment, nurse work characteristics, and burnout on nurse reported job outcomes, and quality of care, and patient adverse events—A cross-sectional survey. *International Journal of Nursing Studies, 51*(8), 1123–1134.

Wonder, A. H., York, J., Jackson, K. L., & Sluys, T. D. (2017). Loss of Magnet® designation and changes in RN work engagement: A report on how 1 hospital's culture changed over time. *Journal of Nursing Administration, 47*(10), 491–496.

Wong, C. A., Cummings, G. G., & Ducharme, L. (2013). The relationship between nursing leadership and patient outcomes: A systematic review update. *Journal of Nursing Management, 21*(5), 709–724.

Wooten, L. P., & Crane, P. (2003). Nurses as implementers of organizational culture. *Nursing Economic$, 21,* 275–279.

Zimmerman, S., Bowers, B. J., Cohen, L. W., Grabowski, D. C., Horn, S. D., & Kemper, P. (2016). New evidence on the green house model of nursing home care: Synthesis of findings and implications for policy, practice, and research. *Health Services Research, 51*(Suppl.), 475–496.

4

Managerial Decision-Making

Betsy Frank

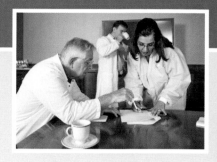

 http://evolve.elsevier.com/Huber/leadership

All nurses make decisions. Decisions can be categorized as clinical, involving direct care, or managerial. Decision-making is central to all managerial roles (Clark-Burg & Alliex, 2017). Managerial decisions range from managing groups of patients at the unit level to the organization or community or health care delivery system levels (see Fig. 4.1). In order for nurses to make effective decisions, they need the analytical skills that account for individual staff and patient care needs and an understanding of ethical frameworks and human resource and financial considerations. Whether at the point-of-care, unit, or organizational level, all decisions affect the level of quality and safe care that is delivered and the climate of the work environment in which nurses and other health professionals work. Furthermore, all decisions need to be made with the entire system in mind.

In an era of corporate mergers, changing reimbursements, value-based purchasing, and expanded roles for nursing in the health care delivery system, decision-making is an important skill for nurses caring for patients and for nurse leaders and managers. Both the American Nurses Association's (2016) and the American Organization for Nursing Leadership (2015) standards for practice and competencies for nurse managers support the fact that in a fast-paced health care delivery environment, staff nurses, leaders, and managers all must be able to analyze and synthesize a large array of information, make decisions to deliver effective day-to-day patient care, and solve multifaceted problems that occur in complex health care delivery systems. Furthermore, the Magnet Recognition Program® (American Nurses Credentialing Center, 2020) and the *Future of nursing* report (2011) of the Institute of Medicine (IOM, now called the National Academies of Sciences, Engineering, and Medicine, Health and Medicine Division) highlighted the need for nurses to be able to be fully involved and even take the lead in decision-making from the unit level to the larger health care delivery system, including on health care institution governing boards (Thew, 2019).

DEFINITIONS

Decision-making is the process of making the best evidenced-informed choice, while taking into the context of the decision (Krishnan, 2018; Spiers et al., 2016). For example, if a nurse calls in sick, staff coverage decisions have to be made immediately. However, a union contract may influence how the manager adjusts the unit's staffing model in the short run, as well as the long term, if the unit is chronically understaffed. Decisions about staffing assignments greatly affect nurses' work life and patient outcomes. These include skill mix, patient-to-nurse ratios, and specific patient assignments.

The process of selecting one course of action from alternatives forms the basic core of the definition of decision-making. Nibbelink and Brewer (2018) noted that decisions made at the unit level are influenced by a unit's culture, patient acuity, and nursing staff expertise. In a chaotic health care delivery environment, where regulations and standards of care are always changing, any decision may cause unanticipated consequences. For example, a decision may be made to implement team-based delivery of care. However, if this new staffing model is made without considering availability of staff of various skill levels, the model might fail.

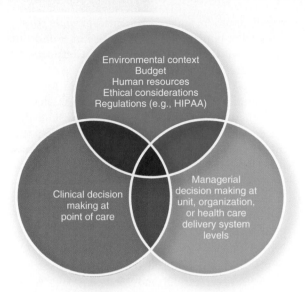

Fig. 4.1 The relationship between clinical and managerial decision-making.

Decision-making environment is the context in which decisions are made. The complexity of patient care needs, staffing expertise, budget allotted to care for patients, union contracts, reimbursement regulations, and leadership styles all affect the decisions that are made. Ultimately all these factors affect the quality of the patient care that is delivered.

Clinical judgment involves forming, refining, and evaluating hypotheses based upon recognizing and analyzing cues (National Council of State Boards of Nursing, 2019).

Clinical reasoning is the decision-making process that is grounded in the professional thought process (Gummesson et al., 2018).

Clinical decision-making involves clinical judgments that result in interventions at the point of patient care (Johansen & O'Brien, 2016; Razieh et al., 2018).

Managerial and organizational decision-making involves decisions for groups of patients at the unit, organizational, or health system levels.

BACKGROUND

Decision-Making Models

All nurses, whether managers or not, use models to help them make decisions. Many of the models include step-by-step frameworks that can guide decision-making. In reality, however, decision-making is an iterative process that may include an intuitive component (Benner, 1984; Tanner, 2006). Yet models can help the staff nurse and manager make some sense of the complex environment in which all decisions are made.

Such models are more than just for immediate problem solving. Decision-making may also be the result of opportunities, challenges, or more long-term leadership initiatives, as opposed to being triggered by an immediate problem. In any case, the processes are virtually the same, but their purposes may be slightly different. Nurse managers use decision-making in managing resources and the environment of care delivery. All decision-making involves an evaluation of the effectiveness of the outcomes that result from the decision-making process itself.

The nursing process is an example of one well-known model for clinical decision-making. However, the nursing process does not truly capture the important component of how the staff nurse or nurse manager makes the choice between competing alternatives for action. Other models may be more appropriate.

Moving beyond the nursing process, Tanner's (2006) model has formed the basis for understanding how clinical decisions are made. Her clinical judgment model involves noticing patient cues, interpreting those cues and responding to (acting on) them, and finally reflecting on the course of action chosen so that clinical learning occurs. The National Council of State Boards of Nursing (2019) published a model of clinical judgment that takes into account not only individual patient assessment but also environmental factors including resources, task complexity, and cultural considerations when making decisions about patient care. Furthermore, this model considers the nurse's knowledge and experience.

Nurse managers consider the environment and their own knowledge and experience when making decisions as well. For example, a nurse manager might want to implement a mentorship program for all new staff on the unit. However, the budget might cause the manager to only assign mentors to new graduates, not all new staff.

Guo's (2008) DECIDE Model is a model that is useful for managerial as well as clinical situations (Aitamaa et al., 2019b; Esan et al., 2016). Using this model can help prevent cognitive bias in high-stress environments because it can help prevent the missing of cues and thus choosing the wrong course of action.

Nurse managers also can use the decision-making dependency (DMD) model to assist in their decision-making processes (Chisengantambu-Winters et al., 2020). This model emphasizes the importance of consulting with personnel at all levels of an organization when a manager makes a decision.

The model outlined here is a combination of the models of Guo (2008) and Chisengantambu-Winters et al. (2020):

- **D**efine the problem or need and its urgency. Does the problem require immediate action (Chisengantambu-Winters et al., 2020)?
- **E**stablish desirable criteria for what you want to accomplish. What should stay the same and what can be done to avoid future problems? Predict how long it will take to respond to the changing environment.
- **C**onsider all possible alternative choices that will accomplish the desired goal or criteria for problem solution. In other words, what is a desirable outcome?
- **I**dentify the best choice or alternative based on expe-

rience, intuition, and experimentation while considering what human and material resources and time are needed to implement the choice. Consider what impact the decision will have.

- **D**evelop and implement an action plan for problem solution taking into account policies that influence the decision-making process. Consider does the decision have to made immediately or can it be made when the manager can carefully consider all the criteria in the process such ethical and financial factors.
- **E**valuate decision through monitoring, troubleshooting, and feedback. This step involves the reflective process emphasized by Tanner (2006).

Notice how these steps are somewhat similar to the nursing process well known to all nurses.

Thus decision-making is used to solve problems. Table 4.1 displays the use of the DECIDE model to

TABLE 4.1   Possible Formation of an Inpatient Hospice Unit Using the DECIDE Model

D—Define the Problem	E—Establish the Criteria	C—Consider All the Alternatives and Steps to Be Taken	I—Identify the Best Alternatives	D—Develop and Implement the Action	E—Evaluate and Monitor the Solution
The Federal government mandates inpatient hospice care. Nurses on med-surg units are not equipped to provide hospice level of care. Therefore a non-profit hospice agency must decide how to provide inpatient care when needed.	The inpatient unit must meet all Federal and State regulations for operation, and census has to be high enough to meet costs. Death certificates must be analyzed to determine which deaths have a hospice diagnosis in order to determine potential census. The competition must be determined. An assessment showed no other inpatient hospice unit is within 60 miles.	Two alternatives exist. One is to construct a free-standing inpatient hospice facility. The second alternative is to remodel a vacant unit at a local hospital and share services such as dietary and maintenance, but rent must be paid to the hospital.	The inpatient hospice unit in the existing local hospital was chosen because total cost was less than a free-standing unit	The Board of Directors of the hospice agency, patients, families, and the medical director must all agree on the plan for the hospice unit. The hospital's architect must be hired to design the unit. Fund raising to remodel the vacant unit for hospice services must occur.	The State Board of Health must give approval to open the unit. Costs must not exceed revenue if the unit is to remain viable. If costs exceed revenue, the hospice agency must determine how to make up for the difference through fundraising and other means.

Acknowledgement: Trudy Rupska MSN, RN, CEO of VNA Homecare and Hospice of the Wabash Valley.

analyze whether to establish an inpatient hospice unit. The DECIDE model depicted in Table 4.1 shows information to consider in making a decision regarding the inpatient unit.

The person at the next level may look at the chosen alternative in a different context. For example, the chief executive officer may frame issues as a competitive struggle not unlike a sports event. The marketing staff may interpret problems as military battles that need to be won. Nurse executives may view concerns from a care or family frame that emphasizes collaboration and working together. Learning and understanding which analogies and perspectives offer the best view of a problem or issue are vital to effective decision-making. It may be necessary for nurse managers to expand their frame of reference and be willing to consider even the most outlandish ideas. Effectiveness is tied to mirroring and messaging language that fosters shared understanding.

Chisengantambu et al. (2018) developed a sandwich support model that can be integrated into the DECIDE and DMD model (Chisengantambu-Winters et al., 2020). Both models demonstrate the importance of having environmental support for the nurse manager from staff as well as the executive level. The models define support in terms of environmental, technical, and financial resources. With support, nurse managers can implement organizational policies while at the same time supporting the staff nurses who work within the organization. Nurse executives can guide the nurse manager in how to effectively support staff during the decision-making process. With support work performance is enhanced and ultimately quality and safe patient care can be delivered.

One note of caution is that no matter the model used or the organizational level where the decision is made, cognitive bias can occur. Fig. 4.2 is an illustration of what can happen in a faulty decision process when data are ignored or biases are present in the process. According to Sherman (2015), by allowing others to question your thinking you can avoid cognitive bias.

DECISION-MAKING PROCESS

Decisions are the visible outcomes of the leadership and management process. Decision-making is essentially the process of selecting one course of action from alternatives. Decisions are made at all levels, but it is important to know who the decision maker is and what the process and timeline of decision-making is. Nurses' control over decision-making may vary as to amount of control and where in the process they can influence decisions. The basic elements of decision-making are identifying the goal for decision-making and making the decision.

The process follows the basic problem-solving process but also involves an evaluation of the effectiveness of the outcomes that result from the decision-making process itself. The seven steps of the problem solving process are (1) define the problem, (2) gather information, (3) determine the overall goal or desired outcome, (4) develop solutions, (5) consider the consequences, (6) make a decision, and (7) implement and evaluate

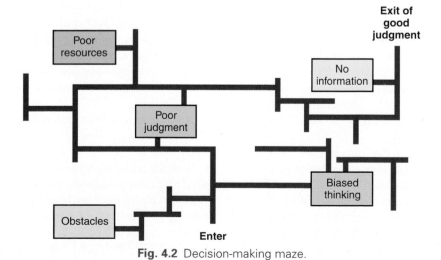

Fig. 4.2 Decision-making maze.

the solution. The decision-making process adds a final step of testing or assessing the solution and the decision-making process itself. Nurses may be sole decision makers or may facilitate group decision-making. Decisions are often made within the structure of shared governance or by using interprofessional teams for problem solving and decision-making.

CLINICAL DECISION-MAKING

Clinical decision-making is the heart of nursing practice. Point-of-care decisions ultimately have an impact on the total organization's performance and, consequently, its financial viability. Delivering quality and safe patient care is a goal for all health care organizations. Thus effective clinical decisions must be made.

Clinical reasoning is a career-long development process. This process must carry over from skills learned during a nurse's education to the workplace. Nurse residency programs are one way to help newly licensed nurses develop their clinical decision-making abilities. Kramer et al. (2012) found that newly licensed nurses identified that autonomous decision-making and prioritization were challenging for them. New graduates often felt that they needed to verify their decisions with others more competent than themselves. The graduates noted they could identify what care needed to be implemented but needed support to develop confidence in making the right decisions regarding care. The use of preceptors and/or coaches and didactic presentations in the residency program helped the new graduates develop their confidence to make autonomous decisions. Staff nurses must continually make autonomous decisions regarding patient care delivery. Therefore nurse residency programs could promote the new graduate's ability to make the necessary decisions when delivering nursing care autonomously. Some examples of decisions nurses make involve such day-to-day activities as documentation, medication administration, intravenous drug therapy, and prioritization for what care is delivered to a group of patients such as by triage.

In the course of their day, nurses make many decisions from what to chart, how and when to give medications, or when to call a rapid response team. All these decisions have consequences for patient safety.

Medication administration involves many decisions. All nurses know that giving medications involves giving the right patient the right medication, the right dose, the right route, at the right time. If anyone of these rights is wrong, the nurse must take appropriate action. For example, if the dose is wrong, the nurse must contact the prescriber for a new medication order. Medication administration takes place in an environment prone to interruptions which can disturb the nurse's decision-making processes. In fact, Reed et al. (2018) found that medication administration, including preparation of the medication to be administered, was interrupted 39% of the time. Such interruptions have the potential to compromise patient safety.

In addition to distractions other factors can contribute to medication errors ultimately caused by faulty decision-making during medication administration (Keers et al., 2018). Keers and colleagues interviewed 20 nurses who described medication errors, including near misses. They found that a stressful work environment that includes short staffing, improper skill mix, and multitasking all impact decision-making during medication administration. The five "rights" of medication administration are just the beginning of a complex decision-making process.

Triage decisions occur in a very complex environment, and a computerized system can assist in this process (Chang et al., 2017). Using a computerized system, the nurse can enter assessment data to determine the level of triage or urgency. Chang and colleagues interviewed 15 Taiwanese emergency department triage nurses in order to gain an understanding of the clinical decision-making process during triage. Although the computerized data assessment was used, the nurse's experience, the patients' overall health status, and environmental factors such as available equipment and conflict with staff and patients also affected the triage decision. For example, if a patient required a procedure that might indicate a lower level of triage as determined by the computer, but the nurse thought the procedure was more urgent, the nurse would "up" the level of triage.

Prioritization occurs not only in triage situations but also across the care spectrum. Nurses take care of more than one patient at a time. Thus decisions have to be made regarding what care has to be delivered and what care can possibly be omitted (Harvey et al., 2018). Ethical frameworks may be unconsciously used when making decisions (see Chapter 7). Some patient care activities can be delegated, but on a busy day even thinking about delegation can be challenging.

Clinical decision-making is complex and step-by-step processes are helpful, but not all situations lend themselves to such processes. A more holistic approach is often needed as priorities can rapidly change (Benner et al., 2010). Therefore leaders and managers at all levels of an organization need to foster a culture where effective, evidence-based clinical decision-making can occur.

MANAGERIAL AND ORGANIZATIONAL DECISION-MAKING

All nurse managers and leaders need to consider the implications of their decisions. Each decision made involves financial, ethical, and human resources. Furthermore, reimbursement and other regulations must be considered. Nurse managers, for example, make staffing decisions and thus commit financial resources for the purpose of delivering patient care. Hospital administrators may decide to add additional services to keep up with external forces. These decisions subsequently have financial implications related to reimbursement, staffing, and human resources deployment.

Nurse managers work in a complex environment that causes stress that may ultimately hamper their cognitive decision-making abilities (Shirey et al., 2013). In any situation, a nurse manager's experience, level of work complexity, and situation factors such as uncertainty and role overload influence how he or she recognizes environmental patterns and cues and the subsequent questions asked. The decisions that result have wide impact on the organization. If a manager is stressed, important factors in the cognitive decision-making process may be missed and organizational outcomes adversely affected. Not only does stress impact organizational outcomes, but the nurse manager's own mental and physical health can be impacted (Udon et al., 2017). Lack of autonomy in decision-making is one stressor that can adversely impact a manager's health (Fallman et al., 2019). On the other hand, support from staff and upper level management can mitigate some of the stress in the work environment (Chisengantambu et al., 2018).

Ethical decision-making is inherent in the role of the nurse manager. When decisions involve an ethical dilemma, nurse managers may experience stress (Ganz et al., 2015). Aitamaa et al. (2016) interviewed nine nurse managers and found that ethical dilemmas occur in four areas: conflicts with staff, patients, and administration; lack of appreciation for the value of nursing

as a profession; disregard of problems that had to be ignored because the problems were considered "normal" in the organization; inability to carry out the job due to obstacles such as financial and limited power within the organization. How the nurse manager deals with these dilemmas has an effect on the quality of the work environment.

One way to deal with ethical dilemmas is through moral case discussions between staff and managers (Weidema et al., 2015). In an open and safe environment, a case study is presented for full debate, analysis, and sharing of possible action steps for resolution. However, using this participatory management technique is hard to incorporate in the workflow when there is a heavy day-to-day workload. Furthermore, conducting case discussions between staff and managers could inhibit free discussion between the two groups just because of the presence of hierarchal relationships (Weidema et al., 2015). Weidema and colleagues suggested that if staff nurses feel empowered to make autonomous decisions, then communication in the case discussions could actually occur without the presence of the manager.

Nurse managers need to develop ways of being that strengthen their ability to make ethical decisions (Roshanzadeh et al., 2019). Nineteen nurse managers were interviewed, and data analysis showed that assertiveness, commitment, and insight promoted sound decision-making. If a nurse manager is assertive, then the manager has confidence in their ethical decision-making ability. A nurse manager who has commitment takes responsibility for decision-making and aims to prevent errors. A manager who has insight is self-aware, logical, intelligent and is fair in the decision-making process.

On an organizational level, Aitamaa et al. (2019a) suggested that a values-based organization can mitigate the severity of ethical problems. They also stated that ethics education could enhance the nurse manager's ability to make ethical decisions.

A nurse manager's leadership style may affect how decisions are made throughout the organization. Leadership style influences decision-making by promoting structural empowerment and engagement in the work (Garcia-Sierra & Fernández-Castro, 2018).

Praising employees affects a nurse's job satisfaction (Sveinsdóttir et al., 2016). This in turn contributes to a healthy work environment wherein nurses are free to make autonomous decisions that contribute to positive patient outcomes. Dans and Lundmark (2019) noted that autonomy is one of the most important influences on patient outcomes. Furthermore, Kowalski et al. (2020) integrative literature review confirms that autonomy in decision-making is a key component of a practice environment that promotes positive patient outcomes. Transformational leaders are the key to achieving these positive outcomes (Moon et al., 2019).

Patient Acuity and Staffing: An Example of Decision-Making

An example of decision-making in nursing practice is staffing and assignment decisions. Patients need nursing care. Needs for care are not uniform. The need severity (physical and psychological) is called *patient acuity*, which is a rating of the complexity of the patient's condition. The degree of work needed for any patient is called *nursing intensity* and is a combination of the severity of illness, the patient's dependency, the complexity of care, and the amount of time needed. The organization staffs a set number of nurses and assistants to deliver care to patients. Both patients' needs for nursing care and the amount of nurse time that is required to meet patients' needs for care must be matched up and caregivers deployed, sometimes 24/7.

Frontline nurses are responsible for the decision-making about patient acuity and nursing intensity. Managers are responsible for the decision-making about staffing and scheduling. The individual nurse experiences this decision-making as workload (nursing work activities), nurse-to-patient ratios, and patient assignments. In theory, the nursing interventions required to support the patients' needs should be in proportion to the levels of severity and degrees of intensity (Gray & Kerfoot, 2016). However, for a variety of reasons, decision-making around staffing, scheduling, patient assignments is imprecise and creates tension and stress for both nurses and managers. For example, data-driven acuity systems often do not consider experience levels of staff, and the systems, themselves, often rely on subjective data when calculating the acuity score (Gray & Kerfoot, 2016).

Allen (2015) interviewed 14 charge nurses in order to explore how staffing decisions were made. Findings showed that nurse-patient assignments involved a complex process that included not only patient factors, such as acuity; the nurse, including expertise; and the environment, including nurse patient ratios and location of patients on the unit. Given the complexity of staffing

decisions, the nurse manager needs to think about what unanticipated and adverse consequences could occur as a result of staffing decisions.

DECISION-MAKING TOOLS

Both nurses at the point of care and nurse managers need a variety of tools to facilitate effective decision-making. For example, there are a variety of clinical decision-making tools such as algorithms, policies, procedures, clinical protocols, standard order sets, and smart alerts.

Although trial and error or a shoot-from-the-hip approach can work, direct patient care nurses and managers have a variety of other approaches that can be used to make decisions that promote quality and safe care. For example, by analyzing the data in Table 4.2, the nurse can help decide if an additional medical assistant should be hired in a small rural health clinic. The nurse must also decide if the assistant should be hired full or part-time.

Shared Governance

Another decision making approach is shared governance. Although this topic is discussed more fully in Chapter 13, a brief discussion is warranted here. Shared governance is an organizational structure that promotes empowerment and autonomous decision-making at the point of care, accountability that is shared among all parties in a decision, and organizational processes that promote an egalitarian environment in decision-making processes. Shared governance promotes staff nurses' responsibility and accountability for patient outcomes (Medeiros, 2018). For example, a committee within a shared governance organization could develop and test a new fall-prevention protocol, exhibiting nursing practice empowerment. Nurse leaders have a critical role in promoting the success of the decisions that arise out of shared governance. They can use their expertise to coach staff on how to implement their decisions, as well as facilitate effective group functioning when group process within the governance structure goes awry.

Evidence-Informed Decision-Making

Nurses are familiar with evidence-based practice for clinical standards of practice. In the management realm, using evidence to make decisions is as important as is using evidence for clinical decisions. One example is the evidence-based protocol that is widely used by staff

TABLE 4.2 Desired Objectives Analysis			
Objective	Alternative A Full-time Hire	Alternative B Part-time Hire	Alternative C No Hire
Increases workflow	5	4	1
Enables more examination rooms to be filled at one time	5	3	1
Decreases patient wait time	4	3	1
Increases the number of patients seen in a day	4	3	1
Revenue minus personnel costs increase	4	5	5
Total score	22	18	9

1, Does not meet objective; 2, meets some aspects of objective; 3, meets objective; 4, exceeds objective; 5, significantly exceeds objective.

nurses to prevent catheter acquired urinary infections (American Nurses Association, 2017). But what about managers? Jansson and Forsberg's study (2016) revealed that nurse managers have a critical role in facilitating the use of evidence at the point of care.

Specific interventions at the organizational level can promote better decision-making. Thomson and colleagues (2017) conducted an educational program for primary health providers in Britain's national health care system (NHS). Participants were divided into three groups: Group 1 attended a full day educational session, Group 2 a half-day session, and Group 3 six 2.5-hour sessions. All groups found a self-reported increase in understanding of the theory of decision-making following the educational sessions. The educational intervention appeared to have little impact on application to practice. The researchers posited that perhaps the self-reported questionnaire could not detect small differences in improvement in decision-making in practice (Thomson et al., 2017). Another factor may have accounted for this finding. Perhaps a longer term follow-up using observations of clinical practice rather than self-report may have more precisely captured any changes in decision-making following the educational program.

Pilot Projects

Pilot projects are critical for implementation for evidence-informed decision-making. Pilot projects or carefully defined trials are used to try out a solution alternative on a small or restricted basis to reduce risk and to see whether major problems will occur. Pilot project strategies may resemble research projects, and

these projects may also be linked to quality improvement initiatives. One example of a pilot quality improvement project was reported by Massarweh and colleagues (2017). An eAssignment sheet for nurse staffing was developed at a California multi-hospital system to replace multiple paper records of assignments. This decision support tool for staffing considered such things as union contract requirements, legislated nurse-patient ratios, and nurse competency. If a less experienced nurse was assigned to a complex patient, the system alerted the nurse manager who reached out to that nurse to assist in problem solving when necessary. The system also alerted the nurse manager if care hours assigned did not conform with the expected care hours based on acuity. Nurse managers agreed that patient care assignments were more data-driven and took less time than did the paper system. Furthermore, the data collected through the eAssignment system was used for financial management.

SBAR

SBAR is a communication technique that helps members of the health team communicate effectively so that appropriate decisions can be made. Because hand-off communication is so crucial to decision-making about patient care, SBAR is used to clarify and organize essential but complex patient care information (see Chapter 2). The acronym stands for Situation, Background, Assessment, Recommendation (Stewart & Hand, 2017). Teaching SBAR to students helps them to develop their clinical judgment skills and can also be used to help new nurses further develop their autonomous decision-making.

SBAR has been demonstrated to be particularly useful in a rapid paced emergency department where incomplete reporting can result in errors being made (Campbell & Dontje, 2019). Therefore all providers need a way to communicate in order to guide effective clinical decision-making. When SBAR was used as a framework for bedside reporting at change of shift in the emergency department, as part of a quality improvement project, nurses reported that SBAR helped to reduce the number of poor patient outcomes that were due to incomplete communication between shifts (Campbell & Dontje, 2019).

Simulation

Simulation is a well-known technique for developing and maintaining clinical decision-making. It is used to teach skills and verify competencies. Simulation could also be used to improve management decision-making. A meta-analysis conducted by Orique and Phillips (2018) showed that simulation was effective in improving knowledge and skills in recognizing clinical deterioration. Likewise, simulation is a useful strategy for practicing interprofessional collaboration (Blondon et al., 2017).

Simulation is also useful for nurse leaders to practice skills particular to their role. Junious (2020) used simulation in a master's in nursing administration program to help future nurse leaders learn root cause analysis for errors that could "lead to a sentinel event" (Junious, 2020, p. 57). Students had to work through the root cause analysis procedure and identify flaws in the system of care. Debriefing is an important and necessary part of instruction using simulation. Junious (2020) described this post-simulation evaluation by debriefing as all students and faculty participating in a roundtable debriefing discussion done immediately after completing the scenario and focused on students' initial thoughts and feelings. Faculty critiques included positive and negative feedback and advice. Students used this to develop a presentation on the process.

Data Analytics and Decision Support Systems

Decisions need to be data driven. Nurses and nurse managers have a wide array of data—including electronic health records, human resource data, and financial data—available to them for use in making decisions (Murphy et al., 2013). Making sense of these data is necessary but often a challenge.

By analyzing big data sets, nurse managers can improve staff performance. For example, Loresto and colleagues (2019) studied patterns of medication delivery to individual patients. The data were used to look, in particular, at delays in medication administration. Over a million medications were given to over 29,000 by patients by 704 nurses on 18 hospital units. Although nurse and patient characteristics had little effect on the delays, Loresto and colleagues (2019) suggested that patient mix and nurse staffing could have affected the medication delays.

Data analytics can also be used to promote financial success across the health care delivery system. Polancich and colleagues (2017) described how data analytics helped to improve the financial performance of nurse-led clinics that served patients with diabetes and heart failure. The measure of success was the number of inpatient days avoided and the resultant cost avoidance, or costs that did not occur. The clinic that served the patients with diabetes avoided $300,000 in annualized costs through decreasing inpatient days by 50%. For the patients with heart failure, inpatient days decreased by 18% after the nurse-led clinic was instituted. Cost avoidance was over $47,600. By analyzing data such as these, nurse managers can justify their return on investment for new or continuing patient care delivery models.

In addition to the use of data analytics to help decide if a particular patient care delivery system is justified, nurse managers can use decision support systems to make day-to-day decisions concerned with patient care unit operation. Staffing is one of the primary decisions that managers make. In addition, determining supply availability and patient flow are other uses for decision support systems. Peltonen and colleagues (2019) surveyed nurse managers in Finland to determine whether or not the information systems in their hospitals assisted them in day-to-day decision-making. Results showed that respondents were fairly satisfied with access to information, but the information was not always useful in decision-making. The respondents noted that multiple systems of information had to be accessed in order to make decisions. In another study by Peltonen and colleagues (2018), respondents noted the need for information to be shared with all stakeholders in the decision-making process. For decision supports systems to be useful, all stakeholders, including nurse managers, need to have a say in the systems' design.

Using a personal device such as a smartphone has the potential for assisting nurse managers and beside clinicians in making decisions. Martinez and colleagues (2017) interviewed 10 Canadian nurse managers for the purpose of studying the acceptance of personal devices, such as smartphones and tablets, in the clinical setting. One advantage was ready access to evidence-based information to use in patient care decisions. One big disadvantage identified was concerns for patient privacy and data security. As the use of mobile technology expands, nurse managers and leaders will need to take the lead in determining how best to use this rapidly expanding information system.

Artificial intelligence also has possibilities for improving decision-making for clinicians and nurse leaders (Clancy, 2020). Artificial intelligence could help analyze patterns of data and suggest courses of action. Robots could deliver supplies, saving human resources for more important tasks (Clancy, 2020).

Six Sigma is a quality and decision support technique that uses data to build process-improvement models. The goal is to eliminate defects in safety and quality in health care delivery (American Society for Quality, n.d.). Essentially Six Sigma is a variant of the plan-do-study-act (PDSA) cycle promoted by the Institute for Healthcare Improvement (n.d.). For example, data may be used to identify ways to decrease health care acquired infections. Improta and colleagues (2018) used an interprofessional team to investigate how Six Sigma could be used to decrease infections. Through the Six Sigma process, needed corrections in processes were identified, which led to a decreased infection rate across a variety of patient care units. Thus Six Sigma and Lean quality improvement techniques can be used for clinical and managerial decision-making as well (see Chapter 18).

Data analytics are most useful in assisting in decision-making, and an expanded discussion of the use of data analytics is found in Chapter 25. However, use of data to make decisions can have unintended consequences. Aron and colleagues (2019) examined data from Veteran's Affairs hospitals and discovered that many patients with diabetes were overtreated. However, when reduction in overtreatment was promoted, an increase in patients who were undertreated occurred. Nurse managers and leaders need to recognize that decision based on data analysis can lead to better or worse organizational outcomes.

LEADERSHIP AND MANAGEMENT IMPLICATIONS

All health care is delivered in complex and sometimes chaotic organizations. Decisions made using a variety of tools and strategies can lead to safer care delivery environments. However, the rapid pace of decision-making may hamper the use of available evidence to assist in that decision-making. Furthermore, the time for reflection about clinicians' and managers' actions may hamper development of clinical judgment and managerial decision-making abilities.

Strategies for Decision-Making

The focus of leadership and management decision-making is more closely related to the nurse's role as care coordinator and systems problem solver. Some decisions, such as those requiring disciplinary action, do require the manager's *direct intervention*. In conflicts between staff members or between family and staff members, the manager might use negotiation and other forms of conflict management that could be viewed as *indirect intervention* because the manager does not actually decide what should be done to deal with an issue but rather persuades others to solve the problem themselves. The nurse manager might *delegate* the decision-making to others. For example, a unit manager might ask a team of staff nurses and the unit secretary to figure out when the best time is to order supplies for the unit.

Sometimes the nurse manager might choose *watchful waiting*. A particular staff member might be causing some interpersonal difficulties. If the staff member has submitted his or her resignation, dealing with the behavior might not be worth the energy.

Most decision-making should take place within the confines of *collaboration and consultation*. That collaboration often takes place within an interprofessional context. Patient care requires a team approach among nursing, medicine, and other disciplines such as physical therapy. Working in an interprofessional context is an essential skill for both clinicians and managers (Interprofessional Education Collaborative, 2016).

Shared governance initiatives have shown that collaboration and consultation result in high-quality patient care delivery systems (Dans & Lundmark, 2019). Therefore a critical role for nurse managers and leaders is *facilitation* by fostering a climate that encourages creativity and interdependence.

Modeling desired decision-making behaviors is also important. For example, in hospitals, nurse leaders and managers can use change-of-shift reports to promote deep clinical reasoning using the Socratic method and asking who, what, when, and where questions such as "What nursing interventions have been effective?" or "What will happen if this course of action is chosen?" An organizational climate that fosters patient safety can enhance nurses' clinical reasoning skills. Fig. 4.3 summarizes global strategies used for decision-making that contribute to quality and safe patient care.

Clearly all nurses are on information overload. Ways to capture the available data and use it for effective problem solving and decision-making are critical. The use of computerized informatics applications to aid decision-making is on the rise. For example, hospital information systems can be used to capture data such as length of stay, skill mix, case mix, patient and employee job satisfaction, and other variables that can be important when decisions need to be made (Peltonen et al., 2019). Refinements such as smart alerts show promise to ease the complexity and information overload of care delivery and thus reduce errors.

Nurse managers and leaders solve problems in complex systems where all decisions carry some amount of risk (Shirey et al., 2013). Understanding a manager's cognitive workflow has the potential for use in decision support tools (Effken et al., 2011). Cognitive workflow analysis includes work domain, decision-making procedures, personnel skill level, and social organization and collaboration patterns.

Braaten (2015) used qualitative methods to investigate barriers to workflow using the example of when to call a Rapid Response Team (RRT). The results indicated that human resources in the form of appropriate staffing helped to identify patients in need of an RRT. Nonhuman resources included the electronic medical record and policies related to the RRT. Respondents had to justify calling the RRT within the framework of policies and enough staffing to recognize the change, which was often subtle, in the patient's condition as observed and not from data in the medical record. If policies were unclear, the nurse's decision-making was hampered. Based on the findings of this study, Braaten noted the critical importance of managerial support so that appropriate decisions could be made.

Just like complex patient-care scenarios, complex social organizations such as hospitals can produce the best outcomes when creativity and ability of the staff at all levels of the organization are enabled (Belrhiti et al., 2018). Expert nurse leaders need to understand the system they work in is often unordered and rapidly changing. Because change is occurring so rapidly, nurse managers may feel stressed when past practices no longer apply. Therefore decentralized decision-making is essential.

Inevitably some mistakes will be made, but nurse managers and leaders who view mistakes as learning opportunities help promote effective organizations. Such an attitude fosters the concept of a learning organization (see Chapter 2), where organizations stay vital by learning and growing. Leaders can foster a climate wherein new communication patterns emerge, bottom-up communication changes the organization, and differences in talents, structures, and communication networks come forth and promote high-performing organizations.

CURRENT ISSUES AND TRENDS

Creativity and innovation will be the cornerstone of nurses' participation in the health care system of the future. An IOM report (2011) and the 2015 update (Altman et al., 2015) noted that nurses should and must take the lead in providing care for patients in a complex, rapidly changing health care system. An additional role for all nurses, including leaders, is to get nurses on various health care and community boards of directors (Nurses on Boards Coalition, 2020). New roles have

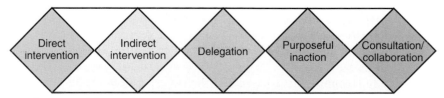

Fig. 4.3 Global decision-making strategies that contribute to quality and safe patient care.

emerged, such as the clinical nurse leader, who is a bedside leader and coordinator of complex care. Nurse leaders are in a unique position in the implementation of Accountable Care Organizations (ACOs), which will coordinate primary care for groups of patients. These leaders understanding and skills necessary to coordinate the continuum of care across the full spectrum of the health care delivery system will be critical to the success of the ACOs (Morrison, 2016). Cost savings will be critical, therefore nurse managers need to take the lead in delivering quality, cost efficient care.

The emphasis on quality and safety will be the focus of much of nurse managers' and leaders' planning and resultant decision-making. The seminal report *To err is human* (IOM, 1999), pointed out that human error was rampant in the health care system, causing lives lost and increasing health costs. Makary and Daniel (2016) and many others have pointed out that medical errors are the third leading cause of death in the United States. However, Mazer and Nabhan (2019) questioned the accuracy of these statistics. Nevertheless, nurse leaders and managers can foster team decision-making in a shared governance environment in order to improve processes of care delivery and mitigate errors (Fischer et al., 2018).

Although financial considerations in an organization are important, quality and safe care that is patient- and family-centered is equally important. The Quality and Safety Education for Nurses (QSEN, 2020) competencies will continue to serve as a guide for clinicians and managers alike as they strive to increase personal and organization performance.

Changing reimbursement patterns as a result of the attempts to modify the Patient Protection and Affordable Care Act (2010) and changing reimbursement regulations from the Centers for Medicare & Medicaid Services (CMS) (2020) will challenge nurse leaders and managers to find creative ways to facilitate the delivery of safe and quality care. More than likely costs will go up, but reimbursements may not keep pace with costs.

Despite the need for creativity, a certain amount of standardization must occur if safe patient care is to happen in complex care environments. Evidence-based management is the ideal, but barriers to implementation do exist, including communication gaps between those who develop guidelines and decision makers (Hasanpoor et al., 2019). Nurse managers have a critical role in incorporating evidence along with patient-centered care and clinical experience in their decision-making (Karlsson et al., 2019).

Nurse leaders need to advocate for a preferred future for nursing and evaluate the effectiveness of decision-making in practice. Both are aimed at making careful projections about what decisions to make—given uncertainty—to improve organizational and system performance. In times of change, nursing has an opportunity to make decisions that proactively direct the future. Nursing has demonstrated its value to the health care system. Therefore nurse leaders must be a party to all decisions regarding how care is delivered in health care organizations via shared governance arrangements (Medeiros, 2018).

Many hospitals are applying for Magnet recognition from the American Nurses Credentialing Center (ANCC, 2020). One of the 14 Forces of Magnetism from the old model that is incorporated in the new model of five domains involves management style and another promotes interdisciplinary collaboration. These two elements—a management style that is collaborative and the promotion of interdisciplinary staff input in decision-making—are evidence-based "best practices" (ANCC, 2020).

The efficiency, efficacy, and effectiveness of health care decisions will continue to enjoy a strong focus in nursing, with shifts toward outcomes specification. As performance improvement specialists, nurses will be challenged to make decisions that directly affect quality, access, cost, productivity, and the "bottom line." Effective approaches to decision-making are needed when care is delivered in a complex system in which multiple stakeholders need to be served, time is constrained, and the amount of information is overwhelming. The decisions that nurse managers and leaders make must be translated from the corporate "lingo" into terms that the clinicians understand if true buy-in is to be achieved (Porter-O'Grady, 2015). Furthermore, all nurses need to have leadership competencies, including the ability to make effective decisions (IOM, 2011). Nurses need to be at the forefront of all decision-making in health care, including at the governing board level.

RESEARCH NOTE

Source

Fischer, S. A., Horak, D., & Kelly, L. A. (2018). Decisional involvement: Differences related to characteristics, role, and shared leadership participation. *Journal of Nursing Care Quality, 33*(4), 354–360.

Purpose

The purpose of this study was to investigate the relationship between nurse attributes, role, and shared leadership participation in their perceptions of decisional involvement that affect their practice (p. 356).

Discussion

Staff nurses and managers from one health system in seven states responded to the Decisional Involvement Scale.

Over 1900 nurses and managers responded to the survey, Decisional involvement scale scores were positively correlated with participation in shared leadership councils and years of experience. Managers, however, had higher decisional involvement scores than did staff nurses. Nurse managers perceived that staff nurses had more decisional involvement than did the staff nurses themselves.

Application to Practice

As nurses gain more years of experience, they become more comfortable with sharing their ideas for practice improvement. However, all front-line nurses need to be mentored in the shared leadership model. When decisions are shared by staff and managers, patient care quality improves.

CASE STUDY

Effective decision-making relies, in part, on analyzing alternative levels of uncertainty or risk. Staffing and scheduling decisions exemplify this. In addition to making "apples to apples" comparisons through such tools as staffing matrices recommended by professional bodies, daily and monthly patient census data, and patient acuity and nursing intensity data can guide unit managers in their analysis, which might precede a request for more staffing. In addition, the nurse manager needs to have an awareness of the environment in which care is delivered in order to make the analysis complete.

Fig. 4.4 is an example of a decision tree. A nurse manager in a home care agency could use a decision tree to justify hiring more licensed practical nurses or more registered nurse case managers. The tree has several branches, and, depending on the end point, an increase in needed personnel could be handled in several ways. Diagrams such as decision trees can be invaluable in understanding complicated alternative solutions. These diagrams are useful in assessment and problem definition and in considering the available alternatives for dealing with a problem. Once the alternative is chosen, a plan needs to be formulated for implementing the chosen approach. The choice implemented must be evaluated. Note, however, that the decision tree in Fig. 4.4 only lists three alternatives. A more complex tree could be constructed that includes more alternatives based on a different combination of tree branches.

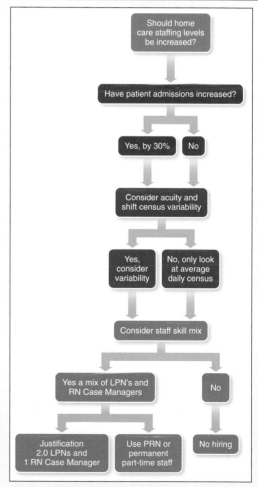

Fig. 4.4 Decision tree for home care staffing.

Acknowledgement: Jessica Wilson, BSN, RN, Clinical Coordinator, VNA Homecare and Hospice of the Wabash Valley.

CRITICAL THINKING EXERCISE

Adam Dean is a new nurse manager on a med-surg unit. One nurse on the night shift is ill and cannot come to work. He contacts the area director, and the director floats a nurse from the mental health unit to his unit to assist. This nurse did work on a med-surg unit until 6 months ago. She and another nurse each have a patient receiving blood transfusions. The float nurse needs another unit of blood, and while the other nurse covers, she goes to the blood bank and signs out the unit of blood. Upon returning to the unit, her colleague is tied up in a procedure and says she will be out in about 20 minutes. After briefly conferring with her colleague, the float nurse hangs the blood on her patient. When her colleague completes her procedure, the two of them are in the process of checking the blood and discover that the blood obtained from the Blood Bank was for the other patient. The blood is stopped, the supervisor is notified as is the patient's physician, and an incident report completed. As it turns out, the patient is a universal recipient. When Adam interviews each nurse individually, the nurse who administered the blood shows no remorse and tells Mr. Dean she cannot understand what the issue is because nothing happened. Adam Dean reviews with her the issue and related policies. She insists that Mr. Dean is upset over nothing. When speaking with the other nurse, she is overwrought, in tears, and asks if Mr. Dean wants her to resign. What actions does Mr. Dean, the manager, take for each nurse and why?

Using the SBAR framework identify:

1. What was the situation?
2. What was the background information?
3. What information does Mr. Dean need to assess the situation?
4. What disciplinary action should Mr. Dean take for each nurse, if any? Should the action be different for each nurse?

As you consider the SBAR scenario, think about what organizational policies you need to consider. What departments in the hospital could assist Mr. Dean in his decision-making process?

Acknowledgement: A. Christine Delucas, DNP, MPH, RN, NEA-BC, Associate Professor and DNP Program Director, University of New Mexico College of Nursing.

REFERENCES

Aitamaa, E., Leino-Kilpi, H., Iltanen, S., & Suhonen, R. (2016). Ethical problems in nursing management: The views of nurse managers. *Nursing Ethics, 23*(6), 646–658. https://doi.org/10.1177/0969733015579309.

Aitamaa, E., Suhonen, R., Iltanen, S., Puukka, P., & Leino-Kilpi, H. (2019a). Ethical problems in nursing management: Frequency and difficulty of the problems. *Health Care Management Review*, Advance online publication. https://doi.org/10.1097/HMR.0000000000000236.

Aitamaa, E., Suhonen, R., Iltanen, S., Puukka, P., & Leino-Kilpi, H. (2019b). Ethical problems in nursing management: A cross-sectional survey about problem solving. *BMC Health Services Research, 19*(417). https://doi.org/10.1186/s12913-019-4245-4.

Allen, S. B. (2015). The nurse patient assignment: Purposes and decision factors. *Journal of Nursing Administration, 45*(12), 628–635. https://doi.org/10.1097/NNA.0000000000000276.

Altman, S., Gubrud, P., Phillips, B., & Salsberg, E. (2015). *Assessing progress on the institute of medicine report: The future of nursing*. Washington, DC: The National Academies Press.

American Nurses Association. (2016). *Nursing administration: Scope and standards of practice* (2nd ed.). Silver Spring, MD: ANA.

American Nurses Association. (2017). ANA CAUTI Prevention Tool. https://www.nursingworld.org/practice-policy/work-environment/health-safety/infection-prevention/ana-cauti-prevention-tool/.

American Nurses Credentialing Center (ANCC). (2020). Magnet model-creating a magnet culture. https://www.nursingworld.org/organizational-programs/magnet/magnet-model/.

American Organization for Nursing Leadership. (2015). Nurse manager competencies. https://www.aonl.org/system/files/media/file/2019/06/nurse-managercompetencies.pdf.

American Society for Quality. (n.d.). *What is Six Sigma?* https://asq.org/quality-resources/six-sigma.

Aron, D. C., Tseng, C. L, Soroka, O., & Pogach, L. M. (2019). Balancing measures: Identifying unintended consequences of diabetes quality performance measures in patients at high risk for hypoglycemia. *International Journal for Quality in Health Care, 31*(4), 246–251. https://doi.org/10.1093/intqhc/mzy151.

Belrhiti, Z., Giralt, A. N., & Marchal, B. (2018). Complex leadership in healthcare: A scoping review. *International Journal of Health Policy and Management, 7*(12), 1073–1084. https://doi.org/10.15171/ijhpm.2018.75.

Benner, P. (1984). *From novice to expert: Excellence and power in clinical practice.* Menlo Park, CA: Addison-Wesley.

Benner, P., Sutphen, M., Leonard, V., & Day, L. (2010). *Educating nurses: A call for radical transformation.* San Francisco, CA: Jossey-Bass.

Blondon, K. S., Maitre, F., Muller-Juge, W., Bochatay, N., Cullati, S., Hudelson, P., Vu, N. V., et al. (2017). Interprofessional collaborative reasoning by residents and nurses in internal medicine: Evidence from a simulation study. *Medical Teacher, 39*(4), 360–367. https://doi.org/10.1080/0142159X.2017.1286309.

Braaten, J. S. (2015). Hospital system barriers to rapid response team activation: A cognitive work analysis. *American Journal of Nursing, 115*(2), 22–32. https://doi.org/10.1097/01.NAJ.0000460673.82070.af.

Campbell, D., & Dontje, K. (2019). Implementing bedside handoff in the emergency department: A practice improvement project. *Journal of Emergency Nursing, 45*(2), 149–154. https://doi.org/10.1016/j.jen.2018.09.007.

Centers for Medicare & Medicaid Services (CMS). (2020). *CMS releases proposed notice of benefit and payment parameters rule for 2021.* https://www.cms.gov/newsroom/press-releases/cms-releases-proposed-notice-benefit-and-payment-parameters-rule-2021.

Chang, W., Liu, H. E., Goopy, S., Chen, L. C., & Han, C. Y. (2017). Using the Five-Level Taiwan Triage Acuity Scale computerized system: Factors in decision making by emergency department triage nurses. *Clinical Nursing Research, 26*(5), 651–666. https://doi.org/10.1177/1054773816636360.

Chisengantambu, C., Robinson, G. M., & Evans, N. (2018). Nurse managers and the sandwich support model. *Journal of Nursing Management, 26*(2), 192–199. https://doi.org/10.1111/jonm.12534.

Chisengantambu-Winters, C., Robinson, G. M., & Evans, N. (2020). Developing a decision-making dependency (DMD) model for nurse managers. *Heliyon, 6*(1), e03128. https://doi.org/10.1016/j.heliyon.2019.e03128.

Clark-Burg, K., & Allix, S. (2017). A study of styles: How do nurse managers make decisions? *Nursing Management, 48*(7), 44–49. https://doi.org/10.1097/01.NUMA.0000520721.78549.ad.

Clancy, T. (2020). Artificial intelligence and nursing: The future is now. *Journal of Nursing Administration, 50*(3), 125–127. https://doi.org/10.1097/NNA.0000000000000855.

Dans, M., & Lundmark, V. (2019). The effects of positive practice environments: Leadership must-knows. *Nursing Management, 50*(10), 7–10. https://doi.org/10.1097/01.NUMA.0000580624.53251.29.

Effken, J. A., Brewer, B. B., Logue, M. D., Gephart, S. M., & Verran, J. (2011). Using cognitive work analysis to fit decision support tools to nurse work flow. *International Journal of Medical Informatics, 80*, 698–707. https://doi.org/10.1016/j.ijmedinf.2011.07.003.

Esan, O. T., Akanbi, C. T., Esan, O., Fajobi, O., & Ikenenbomeh, P. I. (2016). Application of quantitative techniques in decision making by healthcare managers and administrators in Nigerian public tertiary health institutions. *Health Services Management Research, 29*(3), 50–61. https://doi.org/10.1177/0951484816662490.

Fallman, S. L., Jutengren, G., & Dellve, L. (2019). The impact of restricted decision-making autonomy on health care managers' health and work performance. *Journal of Nursing Management, 27*(4), 705–714. https://doi.org/10.1111/jonm.12741.

Fischer, S. A., Horak, D., & Kelly, L. A. (2018). Decisional involvement: Differences related to nurse characteristics, role, and shared leadership participation. *Journal of Nursing Care Quality, 33*(4), 354–360. https://doi.org/10.1097/NCQ.0000000000000312.

Ganz, F. D., Wagner, N., & Toren, O. (2015). Nurse middle manager ethical dilemmas and moral distress. *Nursing Ethics, 22*, 43–51. https://doi.org/10.1177/0969733013515490.

Garcia-Sierra, R., & Fernández-Castro, J. (2018). Relationships between leadership, structural empowerment, and engagement in nurses. *Journal of Advanced Nursing, 74*(12), 2809–2819. https://doi.org/10.1111/jan.13805.

Gray, J., & Kerfoot, K. (2016). Expanding the parameters for excellence in patient assignments: Is leveraging an evidence-data-based acuity methodology realistic. *Nursing Administration Quarterly, 40*(1), 7–13. https://doi.org/10.1097/NAQ.0000000000000138.

Gummesson, C., Sundén, A., & Fex, A. (2018). Clinical reasoning as a conceptual framework for interprofessional learning: A literature review and case study. *Physical Therapy Review, 23*(1), 29–34.

Guo, K. L. (2008). DECIDE: A decision-making model for more effective decision making by healthcare managers. *The Health Care Manager, 27,* 118–127.

Harvey, C. L., Thompson, S., Willis, E., Meyer, E., & Pearson, M. (2018). Understanding how nurses ration care. *Journal of Health Organization and Management, 32*(3), 494–510. https://doi.org/10.1108/JHOM-09-2017-0248.

Hasanpoor, E., Belete, Y. S., Janati, A., Hajebrahimi, S., & Haghgoshayie, E. (2019). Nursing managers' perspectives on the facilitators and barriers to implementation of evidence-based management. *Worldviews on Evidence-Based Nursing, 16*(4), 255–262. https://doi.org/10.1111/wvn.12372.

Improta, G., Cesarelli, M., Montouri, P., Santillo, L. C., & Triassi, M. (2018). Reducing the risk of healthcare-associated infections through Lean Six Sigma: The case of the medicine areas at the Federico II University Hospital in Naples (Italy). *Journal of Evaluation in Clinical Practice, 24*(2), 338–346. https://doi.org/10.1111/jep.12844.

Institute for Healthcare Improvement. (n.d.). QI essentials toolkit: PDSA worksheet. http://www.ihi.org/resources/Pages/Tools/Quality-Improvement-Essentials-Toolkit.aspx.

Institute of Medicine (IOM). (1999). *To err is human: Building a safer health system.* Washington, DC: National Academies Press.

Institute of Medicine (IOM). (2011). *The future of nursing: Leading change, advancing health.* Washington, DC: National Academies Press.

Interprofessional Education Collaborative. (2016). *Core competencies for interprofessional collaborative practice 2016 update.* https://nebula.wsimg.com/2f68a39520b03336b41038c370497473?AccessKeyId=DC06780E69ED19E2B3A5&disposition=0&alloworigin=1.

Jansson, I., & Forsberg, A. (2016). How do nurses and ward managers perceive that evidence-based sources are obtained to inform relevant nursing interventions? An exploratory study. *Journal of Clinical Nursing, 25*, 769–776. https://doi.org/10.1111/jocn.13095.

Johansen, M. L., & O'Brien, J. L. (2016). Decision making in nursing practice: A concept analysis. *Nursing Forum, 51*(1), 40–48. https://doi.org/10.1111/nuf.12119.

Junious, D. L. (2020). Collaborative simulation training strategies used to teach root cause analysis leadership competencies. *Nursing Education Perspectives, 41*(1), 57–58. https://doi.org/10.1097/01.NEP.0000000000000404.

Karlsson, A., Lindeborg, P., Gunningberg, L., & Jangland, E. (2019). Evidence-based-nursing: How is it understood by bedside nurses? A phenomenographic study in surgical settings. *Journal of Nursing Management, 27*(6), 1216–1223. https://doi.org/10.1111/jonm.12802.

Keers, R. N., Plácido, M., Bennett, K., Clayton, K., Brown, P., & Ashcroft, D. M. (2018). What causes medication administration errors in a mental health hospital? A qualitative study with nursing staff. *PLOS ONE, 13*(10), Article e0206233. https://doi.org/10.1371/journal.pone.0206233.

Kowalski, M. O., Basile, C., Bersick, E., Cole, D. A., McClure, D.E., & Weaver, S. H. (2020). What do nurses need to practice effectively in a hospital environment? An integrative review with implications for nurse leaders. https://doi.org/10.1111/wvn.12401.

Kramer, M., Maguire, P., Halfer, D., Budin, W. C., Hall, D. S., Goodloe, L., et al. (2012). The organizational transformative power of nurse residency programs. *Nursing Administration Quarterly, 36*, 155–168. https://doi.org/10.1097/naq.0b013e318249fdaa.

Krishnan, P. (2018). A philosophical analysis of clinical decision making in nursing. *Journal of Nursing Education, 57*(2), 73–78. https://doi.org/10.3928/01484834-20180123-03.

Loresto, F. L., Welton, J., Grim, St., Valdez, C., & Eron, K. (2019). Exploring inpatient medication patterns. A big data and multilevel approach. *Journal of Nursing Administration, 49*(6), 336–342. https://doi.org/10.1097/NNA.0000000000000762.

Makary, M. A., & Daniel, M. (2016). Medical error-the third leading cause of death in the US. *BMJ, 353.* https://doi.org/10:1136/bmj.i2139.

Martinez, K., Borycki, E., & Courtney, K. L. (2017). Bring your own device and nurse managers' decision making. *CIN: Computers, Informatics, Nursing, 35*(2), 69–76. https://doi.org/10.1097/CIN.0000000000000286.

Massarweh, L. J., Tidyman, T., & Luu, D. H. (2017). Starting the shift out right: The electronic eAssignment sheet using clinical decision support in a quality improvement project. *Nursing Economic$, 35*(4), 194–200.

Mazer, B. L., & Nabhan, C. (2019). Strengthening the medical error "meme" pool. *Journal General Internal Medicine, 34*(10), 2264–2267. https://doi.org/10.1007/s11606-019-05156-7.

Medeiros, M. (2018). Shared governance councils: 10 essential actions for nurse leaders. *Nursing management, 49*(7), 12–13. https://doi.org/10.1097/01.NUMA.0000538920.83653.9b.

Moon, S. E., Van Dam, P. J., & Kitsos, A. (2019). *Healthcare, 7*(4), 132. https://doi.org/10.3390/healthcare7040132.

Morrison, J. (2016). Nursing leadership in ACO payment reform. *Nursing Economic$, 34*(5), 230–235.

Murphy, L. S., Wilson, M. L., & Newhouse, R. P. (2013). Data analytics: Making the most of input with strategic output. *Journal of Nursing Administration, 43*, 367–370. https://doi.org/10.1097/NNA.0b013e31829d60c7.

National Council of State Boards of Nursing. (2019). The clinical judgment and task model. https://www.ncsbn.org/NGN_Spring19_Eng_04_Final.pdf.

Nibbelink, C. W., & Brewer, B. B. (2018). Decision-making in nursing practice: An integrative literature review. *Journal of Clinical Nursing, 27*(5-6), 917–928. https://doi.org/10.1111/jocn.14151.

Nurses on Boards Coalition. (2020). About. https://www.nursesonboardscoalition.org/about/.

Orique, S. B., & Phillips, L. J. (2018). The effectiveness of simulation on recognizing and managing clinical deterioration: Meta-analysis. *Western Journal of Nursing Research, 40*(4), 582–609. https://doi.org/10.1177/0193945917697224.

Patient Protection and Affordable Care Act 42 U.S.C. 300gg–11. (2010). https://www.hhs.gov/sites/default/files/ppacacon.pdf.

Peltonen, L. M., Junttila, K., & Salantera, S. (2018). Nursing leaders' satisfaction with information systems in the day-to-day operations management in hospital units. *Studies in Health Technology & Informatics, 250,* 203–207. https://doi.org/10.3233/978-1-61499-872-3-203.

Peltonen, L. M., Sirrala, E., Juntilla, K, Lundgrén-Laine, H., Vahlberg, T, Löyttyniemi, E., Aantaa, R., & Salantera, S. (2019). Information needs in a day-to-day operations management in hospital units: A cross-sectional national survey. *Journal of Nursing Management, 27*(2), 233–244. https://doi.org/10.1111/jonm.12700.

Polancich, S., Williamson, J., Selleck, C. S., Talley, M., Frank, J., White-Williams, C., & Shirey, M. (2017). *Journal for Healthcare Quality, 39*(6), 391–396. https://doi.org/10.1097/JHQ.0000000000000112.

Porter-O'Grady, T. (2015). Through the looking glass: Predictive and adaptive capacity in a time of great change. *Nursing Management, 46*(6), 22–29. https://doi.org/10.1097/01.NUMA.0000465397.67041.bc.

Quality and Safety Education for Nurses (QSEN). (2020). QSEN Competencies. https://qsen.org/competencies/pre-licensurc-ksas/.

Razieh, S., Somayeh, G., & Fariba, H. (2018). Effects of reflection on clinical decision-making of intensive care unit nurses. *Nurse Education Today, 66,* 10–14. https://doi.org/10.1016/j.nedt.2018.03.009.

Reed, C. C., Minnick, A. F., & Dietrich, M. S. (2018). Nurses' responses to interruptions during medication tasks: A time and motion study. *International Journal of Nursing Studies, 82,* 113–120. https://doi.org/10.1016/j.ijnurstu.2018.03.017.

Roshanzadeh, M., Vanaki, Z., & Sadooghiasi, A. (2019). Sensitivity in ethical decision-making: The experiences of nurse managers. *Nursing Ethics, 27*(5), 1174–1186. https://doi.org/10.1177/0969733019864146.

Sherman, R. O. (2015). How to avoid biased thinking. *American Nurse Today, 10*(3), 12–14.

Shirey, M. R., Ebright, P. R., & McDaniel, A. M. (2013). Nurse manager cognitive decision-making amidst stress and work complexity. *Journal of Nursing Management, 21,* 17–30. https://doi.org/10.1111/j.1365-2834.2012.01380.x.

Spiers, J. A., Lo, E., Hofmeyer, A., & Cummings, G. G. (2016). Nurse leaders' perceptions of influence of organizational restructuring on evidence-informed decision-making. *Nursing Leadership, 29*(2), 64–81. https://doi.org/10.12927/cjnl.2016.24805.

Stewart, K. R., & Hand, K. A. (2017). SBAR, communication, and patient safety: An integrated literature review. *MedSurg Nursing, 26*(5), 297–305.

Sveinsdóttir, H., Ragnarsdóttir, E. D., & Blöndal, K. (2016). Praise matters: The influence of nurse unit managers' praise on nurses' practice, work environment and job satisfaction: A questionnaire study. *Journal of Advanced Nursing, 72,* 558–568. https://doi.org/10.1111/jan.12849.

Tanner, C. A. (2006). Thinking like a nurse: A research-based model of clinical judgment in nursing. *Journal of Nursing Education, 45,* 204–211.

Thew, J. (2019, March). The Future of Nursing report: Where are we now?. *Health Leaders.* https://www.healthleadersmedia.com/nursing/future-nursing-report-where-are-we-now.

Thomson, C. L., Maskrey, N., & Vlaev, I. (2017). Making decisions better: An evaluation of an educational intervention. *Journal of Evaluation in Clinical Practice, 23*(2), 251–256. https://doi.org/10.1111/jep.12555.

Udon, S. A., Cummings, G., Care, W. D., & Jenkins, M. (2017). Impact of role stressors on the health of nurse managers. *Journal of Nursing Administration, 47*(3), 159–164. https://doi.org/10.1097/NNA.0000000000000459.

Weidema, F. C., Molewijk, A. C., Kamsteeg, F., & Widdershoven, G. A. M. (2015). Managers' views on and experiences with moral case deliberation in nursing teams. *Journal of Nursing Management, 23*(8), 1067–1075.

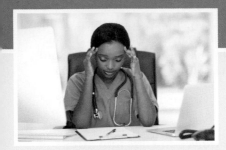

Managing Time and Stress

Susan R. Lacey, Debra V. Craighead

The latest, most comprehensive study of workplace stress calculated that workplace stress, direct and indirect, costs organizations and businesses $300 billion per year in absenteeism, turnover, decreased productivity, and medical and legal fees (Rosch, 2001). Moreover, the Centers for Disease Control and Prevention (CDC, n.d.) estimated that stress is a leading workplace health problem surpassing physical inactivity and obesity. Clearly, workplace stress is a phenomenon that cannot be overlooked.

Stress can manifest as either negative or positive. There are physical, mental, and even professional benefits to good stress (eustress) (Nelson & Simmons, 2004). Good stress provides a feeling of accomplishment, but stressful experiences perceived as negative result in a variety of conscious or subconscious responses to regain stability or homeostasis (Seyle, 1950). The nature of these responses may be physical, mental, psychological, spiritual, or any combination of these. If these responses fail to achieve homeostasis, an individual's resources are depleted, which can threaten general well-being in an acute or chronic way. The warning signs of excessive workplace stress include feeling anxious; being irritable, depressed, or apathetic; or having sleeping problems, social isolation, and use of alcohol or drugs to cope (Segal et al., 2019). Long-term effects of stress may contribute to the development of chronic illnesses such as heart disease, high blood pressure, diabetes, depression, and anxiety (US Department of Health and Human Services National Institute of Mental Health [NIMH], n.d.).

The negative consequences of stress for individuals, organizations, society, and the economy are well

documented (American Institute of Stress [AIS], n.d.). Work-related stress has been called the 21st Century Black Death (Lundberg & Cooper, 2011). In addition, work-related stress affects productivity and effectiveness at work, but it also may negatively affect personal lives and relationships (Rosch, 2001).

Joel Goh and colleagues reviewed more than 200 studies on workplace stress. They found that in some cases workplace stress raises the risk of illness and morbidity more than secondhand smoke (Goh et al., 2015). In addition, they calculated the cost of workplace stress as in excess of $190 billion, with 120,000 annual deaths.

COMPONENTS OF WORKPLACE STRESS

According to the World Health Organization (WHO), work-related stress has two key components: the content and context of work (WHO, 2010). Work content includes workload, work pace, and working hours. Context includes status and pay, role in the organization, and interpersonal work relationships. The content and context of work is perceived on the continuum of positive or negative. Central to this thesis is who is in control of these key components. The further away from control a person is from the context and content of work, the more problematic and stressful work can become. Thus, negative perceptions and lack of control translate into harmful job-related stress.

An article in *The Atlantic* provided a window into the impact and consequences of stress in relation to cost and personal health. The effects of stress are estimated to cost $180 billion or 5% to 8% of annual health care expenditures (White, 2015). Stress:

1. Increases the incidence of chronic and costly conditions, such as diabetes, Alzheimer's, and cardiovascular disease.
2. Increases addiction and mental health conditions associated with job insecurity, unjust dealings with employees, or poor leadership decisions that influence the working conditions of employees.
3. Is linked to over 120,000 deaths per year in the United States from physical and mental health conditions.

Governmental and organizational reports about work-related stress most often reference the work of Paul Rosch, MD, FACP, a leader in the field of occupational stress, specifically, his publication *The quandary of job stress compensation* (Rosch, 2001). Rosch calculated the combined direct and indirect cost of work-related stress to be a staggering $300 billion per year. Although the article is considered dated by academic standards, it remains the most widely referenced publication in support of national discourse, research, and large-scale planning in the area of work-related stress.

DEFINITIONS

Stress is defined as a negative emotional experience associated with biological changes that trigger the body to make adaptations (Rosenthal, 2002). This means stress can be a physical, mental, psychological, or spiritual response to a stressor experience that is evaluated by the individual as taxing or exceeding resources and threatening to one's sense of well-being. Furthermore, chronic stress can lead to acute and chronic health problems.

Job Stress

A seminal report by the National Institute of Occupational Safety and Health (NIOSH) defined job stress as the harmful physical and emotional responses that occur when the requirements of the job do not match the capabilities, resources, or needs of the worker. Job stress can lead to poor health and even injury (NIOSH, 1999).

Time Management

Time management is a deliberative process of identifying and focusing on the activities needed to accomplish tasks and goals in the time available. Since individuals cannot control time, they must learn to manage the available time more efficiently and effectively. This may be difficult, especially when behavior must be changed. At its core, time management is self-management.

BACKGROUND

The Relationship Between Time and Stress in the Health Care Setting

Situational stress and the need to respond in a timely manner are true for most types of work, and particularly in health care. Clinicians and leaders anticipate and even prepare for stressful situations. Time-sensitive care and decision-making may produce mild to severe stress. As if time sensitivity for single events were not stressful enough, it is typically compounded by multiple stressful events that occur at or near the same time. For example, there are specific times designated for medication administration, tests, and procedures, which may be interrupted by unplanned events with patients and/or families. Furthermore, if a clinician fails to complete the treatments or therapies within a defined window of time, a cascade of events may follow, from submitting an incident or variance report to patient harm. In life-threatening emergencies, response time is even more critical. Ineffective or inaccurate interventions may result in lasting consequences for patients—or even death.

The delivery of health care exists in an environment where time is finite and most often related to shift work. Nurses work shifts of time, such as 8- or 12-hour shifts. If time (a shift) is finite, the nurse must make accurate estimates of the amount of time each patient encounter will consume during that shift based on what needs to be done during each encounter.

During real or anticipated budgetary constraints, many organizations seek to reduce labor costs. Because labor expenditures are greatest within nursing, reducing the number of staff nurses on a unit is one strategy to improve the bottom line. However, there is also a need to increase reimbursement for good clinical outcomes and positive patient experiences, and this requires the presence of adequate numbers of nurses to deliver needed care.

The Centers for Medicare and Medicaid Services (CMS), the nation's largest payer, bases 30% of reimbursement on the patient experience and 70% on clinical outcomes (CMS, 2014). If the number of nurses is reduced on a given unit or shift, good outcomes may be compromised, and therefore reimbursement may be compromised. For instance, if normal nurse-to-patient ratios are modified from 1:5 to 1:7 without additional unlicensed assistive support, the time spent on patient encounters will naturally have to be decreased and the availability of nurses will be diminished. Chronic cycles of suboptimal staffing create stress and fatigue.

Evidence has linked lower patient-to-nurse ratios with better outcomes (Aiken et al., 2002). Many believe current staffing models are incongruent with professional practice standards, patient needs, and the organization's ability to maximize reimbursement. This perpetual grind makes it difficult for staff nurses to feel good about nursing or encourage others to join the profession. Many nurses have buyer's remorse for choosing nursing as their career, even more so compared with nurse practitioners and physicians (Peckham, 2015).

Lifecycle: Timing and Stress

"They say timing is everything. But then they say, there is never a perfect time for anything."

Anthony Liccioni (n.d.), poet, author

In life, we all routinely experience change. For generations, the timing of life events has created stress, both anticipated and unexpected. Plans for the work shift or for the future may change abruptly. Acknowledging that these changes are inevitable, and preparing for their occurrence, may make the difference between thriving and struggling to survive.

Timing affects our willingness to seek career advancement. This is often due to the time involved in developing a new work-related skillset. Nurses can prepare for career advancement by knowing about the task expectations involved when moving into new career roles. Sherman and Cohn (2019) examined the role timing plays in life and at work, and noted that demanding careers, coupled with a stressful life event such as caregiving, are common among nurses. Female nurses often feel unrelenting pressure to manage work and caregiving roles effortlessly. Recommended strategies to embrace in order to thrive during hectic life events include balancing life and career ambitions, self-advocacy, leveraging personal strengths, and co-creating work schedules (Sherman & Cohn, 2019).

We all work in a rhythm set by our unique biological clock. In his book *When: The secret to perfect timing*, author Daniel Pink (2018) asserted that timing is a science that can be studied and used to our benefit. He shared that productivity enhancement occurs when we recognize that 80% of us navigate each day in three predictable stages: peak, trough, and recovery. In the peak stage, we can concentrate deeply; in trough stage, we can accomplish routine tasks; and during the recovery stage we relax and therefore gain insight into the problems we face. Night owls move through these stages in the opposite order (recovery, trough, peak). Since our work tasks can be categorized as requiring either an insightful (awareness or creativity) or analytical (deliberate, attention to detail) type of focus, the time of the day chosen to complete a task can affect performance by up to 20% (Pink, 2018).

TIME MANAGEMENT STRATEGIES FOR NURSE LEADERS

Nurse leaders are expected to manage time effectively. The following time management strategies are useful and applicable in any work setting (Chutna & Boothby, 2017). Perform a time audit self-assessment to discover how you are spending your time and how to use small time increments effectively. Do tasks that prepare you in advance of the next workday. Engage in projects that require attention to detail while at your peak and save routine tasks (like answering e-mail) for a trough period. Convene meetings only when necessary, share the agenda in advance, and provide pre-meeting assignments. Moreover, nurse leaders need to model self-care because this augments time management and allows for recovery and rejuvenation (Chutna & Boothby, 2017).

Nurses are required to use time wisely due to facing new challenges hourly. We race to deliver patient-centered care and then chart care completion. Nurses often view time as an unforgiving foe; however, we can learn strategies to get the job done efficiently and effectively (Templeman, 2018). These strategies include cognitive stacking, prioritizing tasks, routinization, and time audits. Box 5.1 contains suggested time-saving strategies for nurses and nurse leaders.

BOX 5.1   Time-Saving Strategies for Nurses and Nurse Leaders

Strategy	Methods
Cognitive stacking	Mental list E-list
Prioritization	CURE: Critical, Urgent, Routine, and Extra Maslow's Hierarchy of Needs ABCs: airway, breathing, circulation
Routinization	Sequence activities and establish a time-frame expectation for routine task
Time audit	Track your time for 24 hours over 1–2 weeks; identify small time gaps (5–10 minutes) where small tasks may be completed

Cognitive stacking (creating mental, electronic, physical lists) is useful to plan the day before starting work. A list of what you need to accomplish should include what routinely needs to be completed on your shift. Prioritize tasks as appropriate using the CURE acronym, which stands for Critical, Urgent, Routine, and Extras. Other nursing prioritization frameworks include ABCs (airway, breathing, and circulation), Maslow's Hierarchy of Needs, and time-sensitive/safety indicators relevant to the care setting (Jesse, 2019). Establish a routine or routinization of work tasks and repeat what works best. Consistency in work routine aids time management (Templeman, 2018). Discover what works for you and use it to configure your daily work routine.

RESILIENCE

Countering the negative aspects of workplace stress is the concept of resilience. Resilience is defined as an ability to bounce back. Resilient people exhibit personal characteristics of an internal locus of control, prosocial behavior, empathy, positive self-image, a sense of optimism, and an ability to organize daily responsibilities (Pines et al., 2012). Several additional factors are associated with resilience, including:

- The capacity to make realistic plans and take steps to carry them out.

- A positive view of yourself and confidence in your strengths and abilities.
- Skills in communication and problem solving.
- The capacity to manage strong feelings and impulses. Empowered people are thought to be more resilient, and for nurses there is an association between stress resiliency and psychological empowerment. Because the behavioral skills needed to manage interpersonal conflict and its feelings of powerlessness and psychological distress can be taught, nurses can learn to resist stressors, manage conflict, and boost resilience (Pines et al., 2012).

Resilience is not a trait that people either have or do not have. It involves behaviors, thoughts, and actions that can be learned and developed by anyone. Today's nurse leader is required to be resilience competent in order to model and assist employees with developing this skill (Bernard, 2019). Nurse leaders model and support resilience development when they promote quality sleep, decompression from work, and assist staff with navigating ethically challenging situations (Bernard, 2019). The *Resilience and professional joy: A toolkit for nurse leaders* contains numerous evidence-based approaches useful for building resilient teams, leaders, organizations, and student nurses (Bernard, 2019).

LEADERSHIP AND MANAGEMENT IMPLICATIONS

Creating an Environment to Prevent and Address Work-Related Stress

To prevent and address work-related stress, creation and innovation are needed. A creation is something new that did not previously exist in that form and occurs in a multitude of fields, not just the arts (Merriam-Webster, n.d.a). Experts who study creativity may differ on the requisite attributes of creative individuals and exact steps in the creative process. However, most agree that intention is the critical first step (Ditkoff, 2010). Without intention, no action is ever taken.

Innovation and innovators in the health care industry are highly sought after, but to innovate is to alter, change, or transform something that exists in a stable system (Marshall, 2013). On the other hand, creativity is less frequently discussed in the industry, and in some cases, is maligned. For example, the term creative accounting is used to describe illegal or unethical activities and does not convey the positive aspect of creativity, which is to produce something needed or valued. Industry leaders prefer to predict the future based on the past and innovate within the current system as opposed to envisioning the future based on what is desired and creating it (Scott, 2003). The former is thought to use hard data, and the latter, subjective or unknown information, inspiration, and feelings. Creativity does not require one to suspend all intellect. Indeed, creative individuals use all of the senses, as well as abstract and concrete thought. Without concrete and abstract thought, it would have been impossible for Salvador Dalí to have painted *The persistence of memory*, or for British scientist Sir Tim Berners-Lee to have written code for the first web browser, which became the genesis of the world wide web (World Wide Web Foundation, 2015).

Getting Started

It is challenging to envision creating a health care organization focused not only on addressing work-related stress when it occurs but also on having structures and processes in place to prevent them from happening in the first place. This is particularly hard while in the midst of persistent demands from payers, consumers, regulators, and even the overarching uncertainty of the Affordable Care Act of 2010 (ACA) mandates. It has always been challenging to secure the necessary resources for prevention, even for patient care. However, failure to do so puts employees at risk, which in turn can jeopardize the lives of patients. It is no longer possible to wait for more evidence about the human and financial costs of work-related stress. Waiting for more stability in the industry, which may never come, wastes precious time. Once that is embraced and there is genuine intention, then design and creation can begin in earnest. This intention and corresponding action will call for bold leaders who reject reactionary quick fixes. Based on the evidence, this can lead to the interconnected outcomes of employees with greater resilience and performance, improved patient outcomes, and measurable and sustained financial benefits.

Strategies

Stress management. Stress management is important for nurses as they cope with stress at work. This is also true for nursing students and new nurses. Among the many stressors are needing to meet professional and academic demands, fear of failure, the workload

of taking care of patients, and insecurity about clinical competence or lack of knowledge. Stress and anxiety are often high during times of education and training when the nurse or student is developing clinical skills. Two low-cost and easily implemented stress-management techniques are mindful meditation and biofeedback. Both were found to decrease anxiety, and mindfulness also significantly lowered stress levels in nursing students (Nowrouzi et al., 2015; Ratanasiripong et al., 2015).

Workplace intervention strategies for stress can be either individual-level stress management and burnout interventions or organizational-level workplace health-promotion programs. For the individual nurse, mindfulness-based stress reduction has evidence of effectiveness; for mental health, psychosocial interventions decrease burnout (Nowrouzi et al., 2015). The Research Note and Box 5.2 also provide some guidance on stress management for individuals suggested by the American Psychological Association (2018) and the CDC (n.d.).

Organization-directed prevention measures can be directed to management style, incentives and career structures, educational opportunities, salaries, and recruitment and retention practices (Nowrouzi et al., 2015). Research on conflict management styles found that nurses who worked in supportive work environments and who avoided conflict (avoidant style of managing conflict) experienced less work stress (Johansen & Cadmus, 2016). In addition, conflict and communicative stress feed off each other in a cycle that contributes to destructive working conditions. Nurses manage conflict and stress through respectful and caring communication and mismanage it through disrespectful communication. Building relationships can be fostered in organizations by formal and informal social gatherings, mentoring, social media, and deliberate culture creation (Moreland & Apker, 2016). Perceived supportive work environments are characterized by perceptions that supervisors are supportive, there is fairness, and there is open communication. Stress is reduced when nurses feel that win–win solutions occur in the work environment (Johansen & Cadmus, 2016).

One example is the implementation of new nurse residency programs. In response to the stress and anxiety ("transition shock") that new nurses feel in the transition from nursing education to nursing practice, organizations are instituting nurse residency programs.

BOX 5.2 Individual Strategies to Manage Stress

American Psychological Association (2018)	Centers for Disease Control and Prevention (n.d.)
• Journaling to track your stressors: record your thoughts and feelings and your reaction to stressful events.	• Reflect on positive experiences and express gratitude.
• Develop healthy responses to stress such as exercise, hobbies, pleasurable activities, adequate sleep.	• Participate in employer-sponsored programs/activities that target healthy lifestyle behaviors.
• Set boundaries by maintaining periods when you are not working or thinking about work (unplug from work e-mail in the evening and on days off).	• Adopt behaviors that promote stress management such as yoga, meditation, mindfulness.
• Take time away to recharge.	• Eat healthy meals, exercise, and get enough sleep.
• Learn relaxation techniques such as meditation, deep breathing, mindfulness (psychological state of moment-to-moment awareness of your current state without feeling inward judgement about your situation.	• Look for satisfaction and meaning in your work.
• Cultivate a social support system including family, friends, co-workers.	• Serve as wellness champion and participate in trainings.

They may be up to a year long. New nurses are mentored and guided during this residency in order to support their coping, reduce their stress, and augment their time-management capabilities. This is a major recruitment and retention strategy. In addition, it is a visible component of a supportive work environment (Rosenfeld & Glassman, 2016; Rush et al., 2013).

Informal nurse leaders can employ a combination of person-directed stress management techniques (for themselves) and organization-directed stress management techniques (for the sake of the work group). Clearly, a supportive work environment is critical, so any interventions that improve nurses' perceptions of the work environment are helpful. Role modeling and setting a tone of respectful and caring communication aids conflict resolution and stress reduction. Informal leaders can take the initiative to address workplace issues in a proactive and evidence-based manner so that nurses see that their issues are being evaluated fully and fairly for problem resolution.

Wellness programs in the larger context. There are a variety of strategies that individuals and organizations need to employ to prevent and address work-related stress. There is no shortage of research, workshops, websites, and blogs about how to reduce stress. Although sources may emphasize the benefits of one strategy over another, most include similar recommendations. Using these strategies can serve as the inspiration for creating this new, vital environment. Instead of employees trying to find their own way through the maze of strategies, the newly created health care environment would provide on-site (or reimbursement for) work-related stress prevention workshops and retreats. Just as the traditional employee health staff conduct new and ongoing physical health screening for risky behaviors such as smoking or substance use, additional screening for resiliency, coping strategies, and support networks needs to be a part of the work structure. Once screened and a profile developed, the employee can use the information to select from wellness options beyond smoking cessation, hypertension, and diabetes management programs in consultation with a wellness professional.

It is common practice to compensate employees who take advantage of preventive health care services. There are some organizations that pay for alternative health care, such as gym memberships, massage, and acupuncture, but that is not the norm. Given the costs of work-related stress, the health care environment of the future will provide full or partial compensation for a much wider array of prevention services that fit the needs of the individual employee. As personalized medicine forges a pathway to realize the potential of matching therapies to an individual's DNA for disease states, wellness offerings should match the employee's needs for work–life balance and prevention of work-related stress. Examples of wellness initiatives and programs might be offered in multiple formats, but could include self-care, setting boundaries, relaxation, and journaling.

Self-care. One of the most important strategies to mitigate individual stress is self-care. Though everyone needs to spend time on themselves, clinicians often put the needs of others ahead of their own. It is difficult to effectively care for patients and their families or be productive at work if clinicians and leaders do not care for themselves. Self-care is unique to each person, but the following are generally accepted as important self-care activities (Fischer & Keenan, 2010): taking personal time each day, getting enough sleep (7–8 hours), nutritious intake and adequate hydration, some form of exercise, and a strong support network, which includes friends, family, and counseling, if necessary. Box 5.2 displays personal strategies for decreasing stress at the workplace.

Setting boundaries. Setting boundaries is one way of engaging in self-care (Gionta, 2009). Family members and even friends faced with a health care question, concern, or crisis call on nurses and other clinicians to provide advice, and in some cases, direct care. To respond and be helpful, clinicians may overextend themselves, sacrificing their own needs or those of their direct family members. In some ways, it is flattering. It validates one's knowledge, skills, and expertise. However, when requests exceed a person's capabilities, it is reasonable to refer them to other experts and services.

Boundaries need not be exceedingly rigid and may change over time. For instance, someone who does not have a husband, wife, partner, or children may seem to have the capacity to take on extra work and may need to set more boundaries than those who have these commitments to others. Clearly, boundaries should be set based on individual needs, not gender, stereotypes, or even where someone is on the lifespan. The most important thing is that setting them should not induce more stress on the individual than not having them at all.

Relaxation. Finding ways to relax can also help one avoid and reduce stress. Because stress can produce both emotional and physical responses, it is important to learn to relax the body and mind, even for short periods. There are numerous relaxation techniques and even apps to download to help a person relax. It is not necessary to devote long periods or find a special

environment to achieve a state of relaxation. One can relax anywhere and for any amount of time (Seaward, 2013). By calming the mind, physiological responses to stress are also reversed, which allows the individual to think more clearly.

Journaling. Keeping a diary or journal was a part of many individuals' lives when they were younger, but most do not continue the practice into adulthood. There are many benefits in keeping a journal. For those who recognize they are experiencing stress but are not fully cognizant of the specific triggers, experts suggest keeping a journal to identify situations that cause stress, the response or action to the stressor, and whether these actions lowered their stress or not (Ullrich & Lutgendorf, 2002).

The work of clinicians and leaders in health care is time sensitive, and time management is, for all intents and purposes, personal management. Journaling about situations that challenge personal time management will provide clarity. This clarity may shed light on learned behaviors that may be sabotaging one's quest for effective time management. Saunders (2013), an international expert and coach in the area of time management, outlined and described secrets to effective time investment. They are priorities, expectations, and routines. Fully understanding these three things can unlock the potential to manage even the most chaotic situation, regardless of the context, at work or home.

Organizational Recommendations

Clearly, organizations are experiencing financial pressures, which make adding the necessary work required to create a new environment that prevents and addresses work-related stress a challenge. However, either way, employees will experience work-related stress, which will negatively affect the organization in one way or another. Therefore, it is a matter of which approach (proactive or reactive) an organization wants to take, either being up front with prevention and early intervention or after the fact with employee loss of productivity, increased sick days, and/or turnover. If an organization chooses the proactive approach, beginning the work to create this environment does not seem as daunting and is a prudent business decision. Box 5.3 displays a list of institutional strategies to decrease stress in the workplace, suggested by Segal et al. (2019). This is not an exhaustive list, nor is it intended to be prescriptive. Instead, it is meant to generate discussions while this new environment is planned. Related evidence-based management strategies to address work-related stress include healthy work environment standards and empowerment strategies.

Healthy Work Environments Standards. A healthy work environment (HWE) is one that is safe, empowering, and satisfying. HWE standards are further discussed in Chapter 3. The American Association of Critical-Care Nurses (AACN) has established six standards that support healthy work environments (AACN, 2005). Although developed for nurses, they are applicable for all types of employees. Emerging research supports the positive effect of these standards to enhance critical-care nurses' work environments (Ulrich et al., 2019). These standards and supporting statements are displayed in Table 5.1.

Empowerment. Employees who are empowered in their jobs are also more engaged and satisfied. Research indicates that structural empowerment leads to higher productivity and satisfaction for the employee, which translates to more satisfied customers. Customer satisfaction stems from the empowered employee's ability to correct a problem at the time it occurs. This leads to better fiscal health for the organization in both direct and indirect labor and benefit costs (Woods, 2005). Empowerment for nurses is manifested in shared governance structures where nurses are engaged and participate in solving clinical practice issues. Shared governance structures are a hallmark of the Magnet Recognition Program®. There is a growing body of evidence that links Magnet hospitals to better clinical and patient level outcomes, as well as to better nursing outcomes (e.g., lower turnover and higher satisfaction), compared with non-Magnet hospitals (Aiken et al., 2008). Improved clinical and organizational outcomes translate to improved financial health.

Clinicians are also empowered by gaining new knowledge and skills beyond required clinical competence. In addition, if these new skills also allow them to be a part of developing solutions to clinical and organizational problems, this can lead to even greater engagement and satisfaction. For example, the Clinical Scene Investigator Academy is currently administered by

TABLE 5.1 AACN Standards for Establishing and Sustaining Healthy Work Environments

Standard	Statement
Skilled communication	Nurses must be as proficient in communication skills as they are in clinical skills.
True collaboration	Nurses must be relentless in pursuing and fostering true collaboration.
Effective decision-making	Nurses must be valued and committed partners in making policy, directing and evaluating clinical care, and leading organizational operations.
Appropriate staffing	Staffing must ensure the effective match between patient needs and nurse competencies.
Meaningful recognition	Nurses must be recognized and must recognize others for the value each brings to the work of the organization.
Authentic leadership	Nurse leaders must fully embrace the imperative of a healthy work environment, authentically live it, and engage others in its achievement.

American Association of Critical-Care Nurses (AACN). (2005). *AACN standards for establishing and sustaining healthy work environments: A journey to excellence.* Aliso Viejo, CA: AACN.

AACN (Lacey et al., 2012, 2017). This program teaches staff nurse teams skills in advanced leadership, quality improvement methods, project management, accurate data management, and how to translate nursing care into fiscal terms. To date, the national program has significantly improved nurse-sensitive outcomes, such as pressure ulcers, catheter-associated infections, ventilator-associated pneumonia, and patient satisfaction (Lacey et al., 2017).

Special Considerations for Nurse Managers

With any unit or department, workflow modifications creep into the manager's routines, creating chaos in a well-planned day. The unit manager has one of the most difficult jobs in meeting the challenges of managing and leading employees, as well as meeting priorities that flow from higher management. The challenge of meeting the expectations of the multiple roles of the nurse manager can produce stress that reveals itself as role strain, which is an unpleasant feeling of frustration and an intense labile emotional state (Richmond et al., 2009). This may lead to communication breakdowns, the sense of failing, and intense anxiety about job performance.

There is a scarcity of evidence about how stress affects the nurse manager role. However, Shirey et al. (2010) have provided a rich source of qualitative evidence about sources and factors related to stress, outcomes of this stress, and coping strategies used to decrease stress. In their study, nurse manager participants reported key sources of stress to include dealing with people (specifically related to people with negative attitudes or employees with subpar work performance); patient and family complaints; physician interactions; and working within the political nature of the hospital with a lack of transparency and collaboration. Staffing was noted as the most stressful part of their role. High stress is experienced by nurse managers and stems from the challenges of a multifaceted job with myriad sources of stress (Kath et al., 2012). Although there is a relationship between job satisfaction and intent to quit, when stress is high for nurse managers, other factors show strong relationships with stress (Kath et al., 2012). Having support from others (e.g., supervisors, co-managers, and co-workers) is a factor that decreases stress (Kath et al., 2012; Shirey et al., 2010). The amount of autonomy and predictability in the job mitigates the negative effects of stress as well (Kath et al., 2012).

There is nothing stopping us from creating this new environment that addresses work-related stress, except for the limits (real and imagined) placed on ourselves and organizations. It takes leadership and vision to see the business case for being proactive. Some of the most brilliant minds work in health care. Together nurses can build a preferred future state that results in managed stress and promotion of healthy work environments where all employees flourish.

CURRENT ISSUES AND TRENDS

Health care delivery environments are characterized by chaos, complexity, high risk, and high stress. This is not likely to change. Clinicians and leaders function in environments with increasing unknowns while trying to take appropriate daily actions as well as predict and plan for the future. This is a highly stressful situation. Individuals respond to unknowns in a fairly predictable pattern, which happens rapidly and primarily in one's subconscious. The process includes mentally triaging proven strategies used in similar situations, selecting and modifying the strategy, and evaluating the strategy in real time or as needed.

There is long-standing evidence that fear of the unknown is a normal part of human nature (Öhman, 2000). It is also known that fear is linked to the feeling of danger. A recently published study found that subjects presented with certain danger had significantly lower stress than subjects presented with potential danger (de Berker et al., 2016). In this study one group of participants, the certain danger group, was told when they picked up a rock a snake would be under it. The other group, the potential danger group, was told a snake may or may not be there. The researchers concluded that when participants knew something would occur ahead of time, they were able to mentally and physically prepare. In addition, physiological responses such as heart rate and breathing were significantly higher for participants in the potential danger group than those in the certain danger group.

Scientists in the field of psychology have studied a person's ability to predict or envision the future in normal and uncertain times. Noted psychologist Daniel Gilbert (2007) outlined his thesis in *Stumbling on happiness*, using scientific evidence coupled with analogies and real-world examples. What he and other social scientists found is that the need to control and predict the future is central to the human condition. It is part of what distinguishes us from other species. In addition, he offers compelling evidence that even those with a great deal of experience, expertise, and cultural wisdom find it difficult to accurately predict the future and make good choices when presented with new and uncertain situations. Specifically, prior experiences coupled with current realities do little to help accurately predict or envision the future, especially when the stakes are high. He extends the logic with additional evidence that in a person's struggle to gain control, make better predictions, and thus make effective plans and choices, individuals fill in details of missing information even if these details are inaccurate. As the brain is filling in inaccurate details from memories, perceptions, and emotions, it allows people to reweave the narrative to one they believe or want to be true.

The research supporting Gilbert's logic is applicable to the current health care industry. Clinicians and leaders make efforts to predict the future and make decisions based on their predictions. Unfortunately, just as Gilbert's work has proven, historical evidence supports the reweaving of narratives and undesirable outcomes. Organizations introduce new initiatives or cut services in response to expert predictions, only to realize when the future becomes the present that it looks nothing like the prediction, rendering the initiatives and related expenditures relatively useless.

An example of significant scale occurred in the 1980s. In response to payer demands, specifically the introduction of diagnosis-related groups (DRGs), reimbursements declined significantly (Fetter et al., 1980). Hospital leaders and external experts predicted vastly reduced margins, and experts recommended reducing expenditures as the best way to address the negative financial impact of DRGs. On face value, that was prudent, and a common business practice given the anticipated loss of revenue. They recommended consolidating organizations, reducing or eliminating services, and closing facilities, primarily within a defined geographical region. Nurse layoffs occurred. These recommendations led to a frenzy of mergers, acquisitions, and closings (Federal Antitrust Policy in the Health Care Marketplace, 1997). Some mergers created complicated partnerships. Many were ill conceived with little or no input from staff, referring physicians, or the communities served. Faith-based and secular hospitals

merged, buildings were shuttered, and hybrid names and slogans emerged. Stark philosophical differences, disruption or elimination of services, and disgruntled staff and physicians made sustaining such mergers difficult. To make matters worse, loyal consumers of one hospital or another felt betrayed. It did not take long for many of these hospitals and systems to unmerge, costing even more money, all because experts inaccurately predicted the long-term consequences of this strategy. Some mergers did survive but rebuilding trust with providers and consumers took many years.

The current example is the odyssey surrounding the fate of the ACA, which has added formidable uncertainties not only for clinicians, leaders, organizations, and systems, but also for the industry's key drivers: payers, consumers, and regulators. The ACA passed along party lines and was signed into law on March 23, 2010 (US Department of Health and Human Services, 2014). Legal challenges were swift and aggressive. The Supreme Court upheld the constitutionality of the law, specifically the individual mandate, on June 28, 2012, after hearing arguments in the National Federation of Independent Business v. Sebelius case (Barnes, 2015). Nevertheless, challenges continue. These continued challenges create speculation regarding how decisions about the ACA will influence current external health care drivers and compound stress in the environment.

Even with the compelling evidence that we lack the ability to accurately predict the future, there is no evidence suggesting we cannot create our desired future. In fact, this advice is often suggested to nurses.

Predictions and Risk

A prediction is a statement or thought about a future event based on past experiences and knowledge (Merriam-Webster, n.d.b). Everyone makes predictions or forecasts about the future many times a day, most of which are made subconsciously. Some predictions involve low risk. Thus, an inaccurate prediction may cause a temporary inconvenience, but not stress. For example, a person driving to work who failed to listen to the current traffic report takes the regular route but is soon stuck for an hour behind an overturned vehicle.

Nurses make predictions in clinical practice based on assessment and clinical judgment. For example, a nurse may predict that following a standardized protocol will result in desired outcomes such as avoidance of catheter-associated urinary tract infections. If the protocol is evidence based, then prediction is low risk.

Other predictions would be considered high risk. If high-risk predictions are inaccurate, the consequences may cause intense stress, anxiety, depression, and even financial loss. Examples of personal situations that require high-risk predictions include choosing or leaving a job, selecting a partner, and buying or selling a large amount of company stock. Nurses are often faced with high-risk predictions in practice, and this is a source of work stress. For example, unstable patients, code situations, or rapid decompensation may result in the need for instant reactions and/or high-risk predictions about treatment.

One additional important aspect of making predictions is that predictions may affect others in positive or negative ways. When clinicians and leaders in health care initiate actions based on predictions, the actions often affect others in small and large ways. Clinicians make predictions every day based on tacit and empirical knowledge. Most would prefer using the term prognosis, not prediction, but they are similar. For example, a nurse predicts that if the patient has difficulty swallowing when provided a sip of water, then he may have difficulty eating solid food; recommendations and interventions occur based on this prediction. Likewise, when leaders make predictions and take subsequent actions about real or anticipated changes in demand from key drivers (e.g., payers, consumers, regulations, and the fate of the ACA), many people may be positive or negatively affected.

RESEARCH NOTE

Source
Chesak, S., Cutshall, S., Bowe, C., Montanari, K., & Bhagra, A. (2019). Stress management for nurses: Critical research review. *Journal of Holistic Nursing 17*(3), 288–295. https://doi.org/10.1177/0898010119842693.

Purpose
This systematic review examined current evidence on stress management interventions for nurses. The authors presented levels of evidence, findings, and instruments used to measure nurse stress.

Discussion
Evidence reviewed ($n = 90$) identified a wide variety of holistic interventions for nurse stress management. However, psychological skill training (coping, stress resilience, and cognitive behavioral therapy; $n = 21$) and mindfulness

and meditation training ($n = 24$) were prevalent. Most interventions focused on handing individual stress, not workplace environmental stress. The authors identified a gap in the literature regarding system-level interventions. Randomized controlled trials are needed at the individual and system-level to add to the body of knowledge to support efficacious and cost-effective interventions.

Application to practice
This systematic review highlighted findings from evidence regarding stress management interventions for nurses. Holistic specialty nurses and the American Nurses Association have called for nurses to adopt self-care activities to promote personal health and well-being. Nurse leaders need to advocate for system-level interventions by demonstrating the significant return-on-investment to the organization.

NEXT-GENERATION NCLEX® EXAMINATION-STYLE CASE STUDY

Caitlin has been working on 2 North for 6 months since graduation from nursing school. Every day seems stressful, and every new situation makes her feel like she does not have what it takes to be a nurse. She often feels overwhelmed. There are very few senior experienced nurses on the unit, and they are burned out from constantly orienting new nurses. Productivity and effectiveness are low. Caitlin is concerned about her own coping yet also wants to build a higher functioning and more resilient team. There are lots of recommended stress reduction techniques. Key to success is choosing techniques that are practical and able to be accomplished by a busy nurse daily.

Choose the most likely options for the information missing from the question below by selecting from the list of options provided.

NEXT-GENERATION NCLEX® EXAMINATION-STYLE CASE STUDY—cont'd

Question

Caitlin spent two days observing the employees on the unit and noticed that they were always busy, skipped breaks and lunch, drank lots of coffee, and never had down time, confirming her personal perceptions. The top 3 strategies an employee may use while at work to relieve stress are:

1) _____

2) _____

3) _____.

Options for Strategies

Getting a massage at the massage parlor 10 mts from work

Eat French fries

Drink 8 glasses of water a day

Taking scheduled lunches

Taking a long walk in nature

Taking yoga classes in your neighborhood

Eat at your desk

Use your getaway place

CRITICAL THINKING EXERCISE

Cindy and the unit council decide to explore strategies for stress reduction and resiliency in the document, *Resilience and professional joy: A toolkit for nurse leaders* (https://www.nurseleader.com/article/S1541-4612(18)30283-0/fulltext). They decide to select two interventions from Leading Self Individuals and Leading Teams for staff nurses and two strategies from Leader Leaders for the charge nurses.

1. What barriers should Cindy anticipate?

2. How should she address these barriers?
3. What should Cindy do first?
4. How should Cindy implement the interventions with the least impact on her unit budget?
5. Should Cindy engage staff and charge nurse champions to promote these interventions?
6. What factors should she continue to assess and analyze throughout the intervention phase?
7. How might Cindy use the $8000 for these efforts?

REFERENCES

Aiken, L. H., Clarke, S. P., Sloane, D. M., Lake, E. T., & Cheney, T. (2008). Effects of hospital care environment on patient mortality and nurse outcomes. *Journal of Nursing Administration, 38*(5), 223–229. https://doi.org/10.1097/01.NNA.0000312773.42352.d7.

Aiken, L. H., Clarke, S. P., Sloane, D. M., Sochalski, J., & Silber, J. H. (2002). Hospital nurse staffing and patient mortality, nurse burnout, and job dissatisfaction. *The Journal of the American Medical Association (JAMA), 288*(16), 1987–1993. https://doi.org/10.1001/jama.288.16.1987.

American Association of Critical-Care Nurses (AACN). (2005). *AACN standards for establishing and sustaining healthy work environments: A journey to excellence.* Aliso Viejo, CA: AACN.

American Institute of Stress (AIS). (n.d.). *Workplace stress.* http://www.stress.org/workplace-stress/.

American Psychological Association. (2018). *Coping with stress at work.* https://www.apa.org/helpcenter/work-stress.

Barnes, R. (2015, June 25). Affordable Care Act survives Supreme Court challenge. *Washington Post.* https://www.washingtonpost.com/politics/courts_law/obamacaresurvives-supreme-court-challenge/2015/06/25/af87608e-188a-11e5-93b7-5eddc056ad8a_story.html.

Bernard, N. (2019). Resilience and professional joy: A toolkit for nurse leaders. *Nurse Leader, 17*(1), 43–48. https://doi.org/10.1016/j.mnl.2018.09.007.

Centers for Disease Control and Prevention (CDC). (n.d.). *Mental health in the workplace. Workplace health promotion.* https://www.cdc.gov/workplacehealthpromotion/tools-resources/pdfs/WHRC-Mental-Health-and-Stress-in-the-Workplac-Issue-Brief-H.pdf.

Centers for Medicare & Medicaid Services. (CMS). (2014). *HCAHPS: Patients' perspectives of care survey.* https://www.cms.gov/Medicare/Quality-Initiatives-Patient-Assessment-instruments/HospitalQualityInits/HospitalHCAHPS.html.

Chesak, S., Cutshall, S., Bowe, C., Montanari, K., & Bhagra, A. (2019). Stress management for nurses: Critical research review. *Journal of Holistic Nursing, 17*(3), 288–295. https://doi.org/10.1177/0898010119842693.

Chutna, K., & Boothby, J. (2017). Time management strategies for nurse leaders. *American Nurse Today, 12*(11), 10–11.

de Berker, A. O., Rutledge, R. B., Mathys, C., Marshall L., Cross G. F., Dolan R. J., et al. (2016). Computations of uncertainty mediate acute stress responses in humans. *Communications, 7,* 10996. https://doi.org/10.1038/ncomms10996.

Ditkoff, M. (2010). Intention: The root of creativity. *Innovation Excellence.* http://www.innovationexcellence.com/blog/2010/07/12/intention-the-root-of-creativity/.

Federal antitrust policy in the health care marketplace: Hearing before the committee on judiciary, senate, 105th Congress. 84. (1997). (Prepared statement of John C. McMeekin on behalf of the American Hospital Association). https://books.google.com/books?id=uwm1sG4a2_4C&dq=Federal+Antitrust+Policy+in+the+Health+Care+Marketplace:+Hearing+before+the+Committee+on+Judiciary,+Senate,+105th+Congress&source=gbs_navlinks_s.

Fetter, R. B., Shin, Y., Freeman, J. L., Averill, R. F., & Thompson, J. D. (1980). Case mix definition by diagnosis related groups. *Medical Care, 18*(2), 1–53.

Fischer, J., & Keenan, N. (2010). *Prioritizing self-care: The key to stress management.* http://ezinearticles.com/?Prioritizing-Self-Care:-The-Key-to-Stress-Management&id=5499316.

Gilbert, D. (2007). *Stumbling on happiness.* New York, NY: Vintage Books.

Gionta, D. (2009). Setting boundaries at work: Steps to making them a reality. *Psychology Today.* https://www.psychologytoday.com/us/blog/occupational-hazards/200901/setting-boundaries-work-steps-making-them-reality.

Goh, J., Pfeffer, J., Zenios, S. A., & Rajpal, S. (2015). Workplace stressors & health outcomes: Health policy for the workplace. *Behavioral Science and Policy, 1*(1), 43–52.

Jesse, M. (2019). Teaching prioritization: "Who, what, and why." *Journal of Nursing Education, 58*(5), 302–305.

Johansen, M. L., & Cadmus, E. (2016). Conflict management style, supportive work environments and the experience of work stress in emergency nurses. *Journal of Nursing Management, 24*(2), 211–218.

Kath, L. M., Stichler, J. F., & Ehrhart, M. G. (2012). Moderators of the negative outcomes of nurse manager stress. *Journal of Nursing Management, 42*(4), 215–221. https://doi.org/10.1097/NNA.0b013e31824ccd25.

Lacey, S. R., Goodyear-Bruch, C., Olney, A., Hanson, D., Altman, M. S., Varn-Davis, et al. (2017). Driving organizational change from the bedside: The AACN Clinical Scene Investigator Academy. *Critical Care Nurse, 37*(4), e12–e25. https://doi.org/10.4037/ccn2017749.

Lacey, S. R., Olney, A., & Cox, K. (2012). The Clinical Scene Investigator Academy: The power of staff nurses improving patient and organizational outcomes. *Journal of Nursing Care Quality, 27*(1), 56–62.

Liccioni, A. (n.d.) Goodreads. https://www.goodreads.com/quotes/7167475-they-say-timing-is-everything-but-then-they-say-there.

Lundberg, U., & Cooper, C. L. (2011). *The science of occupational health: Stress, psychobiology and the new world of work.* Chichester, UK: Wiley-Blackwell.

Marshall, D. (2013). There's a critical difference between creativity and innovation. *Business Insider Australia.* http://www.businessinsider.com.au/difference-between-creativity-and-innovation-2013-4.

Merriam-Webster. (n.d.a.). Creation. *Merriam-Webster's online dictionary.* http://www.merriam-webster.com/dictionary/creation.

Merriam-Webster. (n.d.b.). Prediction. *Merriam-Webster's online dictionary.* http://www.merriam-webster.com/dictionary/prediction.

Moreland, J. J., & Apker, J. (2016). Conflict and stress in hospital nursing: Improving communicative responses to enduring professional challenges. *Health Communication, 31*(7), 815–823.

National Institute for Occupational Safety and Health (NIOSH). (1999). *Stress…at work.* https://www.cdc.gov/niosh/docs/99-101/default.html.

Nelson, D. L., & Simmons, B. L. (2004). Eustress: An elusive construct, an engaging pursuit. In P. L. Perrewé, & D. C. Ganster (Eds.). *Research in occupational stress and well-being* (3, pp. 265–322). Oxford, UK: Elsevier.

Nowrouzi, B., Lightfoot, N., Lariviere, M., Carter, L., Rukholm, E., Schinke, R., et al. (2015). Occupational stress management and burnout interventions in nursing and their implications for healthy work environments. *Workplace Health & Safety, 63*(7), 308–315.

Öhman, A. (2000). Fear and anxiety: Evolutionary, cognitive, and clinical perspectives. In M. Lewis, & J. M. Haviland-Jones (Eds.), *Workplace health & safety, handbook of emotions* (pp. 573–593). New York, NY: The Guilford Press.

Peckham, C. (2015). Nurses tell all! Salaries, benefits, and whether they'd do it again. *Medscape.* http://www.medscape.com/viewarticle/854372.

Pines, E. W., Rauschhuber, M. L., Norgan, G. H., Cook, J. D., Canchola, L., Richardson, C., et al. (2012). Stress resiliency, psychological empowerment and conflict management styles among baccalaureate nursing students. *Journal of Advanced Nursing, 68*(7), 1482–1493. https://doi.org/10.1111/j.1365-2648.2011.05875.x.

Pink, D. H. (2018). *When: The scientific secrets of perfect timing.* New York: Riverhead Books.

Ratanasiripong, P., Park, J. F., Ratanasiripong, N., & Kathalae, D. (2015). Stress and anxiety management in nursing students: Biofeedback and mindfulness mediation. *Journal of Nursing Education, 54*(9), 520–524.

Richmond, P. A., Book, K., Hicks, M., Pimpinella, A., & Jenner, P. A. (2009). C.O.M.E. be a nurse manager. *Nursing Management, 40*(2), 52–54. https://doi.org/10.1097/01.NUMA.0000345875.99318.82.

Rosch, P. J. (2001). The quandary of job stress compensation. *Health and Stress, 3,* 1–4.

Rosenfeld, P., & Glassman, K. (2016). The long-term effect of a nurse residency program, 2005–2012: Analysis of former nurse residents. *Journal of Nursing Administration, 46*(6), 336–344.

Rosenthal, M. S. (2002). *50 ways to prevent and manage stress.* New York, NY: McGraw-Hill.

Rush, K. L., Adamack, M., Gordon, J., Lilly, M., & Janke, R. (2013). Best practices of formal new graduate nurse transition programs: An integrative review. *International Journal of Nursing Studies, 50*(3), 345–356. https://doi.org/10.1016/j.ijnurstu.2012.06.009.

Saunders, E. G. (2013). *The 3 secrets to effective time investment: Achieve more success with less stress.* New York, NY: McGraw-Hill.

Scott, D. L. (2003). *Wall Street words: An A to Z guide to investment terms for today's investor.* Boston, MA: Houghton Mifflin.

Seaward, B. L. (2013). *Essentials of managing stress* (3rd ed.). Burlington, MA: Jones & Bartlett Learning.

Segal, J., Smith, M., Robinson, L., & Segal, R. (2019). *Stress in the workplace.* HelpGuide.org. https://www.helpguide.org/articles/stress/stress-in-the-workplace.htm.

Seyle, H. (1950). Stress and general adaption syndrome. *British Medical Journal, 1*(4667), 1383–1392.

Sherman, R., & Cohn, T. (2019). Leadership challenge: The role of timing in work and life. *American Nurse Today, 14*(10), 15–17.

Shirey, M. R., McDaniel, A. M., Ebright, P. R., Fisher, M. L., & Doebbeling, B. N. (2010). Understanding nurse manager stress and work complexity. *Journal of Nursing Administration, 40*(2), 82–91. https://doi.org/10.1097/NNA.0b013e3181cb9f88.

Templeman, J. (2018). Time: A nurse's friend or foe. *American Nurse Today, 13*(6), 54–55.

Ullrich, P. M., & Lutgendorf, S. K. (2002). Journaling about stressful events: Effects of cognitive processing and emotional expression. *Annals of Behavioral Medicine, 24*(3), 244–250.

Ulrich, B., Barden, C., Cassidy, L., & Varn-Davis, N. (2019). Critical care nurse work environments 2018: Findings and implications. *Critical Care Nurse, 39*(2), 67–84. https://doi.org/10.4037/ccn2019605.

US Department of Health and Human Services. (2014). *Key features of the Affordable Care Act.* http://www.hhs.gov/healthcare/facts-and-features/key-features-of-aca/index.html.

US Department of Health and Human Service National Institute of Mental Health. (n.d.). *Five things you should know about stress.* Mental Health Information. NIH Publication No. 19-MH-8109. https://www.nimh.nih.gov/health/publications/stress/index.shtml#pub3.

White, G. B. (2015). The alarming, long-term consequences of workplace stress. *The Atlantic.* http://www.theatlantic.com/business/archive/2015/02/the-alarming-long-term-consequences-of-workplace-stress/385397/.

Woods, E. (2005). *Employee development at the workplace: Achieving empowerment in a continuous learning environment* (2nd ed.). Dubuque, IA: Kendall Hunt.

World Health Organization (WHO). (2010). *Stress at the workplace.* https://www.who.int/occupational_health/topics/stressatwp/en/.

World Wide Web Foundation. (2015). *Sir Tim Berners-Lee.* http://webfoundation.org/about/sir-tim-berners-lee.

Role Management

Veronica Rankin

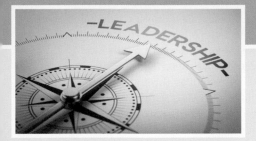

 http://evolve.elsevier.com/Huber/leadership

Health care organizations in the United States continue to experience persistent nursing shortages with increasing demand for complex, low-cost health care services for a higher acuity patient population. Nurse leaders of today need to serve as change agents to innovatively approach practice in a way that will recruit, develop, and retain the nurses of tomorrow through role management. With the impending exodus of the baby boomer population from the health care workforce, leaders must also begin preparing nurse leaders of tomorrow who do not have as many years of nursing experience as those leaving the workforce.

According to the Institute of Medicine (2010) and other sources, these significant nurse staffing deficits are expected to worsen within the next decade as more nurses, belonging to the baby boomer generation, prepare for retirement (Beck & Boulton, 2016; Yeager et al., 2016). These factors, coupled with the highly competitive nurse recruitment environment, require nurse leaders to approach practice differently than ever before. Chism (2016) described nursing as dynamic, noting that nursing continues to evolve to meet the needs of society by caring for its people and maintaining health and well-being. With this in mind, nurse leaders need to be transformational and effectively manage the various roles of nursing in a way that promotes engagement, empowers innovation, builds long-lasting relationships, and supports continued growth and development of nurses. This chapter will explore the nurse staffing issues plaguing health care and provide insight into how nurse leaders can successfully overcome these challenges,

while adapting to the ever-changing world of health care. Strategies are presented to help nurse leaders achieve success and combat challenging factors such as nurse leader vacancies and the reality of an expected influx of less experienced nurse leaders to guide frontline nursing staff. Nurse leaders cannot successfully manage the many roles within nursing without exploring ways in which to address the challenges of health care.

Although a definition of role management was not found in the literature, the definition to be used in this work refers to the activities necessary for leaders to successfully develop and maintain role definitions over time. In order to effectively manage roles, one must define the role, educate others, select the right person to implement the role, provide adequate support, master role development, and continuously evaluate the role for needed changes and sustainment purposes.

DEFINITIONS

Effective leadership, regardless of the discipline type, requires mutual understanding of the meaning and context of concepts used. Role management, and any other leadership function, cannot be accomplished if professionals lack the ability to speak and understand the same language. The following are definitions used in this chapter.

Change agent: an individual who effects change within themselves and builds the capacity for change in others to transform organizational systems (Stefancyk et al., 2013).

Change coach: an individual who alters human capabilities while supporting and influencing others towards change (Stefancyk et al., 2013).

Health care innovation: the process of rethinking and re-creating health care methods of practice and care delivery that extends farther than creating an electronic medical record (Porter-O'Grady & Malloch, 2018).

Innovation: the incessant adaptation to an ever-changing environment and available resources, which requires the creation of new business models and strategies to ensure that the organization survives and thrives in the future (Porter-O'Grady & Malloch, 2018).

Leadership: the science and skill of influencing or guiding a group of individuals towards the achievement of set goals (Carmen, 2002; McArthur, 2006). Leadership denotes accompaniment, whereas management denotes control and supervision.

Management: a guiding influence on an organization and its unit's market, production, and/or resource operations that may address human and non-human problems and is exerted by many individuals through either anticipatory norm-setting or situational intervention with a goal of achieving set objectives (Kaehler & Grundei, 2019).

Nursing: a dynamic practice that continues to evolve to meet the needs of society by caring for its people and maintaining health and well-being within various stages of health and illness (Chism, 2016).

Nursing practice: the independent, yet collaborative care of diverse populations through the use of health promotion, illness prevention, and care of the sick, disabled, and/or dying (International Council of Nurses, 2014).

Role management: the activities necessary for leaders to successfully develop and maintain role definitions over time, based on standardized expectations within an organization.

Transformational coaching: a method of activities used to transport individuals through the process of accepting change and accomplishing desired outcomes (Porter-O'Grady & Malloch, 2018).

BACKGROUND

Role Management

As the complexities of health care continue to evolve, the role of nurse leader must also continue to evolve to meet the needs of the patient population and the staff. Nursing literature lacks a definition of role management; therefore, a concept analysis was conducted to create a definition for the purpose of this chapter.

Classic role theory suggests that roles are created based on standard expectations and are associated with distinguishable positions within an organization (Biddle, 1986). Management, as described in the literature, implies control of resources through supervision and training to achieve set goals (Carmen, 2002; Garrison & McBryde-Foster, 2004). For the purpose of this chapter, role management is defined as the activities necessary for leaders to successfully develop and maintain role definitions over time, based on standardized expectations within an organization. Leaders must think proactively, exceeding the basic definition of management by taking a more creative approach in effective role management. In order to function in this capacity, leaders must fully understand and practice the following activities:

- defining the role
- educating others
- selecting the right personnel
- providing adequate support
- mastering role development
- constantly evaluating the role to ensure maintenance

Defining the Role

There are many roles within nursing that can be categorized in many different ways. Regarding practice, the categories could include administration, clinical, and educational. Within education categories, nurses can be grouped by such education levels as diploma, associates, bachelor's, master's, or doctorate. Regarding specialty training, the opportunities are endless. Furthermore, each category previously mentioned contains its own subcategories and variations posing the potential for what Stanley (2006) refers to as role confusion due to the lack of clarity to delineate one nursing role from another. This confusion further intensifies chaos between nursing staff within a workplace and hampers collaboration and productivity.

Identity plays a critical role in the realm of individual engagement because it serves as the fundamental way in which people define, label, and find themselves within an environment (Armstrong et al., 2018). Role theory postulates that teammates within an organization take on different responsibilities and roles within the organization (Biddle, 1986). Matta et al. (2015) argued that according to role theory, an individual's acted-out behavior is centered on the definition and evolution of their role. Consequently, when clear definitions of duties and role expectations are not provided, the individual may experience ambiguity that increases dissatisfaction, hesitation to practice, confusion, and ineffective performance (Biddle, 1986; Kahn et al., 1964). It is therefore very important for the nurse leader to define the nurse's role and scope of practice prior to implementation, setting expectations, or attempting to educate others about the role. Nelson (2017, p. 407) supported this premise by strongly advising leaders to define and ensure that definitions are created, kept clear, and thoroughly communicated repetitively to avoid "a blurring of the boundaries."

Furthermore, although defining the role is important, equally important is the need to identify the team to which the role will belong. Foster (2017) supported this premise by noting that team identification is critical because the nature of the new role is ultimately determined by the skills and competencies that are required from the clinical team to which the role belongs. Through completely defining a role, all parties involved enter the partnership with a clear understanding of group dynamics to enhance collaboration and teamwork.

Educating Others

The natural progression after defining a role is to educate others regarding the findings. This act is important for not only those partaking in the education, but also to build confidence and personal understanding for the individual. It is also important while educating to explain the role's impact or fit within the team. Armstrong et al. (2018) noted that the interpretation of new information is grossly affected by the way in which individuals align themselves with the responsibilities and purpose of their group. This means that the individual filling the role and the team should be clearly educated on each entity's purpose, goals, objectives, and collaborative expectations (Foster, 2017). Since defining the role was already completed prior to this step, this information should be readily accessible. Education to the team must be provided frequently, as new members join the team, responsibilities or duties of the team change, or group dynamics evolve over time.

Chism (2016) noted the importance of effective education in role management based on findings from the literature that the perceptions of patients, nurses, and other professionals are significantly influenced by previous experiences. A study by Gooden and Jackson (2004) revealed that nurses' attitudes about other nurses

in the health care environment could affect the patient's attitudes and impact health care outcomes. Richmond and Becker (2005) recommended that although attitudes about nurses were positive, these attitudes needed to be cultivated by nurses for sustainment. These authors recommended that nurses take on characteristics that are helpful in promoting credibility and trust that lead to understanding of the role and building of mutual relationships. Important characteristics include clarity in role and vision, commitment to practice, effective communication, collaboration, credibility through credentialing, contributions to patient outcomes, self-confidence, and solution-oriented practice (Richmond & Becker, 2005).

Role modeling is an effective way to educate through demonstration, which can be more impactful than verbal explanation. Chism (2016) noted that effective education depends on consistent demonstration of the value and expertise the nurse brings to health care delivery. The author explained that through role modeling, the nurse develops leadership abilities and interprofessional collaboration skills that enhance success in practice. Furthermore, other health care providers will be more receptive to the role and education offered about the role when evidence in the form of demonstrated outcomes is actualized.

Selecting the Right Personnel

A critical component of role management begins with selecting the right individual for the role. This may require leadership training and coaching for new leaders because an individual's clinical knowledge base or performance at the bedside does not predicate automatic selection for all nursing roles. Contrary to popular belief, the habit of hiring the highest performing nurse who is the most experienced on the unit into a nurse leader role may result in confusion, personal struggles, and poor leadership that ultimately potentiates poor care quality and patient outcomes (Stanley, 2006). It is critical for leaders to learn how to recruit, transition, and retain upcoming leaders more effectively for not only the organization but also for the future of nursing (Sherman & Saifman, 2018).

Koehn (2017) described the lives of five influential leaders in history. This author noted that all of the leaders discussed in the work were made into leaders, meaning they were not born leaders. Koehn postulated that although each leader was gifted in various skills, they each lacked something that was cultivated or had to be learned to become the successful leader that they were. Koehn (2017) listed the following attributes that successful leaders must possess:

1. Be accountable and willing to self-improve.
2. Be able to reflect on their actions and encounters to seek learning.
3. Be able to take instruction.
4. Take inventory of their strengths and weaknesses and maximize their own capabilities.
5. Excel in emotional intelligence, empathy, and intentionality.
6. Develop resilience.
7. Become comfortable with solitude and detachment.
8. Envision the big picture and potential impact.

The recruitment process also needs to include a thorough assessment of the individual's goals, expectations, and essential retention factors as related to the role. Yeager and Wisniewski (2017) conducted a cross-sectional study that examined recruitment and retention perspectives of more than 3000 nurses and non-nurses who worked in public health arenas. Of the 12 organizational factors included in the survey, results revealed that the top five retention factors the nurses reported were autonomy/employee empowerment, flexibility of work schedule, specific duties and responsibilities, opportunities for training/continuing education, and ability to innovate. Understanding the factors that matter to potential employees is critical to successful recruitment and retention efforts (Beck & Boulton, 2016). Present day leaders expecting to master role management need to be cognizant of their employees' driving forces upfront to combat the nursing shortage issues resulting from excessive turnover that are expected to worsen in the future.

Providing Adequate Support

According to Press Ganey (2018), nurse leader support is a key driver in positively impacting novice nurse intent to stay. The same holds true for experienced nurses whether the interest lies in staying at the bedside in a clinical position or aspiring to the executive board room. Bradley and Moore (2019) noted that nurse leaders are often inadequately prepared, developed, and supported in their roles. This undoubtedly perpetuates turnover and poor interest in nursing leadership positions. As leaders prepare to approach practice differently, multiple methods of support should be explored and implemented within the work setting.

Support can be achieved in various ways. One major method strongly supported in the literature is mentoring or coaching. Mentors are absolutely vital to the success of a new leader (Martin & Warshawsky, 2017). Evidence from the literature validates the positive effects of mentored onboarding for leadership success. Coaching is a commonly used technique implemented to help develop the skills of upcoming inquisitive leaders capable of instigating organizational impact. Roussel et al. (2020) noted that there is growing evidence supporting the use of developmental coaching for all new leaders as it has emerged as a cornerstone of learning organizations. Furthermore, in addition to employee retention and patient outcomes, evidence substantiates the fact that coaching promotes engagement among leaders and staff members, enriches communication skills, and advances motivation and decision-making skills (Blackman et al., 2016).

Through coaching, professionalism can be fostered seamlessly. Blackman et al. (2016) noted that the demonstration of personal excellence, genuineness, and credibility of coaches facilitates sustainable progress and continued learning for those who are coached. Now is the time for coaches to role-model to upcoming leaders the power of open communication, self-reflection, responsibility, respect for humankind, and each nurse's responsibility to advocate for professionalism (Roussel et al., 2020).

The concept of a change coach is introduced in the literature by Stefancyk et al. (2013) as a leader who uses behaviors such as guiding, facilitating, and inspiring followers to elicit change. A change coach is described as someone who can alter human capabilities through support and influence. Although both roles of change agent and change coach result in change, the change coach accomplishes change through influence and inspiration more so than hands-on action as with a change agent. A successful leader is described as being one who can easily move between the roles of change agent and change coach as required by the situation.

Competencies such as those provided by the American Organization of Nurse Executives (AONE, 2015), now the American Organization for Nursing Leadership, can serve as a helpful tool in developing a plan for role development and training. By studying these and other competency and role development tools, one can approach mentorship with a certain level of expectancy by being better prepared with the ability to voice needs to the mentor (Moyo, 2019).

Another way in which support can be provided to nurse leaders to effectively manage the various roles of nursing is relationship building or the formation of alliances. According to Siren and Gehrs (2018), nurse leaders are the connecting link between executive leaders and nursing staff at the bedside. They are also expected to foster relationships with interdisciplinary teammates as well as promote physician engagement and collaborative partnerships with nursing (Nelson, 2017). Alliances are automatically built as health care providers collectively share in meeting the needs of patients, communities, and organizations (Harris et al., 2018). By creating alliances, leaders can leverage differences within the team to achieve goals.

Mastering Role Development

Historically, clinical nurses from the frontline are "cut and pasted" into their new leadership role with little to no prior leadership development or mentoring (Sherman & Saifman, 2018). It sounds contradictory that although nursing leadership is well supported in the literature as being one of the most demanding roles in health care (Goodyear & Goodyear, 2018), more guidance and training is oftentimes devoted to new graduate nurses than new nurse leaders who are held accountable to retain them (Sherman & Saifman, 2018). Strategic planning and succession planning need to be devoted to rectifying this finding.

The literature recommends beginning succession planning with role development activities now to train and prepare the nurses of tomorrow. Although Moyo (2019) provided seven key strategies to help millennial nurse leaders achieve success, the literature shows that these strategies are applicable to all leaders, regardless of their generational category (Roussel et al., 2020). These strategies include:

1. Seek out opportunities to learn.
2. Remain confident and optimistic.
3. Show respect and be unbiased.
4. Work on getting to know and understand your staff early.
5. Be firm, yet fair, and always consistent.
6. Be helpful and supportive to your staff.
7. Reflect on your learning and progress.

Saifman and Sherman (2019) conducted a qualitative study on a national sample of 25 millennial nurse managers to explore their experiences as nurse managers. The purpose of this study was to better understand the organization's influential factors on the nurse manager's job satisfaction, development, intent to stay, and their perspectives regarding their role expectations and support as leaders. Findings revealed seven common themes from the participants: "coming into the role, learning as I go, having the support of my director, making an impact, helping staff succeed, and managing change" (Saifman & Sherman, 2019, p. 367). The findings of this study reveal pertinent opportunities leaders should prepare for in order to develop and retain millennial leaders. This study supports the importance of succession planning and formal standardized leadership development processes. Lastly, findings also suggest innovative approaches to modifying the design of the nurse leader role to enhance the desirability of the role for millennials.

Nurse leader training and preparation needs to be strategically planned to ensure that new leaders are trained, equipped, and empowered to achieve success. Simmers (2019) noted that this process begins with a review of the literature to identify best practices, evidence regarding the role, and barriers and challenges to role development and implementation. Once this process has been completed, role development needs to include adequate training, a needs assessment, relationship building, education, and support groups for sustainment.

A study by Warshawsky et al. (2013) led to the creation of a Nurse Manager Practice Environment Scale that assessed factors affecting nurse manager job performance. This study found that the success of a nurse manager is predicated on the manager's ability to create an innovative work culture, foster relationships, facilitate patient safety, and provide adequate resources and staffing. This tool is one of many that can be used to not only assess nurse leader satisfaction or burnout, but it can also be used to assist in developing action plans or strategies for improvement.

Fischer-Cartlidge et al. (2019) conducted a successful multiphase journey to rebuild a Clinical Nurse Specialist team after years of open vacancies and role confusion. The approach included innovative recruitment strategies, development of a talent pipeline through enhancement of student clinical placements, team and individual development activities, and value identification. As a result of the role development activities, the authors achieved role standardization and optimization, increased representation on hospital-wide committees and councils, and were able to quantify their work.

Yeager and Wisniewski (2017) stressed the importance of clearly defined duties and responsibilities that align within the organization's strategic plan, mission and vision statement, and values to enhance role management. Additional recommendations include detailed job descriptions emphasizing activities that the employee will participate in, benefits from organizations that offer training and continuing education, and partnering with local colleges and universities. Offering opportunities for employees to gain new skills and training on the job not only helps to identify future leaders, but it also helps to strengthen engagement by creating a community of invested partnership (Yeager & Wisniewski, 2017).

Role Evaluation/Maintenance

Adequate leadership is critical to role development and nurse positioning to achieve quality improvement and efficient health care delivery (Kraaij et al., 2020). Long-term maintenance of role management depends on the leader's ability to continue to develop and support the role as well as serve as an influential leader on all levels of nursing. Harris and Roussel (2010) noted that professional values, including such concepts as altruism, accountability, responsibility, human dignity, integrity, and other ethical principles, facilitate successful role implementation and management. These values and principles are essential to nursing practice because they govern how professionals communicate, form relationships, manage conflicts, deliver compassionate care, enculturate diversity, evaluate failures and successes, and handle stress (Harris & Roussel, 2010).

An important component of role management maintenance is reward and recognition along the journey. Stefancyk et al. (2013) advised leaders to celebrate successes and view innovations that may not have been seen initially as successful, as learning opportunities. Leaders need to consistently express confidence in the staff, in the role, and in the organization to encourage continued work and engagement. This action will also motivate followers to seek out bigger issues on the unit that can impact quality care.

In role management, maintenance depends upon direct focus on progress and on challenges and barriers to achieving progress. Porter O'Grady and Malloch (2018) advised leaders to address problems directly by approaching barriers proactively. The importance of proactive approaches to problem solving was stressed to avoid the "firefighting" phenomenon that can easily consume nurse leader's workday. Real-time problem-solving helps to develop leaders and strengthens the transformational impact one can have on a work setting. The recommendation is to avoid the error of finding quick fixes, but to instead drill down to the root of the problem to prevent recurrence.

Many evaluation frameworks exist to assess the success of implementations. These frameworks can be used to understand the phases, stages, and circumstantial factors that may be positively or negatively affecting a role or process. Roussel et al. (2020) provided examples of commonly used frameworks such as Reach X Efficacy-Adoption, Implementation, Maintenance (RE-AIM) and Precede-Proceed framework with the explanation that leaders need to be aware of the differences of such tools to ensure that the correct framework is chosen to meet the assessment needs of the leader. Additional assessment methodologies such as theories and process models can also be used to determine aspects of success with role management. Some of the more common quality and performance improvement strategies used to assess progress include Six Sigma, LEAN, Plan-Do-Study-Act, and standardization in practice (Roussel et al., 2020). Regardless of the strategy used, nurse leaders need to know what measures or metrics the role is expected to impact in order to assess progress. With having some method in which to assess progress of the implemented work, the leader can continuously perform pulse checks of the work to ensure that expectations are being met, adequate support is provided, and that the employee understands their role and what is expected of them.

LEADERSHIP AND MANAGEMENT IMPLICATIONS

Role management is defined as the activities necessary for leaders to successfully develop and maintain role definitions over time, based on standardized expectations within an organization. In order to tackle the nursing shortages as well as all of the other demanding challenges of health care, nurse leaders need to approach practice differently than ever before. Nurse leaders need to serve as change agents, change coaches, mentors, and transformational leaders at the bedside to attract clinical nurses into the worsening nurse leader vacancies expected in the near future. In order to successfully serve as role managers, nurse leaders need to define the role, educate others, select the right personnel, provide adequate support, champion role development, and continuously evaluate the role for maintenance. Succession planning for the nurse leaders of tomorrow need to start now to advance care quality because it is an immediate imperative. In addition to innovative practice approaches, leaders and nursing professionals at all levels need to thoroughly understand and practice delegation and ethical decision making to function effectively within their roles. These foundational components of nursing practice are essential to practice. They provide the capacity for nursing professionals to work within a collaborative team construct, impact health outcomes, and demonstrate compassionate, person-centered care.

Change Agents

Through basic nursing education, nurses are aware of the common change theories used in quality improvement work such as Lewin's 3-step Change Theory, Lippitt's Phases of Change Theory, and Prochaska and DiClemente's Transtheoretical Change Model (Kritsonis, 2005). The literature supports the fact that nurse leaders need to exceed change awareness. They need to understand the theories and be skilled at applying and coaching staff through change (Stefancyk et al., 2013). Stefancyk et al. (2013) noted that regardless of the model or method used, effective change penetrates far beyond the processes and structure of an organization to impact the organization's culture.

Leadership is the science and skill of influencing or guiding a group of individuals towards the achievement of set goals (Carmen, 2002; McArthur, 2006). Nurse leaders inhabit a critical position in creating a culture that is accepting of change. As transformational coaches, leaders are responsible for creating a culture of change and the structure in which change is to be actualized, thereby fostering adaptation and employee engagement (Porter-O'Grady & Malloch, 2018). Leadership, not to be confused with management, denotes accompaniment, whereas management denotes control and

supervision. Through role modeling nurse leaders serve an important part in leading change at the front line of care delivery and therefore can be the most influential change agents in an organization.

Stefancyk et al. (2013) defined a change agent as an individual who transforms themselves and influences the capacity for change within individuals around them for the sake of an organization. Rogers (2003) defined a change agent as an individual who influences another person's innovative decisions towards the desirable wishes of an organization. Both definitions imply alignment with some party or institution's goals or action plan. Rogers (2003) also provides stages in the role of change agent which include:

1. Developing a need for change
2. Disseminating information
3. Identifying the problem
4. Developing the client's intent to change
5. Translating intent into action
6. Hardwiring adoption and preventing noncompliance
7. Achieving termination/adjournment

In order to serve as an effective change agent, nurse leaders must understand and put these steps into practice. Couros (2014) expands this work by defining five characteristics that change agents need to employ to be truly effective: having a clear vision, being patient yet tenacious, exploring tough uncertainties, being knowledgeable and role modeling, and building trusting relationships. Stefancyk et al. (2013) supported this information by noting that successful nurse leaders promote and hardwire a culture of change by strategically homing in on the leadership elements of human resource management, foundational thinking, relationship building, and the power of influence.

Transformational Leadership

Transformational leaders create an environment that allows individuals to contribute their fullest potential to achieve the best outcomes possible (Porter-O'Grady & Malloch, 2018). Leaders of today are responsible for inspiring and motivating staff despite the chaos of an unstable and extremely fast-paced environment. Consequently, it is because of the high demand for health care services to be provided at a faster pace to a sicker population, using fewer resources, that transformational leaders are critical to the success of the nursing profession. Tuuk (2012) noted that transformational leaders obligate individuals to take action, transform followers into leaders, and then change leaders into change agents. The author also noted that these types of leaders do not use power to repress and control, but instead empower individuals to create a vision and then trust them to work towards achieving that vision. The most effective way to tackle the challenges of health care is to enlist transformational leaders who are dedicated to serving as change agents.

Delegation

Effective leadership and role management in health care necessitates delegation in order to complete tasks in an efficient manner and to promote continued development (Bake, 2020). In fact, according to the National Council of State Boards of Nursing (NCSBN, 2019), delegation is a critical competency for nurses in all areas of practice, especially nurse leaders. Hewertson (2015) defined delegation as the planned learning of new skills and opportunities for an individual that transfers duties or tasks to that individual for a purpose that is mutually beneficial for the individual and delegator. As a critical competency, all licensed nurses must fully understand the laws and rules of their specific state or jurisdiction, since they can differ from location to location.

When tasks require delegation, the delegation process and the nurse practice act of that jurisdiction must be thoroughly understood to ensure that the process is handled in a safe and ethically sound manner (NCSBN, 2019). The licensed nurse must make the decision regarding the patient's condition, the competence of the delegatee, and the degree of supervision required and available to guarantee safe practice. Delegation goes beyond the delegatee's basic educational training, permitting the performance of tasks that are not routinely performed by the delegate, and may extend beyond their customary role or basic responsibilities. The delegating nurse is still ultimately responsible for making sure that the task is performed correctly. The national guidelines of the NCSBN (2019) outlined five rights of delegation that include: (1) delegation of the right task, (2) delegation under the right conditions, (3) delegation to the right individual, (4) delegation by providing the right instructions and effective communication, and (5) delegation with the right supervision and assessment. In order to comply with these five important steps, the following criteria by the NCSBN (2019) must be met:

- The delegate must have been trained and validated as competent to perform the task or responsibility.
- The nurse cannot delegate a task that requires nursing judgment or critical thinking.
- Delegation can only occur by an individual that owns delegating authority.
- The delegated task must be within the scope of practice of the delegator and the delegate according to the nurse practice act.

Although the licensed nurse is ultimately responsible for the overall well-being of the patient, once the task has been appropriately delegated and accepted by the delegate, the delegatee is responsible for the delegated task or duty (NCSBN, 2019). The delegation process is multidimensional within every health care setting, beginning at the administrative level. Administrators are responsible for setting the criteria and creating the policies and procedures regarding the delegation of nursing responsibilities. Administrators are also responsible for periodically assessing the delegation process and promoting a healthy working environment. Delegation is infused throughout all aspects of nursing; therefore, all nurses should become well versed in the process.

Nurse leaders need to role-model proper and effective delegation through role management. Effective role management requires skills and knowledge in delegation. The principles of delegation as noted by Hewertson (2015) include:

1. Select the right individual.
2. Demonstrate and teach considering various learning styles.
3. Assign and delegate new work that is challenging, yet rewarding and exciting.
4. Provide adequate time for training and development.
5. Delegate gradually while monitoring progress continuously.
6. Align responsibility and authority to manage delegated tasks.
7. Avoid splitting one job if possible, by delegating a job as a whole unit.
8. Share the expected results and outcomes of the job.
9. Avoid holes and overlaps due to incomplete planning.
10. Trust the delegate and allow autonomy within established boundaries.

These principles align with the activities of role management, which include role definition, education, personnel selection, support provision, role development, and evaluation/assessment. It is especially important to transcribe the plan in writing for future reference and to ensure complete understanding. Hewertson (2015) noted that the delegation plan should be a signed and dated document that includes such details as the names of the delegate and delegator, the delegated job duty, the details of the authority, time frame including time allotted for training and practice, agreed milestones, the plan for communication, performance criteria, risk factors, and needed resources.

Ethical Issues

Effective nurse leadership hinges on a thorough understanding of ethics due to the frequency of ethical dilemmas requiring sound decision-making that nurses find themselves in within the role. A definition provided by Butts and Rich (2008, p. 4) described ethics as "the study of ideal human behavior and ideal ways of being." Roussel et al. (2020) explained the meaning of ethics as an individual's conformity to the standards of a professional group. The premise of these definitions center on personal beliefs and moral philosophy that delineates right actions from wrong actions and an individual's adaptability to change behavior based on perceived good and bad intent.

A code of ethics as described by Pozgar (2010), defined the criteria of behavior and specific principles as they apply to the duties of professionals. The Code of Ethics for Nurses, created by the American Nurses Association (ANA, 2015), is considered to be the standard for ethical nurse behavior, regardless of the nursing position or role (Chism, 2016). This code needs to be role modeled by leaders within the workplace to ensure that nursing practice upholds the four responsibilities of nurses, which are "to promote health, to prevent illness, to restore health, and alleviate suffering" (International Council of Nurses [ICN], 2006, p. 1).

Leaders oftentimes find themselves in situations known as ethical dilemmas in which difficult decisions must be made between equally unfavorable options in clinical practice. These dilemmas develop as a result of conflict between principles and rules regarding socially approved human behavior, professional code of ethics standards, public policies of government agencies, business related ethics of an organization, and personal values held by each individual provider. Chism (2016) pinpointed four ethical principles that serve as the cornerstone of biology and medicine to include autonomy, beneficence, nonmaleficience, and justice. When ethical dilemmas arise, these principles are raised to help examine the situation and find resolution. Many authors have provided definitions of these principles for health care providers (Beauchamp & Childress, 2009; Butts & Rich, 2008; Cooper, 2014; Pozgar, 2010) that include:

- Autonomy is an individual's right for self-governance, free from controlling interference by others.
- Beneficence means doing good by helping others with compassionate care.
- Nonmaleficence means to avoid causing harm to others.
- Justice is the provision of fair and equal treatment, consistent with equal distribution of benefits and burden.

Leaders need to become champions of ethics and ensure that resources are available to help guide staff and themselves through ethical decision-making. Chism (2016) advised leaders to be ethically conscious and competent while being committed to consistently doing that which is right. Leaders are also advised to be courageous enough to abide by their own competence despite uneasiness or what is popular. Leaders are further advised to remain open and straightforward to directly address the ethical issue or dilemma. By accomplishing these recommendations in practice, a culture strong in autonomy, beneficence, nonmaleficence, and justice will be actualized.

CURRENT ISSUES & TRENDS

One concern found in the literature relates to the baby boomer exodus expected to worsen within the next decade, which will weaken the supply of seasoned, well-experienced nurse leaders (Beck & Boulton, 2016; Moyo, 2019; Yeager et al., 2016). This vacancy will require millennial nurses to fill in nurse leader vacancies. In fact, it has been estimated that 50% of the entire nursing workforce will soon be filled by millennials (Holland, 2015). This issue is of further concern because nurse leader recruitment has become extremely difficult over the years as manifested by increasing turnover rates (McCright et al., 2018). A way in which nurse leaders of today can ensure that care quality does not suffer from this unavoidable shift is to serve as change agents and approach leadership practice in an innovative, more strategic way. Porter-O'Grady and Malloch (2018) defined innovation as a continuous adaptation to an ever-changing environment and the availability of resources that require the creation of new business models and strategies to ensure that the organization survives and thrives in the future. The authors further defined health care innovation as the process of rethinking and re-creating health care methods of practice and care delivery extending beyond the electronic medical record (Porter-O'Grady & Malloch, 2018). This requires new leadership mindsets that are skilled in delegation and ethical decision-making to manage the seemingly contradictory expectations of stability and uncertainty within which health care exists today.

RESEARCH NOTE

Source
Siren, A., & Gehrs, M. (2019). Engaging nurses in future management careers: Perspectives on leadership and management competency development through an internship initiative. *Nursing Leadership, 31*(4), 36–49.

Purpose
The purpose of the article is to describe the process of creating a nurse management internship program and also explore the experience of an intern who completed the program. The article explores the intern's perspective regarding the program's competency development and the impact of mentorship support on personal resilience.

Discussion
Nurse managers have an important part in leading change at the front lines of care delivery. They need to manage and empower their team, support healthy and collaborative work environments, maintain patient safety, and address satisfaction concerns of patients and their families. As one of the most challenging roles in health care that continues to evolve over time, the nurse manager is the indispensable connector between senior leadership and staff at the point of care. For this purpose, new nurses preparing for nursing management benefit from a structured approach to preparation. The current state of the economy has caused many nurse leaders of the baby boomer generation to delay their retirement. As these leaders exit the workforce, new less-experienced nurses will need to fill the open leadership positions. The challenge with this situation is the fact that many younger generation nurses do not find nursing leadership roles desirable. They perceive the nurse manager role as requiring too much work and being both time consuming and inadequately compensated for the workload. In order to overcome these challenges and draw younger nurses into this role, organizations need to mentor and begin succession planning for the nurse managers of tomorrow. Orientation plans, support networks, and ongoing educational training need to be appropriately structured and adequately provided to nurse manager candidates.

In this article, a 10-year investment was arranged to create an advanced practice nursing scholarship initiative for 23 individuals employed at the addiction and mental health center. The purpose was to help the center "attract, develop, and retain skilled nurses for management, advanced practice and other relevant leadership roles" (Siren & Gehrs, 2018, p. 39). In addition to these scholarships, two 6-month paid internships were made available for 18 individuals over the 10-year period. The purpose was to "offer a period of enhanced professional nursing leadership development by applying knowledge and skills that foster confidence, critical thinking and leadership competency development…" (Siren & Gehrs, 2018, p. 39). A heterogeneous committee made up of senior nursing leaders and other interprofessional leaders monitored both the scholarship and internship processes over the course of the initiative.

The article provides the following steps of creating a successful nurse manager internship that includes selecting the right individual, selecting the right competency context, operationalizing the intern's development plan, identifying a mentorship network, and transitioning into the role. One lesson learned from the process was that novice-level leadership development content is lacking in the literature. Although this internship was especially designed for a novice leader, most of the evidence found related only to senior-level leadership. Another lesson learned from feedback provided by interns was the need for the intern to be within close proximity of their primary mentor for real-time learning. Other lessons included the benefit of a mentorship network, innovative approaches that inspire young nurses to consider management, and formal networking opportunities between novice nurses and senior leaders. The authors recommended further exploration regarding innovative methods to enhance work–life balance of nurse managers, which is extremely important for younger nurses.

Application to Practice
This article provided steps to consider when seeking to attract, recruit, and retain nurse leaders of tomorrow. Through providing the scholarships and internships, this addiction and mental health center was able to create an effective novice-level nurse management development program. The authors presented feedback from an intern

RESEARCH NOTE—cont'd

who completed the program to help others considering replication of similar processes. The application to practice centers on the need to combat the challenges of nurse leader vacancy, turnover, and ill-prepared leaders to handle the growing demands of health care. By applying evidence found in the future, nurse executives have a better chance of recruiting and retaining competent, satisfied, and effective leaders to manage front line care delivery.

CASE STUDY

You are an Assistant Vice President of the neuroscience division at a Level 1 Trauma Center. You have been informed that the Chief Nurse Executive wishes to discuss a new nursing role with you. In preparation for the meeting, you quickly research new nursing roles but are unable to find anything substantial. In the meeting, your Chief Nurse describes a new nursing role called the Clinical Nurse Leader (CNL). She explains that this role is the newest master's prepared role added to the profession of nursing in more than 30 years. The title and initials of the role are the exclusive property of the American Association of Colleges of Nursing, in that only individuals who have completed the program and passed the certification exam may use them. Within her high-level overview, she describes the advanced clinician role as an "attending nurse." She shares that this role was designed to provide the resource and clinical expertise of nurses at the bedside with advanced education who can coach and mentor nurses in order to improve patient outcomes and maintain patient safety. As a fellow nurse leader of the institution, she reminds you of the current state of opportunities on the medical units outside of the intensive care units. She explains the high influx of inexperienced nurses, the climbing acuity levels of patients serviced by the hospital, and constant pressure from administration to do more with less. She further explains her intent to implement the role at your hospital. She knows that the need for this role is much greater in the medical surgical areas as evidence by internal data and nationwide evidence from the literature. The Chief Nurse explains her plan to apply for grant funding, create a partnership with a local university to provide the CNL track, and recruit a certified CNL to serve as CNL Program Coordinator prior to implementing the role. She has not ironed out the rest of the details, but she would like to assess how you feel about the idea altogether. She would like to assess your ideas regarding role implementation and role management. What are first steps to consider in the process? What are critical components that should go into the planning of this initiative? What are pitfalls you can plan to avoid ensuring success of this role?

CRITICAL THINKING EXERCISE

Situation: You've been asked to implement a new role at your facility that you know very little about. Your executive leader has provided the finances needed to implement the role effectively, but, due to pressing matters, cannot lead the implementation of the role and has therefore delegated the task to you to lead. The leader has provided the return on investment expectations that he expects from the role but has left all other details to you to arrange. What are your first steps? What interdisciplinary teammates must be involved in planning this initiative? Follow the steps provided in this chapter to outline an approach that you can present to your executive leader.

REFERENCES

American Nurses Association (ANA). (2015). *Code of ethics for nurses with interpretive statements*. Silver Spring, MD: Nursebooks.org.

American Organization of Nurse Executives (AONE). (2015). *Nurse manager competencies*. http://www.aone.org/resources/nurse-manager-competencies.pdf.

Armstrong, A. K., Krasny, M. E., & Schuldt, J. P. (2018). Identity. In A. K. Armstrong, M. E. Krasny, & J. P. Schuldt (Eds.), *Communicating climate change:* *A guide for educators* (pp. 43–48). Ithaca, NY: Cornell University Press.

Bake, M. (2020). Health care management. *Radiologic Technology, 91*(3), 297–299.

Beauchamp, T. L., & Childress, J. F. (2009). *Principles of biomedical ethics* (6th ed.). New York: Oxford University Press.

Beck, A. J., & Boulton, M. L. (2016). The public health nurse workforce in U.S. state and local health departments, 2012. *Public Health Reports, 131*(1), 145–152.

Biddle, B. J. (1986). Recent developments in role theory. *Annual Review of Sociology, 12*, 67–92. https://doi.org/10.1146/annurev.so.12.080186.000435.

Blackman, A., Marscado, G., & Gray, D. (2016). Challenges for the theory and practice of business coaching: A systematic review of empirical evidence. *Human Resource Development Review, 15*(4), 459–486.

Bradley, J., & Moore, L. (2019). The perceptions of professional leadership coaches regarding the roles and challenges of nurse managers. *Journal of Nursing Administration, 49*(2), 105–109.

Butts, J. B., & Rich, K. L. (2008). *Nursing ethics: Across the curriculum and into practice* (2nd ed.). Sudbury, MA: Jones & Bartlett.

Carmen, T. (2002). *Love em' and lead 'em: Leadership strategies that work for reluctant leaders*. Lanham, MD: Scarecrow Press.

Chism, L. (2016). *The doctor of nursing practice: A guidebook for role development and professional issues*. Burlington, MA: Jones & Bartlett.

Cooper, R. W. (2014). Legal and ethical issues. In D. L. Huber (Ed.), *Leadership and nursing care management* (5th ed., pp. 94–110). St. Louis, MO: Elsevier.

Couros, G. (2014). *5 characteristics of a change agent*. http://georgecouros.ca/blog/archives/3615.

Fischer-Cartlidge, E., Houlihan, N., & Browne, K. (2019). Recruitment, role development, and value identification. *Clinical Nurse Specialist: The Journal for Advanced Nursing Practice, 33*(6), 266–272.

Foster, C. (November, 2017). Aiming high is the key to role development. *Imaging & Therapy Practice*, 6–10. ISSN: 2052-0727

Garrison, D. R., & McBryde-Foster, M. J. (2004). The baccalaureate nurse as a leader in health care delivery. In L. C. Haynes, H. K. Butcher, & T. A. Boese (Eds.), *Nursing in contemporary society: Issues, trends, and transition to practice* (pp. 504–525). Upper Saddle River, NJ: Pearson/Prentice Hall.

Gooden, J., & Jackson, E. (2004). Attitudes of registered nurses toward nurse practitioners. *Journal of American Academy of Nurse Practitioners, 16*(8), 360–364.

Goodyear, C., & Goodyear, M. (2018). Career development for nurse managers. *Nursing Management, 49*(3), 49–53.

Harris, J., & Roussel, L. (2010). *Initiating and sustaining the clinical nurse leader role: A practical guide*. Sudbury, MA: Jones and Bartlett Publishers.

Harris, J., Roussel, L., & Thomas, P. (2018). *Initiating and sustaining the clinical nurse leader role: A practical guide* (3rd ed.). Sudbury MA: Jones and Bartlett Publishers.

Hewertson, R. (2015). *Lead like it matters, because it does matter*. New York: McGraw-Hill Education.

Holland, C. (2015). Practice and education: Partnering to create a pipeline of nurse leaders. *Nursing Management, 46*(1), 8–10.

Institute of Medicine. (2010). *The future of nursing: Leading change, advancing health*. Washington, DC: National Academics Press.

International Council of Nurses [ICN]. (2006). *Code of ethics for nurses*. http://www.icn.ch/images/stories/documents/about/icncode_english.pdf.

International Council of Nurses [ICN]. (2014). *Definition of nursing*. http://www.icn.ch/about-icn/icn-definition-of-nursing.

Kaehler, B., & Grundei, J. (2019). The concept of management: In search of a new definition. *HR governance: A theoretical introduction*. (pp. 3-23). Cham: Springer. https://doi.org/10.1007/978-3-319-94526-2.

Kahn, R. L., Wolfe, D., Quinn, R., Snoek, J., & Rosenthal, R. (1964). *Organizational stress: Studies in role conflict and ambiguity*. New York: Wiley.

Koehn, N. (2017). *Forged in crisis: The power of courageous leadership in turbulent times*. New York: Simon & Schuster.

Kraaij, J., Oostveen, C., Vermeulen, H., Heinen, M., Huis, A., Adriaansen, M., & Peters, J. (2020). Nurse practitioners' perceptions of their ability to enact leadership in hospital care. *Journal of Clinical Nursing, 29*(3/4), 447–458. https://doi.org/10.1111/jocn.15105.

Kritsonis, A. (2005). Comparison of change theories. *International Journal of Scholarly Academic Intellectual Diversity, 8*(1), 1–7. http://www.nationalforum.com/Electronic%20Journal%20Volumes/Kritsonis,%20Alicia%20Comparison%20of%20Change%20Theories%20IJMBA%20V8%20N1%202005.pdf.

Martin, E., & Warshawsky, N. (2017). Guiding principles for creating value and meaning for the next generation of nurse leaders. *Journal of Nursing Administration, 47*(9), 418–420.

Matta, F. K., Scott, B. A., Koopman, J., & Conlon, D. E. (2015). Does seeing "eye to eye" affect work engagement and organizational citizenship behavior? A role theory perspective on LMX agreement. *Academic Management Journal, 58*, 1686–1708. https://doi.org/10.5465/amj.2014.0106.

McArthur, D. (2006). The nurse practitioner as leader. *Journal of the American Academy of Nurse Practitioners, 18*(1), 8–10.

McCright, M., Pabico, C., & Roux, N. (2018). Addressing manager retention with the pathway to excellence framework. *Nursing Management, 49*(8), 6–8.

Moyo, M. (2019). Millennial nurse manager: Leading staff nurses more experienced than you. *Nurse Leader, 17*(3), 253–256. https://doi.org/10.1016/j.mnl.2018.09.005.

National Council of State Boards of Nursing – American Nurses Association. (2019). *National guidelines for nursing delegation*. https://www.ncsbn.org/NGND-PosPaper_06.pdf.

Nelson, K. (2017). Nurse manager perceptions of work overload and strategies to address it. *Nurse Leader, 15*(6), 406–408.

Porter O'Grady, T., & Malloch, K. (2018). *Quantum leadership: Creating sustainable value in health care.* Burlington, MA: Jones & Bartlett.

Pozgar, G. D. (2010). *Legal and ethical issues for health professional* (2nd ed.). Sudbury, MA: Jones & Bartlett Learning.

Press Ganey Nursing Special Report. (2018). *Optimizing the nursing workforce: Key drivers to intent to stay for newly licensed and experienced nurses.* http://healthcare.pressganey.com/2018-Nursing-Special-Report?s=White_Paper-PR.

Richmond, T., & Becker, D. (2005). Creating an advanced practice nurse-friendly culture: A marathon not a sprint. *AACN Clinical Issues, 16*(1), 58–66.

Rogers, E. M. (2003). *Diffusion of innovations* (5th ed.). New York: Free Press.

Roussel, L., Thomas, P., & Harris, J. (2020). *Management and leadership for nurse administrators.* (8th ed.). Burlington, MA: Jones & Bartlett Learning.

Saifman, H., & Sherman, R. (2019). The experience of being a millennial nurse manager. *The Journal of Nursing Administration, 49*(7/8), 366–371.

Sherman, R., & Saifman, H. (2018). Transitioning emerging leaders into nurse leader roles. *Journal of Nursing Administration, 48*(7/8), 355–357.

Simmers, P. (2019). Development of a new nurse navigator program. *JONS-online, 10*(11), 474.

Siren, A., & Gehrs, M. (2018). Engaging nurses in future management careers: Perspectives on leadership and management competency development through an internship initiative. *Nursing Leadership, 31*(4), 36–49.

Stanley, D. (2006). Role conflict: Leaders and managers. *Nursing Management, 13*(5), 31–37.

Stefancyk, A., Hancock, B., & Meadows, M. (2013). The nurse manager change agent, change coach? *Nursing Administration Quarterly, 37*(1), 13–17.

Tuuk, E. (2012). *Transformational leadership in the coming decade: A response to three major workplace trends.* http://www.cornellhrreview.org/transformational-leadership-in-the-coming-decade-a-response-to-three-major-workplace-trends/.

Warshawsky, N. E., Rayens, M. K., Lake, S. W., & Havens, D. S. (2013). The nurse manager practice environment scale: Development and psychometric testing. *Journal of Nursing Administration, 43*(5), 250–257.

Yeager, V. A., Beitsch, L. M., & Hasbrouck, L. (2016). A mismatch between the educational pipeline and the public health workforce: Can it be reconciled? *Public Health Reports, 131*(3), 507–509.

Yeager, V. A., & Wisniewski, J. M. (2017). Factors that influence the recruitment and retention of nurses in public health agencies. *Public Health Reports, 132*(5), 556–562.

7

Legal and Ethical Issues

(Carol) Susan Johnson

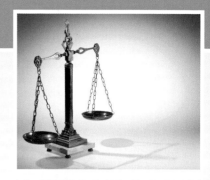

 http://evolve.elsevier.com/Huber/leadership

> *"In civilized life, law floats in a sea of ethics."*
> **Earl Warren, Chief Justice of the United States (1891–1974)**
> **(Pozgar, 2019)**

It takes a special person to consider a career in nursing. Not only is a nurse smart and technically savvy, but there is an essence of caring that simply cannot be taught. Because nursing is known as the profession of caring, society grants nursing autonomy or control over its own practice. The American Nurses Association's (ANA) *Nursing's Social Policy Statement: The Essence of the Profession* (2010, p. 25) indicates "competence is foundational to autonomy: the public has a right to expect nurses to demonstrate professional competence." The profession ensures nursing competence through professional regulation of nursing practice via standards and ethical codes of practice, legal regulation of nursing practice via state licensure requirements and law pertaining to criminal and civil wrongdoing, and self-regulation in which all nurses retain personal accountability for their own practice (American Nurses Association, 2015a).

The practice of nursing is constrained by both legal and ethical boundaries. Law and ethics are two sides of the same coin. Whether a legal mandate or an ethical obligation, the results are the same. Ethics "informs every aspect of the nurse's life" (ANA, 2015b,

p. Preface vii). It is fitting to begin this chapter by addressing how ethics is essential as nurses confront and handle legal issues.

DEFINITIONS

Ethical concepts contain a variety of specific terms requiring definition.

Ethical Terms

The four principles that form the cornerstone of biomedical ethical decision-making are the following: (1) autonomy, (2) beneficence, (3) nonmaleficence, and (4) justice.

Autonomy: The client's right of self-determination and freedom of decision-making.

Beneficence: Doing good for clients and providing benefit balanced against risk.

Nonmaleficence: Doing no harm to clients.

Justice: The norm of being fair to all and giving equal treatment, including distributing benefits, risks, and costs equally (ANA, 2015b).

Biomedical ethics also recognizes a number of rules that are related to the four fundamental ethical principles and, likewise, provide guidance in dealing with ethical dilemmas. Examples of commonly applied rules are fidelity, veracity, confidentiality, and privacy. *Fidelity* means being loyal and faithful to commitments and accountable for responsibilities. *Veracity* is the norm of

---

Photo used with permission from Photos.com.

Disclaimer: The information contained in this chapter is for educational purposes only. It is not legal advice, which can be given only by an attorney admitted to practice in the jurisdiction/state(s) in which you practice.

telling the truth and not intentionally deceiving or misleading clients. Falsification of records is an example of violating veracity in the patient record. *Confidentiality* prohibits some disclosures of some information gained in certain relationships to some third parties without the consent of the original source of the information. *Privacy* is a right of limited physical or informational inaccessibility (ANA, 2015b).

ETHICAL COMPONENTS

Nurses and nurse managers are often faced with ethical dilemmas in connection with decision-making. Ethical dilemmas require that decisions be made about what is right and wrong in situations in which an individual has to make a choice between equally unfavorable alternatives. Like other health care professionals, nurses traditionally have faced ethical dilemmas arising primarily out of clinical practice. These dilemmas have involved conflicts among principles and/or rules attributable to common morality (socially approved norms of human conduct), standards articulated in professional codes of ethics, public policies promulgated by government agencies, and the personal values of the health care professionals themselves. Ethical dilemmas faced by nurses and nurse managers also arise as clashes between the principles, rules, values, and standards of clinical/professional ethics and those of organizational/business ethics.

Although the domain of clinical ethics is the care of clients, the domain of organizational ethics is a facility's business-related activities, including, among others, marketing, admissions, transfer, discharge, billing, and the relationship of the facility and its staff members to other health care providers, educational institutions, and payers. These are activities that also directly affect the care of patients. Organizational ethics reflect a health care facility's basic values that serve as guides for proper and acceptable behavior in decision-making. Together, clinical and organizational ethics reflect a health care facility's concern that, whether related to the continuum of care or the continuum of services related to that care, ethical dilemmas should be resolved based on values-centered principles that focus on doing the right thing and taking the right action.

Professional responsibility is something each nurse must deal with every day in their practice. If an error occurs, but no one knows, is it any less an error? This is the point where ethics and legal mandates come together.

If the nurse accesses a client's record without a valid reason, but does not use the information, it is considered a Health Insurance Portability and Accountability Act (HIPAA) violation. The question is, is it wrong? Or is it wrong only if I get caught? In this author's opinion, it is fundamentally wrong, and accepting responsibility for such errors in judgment and practice are the duty of each and every nurse. "Nurses bear primary responsibility for the nursing care that their patients and clients receive and are accountable for their own practice" (ANA, 2015b, p. 15). Whether nurses are discussing distance practice, medication errors, HIPAA violations, or any other deviation from acceptable nursing practice, it is that accountability that sets nurses apart as the most trusted profession.

Code of Ethics

In addition to these basic moral principles and rules of biomedical ethics, nurses are also provided standards of conduct by professional codes of ethics. For example, the ANA's *Code of Ethics for Nurses with Interpretive Statements* (2015b) provides nonnegotiable standards as to the ethical obligations and duties of those who enter the nursing profession. The ANA indicated that the Code was developed as a guide for carrying out nursing responsibilities to be consistent with quality in nursing care and the ethical obligations of the profession. The focus is not on giving precise answers to specific ethical problems, but rather on providing general guidance as to how to act when faced with ethical dilemmas.

Ethical Decisions

Many of the decisions nurses and nurse managers make on a daily basis have an ethical component and may involve conflicts among ethical responsibilities. These conflicts may involve clashes between the following:

- Two ethical duties to the client (e.g., duty to respect autonomy and duty to benefit the client);
- The client's rights and benefits (e.g., withholding or withdrawing treatment in respect for a client's right to die by forgoing treatment at any time, and treating or continuing treatment that is expected to produce better results for the client);
- Duties to self and duties to the client (e.g., a nurse's desire to remain on the same shift because of parental responsibilities, and the need to advocate for better treatment of the clients by some health care practitioners on that shift);

• Professional ethical provisions and religious ones (e.g., a professional code requiring the recognition of the client's right to self-determination and a nurse's religious beliefs prohibiting abortion).

When ethical dilemmas are encountered in dealing with clinical matters, health care professionals commonly refer to various principles, rules, and standards for guidance in making moral decisions. Principles and rules are normative generalizations that provide guidance in ethical decision-making. Although rules are more specific in content and restricted in scope than principles, neither can fully guide action but instead must be complemented by judgment for a decision to be made (ANA, 2015b, p. 15). Many organizations employ an ethicist and have ethics committees that operate to provide a source of support and guidance for ethical dilemmas faced by nurses in organizations.

All nurses, regardless of position, must apply ethics in their daily practice using the Provisions of the *ANA Code of Ethics for Nurses with Interpretive Statements* (2015b). These Provisions include:

1. Practicing with compassion and respect for every person's worth, dignity, and unique attributes;
2. Demonstrating a primary commitment to the patient;
3. Protecting the patient's rights, health and safety;
4. Making decisions and acting to promote health and provide optimal care;
5. Maintaining own health and safety, integrity, competence, and personal and professional growth;
6. Improving the ethical environment at work and employment conditions conducive to safe, quality health care;
7. Advancing the profession through scholarly inquiry, development of professional standards, and creating nursing and health policy;
8. Collaborating with others to reduce health disparities, protect human rights, and promote health globally;
9. Engaging in professional organizations to communicate nursing values and ethics that promote health and social justice (ANA, 2015b).

Another issue with ethical, as well as legal, implications is bullying within the nursing profession. Incivility and bullying are common in workplace settings. According to the American Nurses Association, incivility is "one or more rude, discourteous, or disrespectful actions that may or may not have a negative intent behind them," whereas bullying is defined as "repeated, unwanted, harmful actions intended to humiliate, offend, and cause distress in the recipient" (American Nurses Association, 2019). Either of these actions are unacceptable and adversely impact the ability of the nurse to care for patients and self. Such actions violate the fifth Provision of the *ANA Code of Ethics for Nurses with Interpretive Statements* (2015b) and result in moral distress and threats to personal integrity. It is essential that such behavior be promptly and thoroughly addressed. Incivility and bullying have no place in any health care facility, and everyone is responsible for ensuring a safe work environment.

LEGAL PERSPECTIVES

Unlike scientific facts, with black and white boundaries, the law provides guidance, mandates, and parameters for lawful practice, and the facts are ever-changing. For example, when nurses see a blood culture result, the result can be placed on a finite range of acceptable norms. However, when examining legal requirements, there may be shades of gray.

No one can practice as a nurse without meeting the legal requirements of the state(s) of licensure. When embarking on a nursing career—or if the nurse has been licensed for some number of years—it is critical that the state board of nursing websites be checked regularly for practice alerts and new laws, as well as legal and regulatory changes for all state(s) in which the nurse practices. A complete list of all state boards of nursing can be found at https://www.allnursingschools.com/how-to-become-a-nurse/state-boards/. Although foundational nursing theory is time honored, it is critical in today's fast-moving digital world that nurses take responsibility for their own knowledge and stay current. The nursing license is a privilege, not a right, which the nurse is given by meeting the licensing requirements throughout their career.

Some laws are designed to protect the nurse, and other laws are there to protect the public from errors or wrong practices done by the nurse. As health professionals, nurses have a duty to perform their practice consistent with all relevant laws, scopes of practice, standards of practice, and codes of ethics consistent with the nurse's education and experience. The concept of title protection, which pertains to who can call themselves "nurse," is designed to provide the public with safe, effective nurses who can be relied on to practice to the current standard of care. By establishing minimum mandatory standards, complemented by specialty certifications and mandatory continuing education, the public can depend on nurses regardless of location or facility where practice occurs. It is imperative that nurses acquire and maintain nursing practice skills and competencies. Patient outcomes rely on competent professional practice.

LEGAL DEFINITIONS

Legal concepts contain a variety of specific terms requiring definition.

Legal Terms

Cross-examination: The opportunity for the attorney to ask questions in court of a witness who has testified in a trial on behalf of the opposing party. The questions on cross-examination are limited to the subjects covered in the direct examination of the witness, but it is important to note that the attorney may ask leading questions, in which he or she is allowed to suggest answers or put words in the witness's mouth (Hill & Hill, 2019). These questions are usually answered with "yes" or "no."

Damages: The amount of money that a plaintiff (the person suing) may be awarded in a lawsuit. There are many types of damages. Special damages are those that were actually caused by the injury and include medical and hospital bills, ambulance charges, loss of wages, property repair or replacement costs, or loss of money due on a contract. The second basic area of damages is general damages, which are presumed to be a result of the other party's actions, but are subjective both in nature and determination of the value of the damages. These include pain and suffering, future problems and crippling effect of an injury, loss of ability to perform various acts, shortening of lifespan, mental anguish, and loss of companionship.

Deposition: The taking and recording of the testimony of a witness under oath before a court reporter in a place away from the courtroom before trial. A deposition is part of permitted pretrial discovery (investigation) set up by an attorney for one of the parties to a lawsuit demanding the sworn testimony of the opposing party (defendant or plaintiff), a witness to an event, or an expert intended to be called at trial by the opposition.

Direct examination: The first questioning of a witness during a trial or deposition (testimony out of court), as distinguished from cross-examination by opposing attorneys, and redirect examination when the witness is again questioned by the original attorney. Questions on direct examination cannot be answered with "yes" or "no."

Expert testimony: Opinions stated during trial or deposition (testimony under oath before trial) by a specialist qualified as an expert on a subject relevant to a lawsuit or a criminal case.

Expert witness: A person who is a specialist in a subject, often technical, who may present their expert opinion without having been a witness to any occurrence relating to the lawsuit or criminal case. This is an exception to the rule against giving an opinion in trial, provided that the expert is qualified by evidence of their expertise, training, and special knowledge. If the expertise is challenged, then the attorney for the party calling the expert must make a showing of the necessary background through questions in court, and the trial judge has discretion to qualify the witness or rule that they are not an expert or are an expert on limited subjects.

Fact witness: A lay witness who has firsthand knowledge of certain facts, having made observations, and can testify to material facts.

Lay witness: A witness who is not an expert witness.

Liable: Responsible or obligated. Thus, a person or entity may be liable for damages due to negligence.

Material fact: A fact upon which all or part of the outcome of a lawsuit depends.

Malpractice: See *professional negligence*.

Negligence: Failure to exercise the care toward others that a reasonable or prudent person would do in the circumstances, or taking action that such a reasonable person would not.

Profession: "Any type of work that needs special training or a particular skill, often one that is respected because it involves a high level of education" (Cambridge Dictionary, 2020a).

Professional judgment: "The application of professional knowledge and experience in defining objectives, solving problems, establishing guidelines, reviewing the work of others, interpreting results and providing and assessing advice or recommendations and other matters which have an element of latitude or decision-making" (Law Insider, 2019).

Professional negligence: An act or continuing conduct of a professional that does not meet the standard of professional competence and results in provable damages to their client or patient. Such an error or omission

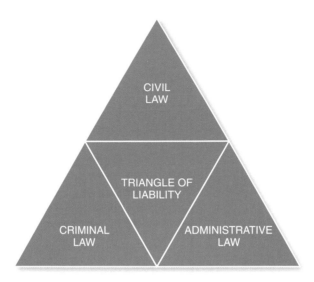

Fig. 7.1 Triangle of liability. From DePietro, S. C. (2016). *Legal and ethical issues in nursing professional development.* In C. M. Smith, & M. G. Harper (Eds.), Leadership in nursing professional development: An organizational & system focus (pp. 78–109). Chicago, IL: Association for Nursing Professional Development (ANPD).

may be through negligence, ignorance (when the professional should have known), or intentional wrongdoing. However, malpractice does not include the exercise of professional judgment even when the results are detrimental to the client or patient.

Types of Law

Administrative and Regulatory Law: These are **regulations** and rules that are created and enforced by federal and state agencies. Regulations about the workplace environment by the Occupational Safety and Health Administration (OSHA) and rules promulgated by the state board of nursing are examples.

Case Law: These are established by courts. **Case** law includes common law and the interpretation of statutes, including civil and criminal laws.

Statutory Law: These are laws passed by **legislative** bodies.

- **Civil:** Private law dealing with lawsuits between private individuals or parties.
- **Criminal:** Public law based on **statute** (enacted by federal or state legislatures) or **common law** (results from rules decided by the judiciary in court cases and referred to as a precedent set by a court), which consists of federal or state laws that make specific behaviors illegal (De Pietro, 2016).

Fig. 7.1 depicts the triangle of legal liability that displays the junctions of responsibility and accountability for health care professionals.

BACKGROUND

State Law and Nursing: Education and Licensure

Part of the way that a profession improves itself is to review its educational requirements and update as appropriate. More than ever, today's nurse is well-educated, because many states and territories are moving toward a minimum educational level of a bachelor's degree in nursing (BSN) for new nurses entering into the profession (NursingLicensure.org, 2019). This trend has been accelerated by *The Future of Nursing,* a report of the Institute of Medicine (IOM, now called the National Academies of Sciences, Engineering, and Medicine, Health and Medicine Division) (IOM, 2011) and its 80% BSN by 2020 challenge. New York was one of the first states to propose "BSN in 10," a concept that would require all nurses with an associate degree in applied sciences/nursing (AAS) or 3-year diploma from a hospital nursing program to obtain a BSN by their 10th year of licensure. Many hospitals, particularly those with the Magnet Recognition Program (R) designation, have established policies that reflect this model, even though states have not yet enacted such laws. Although the National Council of State Boards of Nursing's Licensure Examination (NCLEX) is a national standard, it is also a minimum national standard and may be only one element of the legal requirements for licensure in a state or territory. In addition, advanced practice is another area where state law defines the requirements, both educationally and clinically, for who may practice with a state-issued certification and/or supplemental license (laws and regulations vary by state), especially for nurse practitioners (Advanced Practice Registered Nurses [APRNs]).

"APRNs include certified registered nurse anesthetists, certified nurse-midwives, clinical nurse specialists and certified nurse practitioners. Each has a unique history and context but shares the commonality of being APRNs. While education, accreditation, and certification are necessary components of an overall approach to preparing an APRN for practice, the licensing boards—governed by state regulations and statutes—are the final arbiters of whom is recognized to practice within a given state. Currently, there is no uniform model of regulation of APRNs across the states. Each state independently determines the APRN legal scope of practice, the roles that are recognized, the criteria for entry into advanced practice, and the certification examinations accepted for entry-level competence assessment. This has created a significant barrier for APRNs to easily move from state to state and has decreased access to care for patients"

(APRN Joint Dialogue Group Report, 2008, p. 5).

In each state the nurse practice act, administered by the state board of nursing, is the singular authoritative source to identify the educational, clinical, continuing education, fees, and all other requirements to satisfy the state's licensure requirements.

Administrative Law and State Boards of Nursing

The most well-known administrative laws are regulations that set the minimum standards for a licensed practitioner. These regulations are enforced by the state licensing board for that profession. The scope of practice for nurses is defined by the state and enforced by the state board of nursing. APRNs may be regulated by a separate practice act, or their scope of practice may be included in the state nurse practice act for registered nurses (RNs). Although regulations and state boards of nursing vary by state, the board of nursing can initiate disciplinary actions against nurses in any level of practice for the following:

1. Incompetence or failure to use knowledge, care, skill, and experience of a competent nurse;
2. Gross negligence or departure from standard of care;
3. Unprofessional conduct involving felony conviction, practicing medicine without a license, or possessing or using controlled or illegal drugs; and
4. Crimes such as theft, assault, abuse, fraud, or sexual offenses (De Pietro, 2016).

Disciplinary actions may include probation, suspension, or revocation of the nurse's license.

THE LEGAL SYSTEM AND SOURCES OF LAW

Nurses, nurse managers, and health care facilities are all subject to being found **legally liable** (i.e., legally responsible) for harm caused to others by civil wrongs. More specifically, liability is created when the law imposes a civil obligation on a wrongdoer to compensate an injured party for the consequences of a wrongful act. As shown in Fig. 7.2, there are two sources of legal liability: torts and contracts (Pozgar, 2019).

The most common source of legal liability for nurses and nurse managers is a *tort*. A tort is a wrongful act (other than breach of contract) committed against another person or organization or their property that causes harm and can be remedied by a civil (rather than criminal) lawsuit. Intentional torts are common civil lawsuits and include assault, battery, false imprisonment, property conversion, trespassing, and intentional infliction of emotional distress. In a health care setting, examples of an intentional tort are fear or apprehension of being touched in an offensive manner (assault) or the actual touching of someone without their consent (battery). Nurses should obtain consent before

LEGAL LIABILITY
A civil obligation imposed by law on a wrongdoer requiring compensation of an injured party through money damages or some other legal remedy for the consequences of a wrongful act

"JUDICIAL RISK" FILTER
Various aspects of the litigation process that can introduce further uncertainty and additional cost into the determination of legal liability
- Witnesses' perceptions of the facts can change over time
- Courtroom conditions can influence the jury

TORTS
Tort—a wrongful act (other than a breach of contract) committed by one person that causes harm to another by invading a legally protected right
- **Personal (Direct) Liability**—liability imposed on the person who committed the wrongful act
- **Vicarious Liability**—a person or organization that has not behaved wrongfully can be held legally liable for torts committed by others

CONTRACTS
- **Breach of Contract**—if a party to a contract does not perform as promised, the other party can sue for money damages or seek the remedy of specific performance
- **Hold Harmless or Indemnity Agreements**—one party assumes the liability of another party for damage in situations in which the first party would not otherwise be liable

Types of Torts

Negligence
- An unintentional tort
- Negligence—failure of a person to exercise the degree of care that an ordinary prudent person would have exercised under similar circumstances
- Malpractice—failure of a professional person to act as other prudent professionals with the same knowledge and education would have acted under similar circumstances

Intentional Torts
- A wrongful act that was intended to cause harm

- Examples
  - Assault and battery
  - False imprisonment
  - Defamation—libel and slander
  - Invasion of right of privacy
  - Fraud
  - Intentional torts against property (trespass, conversion)

Strict Liability Torts
- Tort liability imposed when the defendant acted neither negligently nor with intent to cause harm

- May be applied in cases involving dangerously defective roducts—medical devices, use of unlicensed medicines

Fig. 7.2 Sources of legal liability.

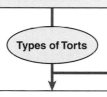

initiating physical contact with clients (De Pietro, 2016). False imprisonment is seen when clients want to leave against medical advice or when they are restrained. An adult who has the capacity to make health care decisions and wants to leave the premises cannot be required to remain. The client must be informed about the consequences of this action, and organizational policies must be followed to address this issue. Nurses must also understand and follow their state's laws regarding clients restrained for psychiatric reasons (prevention of self-harm or harm to others) as these laws vary from state to state (De Pietro, 2016). Although torts most commonly give rise to *personal* (or *direct*) liability for the person committing the wrongful act, in some cases another person or organization may also be held *vicariously* liable for the same wrongful act they did not commit. For example, when a nurse commits a tort, the nurse may be found to be directly liable and the nurse's employer also may be found to be vicariously liable for the nurse's wrongful action (Pozgar, 2019).

As indicated in Fig. 7.2, determination of legal liability as a result of a tort depends on more than just the various technical elements of the tort that must be proved by the injured party (plaintiff), the presentation of various available defenses by the defendant, and the formal rules of the judicial system regarding the litigation process. In the case of torts, the legal outcomes are often influenced also by what may be termed *judicial risk*. This refers to various aspects of the litigation process that can introduce further uncertainty and additional cost into the determination of legal liability. Judicial risk can result in findings with respect to legal liability that are not based solely on the merits of the case nor on the rules of law applicable to the case (Pozgar, 2019).

What we refer to as the legal system is a multifaceted structure of federal, state, and local laws. In addition, there are regulations, which are rules that have full force and effect of law. In other words, in addition to statutes, there is a whole structure of rules created through an enabling statute. Such statutes give authority to an agency, such as the state board of nursing. There are two major divisions in the structure of the law: civil law and criminal law.

Civil Law

There are different standards by which defendants are judged in civil litigation: simple or regular negligence and professional negligence or *malpractice*.

Tort

A tort is a civil or personal wrong, compared with a crime, which is a public wrong. The purpose of tort law is to adjust losses by compensating one person because of the actions of another. Therefore the only remedy available in a civil lawsuit based on tort is monetary damages (i.e., money). Each intentional tort represents a direct interference with a person's physical integrity or right to property. Personal freedom is a fundamental right. One does not waive a fundamental right, such as personal integrity, automatically. On the contrary, a person must be aware that they possess a particular right and can intentionally relinquish it. This is the basis for the concept of informed consent.

Informed consent is a good example of a knowing and voluntary waiver of rights in the medical setting. In the absence of such a waiver of rights, a person touching or keeping another in a clinic, hospital, or any place they choose not to be, may be liable for assault, battery, or false imprisonment. Informed consent is a statutorily created right given to potential recipients of medical treatment. Most state statutes express that it is the duty of the physician to fully inform the patient as to the risks and benefits of a proposed procedure. The physician must also advise the patient of alternative treatments, if any, as well as the option to refuse any treatment. For the patient to be fully informed, the physician must advise the patient of all the potential risks and benefits of each option, including refusing the proposed treatment. Unless there is a specific statute, such as in the case of some APRNs, the physician's duty of informed consent is never transferred or delegated to a nurse.

Intentional torts are deliberate invasions of a person's legal rights and include assault, battery, false imprisonment, and trespassing. Unintentional torts result from negligence. These terms are often confused because they also exist within criminal law. Examples of an intentional tort in health care are forcing unwanted medical care on a patient or holding someone against their will.

Negligence. For a civil lawsuit to be successful in negligence, there are four required elements. These elements are commonly referred to as duty, breach, cause, and harm. All four of the elements must be proven, and the burden of proof is on the plaintiff (the one who brings the complaint). The plaintiff must prove that there was a well-established duty and an obvious breach of such duty. These proofs are not sufficient without also establishing the causal connection to the harm claimed. Proof of damages (harm) is an essential element to a negligence case. Negligence is sometimes referred to as simple negligence, compared with malpractice or professional negligence. This standard is used in cases such as motor vehicle accidents, personal injury (outside the medical setting), and property damage. The *standard of proof* for a simple or regular negligence case is that of a reasonably prudent person.

The concept of negligence is based on the idea that there can be a generally uniform standard of human behavior. The simplest example of this is that when one drives a car, there is a generally accepted expectation that each person will operate the vehicle in a reasonably prudent and careful manner. Each time there is a motor vehicle accident, it is likely that one or more persons deviated from the reasonably prudent person's standard, and liability may attach. However, state statutes may limit or expand a person's ability to bring a cause of action via a lawsuit (De Pietro, 2016).

Professional Negligence (Malpractice). The standard by which a licensed professional nurse (RN) will be judged comes from a governmental standard. The nurse's licensure and scope of practice are derived from the state's nurse practice act. All states and also US territories (Puerto Rico and Guam), have a nurse practice act. Links to all state boards of nursing and those states' nurse practice acts, can be found on individual state board of nursing websites or through the National Council of State Boards of Nursing (NCSBN, 2020a). Nurse practice acts provide broad statements defining nursing practice, delineating the educational and other requirements for licensure and renewal, giving notice to the public of the sort of behavior that can be expected from a nurse, and identifying what unacceptable practices might subject a nurse to disciplinary review or sanctions.

Professions develop a standard for themselves through a complex process of discussion and interaction within the profession and with other professions; knowledge dissemination such as peer reviewed professional journals; meetings; development of standards, guidelines, and statements; networking with colleagues; and the development and refining of academic programs both at the undergraduate and graduate levels for the profession. In addition, each profession has an obligation to monitor its members and self-police the behavior of its own.

For more than 17 years, nursing has been recognized by the general public in a Gallup poll as a highly esteemed profession for ethics and honesty (Brenan, 2018). Nurses have the respect and admiration of the American people and were acknowledged as the most trusted profession. Nurses should take great pride in this recognition. However, it also reminds nurses that they are always being watched by the public and are expected to conduct themselves in a professional, ethical, and truthful manner. Such accolades could easily be lost.

Professional Safeguards

Civil law controls those circumstances when an individual, the plaintiff, feels that he or she has been harmed by another. If the other person, known as the defendant, is a professional, the law provides for *professional liability,* also known as *malpractice.* Professionals are provided with many safeguards to avoid them being wrongfully accused of malpractice. Some of these safeguards include:

Statute of Limitations. A statutory time limit (most commonly 2 years) by which a plaintiff must file a lawsuit against a professional or lose that opportunity forever. In many states, there are exceptions to the time limitation for infants (children under a prescribed statutory age at the time of the alleged event) and an extension of time if the plaintiff was unaware of the injury at the time. One example is if a surgical count was incorrect at the completion of a procedure, an instrument or other substance was left in the patient's abdominal cavity in error, and the nurses "signed off" on the count. The patient is discharged, goes home, and does not have any symptoms or problems for 30 months, at which time it is discovered that the item has encapsulated, become infected, and the patient now requires additional surgery and/or suffers some other harm, even death. It is possible that a lawsuit could be filed as late as 2 years after the discovery of the indwelling item. The standard basis to file a professional liability/malpractice lawsuit is the time when the patient knew or should have known.

Affidavit of Merit. Another safeguard to protect the professional is the requirement of an affidavit of merit. An affidavit of merit is a sworn document by a like kind of professional (a doctor for a doctor defendant and a nurse for a nurse defendant) who reviews the injured patient's chart, and based upon the reviewer's education and experience, makes a statement that the case has merit and should be permitted to go to trial. Their opinion will also include that there is a likelihood of the plaintiff's success at trial. The person who reviews the record and provides the affidavit may never testify or have any other contact with the case.

Sources of Law. Laws are found in case books and online in official reports and legal research services. A reported case is one that can be found in an official reporter. There are state and also federal reporters. When entered into a reporter, the case is printed and becomes part of the ever-growing body of case law. It is important to remember that what is heard on the news, no matter the source, is simply news (maybe entertainment) and is not admissible as evidence at trial (De Pietro, 2016). Official sources of law need to be consulted and used when drawing conclusions.

Under both federal and state rules of evidence, the only way to prove professional negligence is through the use of expert witnesses. Expert witnesses need to be knowledgeable and up to date in their fields and familiar with texts, journals, and the relevant accepted standards of practice. These individuals are often published authors, leaders in the field, or academics.

The Nurse as Witness

There are times when a nurse is called on to testify at a deposition or appear to testify in court. The nurse may have been present in the hospital, clinic, or office setting where they made certain observations. This does not mean necessarily that the nurse is a party to the case; the nurse may not be a defendant. There are two general categories of witnesses who testify at trial: the fact witness and the expert witness.

A **fact witness** is someone who can testify from their own observations. In other words, the nurse can apply their senses to a fact or set of circumstances (e.g., I saw…, I heard…, I smelled…). For example, the nurse might have observed a patient fall in a hospital hallway, but it was not their patient; the person was with another staff member, but the nurse saw the fall. That nurse could testify as a fact witness (sometimes referred to as an eyewitness) to those events that were seen, heard, or felt. A fact witness may not offer an opinion, but must testify only as to personal knowledge.

An **expert witness** is a person with specialized knowledge who aids the judge and jury (in the case of a jury trial) to understand something that is beyond the scope of the average individual. There are multiple standards in determining whether one can be considered

an expert witness. Experts base their opinions and their testimony on their knowledge, education, and experience. State and federal rules of evidence require that a patient claiming that a professional is responsible for their injuries and damages use a "like-kind" expert witness to prove their case (Federal Rules of Evidence 703,704; Legal Information Institute, 2020).

A professional liability case cannot be proven without an expert witness who can testify as to actions or inactions of the professional defendant. Simply put, only a nurse can testify as to the standard of care and scope of practice of another nurse. If the nurse works in a specialty area such as professional case management, the operating room, or the emergency department (ED), a like-kind nurse should be the one to testify as an expert for that particular nurse defendant.

There are typically two experts: one for the plaintiff and one for the defendant nurse. An expert witness is only as good as their education and experience in two critical ways: first by establishing and maintaining credibility by having expertise in the required field, and second by withstanding cross-examination by the plaintiff's attorney. The fastest way to be excluded as an expert witness is to "step outside your sandbox." Any document, text, or other material that an expert refers to in their written report and/or testimony must be available, and in most cases, is admissible into evidence.

It is important to note that if the expert refers to such a document, they must be fully familiar with the entire document. It would be appropriate cross-examination for the nurse to be asked about something in the text or other reference that has nothing to do with the present case and that the expert made no reference to; it goes to the expert's credibility. In other words, did the expert simply "cherry pick" a small portion of a reference that related to the facts, or is that expert fully familiar with the foundational materials? In recent years, some states have permitted professionals whose practice area overlaps with the defendants to testify, although other states interpret the "like-kind" expert strictly. The attorney who seeks a nurse's assistance as an expert should be fully familiar with the criteria in the jurisdiction. However, even those experts who are experienced in courtroom testimony can be enticed to step outside their area of expertise. The next thing that happens is that there is an objection to the witness and their testimony in whole or in part, the expert's credibility is ruined, and an otherwise solid case begins to crumble (De Pietro, 2016).

Criminal Law

Criminal law is based on statutes. Statutes are laws created by the legislature and signed into law by the executive, the governor for state laws, and the president of the United States for federal laws.

Crimes are prohibitions against behaviors that are so egregious that they offend society, not just the individual victim. Crimes are punishable with fines and/or jail, depending on the level of the offense and other factors, and these consequences are delineated in the criminal statute. Nurses can be subject to criminal law for such behaviors as stealing or misusing narcotics, practicing without a license, or intentionally causing physical harm to a person in their care. These criminal offenses violate the public trust and safety and carry serious consequences.

LICENSURE, MULTI-STATE, AND DISTANCE PRACTICE

There is no doubt that the world in which nurses' practice today has been dramatically and forever affected by advances in technology. Gone are the days when the only interaction between nurse and patient was at arm's length. Today, with the advent of electronic health records (EHR), telephonic, e-mail, text, and video connections, nurses and patients can interact from across town or across the country. Distance communications need to be considered with great caution: just because we can, does not mean we should. The law is slow to catch up with technical advances. Although there has been much talk about cost-effective interventions through electronic means, the nurse must adhere to the law. As it stands today, nurses must be licensed in each and every state/jurisdiction in which they practice.

> *"Uniform Licensure Requirements (ULRs) are the essential prerequisites for initial, endorsement, renewal and reinstatement licensure needed across every NCSBN jurisdiction to ensure the safe and competent practice of nursing. ULRs protect the public by setting consistent standards and promoting a health care system that is fluid and accessible by removing barriers to care and maximizing portability for nurses. They also assure the consumer that a nurse in one state has met the requirements of the nurses in every other state. ULRs support the fact that the expectations for the education of*

> *a nurse and the responsibilities of a nurse are the same throughout every NCSBN member board jurisdiction in the United States."*
>
> **(NCSBN, 2019)**

The Nurse Licensure Compact (NLC) allows nurses to have one multistate license, with the ability to practice in both their home state and other compact states. There are currently 34 states in the NLC (NCSBN, 2020b). In 2015 significant revisions were made to the NLC Model Act, requiring all legislatures to revisit the issue. Revisions were made, in part, in response to objections from some states, and it is hoped that the NLC will grow significantly in the coming years to make it easier for nurses to work across state lines. If a nurse lives or works near another state's border, it is often tempting, and may be requested, that the nurse speak telephonically or go in person to deliver care to persons in the neighboring state. Thus it is imperative that nurses be licensed in each state in which they deliver care; otherwise care can only be legally delivered to patients in the state in which the nurse is licensed.

Distance practice is nothing new, but the tools and technologies available today make distance practice far easier and are predicted to become more common. Telehealth, telemedicine, and case management practice are examples where distance practice occurs. There is a two-pronged test to determine if a distance communication is permitted, whether by telephonic, e-mail, or another electronic device. The first test is that the nurse must examine the content of the communication, and the second test is whether that communication constitutes the practice of nursing.

Example #1: Nursing process begins with assessment. Assessment is a "systematic, dynamic way to collect and analyze data about a client, the first step in delivering nursing care. Assessment includes not only physiological data, but also psychological, sociocultural, spiritual, economic, and life-style factors as well" (ANA, 2020). Assessment can start with a simple telephone call, "Good morning. How are you?" If the nurse asks that simple question, "How are you?" and the patient responds with symptoms, then the nurse, based on their knowledge and experience, uses critical thinking, makes professional judgments, and takes action. That is the practice of nursing. To conduct such a dialogue across state lines, the nurse must be licensed in the state where the patient is located. Therefore in this example the nursing process has been established, and licensure is necessary.

Example #2: The caller contacts the patient and says, "Good morning, I'm calling to follow up and remind you of your appointment with Dr. Smith. I've arranged for transportation; the car will pick you up tomorrow morning. Is that ok? Is there anything else I can do for you?" No assessment occurred, no nursing process was initiated, and no nursing skill, based on education and training, was required to conduct this communication. Anyone with minimal training (such as a high school graduate) could perform this task. Review of Chapter 6 on role management will be helpful and provide parameters for appropriate task delegation.

LEGAL DOCUMENTS AND THE NURSE

It is important for the nurse to have a working knowledge of certain legal documents that affect practice. It is not uncommon for the nurse to encounter powers of attorney or advance directives for health care (also referred to as living wills or powers of attorney for health care, depending on the jurisdiction). Patients are asked before admission whether they have a living will or similar document, but what happens to that document varies greatly from facility to facility, even in the same state. The most important thing that the nurse must take away from a discussion of legal documents is that the nurse must actually see the document. It is not enough for an individual to say, "I am the health care representative/proxy" or "I'm the power of attorney," which is simply a misuse of the term.

Power of attorney is the document used for the appointment of another person, referred to as the principal, and empowers that person (the attorney-in-fact or agent) to act on behalf of the principal. In other words, by way of a legal document, one person gives authority to another to act and perform certain functions on behalf of that person. The power of attorney is a document, a writing, prescribed by state law, which can grant very limited or very broad powers to the attorney-in-fact (the agent). It is common to hear people say, "I have power of attorney." That may be a true statement if there is a document that assigns such a power, but it is actually incorrect to say, "I am the power of attorney." Misusing these terms overextends or improperly limits the authority of the attorney-in-fact.

Confusion regarding these terms often stems from those states that permit the use of the term "power of attorney" to extend to health care proxies and directives, commonly called living wills. New York, Michigan, and California are among the states that use a durable power of attorney for health care as the legal document for use as a living will. Other states, like New Jersey, use an advanced directive for health care (*The New Jersey Advance Directives for Health Care Act*, NJ. Stat. §. 26:2H-53–78). No matter what "power" an individual is asserting, without actually seeing the document (or a facsimile thereof where permitted), the nurse may risk a Health Information Portability and *Accountability Act of 1996* (HIPAA) violation or other liability exposure by disclosing information to one who is not entitled to such access (De Pietro, 2016; Pozgar, 2019).

Guardianship

Parents are the guardians of their children until the child reaches the age of majority in the particular state. Typically, this is at 18 years of age, but there are exceptions. Certain states have greatly reduced the age of consent, particularly in the medical setting. It is important to understand the purpose of the rule of law and the requirements in the state(s) in which the nurse practices.

A *guardian* is a person appointed by a court via a judge. In the normal course of events, a parent is the guardian of their child, but all that changes on the child's eighteenth birthday. There are many types of guardians. A *general guardian* is appointed if the court finds that an individual is incapacitated, according to that state's legal definition of incapacity, to govern or manage their affairs. The general guardian exercises all rights and powers of the incapacitated person concerning both the rights of the person and their financial assets, income, and responsibilities (NJ. Stat. §3B:12—24.1). The nurse must pause when any person represents to the nurse, the hospital, or the agency that they are the guardian of a person or custodian of that person's affairs. They *must* provide you with a copy of the specific court order naming them as the guardian over a named person, with any limitations to that guardianship.

Guardian ad litem is a temporary appointment of a person by a court to act on behalf of another for a specific purpose. Typically it is an adult who will take legal action on behalf of a minor child or an adult who is unable to handle their own affairs, even when represented by an attorney. For example, the *guardian ad litem* may file a lawsuit for a child who is injured in an automobile accident or by some other means. *Guardian ad litem* may also be appointed following the death of a person in order to file claim against an estate on behalf of a child or incompetent adult (Phillips & Walsh, 2018).

The Problem of the Adult Child

When a child reaches the age of majority—18 years in most jurisdictions—the parent no longer has access to medical records, nor do parents have the right to make medical decisions for their children. It is difficult for a devoted loving parent to simply stop, when yesterday the privilege and burden of making medical decisions for their child(ren) fell to them, and then the next day, on the eighteenth birthday, this stopped. The problem is further magnified when the child has a disability and special needs. The nurse is in a unique position to have insight and understanding into the child's (now a young adult) needs. In cases where the young adult is not competent to make their own medical decisions, guardianship may be a viable option. In most states, this is a complex procedure requiring an attorney's advice and at least one court appearance.

For a child who is unable to communicate but has the mental capacity to make their own choices, the legal documents described in this chapter are useful tools. It is the nurse's legal and ethical duty to protect the adult "child's" autonomy and not simply accept a parent's intervention, without lawful authority, just because it may seem easier at the moment. Along with incredible advances in prosthetics, electronic aids, and assistive devices, children and adults who were once unable to function in schools, universities, and the workforce are now able to. Thus the limits are being tested with regard to individual autonomy.

Confidentiality and Access to Medical Information

Patient confidentiality has been a central theme to medical and nursing practice for generations, but the rules governing access and release of medical records were solidified about 25 years ago with the advent of HIPAA (Public Law 104–191). Even though HIPAA is federal law and preempts state law, there is great variation from state to state. HIPAA is a minimum mandatory standard. States are permitted to provide additional protections to their residents, but no law can limit or reduce a right provided under federal law. An interactive map is available at: https://medcitynews.com/2017/06/nced-interactive-map-understand-disparity-healthcare-data-sharing-u-s/ and provides a state-by-state comparison.

Iowa, Alabama, and New Hampshire are examples of states whose law was preempted by HIPAA and provides no additional access or rights. California, Colorado, New York, and Nevada provide greater access and protection; they require release of medical records to those who properly make requests in a specific number of days, even though providers are permitted to charge reasonable fees for accessing and copying records (Zaleski, 2017). One of the goals of EHRs was to make provision of medical records to patients who request them easier to access, faster and less expensive to copy, and more accessible to patients (Pozgar, 2019). See the Research Note (Ben-Assuli, 2015) and De Simone (2019) for a discussion of electronic records as important legal documents.

Demonstrating Compliance

Legal compliance is demonstrated by holding and maintaining a professional license in each and every jurisdiction in which the nurse practices, whether in person, telephonically, or through other means of electronic communication. The nurse must maintain up-to-date knowledge through continuing education as mandated by the state(s) of licensure and adhere to all applicable laws and regulations.

Adhering to all applicable federal, state, and local laws and employer policies, is the general principle of necessary compliance, but there is a hierarchy to these duties. Federal law *preempts* state law. Law will always supersede hospital or other employer policies and procedures. Legal compliance is broader than simply following the rules for correct drug dosage, route, and observations of the patient; it starts with patient assessment and goes through full discharge of duties at the standard of care of a reasonable and prudent nurse.

Regulatory Compliance

Regulations are rules that have the same effect as laws. They are created based on a statute, giving authority to an agency or the director of an agency, to create regulations to further the purpose of the enabling statute. HIPAA has now been a part of health care and health care practice for about 25 years. Protecting health information is the core of the law and all the regulations that followed. Nurses need to be familiar with who the privacy officer is in whatever entity they work and use resources to educate and reeducate themselves with the requirements in their state.

The HIPAA Privacy Rule was published on December 28, 2000, with the goal of providing consumers with greater rights for protection of individually identifiable health information, sometimes referred to as personal health information (PHI). In the spring of 2003, there were further modifications to the Final Privacy Rule. The key to HIPAA, and all the changes and improvements over time, is meeting the educational requirement (at minimum, a yearly update) and demonstrating genuine compliance. The Privacy Rule is only part of HIPAA compliance requirements. There are complex regulations controlling the use of electronic communications, including telephone, fax, e-mail, and text messaging, as well as, billing and reporting requirements (Pozgar, 2019).

HIPAA responsibilities come to us as building blocks. The patient privacy rules and access to medical records do not go away when a new responsibility is added. Each new aspect, addition or modification of the law requires that each practitioner have not only a basic understanding of HIPAA (1996), but an ever-enlarging knowledge base regarding HIPAA, the *Health Information Technology for Economic and Clinical Health (HITECH) Act*, which is a portion of the *American Recovery and Reinvestment Act of 2009 (ARRA) 26 USC 1* and the Final Omnibus Rule (2013), and subtle changes that continue to be made. In January 2016, the HIPAA restriction on the disclosure of PHI was modified by agency amendment. "The Department of Health and Human Services issued a final rule expressly permitting certain HIPAA covered entities to provide to the [National Instant Criminal Background Check System] NICS limited demographic and other necessary information about these individuals" (Obama, 2016, p. 1). It is important to obtain and update knowledge of all HIPAA and state privacy and confidentiality mandates.

The Personal Representative

The Department of Health and Human Services (HHS, 2020, p. 1) "recognizes that there may be times when individuals are legally or otherwise incapable of exercising their rights, or simply choose to designate another to act on their behalf with respect to these rights. Under the Rule, a person authorized (under State or other applicable law, e.g., tribal or military law) to act on behalf of the individual in making health care related decisions is the individual's 'personal representative.' Section 164.502(g) provides when, and to what extent, the personal representative must be treated as the individual for purposes of the Rule. In addition to these formal designations of a personal representative, the Rule at 45 CFR 164.510(b) addresses situations in which family members or other persons who are involved in the individual's health care or payment for care may receive protected health information about the individual even if they are not expressly authorized to act on the individual's behalf."

Incident Reports

Incident-reporting systems are set up as a way to report errors, especially safety errors. They are used to gather data and information about patient safety occurrences for organizational learning. There are three types of incidents: a harmful incident, a no-harm incident, and a near miss. Incident-reporting systems are part of risk-management efforts and are voluntary but set an expectation for reporting. Barriers to reporting include personal reasons such as fear, accountability, and nurse characteristics, in addition to organizational factors such as culture, the reporting system, and management behavior (Vrbnjak et al., 2016; Wang et al., 2019). One study found that hospital personnel frequently encounter safety problems that they themselves can resolve on the spot. Fixing and forgetting, instead of fixing and reporting, was the main choice when handling near misses (seen as unworthy of reporting), solving a patient's safety problem (seen as unique or a one-time event), or encountering recurring problems (seen as inevitable, routine events). Although common, fixing and forgetting does not serve as the best organizational handling of patient safety or its risk-management efforts because it does not make patient safety more preventive. This leads to workarounds that may be a set-up for recurring problems (Huber et al., 2019). Nurses may incur liability and risk, with possible ethical implications, if incidents are not properly reported so that investigation and organizational intervention can occur.

LEADERSHIP AND MANAGEMENT IMPLICATIONS

By the very nature of their work, nurses and nurse managers are decision makers who are constantly faced with making choices in personal, clinical, and organizational situations. These decision-making situations are commonly fraught with legal and ethical issues that often become entwined. As members of a profession, nurses and nurse managers are guided by both legal and ethical considerations in making decisions. The legal aspects of nursing management center on decision-making and supervision. Because all nurses retain personal accountability for their own acts and the use of knowledge and skills in the provision of care, personal accountability cannot be assumed by another. Nurse managers keep their own personal accountability for their own specific acts, but they are accountable also for their acts of delegation and supervision (Pozgar, 2019).

Nurse managers carry the major responsibility for developing and upholding the standards of care for the staff. Nurses and nurse managers carry the accountability for the supervision of others, who are often unlicensed assistive personnel. Supervision includes monitoring the tasks performed, ensuring that functions are performed in an appropriate fashion, and ensuring that assigned tasks and functions do not exceed competency or require a license to perform. Nurse managers use their autonomy to make decisions about practice situations. They are accountable for carrying out supervisory responsibilities; proper notification; assessing the competency of staff; training, orientation, and evaluation of staff; reasonable staffing decisions; and monitoring and maintenance of professional treatment relationships with clients, called *non-abandonment* (Pozgar, 2019).

The managers of any health care organization are responsible to the policy-making body of the organization and hold an obligation to comply with the laws of society at local, state, and national levels. Managers are responsible for ensuring that laws are adhered to in the actions of management itself and also in the actions of those employees who assist the managers in carrying out the mission of the organization. Concern for the law involves three general areas: personal negligence in clinical practice, liability for delegation and supervision, and liability of health care organizations (Pozgar, 2019).

Personal Negligence in Clinical Practice

Activities of clinical client care involve corresponding legal accountability and risk. Errors do happen, and some lead to injury to a client. At minimum, nurses have an ethical obligation to nonmaleficence, or to do no harm to clients. This duty is discharged in part by remaining competent in knowledge and skills and the standards of practice. Nursing negligence/malpractice

occurs when the nurse's actions are unreasonable given the circumstances, fail to meet the standard of care, or when the nurse fails to act and causes harm. In nursing, harm related to clinical practice commonly arises from negligent acts or omissions (unintentional torts) and a variety of intentional acts (intentional torts), such as invasion of privacy or assault and battery. To establish legal liability on the grounds of malpractice (professional negligence), the injured client (plaintiff) must prove these four elements:

1. A duty of care was owed to the injured party.
2. There was a breach of that duty.
3. The breach of the duty caused the injury (causation).
4. Actual harm or damages were suffered by the plaintiff.

When errors occur, nurses are advised to work with organizational risk management and establish a strategy for disclosure and apology (Russell, 2018).

Common clinical practice areas that give rise to allegations of malpractice include the general areas of treatment, communication, medication, and the broad category of monitoring/observing/supervising/surveillance. Examples of common negligence allegations in nursing malpractice suits include patient falls, use of restraints, medication errors, burns, equipment injuries, retained foreign objects, failure to monitor, failure to ensure safety, failure to take appropriate nursing action, failure to confirm accuracy of physicians' orders, improper technique or performance of treatments, failure to respond to a patient, failure to follow hospital procedure, and failure to supervise treatment (Pozgar, 2019). Although there is little research into cases where a nurse lost a license or was sued by a patient, there are some case studies recounting specific situations. For example, Wilson (2018) described a long-term care case where the facility was sued for inaccurate recordkeeping and failing to document and report changes in condition. Accurate documentation and prompt reporting by nurses were major issues.

Both nurses and nurse managers have a duty to follow organizational policies and procedures when reasonable. Nurse managers are advised to review policies and procedures carefully, including the language used, in order to adhere to legal and ethical parameters more closely. Clearly management in nursing practice means that nurses must fulfill obligations and duties both to clients and to the organization. This means using knowledge, skill, and decision-making abilities to reduce the incidence of negligence and malpractice by employees as a way to reduce harm to clients and legal risk to the organization. As the primary coordinators of care, nurses need to manage the environment of care delivery. Ensuring staff competence and reporting incompetent practice are key activities. For example, in nursing, legal and ethical issues arise when a nurse is impaired by substance abuse. The overall consideration is protecting the client from harm. Confronting suspected abuse must be done carefully, but when an incident occurs, the nurse manager has a responsibility to intervene (Pozgar, 2019).

Liability of Health Care Organizations

Health care facilities face extensive exposure to legal liability from several sources, in addition to the liability faced by nurses and nurse managers arising out of malpractice in clinical practice, and negligence in the process of delegating and supervising. These sources include negligence of their employees, negligence of independent contractors, corporate negligence arising out of the facility's responsibilities to hire qualified employees and monitor and supervise their activities, and failure to comply with numerous laws and regulations, especially those related to employment issues. Nurse managers have important roles to play in helping their organizations control facility liability arising from each of these sources (Pozgar, 2019).

Nurse managers can help the facility avoid corporate liability by, among other things, ensuring that those who report to them remain competent and qualified and have current licensure. Nurse managers should also report dangerously low staffing levels, incorrect mixes of staff for effectively meeting the health care needs of clients, and report incompetent, illegal, or unethical practices to appropriate authorities. Nurse managers have an important role to play in compliance with human resources (HR) areas of hiring, performance appraisal, management of employees with problems, and termination (Pozgar, 2019).

HR management is a major area for organizational liability. Nursing is a labor-intensive occupation. Some organizations are unionized. Labor and employment law include various laws and regulations that deal with issues related to hiring, firing, employee benefits, compensation, overtime, workplace safety, privacy, drug testing, and preventing discrimination, harassment, and violence. Because of the volume, variety, and complexity of local, state, and federal HR-related laws and regulations, organizations have HR departments whose function is to implement strategies and policies related to employee management.

Mandatory Reporting

Among the many duties under one's professional license to practice nursing is the duty to report. This duty sits firmly on the fence between legal and ethical responsibilities and is a good example of those times when a legal obligation is affected by ethics. This duty to report includes observations of children, elders, disabled, developmentally compromised, and anyone who is at risk or in a vulnerable situation. Licensed professionals have had an affirmative "duty to warn" ever since the 1976 decision of the Supreme Court of California in the case of *Tarasoff v. Regents of the University of California,* 551 P.2d 334 (1976). Since that time, nurses and other health professionals have struggled to identify the triggering point in a patient relationship that rises to the statutory "duty to warn" (Muller & Fink-Samnick, 2015). Initially, the case stood for the concept that if there was a specific threat against an individual, the therapist (in that case) was legally obligated to warn that individual and enable him/her to take steps to protect themselves. In other words, the threat had to be specific to an identifiable individual. Citing previous cases, the court said, "We recognize the difficulty that a therapist encounters in attempting to forecast whether a patient presents a serious danger of violence. Obviously, we do not require that the therapist, in making that determination, render a perfect performance; the therapist need only exercise 'that reasonable degree of skill, knowledge, and care ordinarily possessed and exercised by members of [that professional specialty] under similar circumstances'" (Tarasoff v. Regents of the University of California, 1976, p. 8).

In 2007 the California legislature codified Tarasoff, along with subsequent cases. The then-new law increased the duty to one that is twofold: (1) the duty to inform the potential victim of the risk, and (2) the duty to inform appropriate law enforcement. In the passage of time, states have adopted varying duties for nurses, therapists, social workers, physicians, and other practitioners. It is critical that nurses make inquiry and be fully familiar as to the requirement(s) of the state(s) in which they practice. The National Conference of State Legislatures (NCSL, 2019) lists those states that have laws in place. There are three types of laws: mandatory reporting, permissive reporting, and no reporting requirement at all.

CURRENT ISSUES AND TRENDS

Legal Issues and the Changing Family Dynamic

The ideal American family is no longer a mother, father and 2.6 children (Gao, 2015), and even if the number of children remains constant, the makeup of the family has changed. According to one definition, a family is "a social group of parents, children, and sometimes grandparents, uncles, aunts, and others who are related" (Cambridge Dictionary, 2020b). On June 26, 2015, the US Supreme Court issued its decision in *Obergefell et al. v. Hodges, Director, Ohio Department of Health, et al.* The court held that, "The Fourteenth Amendment requires a State to license a marriage between two people of the same sex and to recognize a marriage between two people of the same sex when their marriage was lawfully licensed and performed out-of-State" (Obergefell v. Hodges, 2015, pp. 3–28).

The traditional US concept of a family is clearly undergoing change. Nurses are confronted with families who may be structured in ways that are completely different from their own life experience and beliefs. Although nurses are entitled to their personal beliefs, those beliefs must remain outside the nurse–patient relationship. The duty as a nurse is to obey the law and act toward all patients, their families, and/or family caregiver with respect, providing them with the care and education that the circumstance requires. This issue is also directly related to the issue of consent and who may give consent for treatment on behalf of the patient. Questions in the practice setting should be referred to supervision, administration, or legal counsel within the facility or practice setting.

Staffing

In view of the significant degrees of change and uncertainty associated with the legal and ethical aspects affecting decision-making in nursing care management, there are important current issues and trends in this area. A major current and continuing issue is the nurse shortage, which for a number of reasons is expected to continue in the foreseeable future. This issue gives rise to a number of legal and ethical challenges for nurse managers and staff nurses. The nurse shortage has resulted in a major problem called short staffing caused largely by increases in cost-cutting measures and other financial constraints, and also from deterioration of working conditions. Short staffing refers to the use of an insufficient nursing staff on a unit or in a facility for the number of patients requiring care at various acuity levels. Consequences commonly associated with short staffing include:

- Deterioration of patient outcomes in terms of increased mortality and failure-to-rescue rates (Needleman et al., 2020; Walker, 2018);
- A general decline in the quality of patient care (Bridges et al., 2019; Carthon et al., 2019);
- Deterioration of nurse outcomes resulting from increased burnout and greater job dissatisfaction (Van Bogaert et al., 2017);
- Increases in organizational costs resulting from increased turnover (NSI Nursing Solutions, Inc., 2019);
- Legal liability.

In an effort to deal with short staffing, nurse managers are often required to do the following: float nurses to areas in which they are not cross-trained, an action that also increases the client-to-nurse ratio closer to staffing requirements; use agency (temporary) personnel; and use unlicensed personnel. Staff nurses, nurse managers, and health care facilities all face numerous possibilities of legal liability—as well as dilemmas involving conflicts between clinical and organizational ethics—as a result of short staffing and actions taken in an effort to temporarily solve this problem (Broadway, 2019).

Nurses need to focus on their use of expert judgment in practicing the highest legal and ethical standards in the quest for high-quality care and services. In some instances, they may also be called on to demonstrate moral courage, which is the courage to honor ethical core values in the face of personal risk. Strategies that are available to the nurse leader chiefly focus on the use of multidisciplinary teams because they can provide an expert group approach to addressing moral and ethical issues. Although not providing definitive answers, the use of a group approach increases the knowledge and ideas that can be brought to bear on the situation and increases analysis that helps to shape the best possible decision under difficult circumstances.

RESEARCH NOTE

Source
Ben-Assuli, O. (2015). Electronic health records, adoption, quality of care, legal and privacy issues, and their implementation in emergency departments. *Health Policy, 119*(3) 287–297.

Purpose
The purpose of this article was to review and analyze proposed and actual uses of electronic health records (EHR) and health information exchanges (HIE) in the emergency department (ED) and the implications and impact of use of these technologies from the clinical and legal standpoint. The focus was on the current body of evidence regarding the status of care quality as Health Information Technology (HIT) implementation becomes more common.

Discussion
The study reviewed use of EHR around the world and found varying degrees of success. One large and successful study was that of the veterans' health system in the United States. This particular study included over 1000 hospitals. Overall, the study found a greater degree of success in non-profit public (government run) hospitals. Training and readiness had a direct impact on the success and compliance with the newly adopted programs. Regulations requiring EHR have a direct impact on compliance and Medicare and Medicaid use, which—although lower at the time of the study—has increased due to regulatory mandates for phased-in implementation. In the ED, ease of use and accessibility of the system may well be a barrier to adoption if the system design does not take into account physicians' busy workflow.

Legal and privacy concerns are significant due to the rapid advancement of technology. Portable devices and security of patient information are paramount in analysis of the costs and benefits of EHR. One concern was that convenience may lead to carelessness, such a "cut and paste." The issue of accidents or mistakes while using these new systems (due to information technology [IT] glitches and bugs) raises new and unanswered questions about potential liability as it relates to professional liability (malpractice). In addition, there is concern that interaction with the IT system may negatively affect the quality of care, thus again exposing medical professionals to liability. Protecting and maintaining patient privacy has always been a nursing responsibility, but with the advent of uploading and sharing of medical information through an electronic system, these burdens take on new concerns.

Application to Practice
Particular concerns were raised with regard to certain practice areas, such as maternity, contraception, and sexual and mental health. Logic would also indicate that other sensitive areas such as drug and alcohol use, HIV/AIDS, sexual orientation, and transgender issues would generate privacy issues. Would patients resist being forthcoming with sensitive information, knowing that their information would be put into "the system"? Nurses need to be sensitive to patient concerns and use interviewing and observational skills to overcome potential gaps in necessary information.

Policies and procedures are critical to framing how nursing will use electronic access, information, and reporting. Safeguards must be established in cooperation with the IT department. Nurses must always be mindful of HIPAA implications and participate whenever possible in the creation and modification of polices affecting patient privacy. Segregating personal information from patient information and protecting patient privacy must never become lax. Compliance with HIPAA and state privacy laws must be at the forefront of practice.

CASE STUDY

Falsification of records is an ethical as well as legal issue. Mary Smith is a registered nurse in a Transitional Care Nursery and one of her responsibilities is to perform heel stick blood glucose determinations for all newborn infants within 1 hour of admission from Labor and Delivery. The patient care assistant assigned to the unit notices that some neonates have no heel stick marks. All documentation in the electronic medical record shows acceptable glucose readings. The patient care assistant reports her concerns to the nursing supervisor who checks the heels of several infants with charted glucose readings by the registered nurse. There is no evidence that the heel sticks have been performed.

1. What actions does the nursing supervisor take and why?
2. What ethical principle has been violated?
3. What ethical rule has been violated?
4. How has ANA's *Code of Ethics for Nurses with Interpretive Statements* (2015) been violated?

CRITICAL THINKING EXERCISE

Michael Jones is the nursing professional development coordinator who is orienting eight newly employed nurses. Five are new graduates and three are experienced nurses who are transitioning to positions in the hospital. This is the third day of orientation. Michael notices that one of the experienced nurses (Amy) constantly corrects one of the new graduates and the graduate nurse (Beth) is no longer asking questions or offering comments. At the end of the day, Michael is in his office preparing for tomorrow's class. Beth asks to speak to him. It is obvious that she has been crying. Michael asks what he can help her with, and she says she overheard Amy tell her experienced colleagues that Beth would never succeed as a nurse. Beth's self-confidence is clearly shaken, and she doesn't know what to do.

1. What action should Michael take?
    a. Tell Beth that she will have to deal with negative people and not take what she hears personally.
    b. Talk with Beth about approaches she can use to diffuse negative comments.
    c. Ensure that Beth is safe to go home and plan to talk with Amy privately before the next class.
2. How can Michael address bullying behavior?
    a. Ask Amy to explain why she is picking on Beth.
    b. Discuss with Amy why such bullying behavior cannot be tolerated in the organization and explore approaches with her to resolve this issue.
    c. Tell Amy that you don't want to hear any more complaints during orientation.
3. What is Michael's responsibility when bullying or incivility occurs?
    a. Maintain a safe positive learning environment.
    b. Avoid calling attention to negative behavior.
    c. Tell both parties to deal with the issue outside class.

REFERENCES

American Nurses Association. (2010). *Nursing's social policy statement: The essence of the profession* (3rd ed.). Silver Spring, MD: American Nurses Association.

American Nurses Association. (2015a). *Nursing: Scope and standards of practice* (3rd ed.). Silver Spring, MD: American Nurses Association.

American Nurses Association. (2015b). *Code of ethics for nurses with interpretive statements* (2nd ed.). Silver Spring, MD: American Nurses Association.

American Nurses Association. (2019). *Violence, incivility, & bullying*. https://www.nursingworld.org/practice-policy/work-environment/violence-incivility-bullying/.

American Nurses Association (ANA). (2020). *The nursing process*. Silver Spring, MD: American Nurses Association. https://www.nursingworld.org/practice-policy/workforce/what-is-nursing/the-nursing-process/.

APRN Joint Dialogue Group Report. (2008,July 7). *Consensus model for APRN regulation: Licensure, accreditation, certification & education*. http://www.nursingworld.org/ConsensusModelforAPRN.

Ben-Assuli, O. (2015). Electronic health records, adoption, quality of care, legal and privacy issues, and their implementation in emergency departments. *Health Policy, 119*(3), 287–297.

Brenan, M. (2018). Nurses again outpace other professions for honesty, ethics. https://news.gallup.com/poll/245597/nurses-again-outpace-professions-honesty-ethics.aspx.

Bridges, J., Griffiths, P., Oliver, E., & Pickering, R. M. (2019). Hospital nurse staffing and staff-patient interactions: An observational study. *BMJ Quality & Safety, 28*(9), 706–713. https://doi.org/10.1136/bmjqs-2018-008948.

Broadway, M. A. (2019). Legal and ethical issues. In P. Yoder-Wise (Ed.), *Leading and managing in nursing* (7th ed.) (pp. 32–61). St. Louis, MO: Elsevier.

Cambridge Dictionary. (2020a). *Profession*. https://dictionary.cambridge.org/us/dictionary/english/profession.

Cambridge Dictionary. (2020b). *Family*. https://dictionary.cambridge.org/us/dictionary/english/family.

Carthon, J. M., Hatfield, L., Dierkes, A., Davis, L., Hedgeland, T., Sanders, A. M., et al. (2019). Association of nurse engagement and nurse staffing on patient safety. *Journal of Nursing Care Quality, 34*(1), 40–46.

Department of Health and Human Services (HHS). (2020). *Personal representatives*. http://www.hhs.gov/hipaa/for-professionals/privacy/guidance/personal-representatives/.

De Pietro, S. C. (2016). Legal and ethical issues in nursing professional development. In C. M. Smith, & M. G. Harper (Eds.), *Leadership in nursing professional development: An organizational & system focus* (pp. 78–109). Chicago, IL: Association for Nursing Professional Development (ANPD).

De Simone, D. M. (2019). Data breaches are not just information technology worries! *Pediatric Nursing, 45*(2), 59–62.

Gao, G. (2015, May 8). *Americans' ideal family size is smaller than it used to be.* https://www.pewresearch.org/fact-tank/2015/05/08/ideal-size-of-the-american-family/.

Hill, G., & Hill, K. (2019). Cross examination. *LAW.COM.* https://dictionary.law.com/Default.aspx?selected=408.

Huber, D. L., Bair, H., & Joseph, M. L. (2019). Roadmap to drive innovativeness in health care. *Nurse Leader, 17*(6), 505–508.

Institute of Medicine (IOM). (2011). *The future of nursing: Leading change, advancing health.* Washington, DC: National Academies Press.

Law Insider. (2019). Definition of professional judgement. https://www.lawinsider.com/dictionary/professional-judgement.

Legal Information Institute. (2020). *Federal rules of evidence.* https://www.law.cornell.edu/rules/fre.

Muller, L. S., & Fink-Samnick, E. (2015). Mandatory reporting: Let's clear up the confusion. *Professional Case Management, 20*(4), 199–203.

National Council of State Boards of Nursing (NCSBN). (2019). *Uniform licensure requirements.* https://www.ncsbn.org/3884.htm.

National Council of State Boards of Nursing. (2020a). *Contact a U.S. member.* https://www.ncsbn.org/contact-bon.htm.

National Council of State Boards of Nursing. (2020b). Nursing licensure compact. https://nursinglicensemap.com/resources/nursing-licensure-compact/.

National Conference of State Legislatures (NCSL). (2019). *State legislative websites directory.* www.ncsl.org/aboutus/ncslservice/state-legislative-websites-directory.aspx.

Needleman, J., Liu, J., Shang, J., Larson, E., & Stone, P. W. (2020). Association of registered nurse and nursing support staffing with inpatient hospital mortality. *BMJ Quality & Safety, 29*(1), 10–18. https://doi.org/10.1136/bmjqs-2018-009219.

NSI Nursing Solutions, Inc. (2019). *2019 National health care retention & RN staffing report.* www.nsinursingsolutions.com.

NursingLicensure.org. (2019). *LPN/LVN and registered nurse license requirements by state.* NursingLicensure.org: https://www.nursinglicensure.org/.

Obama, B. H. (2016, January 6). *New executive actions to reduce gun violence and make our communities safer.* https://www.whitehouse.gov/the-press-office/2016/01/04/fact-sheet-new-executive-actions-reduce-gun-violence-and-make-our.

Obergefell v. Hodges, 576 U.S. __ (2015) (U>S> Supreme Court, 2015). https://supreme.justia.com/cases/federal/us/576/14-556/

Phillips, J., & Walsh, M. A. (2018). Teaming up in child welfare: The perspective of guardians ad litem on the components of interprofessional collaboration. *Children and Youth Services Review, 96*(2019), 17–26.

Pozgar, G. D. (2019). *Legal Aspects of Health Care Administration* (13th ed.). Burlington, MA: Jones & Bartlett Learning, LLC.

Russell, D. (2018). Disclosure and apology: Nursing and risk management working together. *Nursing Management, 49*(6), 17–19.

Tarasoff v. Regents of the University of California, 17 Cal.3d 425, 131 Cal. Rptr. 14 (California Supreme Court 1976).

Van Bogaert, P., Peremans, L., Van Heusden, D., Verspuy, M., Kureckova, V., Van de Cruys, et al. (2017). Predictors of burnout, work engagement and nurse reported job outcomes and quality of care: A mixed method study. *BMC Nursing, 16*(5), 1–14. https://doi.org/10.1186/s12912-016-0200-4.

Vrbnjak, D., Denieffe, S., O'Gorman, C., & Pajnkihar, M. (2016). Barriers to reporting medication errors and near misses among nurses: A systematic review. *International Journal of Nursing Studies, 63*, 162–178.

Walker, A. (2018, March 2). *Nursing satisfaction impacts patient outcomes, mortality.* Nurse.org: https://nurse.org/articles/nursing-satisfaction-patient-results/.

Wang, Y., Coiera, E., & Magrabi, F. (2019). Using convolutional neural networks to identify patient safety incident reports by type and severity. *Journal of the American Medical Informatics Association, 26*(12), 1600–1608.

Wilson, W. C. (2018). Inadequate nurse's notes lead to lawsuit. *Caring for the Ages, 19*(3), 14–15.

Zaleski, A. (2017). *You need a (interactive) map to understand the disparity of healthcare data sharing in the U.S.* https://medcitynews.com/2017/06/need-interactive-map-understand-disparity-healthcare-data-sharing-u-s/.

Communication Leadership

Bob Dent

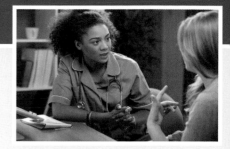

Communication is a process by which meaning is assigned to the needs, feelings, perceptions, and interpretation of what is brought to our awareness. There are several variables that influence how we assign meaning to our experience and thus affect how we communicate. Successful health care outcomes are dependent on clear communication; therefore all nurses need proficiency in interpersonal skills. Nurse leaders and managers need to be mentors, coaches, and role models for effective interpersonal and team communication in order to ensure safe patient outcomes, effective teamwork, and staff satisfaction.

The purpose of this chapter is to enhance nurse leaders' understanding of the pivotal role that communication plays in health care by elucidating the complexities present in human communication, by addressing current key communication issues in health care, and by offering pragmatic strategies using communication models that can be applied to a variety of health care settings.

DEFINITIONS

Communication is based on mutual understanding. Clarity of meaning is derived from a clear definition of terms related to communication. Relevant definitions are as follows:

- **Interpersonal communication:** Communication between two or more individuals involving face-to-face interaction while all parties are aware of the others on an ongoing basis. Each person sends and receives information while continually adapting to the other actors.

- **Interprofessional communication:** Communication between two or more members of the interdisciplinary care team.
- **Intercultural communication:** Communication across cultural contexts. It applies equally to domestic cultural differences such as ethnicity and gender and to international differences such as those associated with nationality or world region (Bennet, 2013).
- **Non-verbal communication:** Unspoken, this communication is composed of affective or expressive behavior.
- **Persuasion, negotiation, and bargaining:** Persuasion is the conscious intent by one individual to modify the thoughts or behaviors of others. Negotiation is a dialogical discussion between two or more parties to arrive at an agreement about some issue. To bargain is to make a series of offers and counteroffers about what each party will do, give, receive, etc., until an agreement is reached to the satisfaction of all. All three of these involve communication. Persuasion uses argumentation and appeals to logic, whereas negotiation and bargaining may involve some sense of compensation and perhaps coercion, such as bullying or condescending behaviors.
- **Verbal communication:** Includes both written and spoken communication.

BACKGROUND

The literature supports the importance of effective team and interpersonal communication at all levels of an organization. Not only is this key in preventing medical errors, but effective communication and team functioning have also been shown to contribute to patient and staff satisfaction (Nicotera et al., 2014). Over 20 years ago, the Institute of Medicine (IOM, 2001) reported that 98,000 patient deaths per year stemmed from preventable medical errors. Not much has changed in the past 20 years. Health care still has a prevalent culture of silence. Frontline workers worried about litigation or job loss cover up mistakes, and leaders fail to address medical errors even in a preemptive fashion, almost as if not to jinx their luck (Aguilar, 2019).

Furthermore, individual, team, and interprofessional communication is influenced by organizational climate and culture (see Chapter 3). An organization with a rigid bureaucratic one-way communication network or lack of transparency will impede effective communication among all levels of the organization. A less rigid, more open, transparent structure will encourage creative problem-solving and healthy conflict resolution, elements that are needed for healthy organizations. Open communication practices are important because this builds trust. Trust, respect, and empathy are three ingredients that foster positive communication outcomes. The Joint Commission (2015) recognized that the leading causes of sentinel events—a patient safety event that reaches a patient and results in death, permanent harm, or results in severe temporary harm and interventions required to sustain life—relate to poor communication and leadership (The Joint Commission Online, 2015).

Stephen R. Covey (2004), the author of *The 8th Habit: From effectiveness to greatness*, discussed the emotional bank account derived from relationships built with each other. He explained the concept with the metaphor: "It is like a financial bank account into which you make deposits and withdrawals—only in this case, you make emotional deposits and withdrawals in your relationships that either build or destroy them" (p. 165). If a nurse leader breaches the trust of their staff, other leaders, or the medical staff, they may not ever be able to make enough deposits to get out of debt.

Proficiency in verbal, non-verbal, and written communication is a core leadership competency. Leaders need to possess the skills necessary to inspire a shared vision, ensure the mission, and establish a culture where this can be achieved. Leaders also need special communication skills in order to implement change.

Interpersonal relationship skills—including the ability to communicate—are as essential to a leader's personal set of leadership skills as psychomotor skills are for a clinical nurse. Leadership ability is predicated on a facility for communication. Human interaction issues are an area where leaders can spend a considerable amount of time. Power and conflict become important focal points of human interaction in organizations that may need managerial intervention or resolution through persuasion or negotiation. Because nurses may frequently be in situations in which they need to persuade others to cooperate, proficiency in managing conflict, bargaining, negotiating, and the art of "crucial conversations" is essential for nurses and nurse leaders. The foregoing skills require practice, experience, assertiveness, and confidence, which are necessary elements in the nurse leader's armamentarium.

Nurses need to be able to feel safe enough to articulate needs, viewpoints, and ideas for improvement of health care and the work environment. Feeling that one has not been heard can be a source of true frustration, anger, and conflict.

Nurse leaders play a crucial role in the management of information and communication for the purpose of effective care coordination and to prevent unsafe and error-prone care situations. Providers need high-quality information and access to health care information systems and effective communication models. Nurse leaders are responsible for developing care delivery systems with adequate structure and an effective communication system that enhances care coordination. These systems of communication need to enable patient rescue and safety by coordinating care, preventing information loss, and improving methods of surveillance. For example, there is a distinction between interprofessional collaboration and merely working on the same task together. This occurs when multiple health care providers are taking care of the same patient, but in a mode where multiple providers are simultaneously doing different jobs rather than there being collaborative efforts.

Successful nurse leaders are effective communicators establishing trust and respect. Nurse leaders need to model behavior and language that sets the tone for a positive and supportive work environment. Equally critical is the development and fostering of similarly effective communication skills in all nurses for peer-to-peer, interprofessional, intercultural, and followership interactions.

COMMUNICATION THEORIES AND MODELS

Communication is a process in which information, perception, and understanding are transmitted from person to person. It is important to nurses and is an integral part of any relationship. Nurse leaders and managers can view communication as a tool to accomplish work and meet goals. The significance of communication revolves around its effectiveness and the climate in which communication occurs. Effective communication is enhanced by clear, direct, straightforward, and frequent message transmission. Trust, respect, and empathy are the three ingredients needed to create and foster effective communication.

Much of what was written in the past with respect to communication in health care was about teaching techniques and skills such as interviewing and how to elicit information from patients. These works also included explanations regarding how to reflect, clarify, summarize, provide feedback, use silence, and actively listen. Learning communication techniques is not enough. Communication is more than messages, and human beings are more than senders and receivers. Further, communication models specifically written for nursing are limited, and rigorous studies using randomized controlled trials or systematic reviews to determine the effectiveness of models applicable to nursing practice are not well documented.

Communication is a process that is affected by several internal and external variables, takes place on multiple levels of complexity, is difficult to measure, and for which standardized instruments are lacking (Foronda et al., 2015).

COMMUNICATION TO FACILITATE CHANGE: KOTTER

In alignment with the goals of the Institute of Medicine's (IOM, 2011) report on *The Future of Nursing*, nurses are called upon to "lead change to advance health," yet the report acknowledges that several barriers exist that prevent nurses from responding to this call and participating fully in the rapidly changing health care environment. In a classic work, Kotter (1996) proposed a model in business for making change in organizations. This framework underscores that all change is made by communication, and the effectiveness and sustainability of the change is based on the skilled communication of the leadership and stakeholders endorsing the change process.

> **BOX 8.1   Kotter's Eight-Stage Process of Creating Major Change**
>
> 1. Establishing a sense of urgency
> 2. Creating the guiding coalition
> 3. Developing a vision and a strategy
> 4. Communicating the change vision
> 5. Empowering broad-based action
> 6. Generating short-term wins
> 7. Consolidating gains and producing more change
> 8. Anchoring new approaches in the culture
>
> From Kotter, J. (1996). *Leading change* (p. 21). Boston, MA: Harvard Business School Press.

Kotter (1996) suggested the following are needed to empower people to make change: communicate the vision to employees, make structures compatible with the vision, provide the training employees need, align information and personnel systems, and confront supervisors who undercut needed change. Further, he suggested that structures, skills, systems, and supervisors are generally the four barriers to any transformational process. Before implementing change, the nurse leader is well advised to first analyze the communication pattern currently in place at the macro and micro level and to be cognizant of the organization's general culture, climate, and politics. Box 8.1 outlines the points of Kotter's change process.

Leadership needs to be part of the guiding coalition in all of these stages to be supportive and communicate needed change. Kotter stated that the barriers that can interfere with change are as follows: "inwardly focused cultures, paralyzing bureaucracy, parochial politics, a low level of trust, lack of teamwork, arrogant attitudes, a lack of leadership in middle management, and general human fear of the unknown" (p. 20). He also stated that organizations that are more manager versus leader oriented will not produce needed change that is sustainable, because managers "plan, organize and control," whereas leaders "establish direction, align people, and motivate and inspire," qualities that are needed to "produce extremely useful change" (p. 26).

Intrapersonal and Interpersonal Communication

Decades ago, Abraham Maslow developed a model for understanding human needs. He identified that how we respond, react, and behave is based on our needs and whether they are being met. Thus this model is still relevant and is a useful framework for understanding human communication. At the bottom of Maslow's pyramid of human needs are our most basic needs for survival, followed by safety and security, love and belonging, esteem and appreciation, and finally altruistic needs, like fulfillment by helping others and reaching psychological maturity.

Our most basic needs will not be met if we are not able to communicate. Babies cry when they are hungry, tired, uncomfortable, and in need of safety and security. They do not usually speak until about age 1 year, and then they start to form words, yet their caregivers know what they want and provide for them in their preverbal state. This happens because we use body language, facial expressions, and other sounds to communicate. Thus, as a species, we would not survive without communication between and among us, and unmet needs can be a source of conflict, misunderstanding, and anger. There are several factors that can influence how we respond.

Words and language are powerful tools that can be used to harm or heal (Sears, 2010). Non-verbal communication, such as use of the body and face, can also convey a strong message. To be most direct and straightforward, verbal and non-verbal communication should be congruent, meaning that our verbal and non-verbal are consistent. Communication problems in interpersonal relationships, whether personal or occupational, can be a source of conflict due to misinterpretation of what was said or meant. Conflict is natural, inherent, and inevitable in hospitals, and can arise in the work environment with heavy workloads, limited resources, unclear policies, organizational changes, poor communication, and differences in employees' abilities, skills, and personalities (Mosadeghrad & Mojbafan, 2019). However, there is an optimum conflict level necessary and beneficial for individual growth and organizational productivity.

Unresolved conflict can lead to resentment, backbiting, bullying, and other dysfunctional behaviors. A supportive work environment, positive communication between staff nurses and leadership, and frequent feedback on job performance, facilitate nurse job satisfaction. Setting a positive and cooperative tone within a work group is each member's responsibility. Moreover, it is incumbent upon nursing leadership to set the tone of the work environment (such as promoting a healthy work environment) and model impeccable interpersonal communication for the staff.

Tools for Improved Communication

Many times individuals get caught in a situation and are just at a loss for words or cannot come up with the response that feels just right at the time. Effective communication tools can help.

Tools for effective communication and speaking up. Poor communication has consequences for patient safety and can be deadly. Medical errors can be avoided, and work environments can become healthier if health care professionals acquire the ability to speak up and discuss emotionally or politically risky topics. Communication breakdowns can be either honest mistakes or undiscussables. Honest mistakes are accidental or unintentional slips and errors such as confusing labels, competing tasks, language barriers, distractions, or gaps during handoffs. Undiscussables occur when someone knows of risks or something being wrong, but does not speak up or chooses to ignore or avoid it. A person may back down from the conversation (Maxfield et al., n.d.).

VitalSmarts, the Association of periOperative Registered Nurses, and the American Association of Critical-Care Nurses worked on research to address communication failures and avoidable medical errors. Their 2005 study called Silence Kills was followed by the 2010 study The Silent Treatment, which confirmed that poor communication is harmful and that despite encountering resistance, nurses need to be enabled to speak up about dangerous shortcuts, incompetence, and disrespect. A safety culture where people speak up when there is a strong suspicion of risk needs to be developed using the communication skills of exceptional nurses and organizational strategies (Maxfield et al., 2010).

There are useful tools developed by the Agency for Healthcare Research and Quality's TeamSTEPPS program (AHRQ, 2020) (discussed later in this chapter). With scripting, these tools help nurses and interprofessional teams to communicate fully and clearly as well as speaking up when appropriate. For example, AHRQ has developed a pocket guide (https://www.ahrq.gov/teamstepps/instructor/essentials/pocketguide.html#passbaton) that presents CUS assertive statements. The CUS model is a tool to help nurses speak up/speak out in uncomfortable situations. A script is presented, using "I am concerned," "I am uncomfortable," or "This is a safety issue." "Stop the line" is one script used. A constructive approach for managing and resolving conflict is the DESC script: *D*escribe the situation, *E*xpress how the situation makes you feel,

Suggest other alternatives, and state Consequences in terms of impact on team goals.

Another helpful tool for effective communication and speaking up is called crucial conversations, which gives guidance on providing constructive feedback. Based on a book by Patterson et al. (2011), a crucial conversation is defined as a discussion between two or more people where the stakes are high, opinions vary, and emotions run strong. Billed as tools for talking when the stakes are high, the focus is on alleviating failure to communicate. The choices when facing crucial conversations are to avoid them, face them but handle them poorly, or face them and handle them well. Examples of crucial conversations range from ending a relationship, to talking to a team member who is not keeping commitments or has a personal hygiene problem, to giving an unfavorable peer or performance review. Dialogue skills are learnable. The book and training courses help people learn how to create conditions that make dialogue the path of least resistance; how to use key skills related to talking, listening, and acting together; and how to master tools for talking when the stakes are high. For nurses, this training promotes a culture of safety because team members can then talk about issues and concerns openly even when they touch on areas of silence in health care—such as incompetence, poor teamwork, and disrespect—or are difficult, risky, or emotionally charged. Some organizations have crucial-conversations training for staff to build skills in how to speak and be heard.

Evidence-Based Practice and Communication

Evidence-based practice (EBP) was developed following several reports by the Institute of Medicine (IOM), now called the National Academies of Sciences, Engineering, and Medicine, that cited staggering numbers of poor patient outcomes related to preventable medical errors. EBP is the preferred model of nursing care now and for the future. EBP encompasses clinical knowledge coupled with research evidence and patient preference to develop best practices, and it is supported by a number of regulatory organizations. However, despite growing evidence for support of EBP, incorporation of this model into daily clinical practice "remains inconsistent and presents complex challenges" (Pryse et al., 2014, p. 244). For EBP to work in an organization, nurse leaders and those in the work environment must be well informed and supportive of individual nurses who wish to incorporate EBP principles into their nursing care. Pryse et al. (2014) developed and tested two psychometric instruments, the EBP Nursing Leadership Scale and the EBP Work Environment Scale that can be used by nurse leaders to determine support for EBP within their organization.

One example of EBP that can be readily learned and implemented by nurses is moving shift report to the bedside. McAllen et al. (2018) completed a literature review finding numerous studies supporting the positive impact of bedside shift report (BSR) on nurse-sensitive outcomes including patient falls, and patient and nurse satisfaction. The results of the quality improvement project were positive. Patient falls decreased by 24%. Patient satisfaction showed statistically significant improvements ($P = .03$) in their general surgery unit after BSR implementation. Implementation of BSR did not increase the average total time required for change of shift report. Earlier identification and correction of potential errors during BSR may have improved the quality of patient care.

Recent research highlighted the complexity of providing quality nursing care with regard to fulfilling patients' expectations (Sharifabad et al., 2019). Effective communication impacts how care is provided to patients and impacts patients' expectations and the perceptions of the quality of nurses' services. Their five service quality of care factors were (1) tangibles: the appearance of the physical environment, equipment, and nurses; (2) reliability: nurses'/organization's ability to provide the right services in a timely fashion; (3) responsiveness: nurses' willingness and urgency in helping patients; (4) assurance: nurses' ability to earn patients' trust with task competence and humility; and (5) empathy: nurses' ability to demonstrate an interest in patients and their care. How care is provided communicates to patients other messages that impact their perceptions and ultimate well-being.

Transformational Leadership and Communication Style

Transformational leadership is a leadership style of communicating that relates to systematic variants such as job satisfaction, change commitment, leadership trust, cooperative conflict management, and market orientation (Yang, 2012). The basic goal of transformational leadership is to empower staff to take ownership of their own development (see Chapter 1).

The American Nurses Credentialing Center's (ANCC) Magnet Model (ANCC, 2020) recognized transformational leadership as one of the five core model components of a Magnet organization. ANCC describes the following to describe transformational leadership:

It is relatively easy to lead people where they want to go; the transformational leader must lead people to where they need to be in order to meet the demands of the future. This requires vision, influence, clinical knowledge, and a strong expertise relating to professional nursing practice. It also acknowledges that transformation may create turbulence and involve atypical approaches to solutions.

The organization's senior leadership team creates the vision for the future, and the systems and environment necessary to achieve that vision. They must enlighten the organization as to why change is necessary, and communicate each department's part in achieving that change. They must listen, transformational way of thinking should take root in the organization and become even stronger as other leaders adapt to this way of thinking.

The intent of this Model Component is no longer just to solve problems, fix broken systems, and empower staff, but to actually transform the organizations to meet the future. Magnet-recognized organizations today strive for stabilization; however, healthcare reformation calls for a type of controlled destabilization that births new ideas and innovations (ANCC, 2020).

Kouzes and Posner (2017) identified the Five Practices of Exemplary Leadership model. This model continues to prove its effectiveness as a clear, evidence-based path to achieving the extraordinary for individuals, teams, organizations, and communities. These leaders:

- **Model the way.** Leaders establish principles concerning the way people should be treated and the way goals should be pursued.
- **Inspire a shared vision**. Leaders passionately believe they can make a difference and enlist others in their dreams.
- **Challenge the process**. Leaders search for opportunities to change the status quo.
- **Enable others to act**. Leaders foster collaboration and build spirited teams.
- **Encourage the heart**. Leaders recognize the contributions of individuals and teams.

ORGANIZATIONAL CULTURE AND CLIMATE

Health care organizations are complex, and role expectations and responsibilities of leadership can change from facility to facility. Some health care organizations are moving away from bureaucratic and hierarchical organizational structures to more facilitative professional governance models. Some have even adopted the model of servant leadership.

Because nurses make up the bulk of the health care workforce, having nurse leaders strategically positioned within the organization to effectively influence other executive stakeholders, including the board of directors or board of trustees, is imperative to achieve the level of influence required to lead others.

Dent and Tye (2018, p. xi) stated, "The first responsibility of the nurse leader is to be clear about his or her own values, and to make a concerted daily effort to assure that these values are reflected in the attitudes they bring to work, the way they treat people, their approach to dealing with conflict, the criteria they use for making decisions, and how they deal with obstacles and setbacks. The second responsibility – the one that more than any other single quality defines the heart of a nurse leader—is to help the people whom they lead do the same thing."

According to workplace specialists, job satisfaction has been found to include much more than salary increases, decreased overtime, and tangible rewards. Appreciation, trust, and respect are not quantifiable but are extremely valuable. These, as well as support for individual growth and a sense of purpose, have been identified as important factors in job satisfaction. Job satisfaction means having a leader who is fair and honest, listens to concerns, and helps the team to develop knowledge, attitudes, and skills to advance their careers. Some have suggested that nurses probably do not leave agencies; they leave dehumanizing nursing leaders. Nurse leaders need to be in touch with the degree to which nursing staff are satisfied. Job satisfaction remains an important issue in the workplace environment, given nurse shortages and high reported levels of burnout.

Nurse leaders set the tone and expectations with every interaction. Much has been written about the effectiveness of informal power and that often, those without official title and position have more influence among leaders and peers than those with formal title and position. Therefore any nurse can exert influence on the cultural norms and climate of the organization, and nurse leaders should model this empowerment approach for all nurses.

Registered nurses (RN) form the backbone of health care in the United States, providing critical health care to the public wherever it is needed, and recognized as the key to the health of our nation. There are over 4 million RNs in the United States today. That means that one in 100 people is an RN. It is forecasted that there will be a shortage of RNs across the country between 2009 and 2030 (American Nurses Association [ANA], 2020). It is imperative then for nurse leaders to establish positive and healthy workplace environments to attract and retain nurses.

Communication in Patient and Family Engaged Care

Patients and their families are the reasons nurses exist in health care. Nurses and nurse leaders need to create an environment with structures and processes to improve patients' care and experiences. Patient and family engaged care (PFEC) is care planned, delivered, managed, and continuously improved in active partnership with patients and their families (or care partners as defined by the patient) to ensure integration of their health and health goals, preferences, and values. It includes explicit and partnered determination of goals and care options, and it requires ongoing assessment of the care match with patient goals (Frampton et al., 2017). Fig. 8.1 depicts the framework of PFEC with

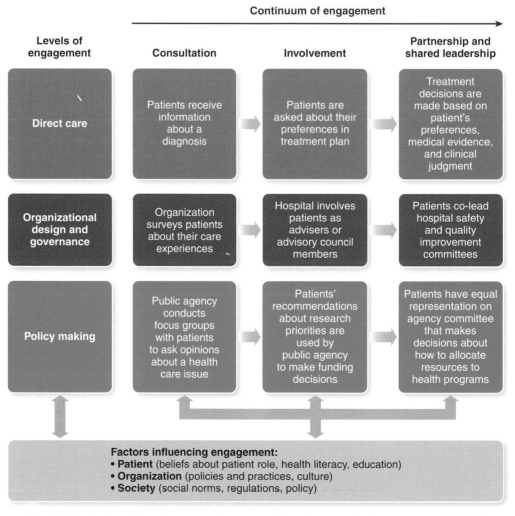

Fig. 8.1 Patient and family engaged care: a guiding framework (Frampton et al., 2017).

many of the key elements identified for improved engagement outcomes such as better culture, better care, better health, and lower costs.

The IOM defined patient-centered care as "providing care that is respectful of and responsive to individual patient preferences, needs and values, and ensuring that patient values guide all clinical decisions" (IOM, 2001, p. 40). Berwick (2009, p. 560) defined patient-centered care as "the experience (to the extent the informed, individual patient desires it) of transparency, individualization, recognition, respect, dignity and choice in all matters, without exception, related to one's person, circumstances, and relationships in health care."

Fooks et al. (2015) described three concepts that represent the principles of good patient relationships (see Box 8.2). Recognizing partnerships, equality, communication, trust, and respect are crucial levers for change. Carman et al. (2013) provided a multidimensional framework for patient and family engagement in health and health care as depicted in Fig. 8.2. The Joint Commission (R³ Report, 2011) has patient-centered communication standards for hospitals. The standards assure hospitals lead by example every day, as hospitals and health care providers demonstrate what it means to honor people's needs and their differences, providing health equity. Effective communication is critical to the successful delivery of health care services. The Joint Commission requires hospitals to effectively communicate with patients when providing care, treatment, and services by (1) identifying the patient's oral and written communication needs, including the patient's preferred language for discussing health care, and (2) communicating with the patient during provision of care, treatment, and services in a manner that meets the patient's oral and written communication needs (R³ Report, 2011).

LEADERSHIP AND MANAGEMENT IMPLICATIONS

Spears (2019, p. 1) stated, "[A]lmost all successful leaders understand that effective leadership really comes down to influence: influencing outcomes, influencing direction, influencing decisions, influencing atmosphere, and influencing people. The degree to which a leader can successfully influence people and teams becomes the 'lid' in his or her role. The only reliable tool we have to influence others is communication."

Effective leadership starts with communication, and progressive leaders need to understand how to ensure that their interventions lead to positive outcomes (Spears, 2019). Box 8.3 displays four conversations for the leader to get right. Strong communication is critical to supporting, guiding, and influencing; a leader's connections with others heighten the ability to influence, as well as the quantity and quality of work performance (Pater, 2016). The leader's communication has implications for success in achieving the organization's mission, vision, and strategic objectives. It is important for nurse leaders to be self-aware of their communication styles and know how to leverage their own and those of their teams. There are many valid and reliable tools to assess their own personality type and the personality types of their teams. These include Meyers-Briggs Type Indicator (MBTI) (https://www.myersbriggs.org/my-mbti-personality-type/mbti-basics/home.htm?bhcp=1), StrengthsFinder (https://www.gallup.com/cliftonstrengths/en/strengthsfinder.aspx), DISC (https://www.discprofile.com/what-is-disc/overview/), HBDI (http://www.hbdi.com/WholeBrainProductsAndServices/programs/thehbdi.php), and others.

For example, one's top five strengths are learned from taking the Strengths Finder survey. Experienced nurse leaders recognize that in all groups there is at least one person who has the positivity strength. When delivering bad news (e.g., outcomes, changes), the leader has to add in something positive to avoid demoralizing the

---

BOX 8.2 Principles of Good Patient Relationships

1. **Patient-centered care** is an overall philosophy and approach that ensures that everything individual providers or health care organizations do clinically or administratively is based on patient needs and preferences.
2. **Patient engagement** is the way in which individual providers or health care organizations solicit patient needs and preferences to ensure they are delivering patient-centered care.
3. **Patient experience** is how patients perceive and experience their care. This involves the ability to hear what is being said, measure the experience, and develop the capacity to use the information to change practice, policies, and rules.

From Fooks, C., Obarski, G., Hale, L., & Hylmar, S. (2015). The patient experience in Ontario 2020: What is possible? *Healthcare Papers, 14*(4): 8–18.

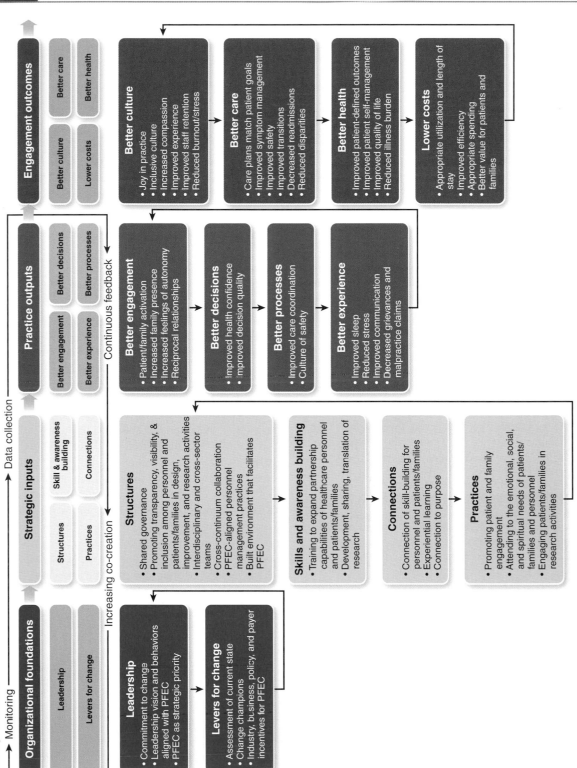

Patient and Family Engaged Care
A Guiding Framework

Fig. 8.2 Framework for patient and family engagement in health and health care (Carman et al., 2013). Note: movement to the right on the continuum of engagement denotes increasing patient participation and collaboration.

1. **The Timely Talk**. A must-have conversation for specific situations.
2. **The Rock Star Reminder**. An opportunity to influence growth and development and ultimate success with someone who has amazing potential.
3. **The Now or Never Conversation**. This conversation should always follow a failed Timely Talk (#1). The person knows that the performance or behavior or other issue cannot continue and has had some time to make changes. This person is now at risk.
4. **The Stay Interview**. A conversation with a proven and valued team member whom you very much want to stay. Add these to your calendar quarterly.

From Spears, T.L. (2019). *The four conversations you must get right as a leader.* American Association for Physician Leadership. https://www.physicianleaders.org/news/the-four-conversations-leader

person. Often the person with a positivity strength will chime in with something positive.

HBDI helps identify how the leader and the team would respond under normal circumstances and under pressure. On any given day, it helps to know how teammates are responding. Noting the responses reveals they are under pressure.

Understanding the different needs and expectations of others in communication requires leaders to customize their approach to communication, including listening and speaking (Fitzgerald & Kirby, 1997). Plonien (2015) discussed how to approach the MBTI in a perioperative setting to improve communication. For the nurse leader, knowledge of personality type provides an opportunity to enhance communication and improve team dynamics. Personality indicators such as the MBTI provide insight into the type of communication needed to connect with personnel, as well as within the interdisciplinary team.

It is imperative for nurse leaders to assess the workplace environment including observing the interactions of their teams regularly, recognizing top performers and addressing negative interactions quickly. No one is exempt from communicating effectively and working as a team. Leaders need to set realistic goals and model appropriate communication practice in establishing a more positive and healthier workplace environment. The next section discusses models that can be employed by nurse leaders to address issues in the health care environment resulting from ineffective communication.

Promoting Healthy, Inclusive Work Environments

In September 2017, the Tri-Council for Nursing (American Association of Colleges of Nursing [AACN]; American Nurses Association [ANA]; American Organization of Nurse Executives [AONE]; and the National League for Nursing [NLN]) issued a press release on the Proclamation on Nursing Civility. To emphasize how critical civil behavior is to excellence in nursing practice and to outstanding congruent care for all patients, the Tri-Council for Nursing issued a bold call to advance civility in nursing. The resolution called upon "all nurses to recognize nursing civility and take steps to systematically eliminate all acts of incivility in their professional practice, workplace environments, and in our communities" (Tri-Council for Nursing, 2017, para. 2). The Tri-Council urged that nursing civility be practiced throughout the United States "to establish healthy work environments that embrace and value cultural diversity, inclusivity, and equality" (Tri-Council for Nursing, 2017, para. 2). It noted that people of all racial, religious, ethnic, sexual orientation, socioeconomic, political, geographic, and other differences are to be treated respectfully. "It's no secret that acts of disrespect, and other overt or subtle negative emotional behavior create a toxic work environment which contributes to burnout, fatigue, depression and other psychological stresses. Eliminating assaults to anyone's self-esteem is essential to providing a healthy work and learning environment," noted Alexander (Tri-Council for Nursing, 2017, para. 3). "The Tri-Council recognizes that instilling an ethic of civility from the very beginning of a nurse's education and throughout the profession will begin to eliminate the dangers that inevitably arise when it is lacking." "Manifesting civility is key to enhancing the patient care experience and ensuring quality team-based care," said Sebastian (Tri-Council for Nursing, 2017, para. 4). "As the most trusted healthcare provider, registered nurses understand the connection between treating patients with respect, establishing open lines of communication, and realizing positive care outcomes" (Tri-Council for Nursing, 2017, para. 4).

"AONE (AONL) is committed to providing nurse leaders with the tools and resources to prevent workplace violence and ensuring the safety of all health care workers and patients. Through its work with the American Hospital Association, AONL is partnering to increase awareness of the issue and support AHA's

Hospitals against Violence initiative," stated Clark (Tri-Council for Nursing, 2017, para. 5). "Civility forms the foundation of a culture of respect for one another and is non-negotiable for a healthy, safe and ethical work environment" (Tri-Council for Nursing, 2017, para. 6). "The ANA has zero-tolerance for any form of incivility, violence, or bullying in the workplace in order to safeguard patients, nurses, and other healthcare team members" (Tri-Council for Nursing, 2017, para. 6). The Tri-Council identified other potential measurable hazards to health care of incivility, intolerance, and disregard for emotional health: difficulty in nurse recruitment and retention, aggravating the persistent shortage of nurses, and poor communication and teamwork giving rise to preventable errors that risk patient safety. Noting that nurses currently enjoy a reputation as the most ethical and honest profession in the country, the council's statement articulates a nurse's ethical obligation to care for others and themselves (Tri-Council for Nursing, 2017, para. 7).

There is support on a national level to promote effective communication and collaboration. It is important that positive interdisciplinary relationships are established and are active in the organizational culture. The workplace does not have to be hostile. Nurse leaders have a responsibility to communicate zero tolerance for bullying and a hostile environment. The ANA (2015) developed a position statement on incivility, bullying, and workplace violence: "ANA's Code of Ethics for Nurses with Interpretive Statements states that nurses are required to 'create an ethical environment and culture of civility and kindness, treating colleagues, co-workers, employees, students, and others with dignity and respect.'" Similarly, nurses must be afforded the same level of respect and dignity as others (ANA, 2015). Thus the nursing profession will no longer tolerate violence of any kind from any source. All registered nurses and employers in all settings, including practice, academia, and research, need to collaborate to create a culture of respect, free of incivility, bullying, and workplace violence. Best practice strategies based on evidence need to be implemented to prevent and mitigate incivility, bullying, and workplace violence; to promote the health, safety, and wellness of registered nurses; and to ensure optimal outcomes across the health care continuum. This position statement, although written specifically for registered nurses and employers, is also relevant to other health care professionals and

stakeholders who collaborate to create and sustain a safe and healthy interprofessional work environment. Stakeholders who have a relationship with the worksite have a responsibility to address incivility, bullying, and workplace violence.

According to the Workplace Bullying Institute (2019), although many good nurses have been driven out by toxic environments, many other nurses have just accepted those environments. Decoster, a cultural anthropologist in Cusco, Peru, described culture as a people's adaptation to an environment (Dent, B., A personal interview of Dr. Jean-Jacques Decoster in Cusco, Peru, October, 2018). It is imperative for nurse leaders to establish more positive and healthier workplace environments where nurses can be and perform at their best.

Tye and Dent (2017) described toxic emotional negativity as the name for the whole collection of behaviors that include gossiping, eye-rolling, bullying, and work-shirking. Toxic emotional negativity is so ubiquitous that often it is hardly even noticed it unless making a concerted effort to do so. The emotional climate of the workplace is defined by expected behaviors and tolerated behaviors; over time, the tolerated behaviors will dominate the expected behaviors. Thus it is imperative for nurses and nurse leaders to establish more positive and healthy workplace environments rid of toxic behaviors that erode teamwork and communication resulting in poor outcomes.

Nonviolent Communication

Expanding on nonviolent communication (NVC) concepts developed by Rosenberg (2004) and Sears (2010) critiqued the health care system. In a nutshell, NVC is predicated on the notion that our language, which is based on our culture and experience, is replete with judgment, criticisms, labels, and phraseology that is bound to create defensive reactions in others and is considered violent. Further, and more importantly, "the labels, analyses and judgments of others are tragic expressions of your own unmet needs" (Sears, 2010, p. 56).

Recalling the earlier discussion of Maslow's hierarchy of needs, this makes perfect sense. Unmet needs in the area of belonging—a basic need—can create issues of safety or feelings of insecurity or of feeling threatened. Anger or helplessness are two responses that may be seen in people trying to protect themselves. No one is safe in a hostile work environment. Therefore when someone feels threatened or unsafe, they may regress to an earlier stage of development to when they felt safe and thus respond in a childlike manner. This may account for behavior that we may consider to be immature.

Sears proposed a four-part nonviolent communication process grounded in compassion, empathy, and honesty. She stated, "Empathy is one of the simplest yet most potent technologies on the planet. It is a low-cost, high yield solution that everyone can use" (Sears, 2010, p. 88). The four parts include making an observation, expressing a feeling, expressing a need, and making a request without demanding. Table 8.1 is an adaptation of these four parts of NVC developed by Rosenberg (2004).

Nurses are by and large caretakers of others and thus may be great at making observations. But they may lack the ability to express their own feelings and needs and lack the ability to make a straightforward request. By becoming proficient at expressing their own feelings and needs and communicating requests in a clear, direct manner, nurses are providing for their own self-care. Only in this way can nurses truly care for others.

Team/Group Communication: TeamSTEPPS and SBAR

Nurse leaders need to be familiar with group theory because little is accomplished in a health care facility without individual participation in a team, group, or meeting. Participation in groups is a necessary part of the functioning of the larger organization. In principle, the degree to which individual need satisfaction is achieved differentiates effective from ineffective groups; the greater the individual's satisfaction, the higher the probability of group effectiveness (Hersey et al., 2013).

Group theorists have articulated different stages of group development. One of the most popular theories, first postulated by Tuckman in 1965, contains four stages as follows: forming, storming, norming, and performing. In the forming stage the group needs direction in defining tasks, goals, and objectives. Members are unclear regarding their respective roles in the group. This initial period can be chaotic and confusing. The next stage is storming. As the name connotes, there can be conflict, and indeed there must be conflict for the group to sort through issues such as leadership, power, and roles. Usually there is some willingness to accept the group goals and objectives, but there are still differences of opinion, competition for recognition, and attempts to influence the group. During the norming period, there is greater agreement on the task goals as the group develops cohesiveness and adjusts to the group and task. Finally, during the performing period, the members are thinking as one and willingly performing the task. There is camaraderie and team spirit as the group becomes self-managing (Hersey et al., 2013).

Members assume a variety of roles within the process of a group. Most are constructive in nature, contributing to the discussion, solving the problem, and achieving the group goals. These roles may be questioning, suggesting possibilities, taking notes, and summarizing the group's progress. However, some roles are not helpful. The most disruptive periods in group process are with intergroup dissonance and competition. It is at these levels that members may behave in roles that hinder group effectiveness, such as criticizing, attacking, or name-calling. The leader needs to intervene as appropriate with discussions of goals, standards, and feedback on behavior and progress for individuals or the group, depending on the situation. The degree to which roles are not helpful probably influences member satisfaction, and certainly interferes with communication and collaboration (Hersey et al., 2013). For example, using a generic team-based communication

TABLE 8.1 Four Parts of Nonviolent Communication (NVC)	
Clearly Expressing (Without Blaming or Criticizing)	**Empathetically Receiving (Without Hearing Blame or Criticism)**
1. Making an observation	1. What you observe
2. Expressing a feeling	2. How you feel based on your observation
3. Stating what you need	3. How you feel based on what you are hearing
4. Making a request (without demanding)	4. Hearing the request for an action to be taken

From Rosenberg, M.B. (2004). *We can work it out: Resolving conflicts peacefully and powerfully.* Encinitas, CA: Puddledancer Press.

model, Matzke et al. (2014) analyzed conversations between nurses and physicians. Their findings indicated that although about half of the conversations were considered collegial, communication was status-based rather than team-based. Status-based communications were described as patterns that allow an individual with more perceived power to be more forceful and directive in their communication toward other team members. Unfortunately, this autocratic style of communication does not support team building or promote good working relationships, and this can lead to preventable medical errors.

Research in small task group process has also revealed movement from an initial organization through a period of disorganization or chaos to reorganization at a level that achieves a goal. A group is defined as two or more people, and it exists to meet the needs of everyone in the group so that each will be satisfied. The leader's four major styles of communication used with task groups are similar to those for individuals (telling, selling, participating, and delegating). The process includes moving from defining, clarifying, and involving to empowering according to the leader's assessment of the readiness of the group (Hersey et al., 2013). The relationship styles of defining, clarifying, involving, and empowering suggest the highest probability of success for the manner in which the leader relates to the group.

TeamSTEPPS

The Agency for Healthcare Research and Quality (AHRQ) has collected data regarding patient safety over many years. They continue to show that communication problems are found to be the most common root causes of medical errors. After discovering the staggering number of preventable medical errors and recognizing that communication problems were cited as the number one contributor, the AHRQ partnered with the Department of Defense (DOD) and developed the Team STEPPS program (AHRQ, 2020).

TeamSTEPPS is an evidence-based, comprehensive education and training program designed to improve patient safety by eliminating preventable medical errors related to ineffective team communication. TeamSTEPPS stands for Team Strategies and Tools to Enhance Performance and Patient Safety. TeamSTEPPS has been adapted and implemented effectively in several health care settings and across numerous specialty areas. Much support exists in the literature documenting the

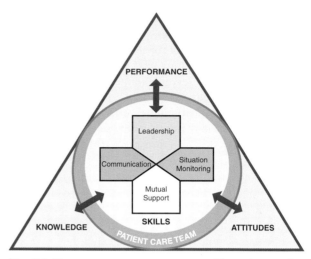

Fig. 8.3 Team competency outcomes. (From Agency for Healthcare Research and Quality. [2020]. *Pocket guide: TeamSTEPPS 2.0: Team Strategies & tools to enhance performance and patient safety.* Rockville, MD: AHRQ. https://www.ahrq.gov/sites/default/files/wysiwyg/professionals/education/curriculum-tools/teamstepps/instructor/essentials/pocketguide.pdf).

utility and effectiveness of TeamSTEPPS. The program consists of five key principles: team structure, leadership, situation monitoring, mutual support, and communication. Fig. 8.3   is a visual depiction of the five key principles of the TeamSTEPPS program. Extensive education and training programs are available on the AHRQ website.

SBAR and Handoff Communication

To address the "communication arm" of the TeamSTEPPS model pictured at the left side of Fig. 8.3, strategies such as SBAR have been created to enhance teamwork communication. One of the strategies that has been well documented and is familiar to nurses is SBAR, which stands for: Situation, Background, Assessment, and Recommendation. Fig. 8.4 demonstrates the four steps involved in SBAR. The SBAR tool provides members of the interprofessional team a great template to enhance communication such as framing conversations on a leadership agenda; framing email communication addressing specific concerns; or for more efficient communication with policymakers (Jurns, 2019).

Tiered daily huddles are becoming the norm in many hospitals and health systems. Hurle (2019),

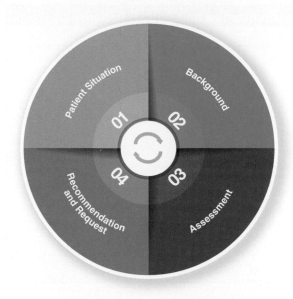

Fig. 8.4 Four steps in the SBAR process.

senior director of enterprise continuous improvement at Cleveland Clinic, built their tiered huddles upon existing practices focusing on patient safety and quality issues, caregiver safety issues, and providing access to care for their patients. They discovered that huddles needed to be smaller, connected, and standardized.

Midland (TX) Memorial Hospital holds daily leadership huddles in the hospital's lobby. These huddles helped drastically increase patient satisfaction, patient safety, and transformed a culture (Thrall, 2020). The huddle lasts no more than about 14 minutes, with information cascading to leaders shortly thereafter to share with employees in departments throughout the hospital.

Emory Healthcare in Georgia also has created leader standard work with tiered readiness huddles performing SMESS checks. SMESS communicates needs associated with Safety, Methods, Equipment, Supplies, and Staffing. Tier 1 Huddles are performed at the unit or department level engaging frontline employees. Unresolved issues or relevant information are escalated to Tier 2 Huddles, which are service line or division-based leaders. Unresolved issues or relevant information from Tier 2 are escalated using the same SMESS process in Tier 3 Huddles, which are organization-wide and include leaders from administration. As Emory Healthcare is a large

health care system, unresolved issues or relevant information is then escalated to Tier 5 Huddles, where senior members of Emory Healthcare lead these huddles to guide resolution for systems-related issues. Huddles improve communication and teamwork resulting in improved outcomes.

CURRENT COMMUNICATION ISSUES AND TRENDS

Teaching Communication

The Research Note at the end of the chapter highlights how important it is to teach team communication strategies. These may be such things as TeamSTEPPS, SBAR, NVC model, and others. There is a need to determine a theoretical and evidence-based approach to teaching communication. It is important that this approach be most effective in developing interpersonal, interprofessional, and intercultural communication skills to ensure that nurses have the highest probability of responding in an empathetic manner with patients in critical life situations. More of this teaching can be done in simulated environments with interprofessional teams. Clearly, communication content builds. Nurses work first on therapeutic communication and then progress to mastering communication as a leader (see Table 8.2).

Patient Privacy

A related concern for the management of information and communication is how to prevent breaches of patient confidentiality. *The Health Insurance Portability and Accountability Act* (HIPAA) provisions have heightened awareness about and presented strategies to protect patients' privacy and data security in health care transactions. For example, fax transmissions need to be secure, and security measures need to be taken to protect computerized databases and electronic transmissions. End-user encryption is commonly used for data security. Health care providers' actions that disseminate confidential information can harm patients. For example, some nurses are uncomfortable performing handover reporting at the patient's bedside because of the risks of sharing patient information where other persons may be within earshot. Discretion and sensitivity are best used in these situations. Systems, processes, and structures can be altered to protect patient privacy.

TABLE 8.2 **Practical Applications to Improve Communication and Build Relationships**	
Application	**Frequency**
1. Safety huddles	Every shift
2. Leadership rounds	Daily
3. Gemba walks	Daily
4. Newsletters (print or electronic)	Weekly/monthly
5. New employee experience (orientation) to receive foundational training and set expectations	Each orientation
6. Performance check-ins	Monthly
7. Professional governance (formal)	Monthly
8. CNO Advisory Councils (frontline staff and frontline nurse leaders)	Monthly
9. Mentoring/coaching	Monthly or as needed
10. CNO town hall meetings (live and virtual using technology)	Quarterly
11. Social media (e.g., Facebook, Yammer, LinkedIn, Twitter, Instagram)	Regularly

Adapted from Dent, B. (Fall 2019) Commentary: Communications. *Frontiers of Health Services Management, 36*(1), 2.

Communication in Emergencies

Communication effectiveness becomes crucial in times of emergency or disaster. In fact, often one of the key outcomes of disaster drills is to identify breaks in the communication system so they can be fixed before a real-time event occurs. TeamSTEPPS was developed to address communication issues between nurses and providers during critical patient events. Communication at these times must be impeccable. The AHRQ offers a plethora of team communication tools on their website for teams to practice and role-play so that they can be prepared to address issues efficiently during emergency situations.

Written Communication

The entire health care system relies on reliable, efficient tools and methods to produce timely and accurate patient documentation. The nursing profession, at the hub of the health care system, is called upon to produce the lion's share of the day-in, day-out documentation that exists in health care facilities. Proficiency and professionalism are imperative in all written documentation. Nurses need to have a command of the English language in order to produce written information that is useful and readable. Patient documentation is only one form of written communication needed by nursing staff. Promotions and awards in the profession are usually based on written documentation of performance and

outcomes endorsing an individual staff member. Grants and funds for projects are based upon extensive written proposals that address specific criteria. Quality improvement initiatives within a hospital can be awarded based on both written proposals and oral presentations, such as those making a business case for a clinically based initiative. Sharing information with colleagues is nurses' professional responsibility, such as by authoring textbooks and journals and providing expertise as peer reviewers and subject matter experts.

Electronic Communication and Social Media

With the advent of e-mail and explosion of social media and cell phones, the avenues of communication have changed. Health care systems have kept pace by developing extensive internal information technology (IT) departments that have engineered electronic medical records, secured e-mail servers for communication between patients and their providers, and developed numerous health care "apps." Electronic communication has assisted nurses in being better informed regarding patients. However, within the professional health care realm, there is a tendency to rely on these modes of communication when other methods would be preferable and more appropriate. For instance, there are definite times when a face-to-face conversation is preferred to an e-mail. Warrell (2012) noted that there are four times you should never use e-mail: (1) when you are angry, (2) when rebuking or criticizing, (3) if there is any chance your words could be misunderstood, or (4) when you are canceling or apologizing. In our busy professional lives, it is easier to send off a quick e-mail than to pick up the phone or walk down the hall; however, e-mail distances us from others and is really only the preferred means of communication when information is simply being conveyed. It is not appropriate for a back-and-forth dialogue where feelings need to be expressed and opinions heard.

Similarly, there is an appropriate use of texting, social media, Facebook, Twitter, and hashtags (#). However, this form of communication can be overused, making face-to-face conversations a thing of the past. Video chatting provides a nice way to have a conversation and actually see the person. There are several very good health care apps that have been produced for downloading on smartphones for free or at a fairly minimal cost. Some of these apps are very useful; some are a waste of time and money. The important thing to remember is to maintain professionalism and appropriate boundaries when using social media and to be judicious in what information is shared about yourself and others publicly. Many organizations have formal social media policies to help nurses navigate around what is appropriate for sharing on social media. Patient privacy, potential HIPAA violations, perceived bullying, and damage to reputations are major concerns.

RESEARCH NOTE

Source

Raley, J., Meenakshi, R., Dent, D., Willis, R., Lawson, K., & Duzinski, S. (2016). The role of communication during trauma activations: Investigating the need for team and leader communication training. *Journal of Surgical Education, 74*(1), 173–177.

Purpose

Fatal errors due to miscommunication among members of trauma teams are two to four times more likely to occur than in other medical teams, yet most trauma team members do not receive communication effectiveness training. The purpose of this study is to demonstrate that communication training is necessary and highlight specific team communication competencies that trauma teams should learn to improve communication during activations.

Study Design

Data were collected in two phases. Phase 1 required participants to complete a series of surveys. Phase 2 included live observations and assessments of pediatric trauma activations using the assessment of pediatric resuscitation team assessments (APRC-TA) and assessment of pediatric resuscitation leader assessments (APRC-LA). Data were collected at a southwestern pediatric hospital. Trauma team members and leaders completed surveys at a meeting and were observed while conducting activations in the trauma bay. Trained research scientists and clinical staff used the APRC-TA and APRC-LA to measure trauma teams' performance and communication effectiveness. The sample included 29 health care providers who regularly participate in trauma activations. Additionally, 12 live trauma activations were assessed.

Discussion

Findings from the study suggest that the medical performance and communication effectiveness of trauma teams seem to be linked. Accordingly, health care providers working in trauma settings have begun to verbalize their concerns about miscommunication between team members. Trauma team members who participated in the study believe communication training is important and necessary, and if given the chance, they would attend this type of training. Team communication training is associated with increases in group cohesion and decreases in communication errors. Nurses and providers believe that communication training may improve patient safety and reduce the number of errors made in emergency settings.

Application to Practice

Although this study focused on communication in a pediatric hospital during trauma activations, communication mishaps in health care settings continue to be a leading cause of patient safety events. Communication training for all teams may help build team cohesion, relationships built on trust, and improve outcomes associated with patient safety.

NEXT-GENERATION NCLEX® EXAMINATION-STYLE CASE STUDY

Nurse Manager Tyler has been in his job for 9 months in a busy academic medical center and is just beginning to settle in. He has noticed a spike in medication errors on the unit. It is difficult to manage health care providers' incoming orders as well as the confusion and complexity of multiple provider teams (e.g., neuro, cardiovascular, oncology) rounding independently and making medication and treatment changes that sometimes conflict. Tyler just got the latest data on his unit's quality and safety measures. The medication error rate has increased. He calls the Chair of the unit's Shared Governance Council (SGC) to help evaluate ideas to address communication breakdowns.

Which communication strategies will Tyler, the nurse manager, use to support effective communication interventions? **Select all that apply.**

_____ **A.** Confrontive communication style
_____ **B.** AHRQ's CUS assertive statements.
_____ **C.** Incident reporting
_____ **D.** Crucial Conversations
_____ **E.** Formal referral to immediate supervisor
_____ **F.** TeamSTEPPS SBAR

CRITICAL THINKING EXERCISE

You are the new nurse leader of a heart and vascular service line. You note the outcomes for this area are poor (e.g., patient experience, quality of care, labor expenses). Interprofessional relationships are strained. The equipment in the area needs to be updated. More than 75% of nurses are contract labor. The team has been unsuccessful in recruiting, leaving some RN requisitions open for up to 2 years. However, you are asked by the senior leaders to accommodate adding additional cardiovascular providers and position your team for growth.

1. What are your priorities for this area as the new nurse leader?
2. What communication strategies would you use with your team?
3. Using the SBAR tool, describe how you would communicate requests to the CNO and other members of the senior leadership team, as needed.

REFERENCES

Agency for Healthcare Research and Quality (AHRQ). (2020). *TeamSTEPPS*. Rockville, MD: AHRQ. https://www.ahrq.gov/teamstepps/index.html.

Aguilar, A. (2019). Culture of silence contributes to lack of progress on patient safety. *Modern Healthcare, 49*(44), 34.

American Nurses Association (ANA). (2015). *Incivility, bullying, and workplace violence. ANA Position Statement.* https://www.nursingworld.org/practice-policy/nursing-excellence/official-position-statements/id/incivility-bullying-and-workplace-violence/.

American Nurses Association (ANA). (2020). *What is nursing?* https://www.nursingworld.org/practice-policy/workforce/what-is-nursing/.

American Nurses Credentialing Center (ANCC). (2020). *Magnet model.* https://www.nursingworld.org/organizational-programs/magnet/magnet-model/.

Bennet, M. J. (2013). *Intercultural communication.* https://www.idrinstitute.org/resources/intercultural-communication/.

Berwick, D. M. (2009). What 'patient-centered' should mean: Confessions of an extremist. *Health Affairs – Web Exclusive.* https://www.healthaffairs.org/doi/pdf/10.1377/hlthaff.28.4.w555.

Carman, K., Dardess, P., Maurer, M., Sofaer, S., Adams, K., Bechtel, C., et al. (2013). Patient and family engagement: A framework for understanding the elements and developing interventions and policies. *Health Affairs, 32*(2), 223–231.

Covey, S. R. (2004). *The 8th habit: From effectiveness to greatness.* New York: Free Press.

Dent, B., & Tye, J. (2018). *The heart of a nurse leader: Values based leadership for healthcare organizations.* Monee, IL: Joe Tye and Bob Dent.

Dent, B. (Fall 2019). Commentary: Communications. *Frontiers of Health Services Management, 36*(1), 2.

Fitzgerald, C., & Kirby, L. K. (1997). *Developing leaders: Research and applications in psychological type and leadership development.* Palo Alto, CA: Davies-Black Publishing.

Fooks, C., Obarski, G., Hale, L., & Hylmar, S. (2015). The patient experience in Ontario 2020: What is possible? *Healthcare Papers, 14*(4), 8–18.

Foronda C. L., Alhusen J., Budhathoki C., Lamb M., Tinsley K., MacWilliams B., et al. (2015). A mixed-methods, international, multisite study to develop and validate a measure of nurse-to-physician communication in simulation. *Nursing Education Perspectives, 36*(6), 383–388.

Frampton, S. B., Guastello, S., Hoy, L., Naylor, M., Sheridan, S., & Johnston-Fleece, M. (2017). Harnessing evidence and experience to change culture: A guiding framework for patient and family engaged care. *National Academy of Medicine Perspectives, 7*. https://doi.org/10.31478/201701f.

Hersey, P., Blanchard, K., & Johnson, D. (2013). *Management of organizational behavior: Leading human resources* (10th ed.). Upper Saddle River, NJ: Pearson Education.

Hurle, N. (2019). How we improved our tiered daily huddles. *The Lean Post.* https://www.lean.org/LeanPost/Posting.cfm?LeanPostId=1095.

Institute of Medicine (IOM). (2001). *To err is human: Building a safer health system.* Washington, DC: National Academies Press (pp. 40).

Institute of Medicine (IOM). (2011). *The future of nursing: Leading change, advancing health.* Washington, DC: National Academies Press.

Jurns, C. (2019). Using SBAR to communicate with policymakers. *The Online Journal of Issues in Nursing, 24*(1). https://doi.org/10.3912/OJIN.Vol24No01PPT47.

Kotter, J. (1996). *Leading change.* Boston, MA: Harvard Business School Press.

Kouzes, J. M., & Posner, B. Z. (2017). *The leadership challenge: How to make extraordinary things happen in organizations* (6th ed.). Hoboken, NJ: John Wiley & Sons, Inc.

Matzke, B., Houston, S., Fischer, U., & Bradshaw, M. J. (2014). Using a team-centered approach to evaluate effectiveness of nurse-physician communications. *JOGNN: Journal of Obstetric, Gynecologic & Neonatal Nursing, 43*(6), 684–694. https://doi.org/10.1111/1552-6909.12486.

Maxfield, D., Grenny, J., Lavandero, R., & Groah, L. (n.d.). *The silent treatment: Why safety tools and checklists aren't enough to save lives.* http://www.silenttreatmentstudy.com/silencekills/.

Maxfield, D., Harmon, H., & McDonald, C. (2010). Crucial conversations for motivating colleagues and patients. *American Nurse Today, 5*(5), 16–18.

McAllen, E. R., Stephens, K., Swanson-Biearman, B., Kerr, K., & Whiteman, K. (2018). Moving shift report to the bedside: An evidence-based quality improvement project. *The Online Journal of Issues in Nursing, 23*(2). https://doi.org/10.3912/OJIN.Vol23No02PPT22.

Mosadeghrad, A. M., & Mojbafan, A. (2019). Conflict and conflict management in hospitals. *International Journal of Health Care Quality Assurance, 32*(3), 550–561.

Nicotera, A., Mahon, M., & Wright, K. (2014). Communication that builds teams: Assessing a nursing conflict intervention. *Nursing Administration Quarterly, 38*(3), 248–260.

Pater, R. (2016). Preventing strained communications. *Occupational Health & Safety, 85*(8), 50.

Patterson, K., Grenny, J., McMillan, R., & Switzler, A. (2011). *Crucial conversations: Tools for talking when stakes are high* (2nd ed.). New York, NY: McGraw-Hill Education.

Plonien, C. (2015). Using personality indicators to enhance nurse leader communication. *AORN Journal, 102*(1), 74–80.

Pryse, Y., McDaniel, A., & Schafer, J. (2014). Psychometric analysis of two new scales: The Evidence-Based Practice Nursing Leadership and Work Environment Scales. *Worldviews on Evidence-Based Nursing, 11*(4), 240–247.

R³ Report. (2011). *Requirement, rationale, reference.* The Joint Commission (pp. 2). February 9, 2011. https://www.jointcommission.org/-/media/tjc/documents/standards/r3-reports/r3-report-issue-1-20111.pdf on March 9, 2020.

Raley, J., Meenakshi, R., Dent, D., Willis, R., Lawson, K., & Duzinski, S. (2016). The role of communication during trauma activations: Investigating the need for team and leader communication training. *Journal of Surgical Education, 74*(1), 173–177.

Rosenberg, M. B. (2004). *We can work it out: Resolving conflicts peacefully and powerfully.* Encinitas, CA: Puddledancer Press.

Sharifabad, M. A. M., Ardakani, M. F., Bahrami, M. A., & Fallahzadeh, H. (2019). Nurses' communication skills and the quality of inpatient services from patients' viewpoints. *Medical Science, 23*(96), 163–167.

Sears, M. (2010). *Humanizing health care: Creating cultures of compassion with nonviolent communication.* Encinitas, CA: Puddledancer Press.

Spears, T. L. (2019). *The four conversations you must get right as a leader.* American Association for Physician Leadership. https://www.physicianleaders.org/news/the-four-conversations-leader.

The Joint Commission. (2015). *Sentinel event statistics released for 2014.* Joint Commission Online. April 29, 2015. https://www.jointcommission.org/-/media/deprecated-unorganized/imported-assets/tjc/system-folders/joint-commission-online/jconline_april_29_15pdf.pdf?db=web&hash=DEFFBC41623A360F1C1428A5E9602773.

Thrall, T. H. (2020). How a 14-minute meeting transformed this hospital. *Hospitals & Health Networks*: Advisory Board Daily Briefing. March 15, 2016, republished on January 10, 2020. https://www.advisory.com/daily-briefing/2016/03/15/14-minutes.

Tri-Council for Nursing. (2017). *Tri-Council for nursing issues proclamation on nursing civility*. http://www.nln.org/docs/default-source/newsroom/tri-council-civility-proclamation-draft-2-krk-bm-tri-092617.pdf?sfvrsn=2.

Tuckman, B. W. (1965). Developmental sequence in small groups. *Psychological Bulletin, 63*(6), 384–399. https://doi.org/10.1037/h0022100.

Tye, J., & Dent, B. (2017). *Building a culture of ownership in healthcare: The invisible architecture of core values, attitude, and self-empowerment*. Indianapolis, IN: Sigma Theta Tau International.

Warrell, M. (2012, August 27). Hiding behind email? Four times you should never use email. *Forbes*. http://www.forbes.com/sites/margiewarrell/2012/08/27/do-you-hide-behind-email/#dc8f0e97bf00.

Workplace Bullying Institute (WBI). (2019). *WBI—the Workplace Bullying Institute*. https://www.workplacebullying.org/.

Yang, Y. (2012). Studies of transformational leadership in consumer service: Leadership trust and the mediating-moderating role of cooperative conflict management. *Psychological Reports, 110*(1), 315–337.

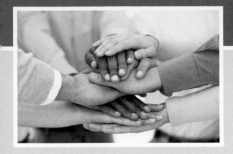

9

Team Building and Working With Effective Groups

Sandra Lynne Swearingen

ⓔ http://evolve.elsevier.com/Huber/leadership

Nurse leaders in today's health care organizations must be skilled communicators, collaborators, and facilitators with an exquisite ability to lead the collective work of individuals. At times they will serve as a leader for a team or group, and at other times they will serve as a member. Being capable of both leading and following are essential skills for nurses. A significant percentage of work completed in organizations today is done through the collaborative efforts of different types of teams or work groups. There is an even greater emphasis on shared leadership in nursing, as well as in working with other health care professionals as part of an interdisciplinary or multidisciplinary team. Understanding the characteristics of teams, groups, and the basic principles for attaining successful outcomes increases the leader's effectiveness.

Health care leaders recognize that an interdisciplinary, team-based approach is essential for high-quality, patient-centered, coordinated, and effective health care. Teamwork allows for greater exchange of information, ideas, and problem-solving to address the complex issues of health care. Engaging teams in this process allows for diverse points of view, creativity, innovation, and an enhanced ability to adapt to continuous or sudden change. The health care environment continues to evolve at an unprecedented rate with new specialized knowledge, scientific and technological advances, and redesign of care processes. A high degree of specialization exists, even within a profession. The nursing profession, for example, includes individuals with a variety of different roles, including direct care registered nurses, clinical nurse leaders, licensed practical nurses, nurse practitioners, clinical nurse specialists, nurse educators, nurse midwives, and nurse anesthetists. Establishing

effective teamwork across various specialties within and across professions is key to interdisciplinary collaboration to address and adapt to the constant state of change in health care.

The ability to collaborate is essential for optimal patient outcomes. The focus of health care organizations today is to achieve the Institute of Health Care Improvement's (IHI, 2016) Triple Aim. The goal is "simultaneously improving the health of the population, enhancing the experience and outcomes of the patient, and reducing per capita cost of care for the benefit of communities." This Triple Aim has been expanded to a fourth "Quadruple Aim" workforce element of improving the experience of providing care (Sikka et al., 2015). The shift in payment methodologies from fee-for-service to value-based purchasing and accountable care has created incentives and penalties for organizations to improve quality, efficiency, and the overall value of health care. The expectation for health care leaders is to continuously improve while delivering safe, high-quality patient care. Changing reimbursement methodologies, increasing governmental regulation, and managing care across the continuum require a high level of engagement between clinical disciplines, non-clinical staff, and senior management. Just as in other industries, rapid information dissemination and the shift to a knowledge worker–based service society are some of the social and economic forces operative in health care. These forces converge to create the tumultuous change currently underway in health care delivery. Teamwork is the solution.

Employees who work in a collaborative manner with others and who can work effectively within a team context can provide the strength, structure, and resiliency to deal with work complexities and changes. Today's health care organizations are considered *learning organizations*, and there is a renewed emphasis on the role of teams. Just as interdisciplinary teams play an important role in delivering mental health, home care, rehabilitation, hospice, and other community-based services, hospitals and large health care systems engage teams as an essential element of their core processes and structure. This is the general way now that business gets done in all health care settings. The Institute of Medicine (IOM, now called the National Academies of Sciences, Engineering, and Medicine, Health and Medicine Division) suggested that working as part of an interdisciplinary team is an essential core competency of health care professionals and that professionals cooperate, collaborate, communicate, and integrate care in teams to be sure that care is continuous and reliable (Altman et al., 2016).

Because health care professionals are specialists, it is incumbent on leaders to bring people together in groups and teams to build on their knowledge and strengths and ultimately to ensure safe, effective care. Leaders have an ever-increasing role to ensure that teams are effective, efficient, and productive. In their book *The wisdom of teams: Creating the high-performance organization*, Katzenbach and Smith (2015) claimed that teams should be the basic unit of organization for most businesses as a way to reach the highest levels of performance.

Team building is a strategy for designing, implementing, developing, and nurturing work teams in organizations. These work teams are a specialized subset of the many types of groups that form or are formed in organizations.

In nursing, group process theory relates to both how to be therapeutic with clients and how to work as an employee within an organization, which is often large and complex. Nursing has an integral role as a member of the health care team. As a caregiver, the nurse serves a key role as a patient advocate and frequently serves as the coordinator of care with other members of the team. The nurse tracks whether different interventions have been effective or whether alternative strategies might be needed. As a care provider spending significant time with the patient, often a nurse will see fine, distinct changes in a patient's condition before other members of the health care team. Nurses oversee the plan of care and are involved more intimately and more proximately than any of the other health care providers in managing the total health care of the patient. Therefore understanding and developing skills in group process and group dynamics is essential within the context of leadership and management in nursing because of the group functioning and coordinative aspects of nursing practice. Equally important is the nurse's role in coordinating multidisciplinary and interdisciplinary teams. Because care is complex and involves the expertise of many disciplines, nurses need strong group process and interaction skills to communicate clearly and collaborate effectively with a variety of colleagues.

DEFINITIONS

A **group** is defined as any collection of interconnected individuals working together for some purpose. Groups are important in organizations, not only because of informal network dynamics, but also because of the multitude of formal committees, task forces, councils, and teams in the contemporary organization. A **committee** is a relatively stable and formally composed group. Committees are a specific type of group in that they are stable, meet periodically, and have an identified purpose that is part of the organizational structure. There is a mechanism for maintaining and selecting members. Typically, committees have official status and sanction within an organization. For example, there are policy and procedure committees, quality and patient safety committees, and ethics committees.

A **task force** is a temporary group of individuals formed to carry out a specific mission or project. Task forces may solve a problem that requires a multidisciplinary approach. A **council** is an advisory group of individuals who may be elected or appointed and that has a defined charter or purpose and meets regularly. In a nursing professional shared governance model, the councilor structure is commonplace. Councils promote collegiality and engagement. Nursing may have unit practice councils, a hospital practice council, and a leadership council, as well as specific areas of focus, such as a nursing research council or education council.

Collaboration is defined as people undertaking harmonizing roles and jointly working to share responsibility for problem-solving and decision-making to formulate and carry out plans (Baggs & Schmitt, 1998; Christensen & Larson, 1993). It is a complex phenomenon that brings together two or more individuals, often from different professional disciplines, who work to achieve shared aims and objectives such as working together toward a common goal for the patient.

Communication is a process by which information is exchanged between individuals through a common system of symbols, signs, or behavior (Merriam-Webster, 2019). It includes the style and extent of interactions both among members and between members and those outside the team. It also refers to the way flows of conflict, decision-making, and day-to-day interactions occur.

Team building is defined as the process of deliberately creating and unifying a group into a functioning team. A **team** is made up of persons working on individual tasks that impact the overall objectives of the group. Team members need to collaborate with each other to combine individual tasks into a cohesive product that meets the goals of the team (Turner et al., 2018). Genuine communication is also a requirement of information exchanges within the team (Kayser, 2011). Finally, if a team is to remain effective in an ever-evolving, complex environment, it also needs to be adaptable (Kozlowski & Ilgen, 2006). Teams are interdependent, with shared responsibility to achieve their goals and for their successes or failures. Teams have the authority to coordinate activities and tasks; team members may have defined roles, duties, or responsibilities.

In today's workplace culture, working in a team is imperative to the success of many health care organizations. Teams tend to demonstrate synergy and therefore make better decisions as a group than as singular individuals. In addition, due to increasing technology, one individual cannot be an expert in all work processes. Health care workers are made up of many experts from many fields and occupations. Each of these team members may have expertise that is beyond the scope of one manager (Belker et al., 2019).

The distinction between a work group and a true team is crucial. Health care leaders may mistakenly assume that simply calling a group a *team* actually makes it a team. As Katzenbach and Smith (2015) emphasized, the group becomes a true team only by doing its collective work. The team goes through a developmental process that takes time and the investment of energy to materialize. Many collective entities in today's organizations are called *teams* yet clearly function more as work groups than true teams.

A **work group** is a collection of individuals who are charged with completing a specific activity or mission. Work groups come together to share information and ideas, and they may make some decisions mutually. However, the members of the work group have individual work products for which they are responsible, and these consume their major focus and effort. For example, in a patient care unit, the unit clerk has certain responsibilities, as do the charge nurse, direct care nurse, and nurse manager. The boundaries remain clearly separated when the collective entity is a work group. Each person may view their role as being individually accountable, but there is little to no collective accountability.

This is in contrast with a true team, which is a collective entity where leadership rotates and is shared by various members of the team, depending on appropriateness and fit of skills and abilities. In a true team, there are collective work products, for example, the provision of quality patient care to all patients housed in the department or seen in the clinic. There is group as well as individual accountability. If one member of the team is having a problem, it is not just that individual's problem; instead it becomes a team problem for all members of the team to pull together to resolve. An example of team thinking is "No one sits down until we can all sit down" or "No one goes home until we all go home." If quality outcomes are difficult for one team member, all team members are affected by this and become engaged in helping the affected team member meet expectations. In the management book *The goal* (Goldratt & Cox, 2016), the author tells a parable about taking a Boy Scout troop on a hike. When it was discovered that Scout Herbie was slowing the whole group down, the weight in his backpack was redistributed, and the troop sped up. This is how a high-performing team works.

BACKGROUND

Group interactions are a pervasive element of the health care environment in which nurses work. A basic understanding of groups helps nurses function more effectively. These principles apply to any group, whether an actual team, a committee, task force, council, or an informal group effort. Team effectiveness has nine core processes composed of the following elements (Turner et al., 2018):

- *Coaching:* The establishment of goals and behaviors in order to accomplish the team's work. This includes any activity performed individually and collaboratively for team effectiveness. It also includes person-to-person interactions that assist in the synchronization and utilization of resources in accomplishing the work of the team.

- *Cognition:* The ability of team members to mutually understand the task of the team. This includes the ability to make appropriate judgments, solve problems, incorporate information, forecast, and acquire information.
- *Cohesiveness:* The degree to which members of the team desire to remain in the team and meet the goals of the team. Feeling that they fit in the team and identify with the group are important to cohesiveness in the group.
- *Collective efficacy:* The team is capable, competent, and empowered to meet the team's goals successfully.
- *Collective identity:* A person's sense of being an individual is replaced by being a team member.
- *Communication:* The process by which people share information within the team. Communication should allow for the mutual exchange of information.
- *Conflict:* Any perceived incompatibility of opinions, benefits, or principles held by team members that are perceived threatening to other members of the team.
- *Cooperation:* Involves the group members working together towards a common goal. It is a structure where the success of one person improves the chances of success of the group.
- *Coordination:* Includes the progressive composition of codependent actions that impact the team's goals. Coordination also references the team's ability to use assets and turn tasks into desired outcomes of the team.

Marks et al. (2001) presented a taxonomy of team processes categorized into three different phases: the transition phase, the action phase, and the interpersonal phase.

- *Transition phase:* This is the phase when team members distribute duties, schedule actions, and allocate assets needed to meet the goals of the team. Three identified processes take place during this phase: mission analysis, goal specification, and strategy formation.
- *Action phase:* This phase pertains to activities relating to the attainment of established goals. There are four processes that take place in the action phase: monitoring goal progress, monitoring systems, monitoring

the team itself, and activities that coordinate the work of the team.

- *Interpersonal phase:* This phase is about relationships between team members and other stakeholders. This is a phase that is typically present throughout the duration of the team and includes three processes: controlling conflict within the group, building the confidence and drive of the team members, and facilitation of emotive equilibrium between team members.

WHY GROUPS ARE FORMED

In nursing, the formation of groups occurs primarily for one of two reasons: (1) to provide a personal or professional socialization and exchange forum, or (2) to provide a mechanism for interdependent work accomplishment. Groups can be social, professional, or organizational in purpose. The following are some reasons why groups would be established in organizations:

- Group activities can create a sense of status and esteem, allowing an individual to be part of something bigger themselves.
- Groups allow an individual to test and establish reality.
- Groups allow engagement of individuals with leaders to share responsibility, decision-making, and accountability for outcomes.
- Groups function as a mechanism for individuals to work collectively and cooperatively to get a job done.
- Groups address complex problems or tasks by a diverse group of individuals with specialized knowledge and/or skill.
- Groups can maximize leaders' strengths and minimize their weaknesses.

A major part of the working environment of nurses is accomplishment of work through group activity. The work group provides an institutional and professional identity for an individual nurse, and work groups become a focus for interpersonal relationships, support, and social integration. Job satisfaction, positive relational leadership, and positive quality outcomes are linked (Wong et al., 2013). Factors related to job satisfaction include working conditions, job stress, role conflict and ambiguity, role perception, role content, and organizational and professional commitment (Lu et al., 2012). In addition, being part of a healthy group or team is related to the level of organizational commitment by the team member. Cultural issues that become barriers to effective teamwork and communication include workplace discrimination, bullying, fear of discipline, lack of feedback, and strong hierarchical models (Teunissen et al., 2020). Individuals with an emotional connection to their work group have lower levels of turnover and higher levels of engagement (Manion, 2009).

Work groups can be disrupted by factors such as downsizing, reorganization, absenteeism, loss of leadership, bullying, and turnover. Work group disruption has been linked to negative outcomes (Kalisch & Lee, 2010). In a study of four hospitals, interpersonal relations were found to be an important part of nurses' job satisfaction. Interpersonal relationships are integral to work group functioning. Things get done because of relationships among people. Nurses need to build successful collaborative relationships among multiple levels of intra- and interdisciplinary colleagues, other members of the organization, and patients. The level of nursing teamwork has been found to be directly linked to missed nursing care (Kalisch & Lee, 2010).

One vulnerable group of nurses are new graduates. There has been extensive research suggesting that workplace bullying occurs particularly with new graduates. Read and Laschinger (2013) found the sense of community and similarity between the ideals and beliefs of the nurses within a work unit affected the perception of bullying. Some of the job characteristics related to workplace bullying include workload, job control, reward, and recognition. Budin et al. (2013) found that support from their leader or a mentor had an impact on the likelihood of a new graduate being a victim of bullying. Bullying may affect trust, communication, and cohesiveness in a group. Furthermore, informal work group norms exert a strong influence on nurses' behavior and functioning within a group. Nurse residency programs for new graduate nurses are an antidote.

Work group relationships can reinforce behaviors and rationalization, thus leading to deviant behaviors such as workarounds that become passively or actively accepted. Debono et al. (2013) conducted an extensive literature search of studies concerning nurse workaround behaviors. There were several themes related to teamwork. First, workarounds may be individual or supported by a group who share the belief that rules are "flexible." When that is the case, there is also an understanding of who will and will not perform a workaround. Second, nurses may justify working around policies and procedures as necessary to benefit the patient. Finally, acceptance or proliferation of workarounds

can be affected by a variety of factors, including group norms, leadership, professional structures, personal relationships, and organizational culture. A culture of innovativeness can be fostered as a fixing and reporting method for broken processes or systems failures so that there are more permanent and precise solutions to workarounds (Huber et al., 2019).

Clearly, there is a strong relationship between work groups, interpersonal relationships, leadership, and outcomes such as nurses' behaviors and perceptions. Work group relationships are a powerful mechanism influencing both good and bad outcomes in nursing practice.

ADVANTAGES OF GROUPS

Groups have the potential for being a driving force for change in an organization. Ronco (2005) identified positive impacts groups can have on an organization:

1. *Synergy:* Groups have potential to perform at higher levels than an individual would on their own.
2. *Positive individual impacts:* Groups have potential to improve every member of the group or at least help each one reach their highest potential.
3. *Motivation:* Groups have potential to motivate their individual members and provide encouragement, constructive criticism, and praise.
4. *Diverse thinking:* Groups have potential to engage in diverse thinking, thereby identifying problems that might otherwise go unnoticed or ignored and exploring solutions.
5. *Linkage to the larger organization:* Groups have potential to make individuals feel more connected to the larger organization.

Working as a team has advantages over working alone relative to solving problems. The main benefit of teamwork is it allows organizations to achieve goals that individuals working alone cannot. This is due to inherent advantages built into teamwork such as (Lumen Learning, 2020):

1. *Increased efficiency.* By combining the skills of individuals, the work effort is increased, allowing the team to accomplish more than an individual can.
2. *Speed.* Since there are many contributors in a team effort, tasks and activities are completed more rapidly.
3. *Reflection in ideas.* Different people have different ideas and perceptions of an issue. Combining such differences can achieve previously unidentified solutions.

4. *Superior effectiveness.* Teams work together and divide the work at hand. Through harmonization of tasks and efforts the work is shared out to better address issues.

5. *Social aspects.* Teamwork improves the work experience for individual team members because they receive support and assistance when they work on mutual tasks. This type of support helps people achieve normally unattainable goals. This also leads to team members having a greater sense of achievement.

Groups are one vehicle for creative problem-solving, stimulating innovation, and building consensus. To be successful, the leader must be skilled at facilitation, ensuring meetings have a clear purpose and are organized, focused, and productive, with balanced participation by team members. An effective meeting will start and finish on time and result in a balanced discussion of pros and cons on a topic or issue, with required next steps, actions, follow-up, and specific member assignments and accountabilities. These practices demonstrate the leader's organizational skills and respect for contributions by all team members and their time. It is imperative that there is a clearly defined purpose for a group, particularly when the group is part of a larger organization. Ideally this is an early discussion by the group and is determined with input from all members. The purpose and value of the group needs to be evaluated periodically in addition to evaluating whether the team is meeting its goals. Is it functional? Is it accomplishing the task to which it was assigned or committed? If not, should the group be disbanded or reorganized?

When the work output of any group is analyzed, meetings can be costly endeavors. For example, when the number of hours spent by all committee members is multiplied by their individual hourly salary along with fringe benefit costs, the sum of costs for the group may be astounding. This is one reason for paying attention to how well the group is functioning. Just as important is assessing whether the group adds value to the organization and the individuals involved. If team members are not actively contributing to the group's charge, their role and time on the team may be wasted energy, resulting in a drain on enthusiasm and effectiveness in the group. The cost of group work can be balanced by calculating benefits such as increased productivity or risk/cost avoidance.

A highly functioning group may have a profound impact on an organization. Such groups often identify and solve complex problems. Participation and involvement in a group decision typically results in individuals being more engaged and committed to a decision, even if there is disagreement. Disagreement and conflict are important elements for the leader to guide teams through and are often productive factors in solving problems. In this way, leaders of teams can demonstrate effective means of resolving differences, which are commonplace in health care.

DISADVANTAGES OF GROUPS

Ronco (2005) identified six potential negative impacts groups can have on an organization, including negativity, passivity, individual focus, groupthink, vocal minority, and the ethical dark side. A seventh is disruptive conflicts.

1. *Negativity:* Research suggests that people working in groups tend to be more negative than if they work individually.

2. *Passivity:* People may become passive participants in a group versus being active participants. Unbalanced participation may lead to feelings of resentment, jealousy, and disillusionment. Some may "slide by" on the work effort of others.

3. *Individual focus and individual domination:* Individuals may have difficulty thinking globally and objectively. They may focus on how a discussion affects them as an individual instead of as a group. Some individuals may also dominate the group, compromising group process. Strong opinions of group members may stifle discussion, creativity, and innovation. As a result, the group or leader may need to divert its energy and productivity into working out interpersonal dynamics rather than moving forward on the group's task.

4. *Groupthink:* Groups may reach quick agreement and be unwilling to challenge or debate. Sometimes decisions result from pressure—by the group, leader, or external deadlines—to complete the work. Groups may influence individual members when most of the group feels a certain way about an issue or task. Minority group members, who may disagree, experience an element of pressure due to psychological dynamics related to subtle pressure for group acceptance and conformity. Creative and innovate ideas may be lost if a group reaches decisions too quickly.

5. *Vocal minority:* Groups tend to allow the most vocal members of a group to represent overall group views even when they are the minority of members. It may be difficult to be a devil's advocate or to adopt the role of bringing alternative critique points to the group for consideration due to a concern about not being socially accepted or fear of conflict. For example, derision and humiliation can occur if members react negatively.

6. *Ethical dark side:* Groups have potential, based on power in the group, to not support ethical choices.

7. *Disruptive conflicts:* If people perceive an adverse effect on a group member or if they feel threatened, conflict emerges. Conflicts can accelerate in a competitive environment when members vest in their own position and are not willing to consider a different point of view. Conflicts about substantive issues actually help the group become more effective in decision-making. However, when conflicts occur over differences in personality, opinions, or values, conflicts can become destructive. Interdisciplinary teams may experience conflict due to team instability or differences in personal and professional priorities (Teunissen et al., 2020). Although it may seem contradictory, conflicts can serve as a control mechanism in a group and may result in far superior outcomes. When group members are comfortable respectfully disagreeing with each other, a premature acceptance of decisions can be avoided since opposing viewpoints are considered.

GROUP DECISION-MAKING

Group work can be—and typically is—a slow process. It takes more time for a group to arrive at a decision than for one person to make the decision.

In addition, a continuum of decision-making power may be vested in a group (Fig. 9.1). A group or committee has certain powers, tasks, and functions, and also certain parameters or latitude in terms of how far to go in deciding. Decision power is a matter of degree, with four distinct points on the continuum of authority for decision-making: authoritative, consultative, joint, and delegated.

On one end of the continuum is *authoritative decision-making*, where the leader makes the decision. In this process there is input, perhaps, but not necessarily a vote. One example of this is in some medical emergencies, such as cardiac arrest: there is no time for discussion, and the leader needs to take control and direct the team. Authoritative style is generally ineffective in non-emergencies because it can generate increased cynicism and employee disengagement.

Consultative decision-making occurs when decisions involve employee participation, but the leader still makes the final decision. Group members may make certain recommendations, to the leader, chairperson, or head of the group, who will make the final decision. There is increased participation in this type of procedure, but the ultimate decision is not under the control of group members. Consultative decision-making is used in nursing with task forces, quality committees, and shared governance councils.

Some decision procedures result in *joint decision-making*. In this approach, the entire group makes a decision by a two-thirds vote, simple majority, consensus, or some other process. In a joint decision procedure, team members have as much influence as the leader. The leader has one voice, one vote. The leader can use persuasion, but when it comes to the final vote, the leader's vote is equivalent to that of any other group member. This is fundamentally different from the leader making the decision with group input. This type of decision-making is used in a high functioning multidisciplinary team. Every team member is heard and valued equally. In nursing, individual unit and hospital councils may

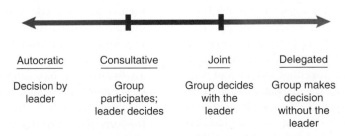

Fig. 9.1 Range of decision powers.

have authority to implement certain decisions related to clinical practice.

At the other end of the decision-making continuum is a *delegated decision procedure*. This occurs when the committee chair or leader allows participants to make the final decision. For example, establishment of a self-directed work team for the purpose of self-scheduling involves decision delegation. The leader may set up basic parameters to follow, such as ensuring an appropriate number of staff by role and experience for a shift or for the entire schedule before it is released. In nursing, many leaders use self-scheduling to engage the team and allow for flexibility in scheduling. The true test of delegation decision-making is whether the leader overrides the followers' decision. Technically, the leader would not have authority to veto or override unless he or she determined the decision made would compromise safety or organizational well-being. For example, new legal mandates supersede group decision-making. If it is truly a delegation situation, the leader would go forward with the approach that the decision is the group's choice. The group then becomes accountable for outcomes and is responsible for resolving any issues. Hersey et al. (2013) labeled these same four procedures as *authoritative, consultative, facilitative*, and *delegative* decision-making styles.

It is advisable for followers in any group to determine who has authority to make decisions. Knowledge about the type of group and the delegation or decision-making to be anticipated is critical to participation. A leadership or conflict moment may occur when a group assumes that they have the authority to make decisions, but the leader disagrees. Clarity before beginning work on an issue prevents unnecessary conflict and augments productivity. However, group members and leaders need to become skilled and comfortable in handling interpersonal dynamics.

Group decision-making may be time consuming. The leader needs to be skilled at allowing appropriate amounts of discussion to occur, ensuring that varying opinions are presented before a decision is made. A decision can be derailed if the leader is not skilled at facilitation, does not have a clear purpose for meeting, or is disorganized, unfocused, or allows unbalanced participation or discussion. Meetings that do not start and finish on time show a lack of respect for participants. When there is limited discussion of pros and cons of a topic or issue, members of the group may feel disenfranchised and limit their attendance or participation.

Leaders need to be skilled at ensuring there is equal participation and ideas and suggestions by all group members are considered. Group members and leaders need to become skilled and comfortable in handling interpersonal dynamics, including conflict.

TEAM BUILDING

There are five stages of team development as defined by Newell and Kirkwood (2020): (1) Forming: This is where ground rules are assessed, set, and discussed by the group. The team begins to gather information about goals in this stage. (2) Storming: This is a period of conflict with and between team members as they work to understand their positions in the team. This stage ends when the team members can agree about issues and resolve conflict. (3) Norming: The team comes together and begins building cohesion between members. The team also agrees about established norms for the group. (4) Performing: The team begins to produce work. This is where the generation and application of problem-solving skills to problems identified in earlier stages is completed. (5) Adjournment is when the team completes their goals and disengages/breaks up the team.

Teams use processes to function. There are different views of ways to study the processes of a team. Einola and Alvesson (2019) discussed three processes often used in the study of teams:

1. *Entity-based process view.* In this view, the team process is seen as the logic applied to explain the relationships or actions of individuals or organizations. The concepts of this process are things such as verbal interactions, alliance building, dispute management, and the sorting of inputs and outputs. Team process is seen as a linear, input-process-outcome framework. This process view also coincides with the form, storm, norm, and perform model.

2. *Dynamic entity-based process view.* In this model, the process is focused on a flow in which entities (team members) travel. The focus is still on input-process-outcome, but the frameworks are more robust and profound. Team processes are categorized as transition, action, or interpersonal processes; these groups are further split into subprocesses. It is felt that this view focuses on structure, function, and how stages follow each other in the team process. Outcomes from one stage are often seen as inputs for successive stages.

3. *Fluid process view.* This view is one where the interest focuses on how teams came to be, are reproduced, how they adapt to the environment, and how stable they are. Under fluid process view a team is not a given entity, but just a possibility. Teams under fluid process view are partial, fragile, shifting, inconsistent, or stable (stable in this view is a temporary state and not a fixed state or definitive outcome). This view is about situational sensemaking (turning complex and confusing situations into something understandable) and relationships in the team. Process refers more to the process of being the team based on team interactions that shift experiences and meanings.

WORKING WITH TEAMS

In health care, multidisciplinary and interdisciplinary care teams are necessary for survival. Teamwork affects clinical performance, and team training is an effective strategy for improving patient safety. Implementation strategies and organizational conditions matter (Salas & Rosen, 2013). Organizational design principles and management approaches that strive to prevent patient injury and improve quality include use of high-reliability theory. High-reliability health care organizations are characterized by an organizational commitment to safety, redundancy of processes, safety measures, and an organizational culture for continuous learning (Riley et al., 2010). These organizations provide safe care and use deliberate design to minimize errors. Applied to nursing, the concept is *high-reliability teams.* Using reliability principles, multidisciplinary and interdisciplinary teams can focus on reducing flaws in care processes, increase the consistency of appropriateness of care delivery, and improve patient outcomes. Team training and system design are the key hallmarks of high-reliability patient care units. Members of high-reliability teams have four key behaviors: situational awareness, use of standardized communication, closed-loop communication, and a shared mental model, which can be enhanced with interdisciplinary team training (Riley et al., 2010). High-performance teams are essential to an organization's efficiency and effectiveness. High-quality work outcomes and cost control suffer without communication, collaboration, and teamwork. Interdisciplinary team members rely on each other's skills in a highly dynamic work environment (Teunissen et al., 2020).

Nurse leaders need to learn how to create, lead, and manage teams; all nurses also need to know how to be effective team players. Skilled leaders listen, invite, and encourage participation by team members. They understand the individual strengths and weakness of each member. Formation of a well-functioning group or team is never the work of just the leader. Members, as followers, give input, participate in decision-making, share responsibility, and hold themselves and each other accountable for group outcomes. A highly skilled and effective professional is not necessarily a highly skilled and effective group member. Distinct skill sets are required and are beneficial for nurses. Leaders and staff members alike should be able to function both independently and interdependently with others. They need to have the judgment to know when and which form of functioning is more appropriate. Regardless of the role as leader or group member, vision, and goals of the group need to be effectively embraced.

Types of Teams

Three types of teams found in health care are: (1) primary work teams, (2) leadership teams, and (3) ad hoc teams (Manion, 2011). Primary work teams include all forms of operational teams, including patient care teams such as a medical intensive care team and teams organized by a focused area, such as the rapid response team or a quality improvement team. In the operating room, teams are often based on the specialty (e.g., a cardiovascular or orthopedic team). The senior executive team is an example of an executive or management leadership team. At the hospital department level there may be a leadership team composed of the nurse manager, charge nurses, and perhaps an educator. Project teams and problem-solving teams are examples of ad hoc teams found across settings and sites. Specific problem-solving teams in departments are other examples of ad hoc teams, frequently referred to as task forces. The chief characteristic of these teams is that they are created to perform a specific piece of work. When work is completed, the team dissolves. Designing, building, and implementing effective work teams requires a specific methodology and process. A primary work team fails if it behaves like a collection of individuals operating from narrowly defined jobs; if it is composed of the wrong mix of members, size, structure, responsibility, or expertise, or if it cannot fluidly shift activities and adapt to changes. Teams need to be designed based on work responsibilities, skills, and competencies required by the work of the team. After the team design is determined, the next step is to build the team by incorporating essential elements needed to function. These include a common purpose, agreed-on performance goals or results-driven structure, competent members, a common approach for the work, complementary skills, collaborative relationships, mutual accountability, standards of excellence, external support, and principled leadership (Manion, 2011). The complementary skills needed in the right mix to do the team's task fall into at least three categories: technical or functional expertise, problem-solving and decision-making skills, and interpersonal skills. These are defined characteristics of *highly effective teams* (Wynia, 2012, pp. 1327–1328) (Table 9.1).

Managing this development process is a key leadership function. The leader guides the team in development of its purpose. Team members are more likely to coalesce into a strong team if they have been given time and opportunity to carefully reflect on their purpose and agree on what they do and for whom they do it. This leads to a unified commitment. A team becomes a true team by doing its work. Specific performance goals give it direction and provide evaluative criteria to measure success. Unnecessary conflict can occur if the leader and team members have not established key processes. Agreement is needed about how things are going to be done and by whom. This ranges from establishment of team behavioral norms to agreement on procedural issues. This step usually requires a significant amount of time and will continue to be addressed throughout the lifetime of the team. When foundations are laid carefully, effective teams can emerge (Manion, 2011).

Team Dynamics

The dynamics of interdisciplinary teams create some unique challenges. When teams are composed of professionals who have been educated, socialized, and are used to a unique vocabulary, professional values, and standards and practices, then it may become challenging for them to work across disciplines. Regrouping people into multidisciplinary groups increases team diversity

TABLE 9.1　Values and Principles of High-Functioning Health Care Teams	
Share Values Among Team Members	**Principles to Guide Team-Based Care**
Honesty Put a high value on open communication within the team, including transparency about aims, decisions, uncertainty, and mistakes.	Clear roles Have clear expectations for each member's functions, responsibilities, and accountabilities.
Discipline Carry out roles and responsibilities even when inconvenient and seek out and share information to improve even when it is uncomfortable.	Mutual trust Earn each other's trust, creating strong norms for reciprocity and greater opportunities for shared achievement.
Creativity Be excited by the possibility of tackling new or emerging problems, seeing errors and unanticipated bad outcomes as potential opportunities to learn and improve.	Effective communication Prioritize and continuously refine communication skills using consistent channels for candid and complete communication.
Humility Recognize differences in training but do not believe that one type of training perspective is uniformly superior; recognize that team members are human and will make mistakes.	Shared goals Work to establish shared goals that reflect patient and family priorities and that can be clearly articulated, understood, and supported by all members.
Curiosity Delight in seeking out and reflecting on lessons learned and using those insights for continuous improvement.	Measurable processes and outcomes Agree on and implement reliable and timely feedback on successes and failures in both the overall functioning of the team and achievement of specific goals.

Data from Wynia, M.K., Von Kohorn, I., & Mitchell, P.H. (2012). Challenges at the intersection of team-based and patient-centered health care: Insights from an IOM working group. *Journal of the American Medical Association, 308*(13), 1327–1328.

and is essential to ensure high-quality, coordinated, reliable care.

Challenges occur when:

- There is confusion about the team's work.
- The team lacks real authority.
- Structural team building is not done.
- Dysfunctional behavior occurs, and team members do not know how to constructively deal with it.
- Team-based outcome measures and coaching are lacking.

Trust and communication are critical elements of building effective work teams. It is not enough to simply structure the team. Team members need to learn to work collaboratively and interdependently. Team performance and effectiveness are important managerial concerns.

Teams form, grow, and mature in stages. Team dynamics change throughout this process. Teams benefit from team building and developmental training. Articulating and negotiating expectations for healthy interpersonal behavior benefits team development. A key characteristic of an emotionally intelligent team is establishment of norms to guide team member behaviors (Cherniss & Goleman, 2001).

Team norms are best established when the team initially forms. They are continually revisited, modified, and expanded throughout the team's life. The process for developing norms is usually leader initiated and begins with a team conversation about how team members behave and contribute. Norms are usually developed during a group meeting in which ideas are shared, refined, and finally negotiated with all team members. Appropriate topics for behavioral norms include, but are not limited to, expectations around communication, both at individual and group levels; how team members treat each other; how support is to be demonstrated; decision-making processes; and how conflict is to be handled. For example, one team developed the following expectations of each other.

I expect you to:

- Communicate in an open, honest, and direct manner with me;
- Give me feedback when my behavior creates a difficult or uncomfortable situation for you;
- Persist and work with me on difficult issues until we reach a mutually agreeable resolution;
- Pitch in gladly, provide help when asked, and look for ways to help each other out;

- Respect confidences and not share sensitive information we discuss with others without my knowledge or permission;
- Be trustworthy as evidenced by honoring and meeting commitments made, including being on time and staying engaged (being present) throughout the meeting;
- Refrain from using technology and "multitasking" during meetings;
- Be loyal to absent team members, and present them in the best light to others.

Often these norms are referred to as the *team operating agreement*, the *code of conduct*, ground rules, or *articulated expectations*. Once the norms are identified, team members sign them, indicating agreement, and the norms often are posted in the workplace. These norms are more than just a paper exercise. They signify that team members agree to live by established expectations and address other team members who do not. As new members join the team, it is important to share team members' expectations. It is also beneficial to revisit defined expectations on a regular basis.

Team effectiveness is dependent not only on how individual team members perform and adhere to norms, but also on the degree of communication, cooperation, and emotional intelligence of individual members and the team's leader. The ability to manage conflict and have self-awareness is essential for a team to reach peak performance. The greater the performance of a team, the greater is the advantage to group members, patients, and the organization.

COMMITTEES

An essential part of any nurse's role is to be involved in committee and group work. Work is accomplished through people, and quality of care is furthered through committee actions. It positively impacts nurses' job satisfaction and autonomy to have an avenue of involvement and participation to actively solve problems and retain autonomy over nursing care. Professional shared governance models incorporate staff nurse participation in groups and committees as a core element of how work gets accomplished.

Some people prefer not to participate in committees because they dislike the time involved or because they are frustrated with psychodynamics of group process and decision-making. However, committees are a mainstay of organizations and can be an important way to make changes in clinical practice. Understanding committee workings facilitates the process of being a more effective nurse.

Committee structures are preferable in two kinds of situations:

1. *Situations in which each member's input is needed to attain a certain goal.* For example, a committee may be set up to review patient safety issues in a department, such as patient falls. If the work cannot be done alone or if there is a need to have everyone's agreement or support, then a committee is probably appropriate.

2. *Situations in which diverse representation facilitates implementation of proposed activities.* To have a diverse group of people provide input in order to get the job done, a committee should be created. For example, a multidisciplinary product committee could be established to develop a process in which existing and new products would be reviewed before large purchases are made. This approach allows nurses to evaluate new products and look at value to patient care, safety, efficacy, and cost. It also provides a disciplined approach to product review, with an aim of preventing duplication of products and promoting good financial stewardship.

Types of Committees

Several types of committees are found in organizations. One kind is the *standing* committee, that is a constant, ongoing part of the organizational mission, performing critical and essential functions. For example, policy committees are standing committees because there always are policies to write and review. The same is true for a patient safety committee because these functions and activities are ongoing and continuous.

Contrasted with a standing committee is the task force, also called a *project team* or *ad hoc committee*. This committee is developed in response to some emergent or immediate need. A task force is not part of the organizational core mission. It is formed in response to a specific circumstance that arises or to study a specific problem. The committee is expected to disband when the issue is resolved. Examples are a search committee to replace an advanced practice nurse or a problem-solving group dealing with emergency department patient throughput and hospital bed availability.

Some groups or committees are structured to gather members *based on organizational position or job position.* For example, all the nurse managers may belong to a group of nurse managers, or staff nurses may belong to a staff nurse council. By holding a position of nurse manager, a person belongs to that committee. Committee involvement provides an opportunity for peer interaction, support, and problem-solving.

There are multidisciplinary interdivisional committees. A *multidisciplinary* committee includes participants from several divisions, locations, or specialties. Participants may be from within the institution or from both inside and outside the organization. These committees are often used to coordinate and eliminate boundary conflicts. Some examples are a product committee, risk management committee, or patient safety committee in which nurses, physicians, and allied health colleagues work together to improve patient care and reduce interprofessional conflicts. In some cases, multidisciplinary teams are formed using a committee structure (e.g., to develop a critical pathway such as sepsis screening). Other committees may be cross-functional (e.g., nurses meeting with members from information technology or facilities management department to discuss and resolve issues).

Within organizations, committees perform a central role in the implementation of the strategic plan. A committee is a group that can assume responsibility and be held accountable for planning, implementing, and evaluating outcomes of a strategic goal translated to the operational level. Committees accomplish some departmental activities and provide a mechanism for increasing staff participation in decision-making. In an environment characterized by complex work, committees become a major vehicle for resolving issues related to the organization's mission. Two elements promote efficient and effective committee decision-making: appropriate representation (by including people affected by changes) and delegation of an appropriate level of authority to the committee (Manion, 2011).

Committees evolve over time. To remain vital, committees need to be evaluated regularly for congruence with organizational mission and contribution to outcomes. The committee's goals and outcomes need to be reviewed annually, with membership reevaluated and changed as necessary. If asked to be on a committee as a department representative, it is advisable for the nurse to explore the nature and characteristics of the committee.

The nurse needs to determine the authority level delegated to this committee, remembering that delegation may be formal or informal. Another factor involves assessing the personal level of interest in the work of the committee. Other factors include whether people on the committee are highly motivated, whether they are task- or relationship-oriented people, and what committee politics exist. Feedback mechanisms and the committee's productivity are key characteristics. The track record of the committee is reflected in its output. These characteristics are important for the nurse to understand before deciding whether to participate. Preparation for followership enhances both personal and committee productivity. It is also helpful to clarify any expectations for the committee role being considered. For example, is the nurse there to share individual opinions or to represent others in the department? The latter role requires more active solicitation of colleagues' opinions and ideas.

EFFECTIVE MEETINGS

Meetings are common occurrences in health care organizations. Whether a meeting involves a group, committee, or team, the leader's role is to maximize the benefits of the meeting. Structuring a meeting for effectiveness requires preparation and effort. To manage effective meetings, the leader needs to consider the meeting's purpose. Some of the most common reasons meetings are ineffective relate to a lack of clarity of purpose, or too many competing issues on the agenda for a single meeting. For example, a brief team huddle would become ineffective if it turned into a decision-making group about a key department issue.

Probably the most common type of meeting is held for *information dissemination or sharing*. For example, the designated leadership person calls the group together to let members review the organization's performance scorecard. That may include organization and individual department performance in financial management, patient experience scores, quality scores, and employee measures such as turnover. A meeting is called to disseminate information about what is happening and to provide time for questions and answers. This also occurs when there has been an organizational change, such as the decision that one unit is going to be consolidating with another unit or that a new building, department relocation, or new service is being planned or implemented.

One familiar form of information sharing is the end-of-shift report. Pertinent, important information about patients is reviewed and discussed by staff members from the outgoing and incoming shift. The shift handoff report is a very common form of this type of meeting. This is a very short meeting at the beginning of shift with all team members to review the upcoming shift or any emergent topics that need to be communicated. These meetings may be called huddles.

Second, there are meetings held for *opinion seeking*. The goal of these meetings is open dialogue to solicit group and individual opinions and ideas on specific topics or issues. This purpose does not imply that decision-making is the prerogative of the group. Seeking opinions is an input strategy and may be used for gathering data or testing group reactions. For example, an opinion-seeking meeting may be called to invite input on equipment purchases for budget requests.

The third type of meeting is held for *problem-solving and/or decision-making*. The meeting is structured to solicit help in clarifying, analyzing, and solving a specific problem. This type of meeting is action oriented. Group participation in decision-making is encouraged. For example, group problem-solving or unit meetings may be called to discuss ways to solve problems related to patient safety issues, or complex and challenging patients or family members. Meetings for problem-solving need to follow a methodical structure, otherwise they are likely either to deteriorate into a complaint session or to result in ineffective or unacceptable recommendations. Effectively leading these groups requires strong facilitation skills and knowledge in problem-solving techniques. It is helpful to focus on common agreed-on goals such as patient safety.

Yet another type of meeting is a *strategy* meeting. These meetings are less frequent—perhaps quarterly or annually—and focus on reviewing the organization's vision and strategic goals, developing future goals and strategies for the department or work group, or tackling one issue in great depth, such as implementing a professional shared governance model or a new model of care delivery. This may be called by executive nursing leaders as a "summit," a "retreat," or "town hall meeting."

Preparing for Meetings

In the most effective groups, all members are clear about the purpose of the meeting they are attending, are prepared, and help the group to stay focused. When the group becomes distracted by other issues (for example, getting side-tracked by operational issues during a strategy meeting), focus is lost, and meeting time is wasted. This is a sign that the meeting structure may need to be evaluated.

In preparing for a meeting, a leader should make certain that the committee's process stays true to the purpose of the meeting. There is a caution about having a mix of items in the same meeting. For example, basic information dissemination is best addressed at a quarterly strategic meeting. This does not mean that any of these items are less important, but introducing them in the wrong venue or with the wrong timing will reduce the effectiveness of the meeting.

A timed agenda may be a helpful way to facilitate the group's process. This involves identifying on the agenda, next to each item, the anticipated amount of time allotted for discussion. It might be beneficial to review proposed time allotments with committee members before meeting to ensure realistic estimates. Time estimates should serve as a guideline rather than a rigid parameter. It is important not to cut off discussion prematurely or force a decision when a discussion is productive but taking longer than anticipated. One effective strategy is to do a time check with members and adjust accordingly. This may require an adjustment in the agenda. Many leaders organize agenda items according to priority topics. Some leaders have a brief agenda and add to it to cover any pressing issues or topics based on the team's input. This can be done at the beginning of the meeting or after planned agenda items are covered. Meetings can rapidly become disorganized without an agenda or a carefully facilitated discussion. The leader must be mindful of the time allotted for the meeting.

Leader Duties

The leader of the group can facilitate meeting effectiveness by preparing and dealing with both the task and people involved. The leader should listen carefully, process interactions, control flow, and keep the meeting directed toward accomplishing objectives. The ideal size of a group depends on work to be accomplished. If group interaction and getting everyone's input is important, then the size of the ideal group needs to be small, ideally 4 to 7 people, with 12 being the upper limit. Members should be carefully selected for providing best input, being representative, and having potential contribution to the work.

The leader needs to start on time and be alert to seating positions. Some leaders assign seating to maximize group participation and prevent disruption. The leader can facilitate effectiveness ensuring that all members of the team have an ability to actively participate. The leader may need to control compulsive talkers, draw out silent members, protect junior members, encourage the respectful clash of ideas, discourage the clash of personalities, prevent squashing of creative ideas, and close on a note of achievement (Jay, 1982). The leader also needs to attend to careful meeting wrap-up. Summarizing the group's accomplishments after the meeting and verifying task assignments are important leader responsibilities. Box 9.1 presents a checklist for leading effective meetings.

Without thought and preparation, people may go into a meeting focused on their own issues, biases, and perspectives; they may not be focused on being productive

---

BOX 9.1   Effective Meetings Checklist for Leaders

- Identify the purpose of the meeting. Is it for:
  - Information dissemination
  - Opinion seeking
  - Problem-solving
- Prepare an agenda and related materials
- Identify time needed for each item on the agenda
- Identify the category of each agenda item. Is it:
  - For information
  - For development
  - For implementation
  - For change in the system
- Identify the number and type of members needed
- Carefully select members (based on skill and expertise)
- Distribute agenda and related materials such as previous minutes well in advance of meeting with instructions for assignments due and materials to be reviewed before the meeting
- Listen carefully and summarize discussion and assignments at the end of the meeting
- Process group interactions to ensure balanced dialogue by all members
- Control the flow of interactions
- Keep the meeting directed toward accomplishing objectives
- Start on time and finish on time

Data modified from Jay, A. (1982). How to run a meeting. *Journal of Nursing Administration, 12*(1), 22–28.

within the meeting. However, even in a negative situation, individuals may choose to participate in a way that assists or enhances the process by making constructive suggestions about how things could be done better. This is an ideal situation, one to be encouraged, structured, and facilitated by the leader.

The duties of the chairperson include preparing the physical environment. Comfort and convenience engineering are part of the leader's responsibility in terms of preparing an environment that is conducive to people being satisfied, productive, positive, and working together. The worst-case situation occurs if the meeting room is uncomfortable, including being too cold, too hot, too noisy, too small, or too large. Another challenge is when technology does not work. The chairperson needs to ensure the meeting room, including technology, is set up appropriately. Consider how to facilitate group work through hosting functions related to breaks, food, and beverages. It is human nature for members to be more relaxed and productive in comfortable surroundings. With the reliance on technology versus the need for people to "be present" during a meeting, many leaders have added mechanisms to foster group interactions.

As all nurses are pressured to do more with less under severe time and travel constraints, conducting meetings assisted by technology has become a major strategy. The prevalence and ease of technology, such as video conference calls, webinars, Internet-based meeting technology, real-time (synchronous) discussion boards, and related audio or video technology strategies are commonly employed. These become useful ways to save time by eliminating travel to a remote site. However, specific problems may occur, such as technology incompatibility, speed of transmission, connection failures, or other delays in transmission that result in inconsistent communication, a lack of interpersonal modulation due to absence of body language, or a tendency to forget about people who are not actually in the room. Ensuring that the agenda, minutes, assignments, and presentations are sent in advance will mitigate some technology difficulties. Despite these known issues, nurses will increasingly experience meetings assisted by technology.

Positive meeting dynamics are a shared responsibility between the leader and group members. A leader has a responsibility to prepare in advance for meetings and provide participants support in preparation. The participants' responsibility is to read and be prepared, show up on time, participate openly and positively, share responsibility for managing the group's dynamics, and attend to the task at hand. Depending on the meeting, the leader needs to prepare an agenda with handouts and background materials and distribute them to the members to give them time to review. A leader who does not distribute materials in advance may limit effectiveness of the meeting because members will not be prepared. Most materials can be sent electronically to members. The better prepared members are, the more they can participate, positively affect the quality of decisions, and feel gratified by their participation.

If the leader's preparation activities include generating an agenda or reviewing the status of agenda topics, questions to ask when organizing and preparing include the following:

- Where are we/what is the current status?
- What else needs to be done?
- What supporting materials might help the committee members?
- Who should be invited?
- Are there other experts or people from other departments that can contribute to this committee's process?
- What do we hope to accomplish?

CONSTRUCTIVE GROUP ROLES AND BEHAVIORS

Savvy group leaders and members understand that people in groups assume a variety of roles. In a now-classic work, Lancaster (1981) identified both group building roles and group maintenance roles as being a part of group interactions. Group building roles include *initiator, encourager, opinion giver, clarifier, listener,* and *summarizer.* Group maintenance roles include *tension reliever, compromiser, gatekeeper,* and *harmonizer.* The group building roles concentrate more on relationship functions than on task functions; the group maintenance roles focus more on task functions than on relationship functions. Effective groups need a balance of members and roles.

Beyond the more general group, roles are specific, structured roles that can help increase the effectiveness of the group. For example, one positive way to handle meetings is to identify a facilitator. This is often the formal group leader or individual in a position of authority, but it does not have to be. If this is a true team, the role of facilitator may rotate among team members. In a committee, the facilitator is probably the committee chairperson. A facilitator conducts the meeting, ensuring that everyone can speak, maintains the focus of the meeting, and ensures group dynamics remain positive.

A group recorder is also needed. The task of taking minutes or summarizing discussion and decisions may need to be delegated to a clerical support person (if possible) if group members are averse to taking on the task of recording outcomes. However, a recorder who is a group member technically can do far more than just take minutes. This person should be in tune with group processing and with inputs and roles of group members. In addition, they can help keep the group on time. The recorder can provide feedback to the facilitator in terms of how to improve the process. One key tip is to construct a standardized meeting agenda and a record (or minutes) to facilitate group process. It is helpful to decide in advance the level of detail required in the minutes to avoid lengthy minutes and potentially unnecessary effort.

One useful way to expedite group work is to use a laptop computer to directly enter draft minutes. It is also valuable to summarize actions and assignments at the end of the meeting. Some leaders choose to allow the recorder to summarize discussion on a topic versus composing detailed minutes on each topic. Sending out minutes and talking points or a summary of items discussed, and decisions made shortly after the meeting can support continued engagement and communication of the group.

Finally, group members who believe they can be active participants—with equal status in the meeting—are generally more engaged and feel empowered. The three components of facilitator, recorder, and group members contribute to the design of a positive working group. All can share in the basic group role functions. As with teams, leaders should establish ground rules for members of the group to facilitate maximum engagement. Some common rules may include:

- Meetings begin and end on time
- Members need to be on time, prepared, and stay for the entire meeting
- No cell phone or computer use during the meeting except on scheduled breaks
- One person speaks at a time
- No sidebar conversations.

DISRUPTIVE ROLES AND BEHAVIORS

Another role that the group leader assumes is that of process facilitator. The leader needs to observe group members' actions and be prepared to control or redirect disruptive behaviors. It is important to focus on behavior that needs to be adjusted and not label an individual in a group. Although the leader has a responsibility to deal with nonproductive behaviors, in a mature team or highly effective group, monitoring of behaviors is also a responsibility of other group members. If the issue is not addressed by a fellow group member, then the leader needs to be prepared to address it. However, it is hierarchical thinking to leave this responsibility solely to the leader and doing so reinforces formal hierarchy in the group. It is also important that the leader, facilitator, or group member avoids embarrassing a member of a group publicly, because the impact on the group will be equally disruptive. Many times, individuals do not have insight concerning their own behavior or its impact on the group. It can be a "teachable moment" to enhance an individual professionally by diplomatically redirecting to positive behavior. The following section delineates types of disruptive group members that are encountered (Jacobs & Rosenthal, 1984), with strategies for the leader to use in managing the behavior of the group member.

Compulsive Talkers

A common disruptive behavior is seen in individuals who are compulsive talkers. Often their behavior can be modified. One suggestion is to thank them for their input and then ask to hear from others on that same topic before they are given the opportunity to speak again. This will serve as a way of guiding and opening up the meeting to be more effective. If this behavior continues to affect the group negatively and the individual is not receptive to subtle feedback, meeting with the person after group work and giving direct, constructive feedback about the negative impact of the behavior may be necessary. There are techniques that can be shared to assist them in future meetings, such as asking them to keep track of the number of times they have spoken on a subject. In a mature team, it would be expected that this issue could be brought up and dealt with by any team member.

Nontalkers

The nontalkers are the quiet ones. They may not be comfortable speaking in front of a group or may process information more slowly than other members of the group. It is important to create a safe environment where their ideas are considered. Some approaches include offering the option of submitting their ideas in writing or directly asking them to share their thoughts on the matter at hand. Anyone in the group can specifically ask them questions to draw them out, thereby encouraging a broader range of group input. Preparing members in advance by distributing the agenda or letting them know where their input will be crucial is also a way to include nontalkers. Sometimes these individuals need time to think through their thoughts before they engage in a conversation, unlike more spontaneous and verbal peers. It is important to understand their communication style and not embarrass them in front of a group if they are not engaged in discussion.

Interrupters

The facilitator must address the interrupter because this person demonstrates a lack of awareness or self-control. The interrupter can be a problem in groups because they can stifle group conversation. Individuals who are interrupted may feel violated and wonder why they are not given the courtesy of finishing a thought and having their full input considered. Anyone in the group can halt the interruption, control, and redirect the interrupter. This can be accomplished by saying, "Let's allow Joan to finish what she was saying." If the group does not intervene, it is the responsibility of the facilitator. One consideration when developing ground rules for the group is to list no interruptions as an expectation. Interrupters may be individuals who process information quickly. It might be beneficial to meet with them privately to give them some examples. They might not have insight concerning their behavior and actions needed to support communication within the group.

Squashers

Squashers try to squash an idea before it is even developed. Suggestions about processes or procedures that have not been proven or even tried are much easier to criticize than are facts or opinions. Persons who are averse to change may have a litany of reasons why a potential solution would never work or why this proposed project simply cannot or should not happen. Often these are people who do not want to take a personal risk or undergo the personal effort of making a change, so it is easier to squash everything and maintain the status quo. Especially during brainstorming sessions, the leader needs to be alert to and have a method for containing the squasher. An easy way to influence this is to set the expectation at the beginning of the session by saying, for example, "For this exercise, please do not engage in analyzing or saying anything negative about the ideas thrown out until we have them all identified." There will be time later that allows dissecting and critiquing a new idea. Negative remarks adversely affect the level of creativity in any group, but the individual may have a wealth of experience and knowledge such that they discern pitfalls and barriers more quickly than others. Careful team discussion guidance is needed.

Distracted or Unreliable Members

Unreliable members really may not be committed to the group's work. They may be distracted, which they exhibit in a variety of ways including arriving late, leaving early, answering phone calls, texting, or reading e-mails during the meeting. They may not be prepared for the meeting. Ultimately, they are not contributing to the ongoing group work or the task at hand nor are they invested in the group's goals. The leader needs to address this issue with them. One possible solution is to meet with them privately and discuss whether they are interested and able to be part of the group. There are times when individuals overcommit, and as a result do not fulfill their obligations to the group. Sharing observed group behaviors and explaining expectations is essential if they wish to be part of the group. If they do, it might be beneficial to give them a specific assignment with accountability. If this does not work, they may need to be released from the group or placed in an advisory role.

MANAGING DISRUPTIVE BEHAVIOR IN GROUPS

The most useful way to have an impact on negative behaviors is to lead the group through clarification of working expectations. When group members have clearly identified what is needed to productively work together in a group setting, they have established norms for acceptable and unacceptable behavior.

The nurse leader can take an active role in structuring group work for positive processing and effective outcomes. It is important to control communication flow to modulate disruptive group members without enhancing conflict. Another way is to structure positive and constructive group roles among members. Peer pressure is a powerful group behavior modification tactic, especially for group members for whom approval of the rest of the group is important. The leader's vision, enthusiasm, interpersonal relationship skills, and empowerment of followers all facilitate group effectiveness.

LEADERSHIP AND MANAGEMENT IMPLICATIONS

Leaders play a significant role in the success of an organization and, specifically, patient safety, quality, and joy at work. The ability to work with a committed collaborative group, team, or committee is essential for an organization to continue to grow and improve, and also retain top talent. It is well documented in the literature that nursing job satisfaction and burnout correlate with the degree of teamwork, work environment, professional practice, and degree of professional and collaborative working relationships with both the nursing team and medical staff. For example, new nurses in nurse residency programs report difficulty in working on project and patient care teams if they have not had prior exposure or background. Because of the growing use of interdisciplinary teams, leaders and managers can structure in mentored experiences so new nurses specifically can grow in knowledge and skill in teamwork. Health care organizations that have managers with an effective management style that allows a degree of autonomy, promotes interdisciplinary relationships, and promotes professional development have a lower turnover among the nursing staff.

The leadership and management roles are essential in ensuring groups, teams, and committees are effective. With limited resources the leader should consider the work to be accomplished, determine the structure most suited to do the work, put the structure in place, and facilitate work processes. This requires a leader who understands basic differences among work groups and teams, committees, and informal groups. A leader also needs to be able to think carefully about the work to be accomplished and determine whether it is primarily collective or individual work.

A leader's role includes selecting the right members, inspiring participation, preparing critical questions, developing agendas and background materials, summarizing minutes and developing talking points, continually coaching the group for effective functioning, and guiding long-range strategy. This is the planning, coordinative, and tracking function. Leaders and managers address questions such as:

- What is the task?
- What is the best way for this task to be accomplished?
- Is collective work involved?
- Do we need a team, or will a good work group or committee suffice?
- How many meetings will it take?
- How much effort is required?
- How can the tasks be divided?
- How can they be delegated?
- What measures will demonstrate success?

In planning for meetings, a good leader puts in time and effort needed to provide preliminary information and documents so that all members are prepared when they come to the meeting, know what the issues are, and are familiar with the background of the task to be accomplished. The leader facilitates the group in agreeing about norms for decision-making, length of discussion, when to vote or use consensus, and processes through which the task is completed efficiently and effectively. This is done as a deliberate agenda item that the leader initiates, opens for discussion, and brings to closure. Sometimes an off-site retreat is used to employ high-relationship and group-forming strategies. Nurses may find the group leader role challenges them to plan, organize, coordinate, and evaluate the work of the group.

An effective leader understands a process is involved in creating effective, engaged work teams, highly functioning groups, and committees. The process requires facilitation and significant amounts of coaching from the leader. The leader's style needs to fit the group development stage. The leader will need to supply more extensive structure and direction in early stages and minimal structure and direction in later stages. The leader needs to support the work and at times coach the team or group. Group skill, capability, and readiness need to be assessed. Ensuring appropriate resources is imperative. Finally, celebrating successes of the group, team, or committee is essential, with the understanding that recognition is related to personal preferences. Although some individuals enjoy public recognition, others prefer private recognition such as a note or private comment about a job well done.

CURRENT ISSUES AND TRENDS

Creating Healthy Workplaces

Creation of a positive and healthy work environment is a key issue in health care. Organizations continue to struggle with attracting and retaining highly qualified nurses and other members of the health care team. They also struggle with motivating employees who are highly engaged and experience joy in work. There is much evidence that confirms that an unhealthy work environment contributes to unsafe conditions that result in medical errors, poorly coordinated and ineffective care, and conflict and stress among members of the health care team (Roth et al., 2015). In 2005 the American Association of Critical-Care Nurses (AACN, 2005) released *AACN Standards for Establishing and Sustaining Healthy Work Environments: A Journey to Excellence.* The six standards are as follows: skilled communication, true collaboration, effective decision-making, appropriate staffing, meaningful recognition, and authentic leadership. These are recognized in nursing as the gold standard for health care organizations.

A healthy work environment assumes relationships a person has with colleagues and co-workers are positive and respectful. Leadership plays an important role in supporting the nursing team. Ensuring adequate staff, an appropriate workload, and mutual respect among the nursing team and other disciplines is critical to creating and sustaining a healthy work environment. A positive work environment for nurses demonstrates problem-solving and resolution of issues resulting in workplace conditions improving. Effective problem-solving groups are a crucial aspect of making this happen.

TeamSTEPPS

In the early 2000s, the Agency for Healthcare Research and Quality (AHRQ), in partnership with the Department of Defense, began working on a patient safety initiative that was directed at improving teamwork in health care settings. TeamSTEPPS was the result (AHRQ, 2016). The acronym stands for Team Strategies and Tools to Enhance Performance and Patient Safety. The premise is quite simple. Anyone who touches a patient (nurse, physician, pharmacist, technician) must work together to ensure the delivery of safe and high-quality care. It is aimed at helping health care professionals work together more effectively as a team. TeamSTEPPS teaches professionals to understand each other's roles and collaborate to improve the quality of care delivered. The aim is to foster a culture where any member of the team has freedom to respectfully question authority when an error may be occurring. It teaches the team that questioning authority need not be threatening. In the airline industry, there is similar training known as crew resource management.

One example is a structured process for communication to ensure information is clearly exchanged between team members. There is a specific training curriculum used to integrate teamwork principles. This program is like a boot camp in teamwork and interdependent relationships. It offers a host of innovations such as team huddles, patient handoff briefings, time-outs before commencement of a surgical procedure, and the SBAR (situation, background, assessment, and recommendation) technique for communicating information in a concise manner. The website http://www.ahrq.gov/teamstepps/index.html offers an impressive number of resources.

Innovation Centers

Fostering innovation is essential as health care continues to transform with targeted focus on continuous improvement and breakthrough novel ideas and approaches to patient care (see Chapter 2). Health care organizations today are being measured on quality results, the patient experience, and cost of care. Innovation groups and committees are engaged in total quality management (TQM) initiatives, continuous quality improvement (CQI) methods using techniques such as Lean, Six Sigma, and rapid response teams.

A common response to problems is to look for an individual to blame. The result of systems thinking is to capture the energy of teams to resolve systems problems. An overall focus on quality has led to adoption of business management concepts such as Lean and Six Sigma. These are customer-focused and data-driven approaches to deriving best practices. The focus is on reducing process variation and improving process capability. Lean focuses on process speed and reduction of waste and inefficiencies; Six Sigma focuses on process quality with the aim of fewer defects.

A current innovation in health care is the MakerNurse project from the Robert Wood Johnson Foundation (https://www.rwjf.org/en/how-we-work/grants-explorer/featured-programs/maker-nurse.html). Nurses are adept at problem-solving, creating workarounds, and suggesting care innovations. MakerNurse is an initiative that listens to and gathers stories to detail the natural abilities of nurses to solve problems in an inventive, creative, innovated manner. From these stories a database of information has been built to support nurses with tools and resources that enable nurses to continue innovation at the patient's bedside.

Many organizations have created innovation centers to discover new ways to address health care challenges. New health care products and services are being tested—and in some cases commercialized—through collaboration with clinicians, scientists, entrepreneurs, and business partners. Innovation centers are focused on disruptive innovation to expedite change. This may involve developing new techniques and approaches to operational efficiency including testing new workflows, patient care redesign, standardization, and teamwork through simulation and hands-on experiential learning.

Leaders are cautioned that creativity and innovation at a team level require diversity in membership and perspective. Diverse teams have freedom to challenge the status quo and engage in creative problem-solving. Nursing leaders play a crucial role integrating with other disciplines in making a commitment to ensure teams feel supported and have freedom to creatively identify new ways to address clinical processes and care redesign. Leaders who understand and use these techniques and processes of innovation can be effective in disseminating and implementing novel approaches to patient care.

Multidisciplinary Quality Improvement Teams

Whether using CQI, TQM, Lean, Six Sigma, or some related quality improvement program, direct care nurses are expected to participate more actively in multidisciplinary quality improvement teams. In an organization that identifies problems as systems problems, the next step is to acknowledge that anyone involved in the system needs to be engaged in solving problems. Therefore coordinating patient care and solving problems through interdisciplinary committees and groups with people of equal status is the strategy best suited to solving systems problems.

The strategy behind systems-based approaches is to bring together interdisciplinary, collaborative groups. This means that if there is a problem in patient care, physicians, nurses, ancillary staff, and other direct caregivers work together to identify issues and possible solutions. Solutions identified can be tested and evaluated through collaboration. The facilitator does not have to be a content expert or have the most expertise in that problem area. In fact, having the most expertise in a problem area can be problematic when functioning as a facilitator because it becomes too tempting to take over the process. The individual's facilitation skills are crucially important.

Establishing equality among peers regardless of status and using expertise and responsibility result in a different way of looking at work. This has implications in terms of how nursing practice may change. It also means nurses are going to continue to be substantially involved in groups, committees, and teams. Multidisciplinary teams are not just for problem-solving and process improvement. The current pace and complexity of the world today also demands that new approaches to care delivery be considered by teams.

RESEARCH NOTE

Source

Miller, C.J., Kim, B., Silverman, A, & Bauer, M.S. (2018). A systematic review of team-building interventions in non-acute healthcare settings. *BMC Health Services Research, 18*:146, 1–21. https://doi.org/10.1186/s12913-018-2961-9.

Purpose

A systematic review was done to identify team-building interventions. The process identified 14 team-building interventions that pertained to nonacute care settings along with 25 documents describing observed studies of the interventions.

Discussion

The authors developed a Team Effectiveness Pyramid as a conceptual model of nonacute health care. The authors proposed that the pyramid was in four levels: (1) Foundational Resources such as leadership support, staffing, space, civility, and respect, (2) Team Building Interventions such as knowledge of team work principles and attitudes towards teamwork, (3) Enhanced Team Functioning demonstrated by shared purpose and goals, coordination and communication, role clarity, increased civility and respect, and capacity to improve process, and (4) Patient Impact including patient outcomes and patient satisfaction. Three authors independently rated a subset of 10 manuscripts using a descriptive approach to report the characteristics of team-building interventions/empirical studies and to catalogue support for each intervention.

Results

Evaluations of team building strategies were mostly positive with mixed results in relation to team functioning and patient impact. Only one study demonstrated statistically significant improvement in teamwork attitudes and knowledge.

Application to Practice

This systematic review found that the evidence base for health care team-building interventions for nonacute

settings demonstrated a paucity of information when compared to short-term team function in acute care settings. One intervention was found to be tested in multiple nonacute settings. The positive findings in relation to team-building interventions were moderated by variables such as few control conditions, inconsistent measures of outcomes, and bias. The results of this study determined a great need for further research in the area of nonacute team building.

CASE STUDY

Developing Leadership Teams to Improve Clinical Metrics

A new C-Suite team was formed to lead a midsized community hospital. Members included the Hospital Chief Executive officer (CEO), Chief of Nursing (CNO), Chief of Finance (CFO), Medical Chief of Staff (COS), various directors of nursing services, directors of ancillary services, and the associate chiefs of staff for various medical/surgical services. The team was established to improve clinical metrics throughout the hospital. Clinical metrics were chosen, thresholds were set to demonstrate needed improvement, and subcommittees were established by the C-Suite to address individual metrics.

Due to the numerous metrics, it was felt that subcommittees would need to be established in order to tackle the enormous amount of data that needed to be reviewed. Nursing was tasked with establishing subcommittees working on metrics that were directly related to nursing; physicians were tasked to established subcommittees to work on metrics directly related to clinical outcomes demonstrated as a result of physician interventions. The Director was tasked to address patient and staff satisfaction indicators. All subcommittees would routinely report the status of their metrics to the C-Suite members composed of the CNO, CFO, COS, and the CEO.

Subcommittee chairs and subchairs were established with the understanding that it was imperative that subject matter experts and stakeholders be on the team and to ensure those chosen would be able to work as a team in improving metrics. Within a month of forming the teams, it was noted that many of the teams were not function-

ing as well as it was hoped they would be. An outside team-building group was commissioned to evaluate and remediate issues affecting team functioning. Issues identified by the team building group included:

- Lack of accountability in some teams leading to some of the team members doing most of the work of the group
- Domination of the group and its processes by one or two people with strong personalities or of higher status
- An overall lack of trust within the group that was undermining group efforts
- Constant conflict between some members who were negatively influencing team performance
- Lack of teaming skills causing an inability to work with others
- Lack of understanding of group goals, roles, tasks, and priorities
- Teams too large to easily come to consensus
- Groupthink was present in some groups causing a limitation of creativity.

The team-building group met with the C-Suite members to discuss their findings and to provide them assistance in forming efficient, effective teams. The first task undertaken was to solidify group goals, roles, tasks, and priorities by clearly delineating them in writing and reviewing them with each low performing team. During this process it was noted that people had been placed on committees who had no concept of the metrics they were supposed to fix, or teams were missing vital specialists on their teams. For example, housekeepers were placed on HEIDIS teams but did have any concept about what they were being asked to do. The Sepsis team was miss-

continued

CASE STUDY—cont'd

ing an all-important clinical pharmacist on their team, and the team working on patient infections did not have an infection disease doctor as a member.

The team building group, with the assistance of the C-Suite, assisted the teams in realigning personnel assigned to each team, sometimes changing chairpersons to those who better understood the issues at hand. Once the teams were reselected, all teams went through formal training to be an effective, efficient team. Team sizes were reduced and conflicts among

members were addressed as part of the team building training. Chairpersons and co-chairs were given special training in how to lead a team, improve team communication, deal with difficult team members, and decrease conflict. Each team was reviewed to assure that the appropriate subject matter experts were part of the individual teams.

After 6 months of monitoring and revising teams as needed, the facility stabilized their metrics and, in many cases, exceeded the thresholds that had been established.

CRITICAL THINKING EXERCISE

Organize into a small group, then select a leader. Take a few minutes to do this, and then select or appoint a process recorder. Here is your assignment:

The leader is a nursing director for hospital services at Deering Hospital. He has been asked to lead a task force to establish the safety of toxic therapeutic drug handling at the staff level. The task force is to create a methodology to identify toxic therapeutic drugs used in the hospital, proper methods to be employed to protect the staff, proper methodologies for disposal of toxic medications, and proper education of staff in relation to the handling and disposal of toxic medications. The leader must select the team members, lead them while preserving teamwork, and produce a viable product that will protect staff from harm. A process recorder is part of the team and will record and report as requested.

1. Observe the process the group uses to select its own leader. Did anyone try to avoid selection? Was someone an enthusiastic volunteer? How long did the process take? Were the selection criteria discussed? What were the selection criteria?
2. What method was used to select/appoint a process recorder? What power strategy was used to make this decision?

3. What is the problem identified in the task?
4. What did the group leader do to handle the situation?
5. What should the group leader do to handle the situation?
6. How did group members respond to the task?
7. What leadership and management strategies might be effective?
8. What could the leader and followers consider changing in the situation?
9. How did group members feel about what happened?

Follow up this exercise with one that tackles a similar problem: this time the leader has just been informed of patient complaints about staff watching TV at night on their phones, ignoring call lights, and keeping patients awake through loud laughing and talking on night shift. There are only a few nurses partaking in this behavior, but they are very intimidating, and most of the staff do not want to get involved in the issue. Evidently this issue has been going on for years, reported continually but never addressed. The staff now exhibits a sense of hopelessness in relation to resolving the issue.

REFERENCES

Agency for Healthcare Research and Quality (AHRQ). (2016). *TeamSTEPPS strategies and tools to enhance performance and patient safety.* http://www.ahrq.gov/professionals/education/curriculum-tools/teamstepps/index.html.

Altman, S., Butler, A., & Shein, L. (Eds.). (2016). *Assessing progress on the Institute of Medicine Report – The Future of Nursing.* Washington, DC: National Academies Press. www.nap.edu.

American Association of Critical-Care Nurses (AACN). (2005). *AACN standards for establishing and sustaining healthy work environments: A journey to excellence.* http://www.aacn.org/wd/hwe/docs/hwestandards.pdf.

Baggs J., & Schmitt, M. (1998). Collaboration between nurses and physicians. *Journal of Nursing Scholarship, 20,* 145–149.

Belker, L., McCormick, L., & Topchik, G. (2019). *Team dynamics.* https://www.amanet.org/articles/team-dynamics/.

Budin, W. C., Brewer, C. S., Chao, Y. Y., & Kovner, C. (2013). Verbal abuse from nurse colleagues and work environment of early registered nurses. *Journal of Nursing Scholarship, 45*(3), 308–316.

Cherniss, C., & Goleman, D. (2001). *The emotionally intelligent workplace: How to select for, measure, and improve emotional intelligence in individuals, groups, and organizations.* San Francisco, CA: Jossey-Bass.

Christensen, C., & Larson, J. (1993). Collaborative medical decision making. *Medical Decision Making, 13,* 339–349.

Debono, D. S., Greenfield, D., Travaglia, J. F., Long, J. C., Black, D., Johnson, J., et al. (2013). Nurses' workarounds in acute healthcare settings: A scoping review. *BMC Health Services Research, 13*(1), 175. https://doi.org/10.1186/1472-6963-13-175.

Einola, K., & Alvesson, M. (2019). The making and unmaking of teams. *Human Relations, 72*(12), 1891–1919.

Goldratt, E. M., & Cox, J. (2016). *The goal: A process of ongoing improvement* (3rd ed.). Abingdon, UK: Routledge.

Hersey, P., Blanchard, K. H., & Johnson, D. E. (2013). *Management of organizational behavior: Leading human resources* (10th ed.). Upper Saddle River, NJ: Pearson Education.

Huber, D. L., Bair, H., & Joseph, M. L. (2019). Roadmap to drive innovativeness in health care. *Nurse Leader, 17*(6), 505–508.

Institute for Healthcare Improvement (IHI). (2016). *Triple aim initiative.* http://www.ihi.org/engage/initiatives/tripleaim/pages/default.aspx.

Jacobs, B., & Rosenthal, T. (1984). Managing effective meetings. *Nursing Economic$, 2*(2), 137–141.

Jay, A. (1982). How to run a meeting. *Journal of Nursing Administration, 12*(1), 22–28.

Kalisch, B., & Lee, K. H. (2010). The impact of teamwork on missed nursing care. *Nursing Outlook, 58*(5), 233–241.

Katzenbach, J. R., & Smith, D. K. (2015). *The wisdom of teams: Creating the high-performance organization* (reprint ed.). Boston, MA: Harvard Business Review Press.

Kayser, T. (2011). *Building team power: How to unleash the collaborative genius of teams for increased engagement, productivity, and results.* New York: McGraw Hill Professional.

Kozlowski, S., & Ilgen, D. (2006). Enhancing the effectiveness of work groups and teams. *Psychological Science of Work Groups and Teams, 7*(3), 77–124.

Lancaster, J. (1981). Making the most of meetings. *Journal of Nursing Administration, 11*(10), 15–19.

Lu, H., Barriball, K. L., Zhang, X., & While, A. E. (2012). Job satisfaction among hospital nurses revisited: A systematic review. *International Journal of Nursing Studies, 49*(8), 1017–1038.

Lumen Learning.com. (2020) *Boundless management. Defining a team.* https://courses.lumenlearning.com/boundless-management/chapter/defining-teams-and-teamwork/.

Manion, J. (2009). *The engaged workforce: Proven strategies to build a positive healthcare workplace.* Chicago, IL: AHA Press.

Manion, J. (2011). *From management to leadership: Strategies for transforming health care.* San Francisco, CA: Jossey-Bass.

Marks, M., Mathieu, J., & Zaccaro, S. (2001). A temporary based framework and taxonomy of team processes. *The Academy of Management Review, 26*(3), 356–376.

Merriam-Webster. (2019). Communication. *The Merriam-Webster.com Dictionary,* Merriam-Webster Inc. https://www.merriam-webster.com/dictionary/communication.

Miller, C., Kim, B., Silverman, A., & Bauer, M. (2018). A systematic review of team-building interventions in non-acute healthcare settings. *BMC Health Services Research, 18*(146), 1–21. https://doi.org/10.1186/s12913-018-2961-9.

Newell, S., & Kirkwood, H. P., Jr. (2020). Teams and teamwork. Adameg, Inc. https://www.referenceforbusiness.com/management/Str-Ti/Teams-and-Teamwork.html.

Read, E., & Laschinger, H. K. (2013). Correlates of new graduate nurses' experiences of workplace mistreatment. *Journal of Nursing Administration, 43*(4), 221–228.

Riley, W., Davis, S. E., Miller, K. K., & McCullough, M. (2010). A model for developing high-reliability teams. *Journal of Nursing Management, 18,* 556–563.

Ronco, W. (2005). *Partnering solutions.* Franklin Lakes, NJ: Career Press.

Roth, C., Wieck, K. L., Fountain, R., & Haas, B. K. (2015). Hospital nurses' perceptions of human factors contributing to nursing errors. *Journal of Nursing Administration, 45*(5), 263–269.

Salas, E., & Rosen, M. A. (2013). Building high reliability teams: Progress and some reflections on teamwork training. *BMJ Quality & Safety, 22*(5), 369–373.

Sikka, R., Morath, J., & Leape, L. (2015). The Quadruple Aim: Care, health, cost and meaning in work. *BMJ Quality & Safety, 24*(10), 608–610. https://doi.org/10.1136/bmjqs-2015-004160.

Teunissen, C., Burrell, B., & Maskill, V. (2020). Effective surgical teams: An integrative review. *Western Journal of Nursing Research, 42*(1), 61–75.

Turner, J. R., Baker, R., & Morris, M. (2018). Complex adaptive systems: Adapting and managing teams and team conflict. *IntechOpen, Chapter 5*, 65–94. https://doi.org/10.5772/intechopen.72344.

Wong, C. A., Cummings, G. G., & Ducharme, L. (2013). The relationship between nursing leadership and patient outcomes: A systematic review update. *Journal of Nursing Management, 21*(5), 709–724.

Wynia, M. K., Von Kohorn, I., & Mitchell, P. H. (2012). Challenges at the intersection of team based and patient-centered health care: Insights from the IOM working group. *Journal of the American Medical Association, 308*(13), 1327–1328.

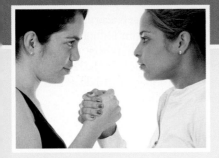

10

Power and Conflict

Mary Louanne Friend

http://evolve.elsevier.com/Huber/leadership

POWER

Nurses are increasingly recognized as leaders who can transform and influence health outcomes by becoming full partners with physicians and other health care professionals to redesign delivery of care in the United States. Several prestigious organizations have acknowledged that nurses are uniquely qualified to lead health care reform, but they must first significantly change their current roles, educational preparation, and responsibilities. The landmark report, *The Future of Nursing: Leading Change, Advancing Health* (Institute of Medicine [IOM], 2011), included recommendations for nurses to improve: (1) access to care, (2) interprofessional collaboration, (3) nursing leadership, (4) nursing education, (5) diversity in nursing, and (6) collection of workforce data. Likewise, in 2010 the Robert Wood Johnson Foundation, in conjunction with the American Association of Retired Persons (AARP) and AARP Foundation, developed the Future of Nursing (n.d.) Campaign to empower nursing to achieve the IOM's recommendations with a nationwide initiative designed to strengthen the power of nursing to help Americans lead longer, healthier lives.

In 2014 the Robert Wood Johnson Foundation requested that the IOM, now called the National Academies of Sciences, Engineering, and Medicine, Health and Medicine Division, assess advancements made since the recommendations of *The Future of Nursing* (IOM, 2011). This follow-up report, *Assessing Progress on the Institute of Medicine Report The Future of Nursing* (National Academies of Sciences, Engineering, and Medicine, 2016), described substantial

improvements including increasing the number of: (1) baccalaureate prepared nurses, (2) nurses with doctoral degrees, (3) states where advanced practiced registered nurses (APRNs) can work to their full capacity, (4) interprofessional educational opportunities, (5) nurses who hold positions on corporate boards, and (6) states that collect nursing workforce data.

However, less progress has been noted in efforts to increase diversity in nursing. Of note, the lack of diversity in nursing has been associated with identified underrepresented groups preferring careers in medicine due in part to the perceived ability to overcome stereotypes, while rejecting nursing to avoid negatively stereotyped careers (Alexander & Diefenbeck, 2020). Additionally, men in nursing have been criticized for being competitive and for receiving preferential leadership opportunities with differential compensation (Brody et al., 2017). These findings are disappointing and suggest the profession has much work to do in terms of improving the image of nursing to increase diversity in both ethnicity and gender.

The authors of the 2016 follow-up report suggested that efforts to increase the numbers of APRNs who practice to the full extent of their education will require ongoing collaboration with other health professions and policy makers to remove scope of practice restrictions. Other recommendations included developing nursing leaders who can (1) lead ongoing reforms to the health care system, (2) direct research on evidence-based improvements to care, (3) translate research findings into practice, (4) be full partners on the health care team, and (5) advocate for policy change (National Academies of Sciences, Engineering, and Medicine, 2016). The accomplishments made thus far are the direct result of nursing leaders working together and collaborating with others to increase their influence. However, nurses also need to learn not only to embrace but also to *value* power if these accomplishments are to be maintained. The process of becoming powerful is not static and will continue to be influenced by societal expectations, emerging technologies, and regulation (Nancarrow & Borthwick, 2005). Both power and conflict have a long history of theoretical development and research primarily found within the business literature. Influential traditions of thought are reviewed in this chapter as they formed the foundation for power and conflict research within nursing.

DEFINITIONS

Power eludes definition but is easy to recognize by its consequences: "the ability of those who possess power to bring about the outcomes they desire" (Salancik & Pfeffer, 1977, p. 3). The general and nursing literature continue to lack a clear definition of power because the construct is often used interchangeably with terms including empowerment, status, leadership, and influence. Power is also defined differently based on the unit of analysis including the individual, groups and institutions. Broadly, **power** is defined as control over resources and is considered to be relational in nature (Fiske, 2010). Power is often described as being either positional (legitimate) or personal.

SOURCES OF POWER

A frequently cited reference related to power is French and Raven's (1959) classic work where power in leadership is defined as the ability of an agent to influence a target within a certain system or context. French and Raven identified five bases of power: (1) reward, (2) coercive, (3) legitimate, (4) expert, and (5) referent (Box 10.1). When reward power is used, people comply because doing so produces positive benefits. Coercive power depends on fear. An individual reacts to the fear of the negative consequences that might occur for failure to comply. Referent power is based on admiration for a person who has desirable resources or personal traits. Legitimate power represents the power a person receives

---

BOX 10.1 French and Raven's Five Sources of Power

1. ***Reward power*** is giving something of value. For example, in nursing, rewards may be a pay raise, praise, a promotion, or a job on the day shift. Reward power is based on the ability to deliver desired rewards.

2. ***Coercive power*** is force against the will. For example, in nursing, coercive power can be the threat of firing, of disciplinary action, or other negative consequences. Coercive power is the power derived from an ability to threaten punishment and deliver penalties. It is a source of power used to apply pressure so that others will meet what is demanded.

3. ***Expert power*** means the use of expertise. It is knowledge, competence, communication, and personal power all combined in a reservoir of knowledge and experience. Expert power is a source of power held by those with some special knowledge, skill, or competence in a particular area. For example, the nurse with the greatest expertise in wound dressings will be sought out by other people in the work environment for this expertise. Expertise is an artful combination of skill and knowledge. It may be founded on depth of knowledge and/or psychomotor skill. There is power in the use of knowledge and skill (i.e., because people need you or can benefit from your expertise, power exists). Therefore the use of expertise can be structured to accomplish or influence movement or action toward certain goals.

4. ***Referent power*** is a little more difficult to understand because it is subtle. It is the use of charisma to influence others. The followers of someone with referent power respond positively to the interpersonal communication and image of the charismatic person. In organizations, this translates into an informal leadership based on liking, charisma, or personal power. Referent power comes from the affinity other people have for someone. They admire the personal qualities, the problem-solving ability, the style, or the dedication the person brings to the work. Referent power can be viewed as an inspirational power because people's admiration for someone allows that person to influence without having to offer rewards or threaten punishments. For example, in the political arena, occasionally there are charismatic political figures or orators. Their influence comes from their followers' liking or identification with them. An example in nursing is Florence Nightingale, who became a symbol of professional nursing. An emotional upsweep is felt by associating with a charismatic person. Referent power is a personal liking and identification experienced by others. Followers attribute referent power to a leader based on the leader's personal characteristics and interpersonal appeal. Physical attractiveness may contribute to referent power.

BOX 10.1   French and Raven's Five Sources of Power—cont'd

5. **Legitimate power** means positional power. It is the right to command within the organizational structure based on the hierarchical position held. The president of the United States has power because of holding the position. Legitimate power is the most common source of power. It is what most often is called *authority*. The authority of position gives the person the right to act, order, and direct others. However, leadership and influence need not be confined to those with authority. Every person possesses the ability to tap different sources of power to use in a variety of situations.

Data from French, J., & Raven, B. (1959). The bases of social power. In D. Cartwright (Ed.), *Studies in social power* (pp. 150–167). Ann Arbor, MI: University of Michigan, Institute for Social Research.

as a result of his or her position in the formal organizational hierarchy. Expert power results from expertise, special skill, or knowledge. This typology is often considered negative because it implies legitimate authority to use positive and negative sanctions (Friend, 2013). Raven later added a sixth base of power, informational or persuasion. *Information power* can stem from any person in the organization and is based on another's perception that the influencer either possesses or has access to information that is valuable to another (Raven, 1965).

Personal power has been associated with social relationships and personal characteristics, including having expertise in knowledge and skills (Yukl, 2013). Yukl suggested that informal power includes referent, expert, or persuasive power. Referent power results from the desire of others to please an agent and is associated with someone who is friendly, charming, and trustworthy. For nurses, clinical competence (expert power) is a considerable source of power because peers will follow a nurse who is perceived to be clinically competent. This personal expertise power is one way that a nurse becomes an informal leader (Mannix et al., 2013). Referent and expert power have reportedly been widely utilized by nurses to implement patient care. *Persuasive power* refers to skill in making rational appeals and is an essential source of personal power (Yukl & Falbe, 1991). It has been suggested nurses' recurrent and direct access to patients increases their informal power in health care settings, yet they continue to lack formal power (Paynton, 2009).

The most recent source of power has been described as capital (Oakes et al., 1998; Ocasio, 2002). There are different types of capital, including economic, cultural, social, and symbolic, which can be used to access valued resources within relationships (Bourdieu, 1985). Bourdieu conceptualized economic capital as material resources that can be converted into money. Cultural capital included cultural and class distinctions acquired through socialization (embodied cultural capital), the possession and display of cultural artifacts that reflect class distinctions (objectified cultural capital), and the acquisition of formal degrees (Ocasio et al., 2020). Social capital is defined by Bourdieu (1985) as resources that can be acquired through access to social relationships and membership in social groups. Symbolic capital included sources such as family names, titles and ranks that provide status and collective recognition. Nahapiet and Goshal (1998) later described three dimensions of social capital including structural, relational, and cognitive social capital. Social capital has been associated with healthy work environments in primary care (DiCicco-Bloom et al., 2007). Social capital theory has also been identified as a framework to understand and measure nurses' contribution to rural health care (Lauder et al., 2006).

SOCIAL CAPITAL IN NURSING

A concept analysis of social capital identified nursing social capital as "nurses' shared assets and way of being and knowing that are evident in, and available through nurses' network of social relationships at work" (Read, 2014, p. 997). Read suggested that future research should include developing tools to measure social capital and that nurse leaders need to focus on strategies to enhance social capital, including improved communication, positive leadership practices, and cultivating a culture of trust among nurses. Laschinger et al. (2014) evaluated the impact of social capital and structural empowerment finding positive correlations between social capital on unit work effectiveness and individual nurses' perception of unit quality. They suggested nursing units that support strong social capital are a value-added investment in patient care quality.

In summary, although power remains an elusive concept, negative connotations of power as individuals imposing their will on another person are still included within nursing textbooks (Catalano, 2019), the constant in many students' lives in relation to literature

(Huntington & Gilmour, 2001). One could even argue that little has changed in nursing since Cohen (1992) wrote the "crises facing nursing today can be summarized under three headings: status and power; economics; and numbers" (p. 113). However, the portrayal of power being absolute or existing only when one agent is dependent upon another is changing, in part due to the scholarship of nursing theorists, who have expanded the characterizations of power as both positive and essential to nursing.

NURSING THEORY AND POWER

The significance of conceptual frameworks of nursing has been well documented (Alligood & Tomey, 2010; Butts et al., 2012; Fawcett, 1999). According to Fawcett, by definition, a profession has unique perspectives and subsequently, requires specific theoretical foundations in order to adequately examine their phenomena of interest. Nurse phenomena of interest are the human as a whole being, the environment, and health (Barrett, 2017). The significance of utilizing nursing knowledge has been increasingly highlighted in the literature because "without theory, nursing becomes a trade who are not professional but instead are ancillary and placed into the despised category of midrange practitioners" (Turkel et al., 2018, p. 186).

Barrett's (1989) Theory of Power as Knowing Participation in Change was developed from a perspective of Rogers' Science of Unitary Human Beings (1970; 1990), and power was identified as one way that human beings participate in patterning their potentials toward well-being. Barrett conceptualized power as a process that can be quantified using the Power as Knowing Participation in Change Tool Version II (PKPCT V II) (Barrett, 2010). Power is making choices, feeling free to act on intention, and creating change. According to Barrett, there are two types of power: power as control and power as freedom, and both are continuously available. Barrett (2017) recommended this framework to be utilized as a structure for strategic planning for the profession.

Sieloff's Theory of Work Team/Group Empowerment within Organizations© (1995) was developed using King's definition of power as a positive resource for nurses within health care organizations, defined as "the capacity to achieve goals" (King, 1981, p. 127). Sieloff's theory defined and measured power at the group level, essential to the work of nurses. The related instrument, The Sieloff-King Assessment of Group Outcome Attainment within Organizations (SKAGOAO) can be utilized to measure the level of nursing group power within organizations (Sieloff, 2003).

Likewise, Chinn's emancipatory theory of Peace and Power (Chinn & Falk-Raphael, 2015) posited that all human relationships involve power that can be used to "create harmony, collective strength, and individual well-being" (p. 62). Chinn rejected the patriarchal view of power as "power over" and instead theorized that power is an exercise to join with others to direct collective energies "toward a future you seek together" (Chinn & Kramer, 1995, p. 8). By incorporating these positive aspects of power, and expanding the concept of power to include groups, nurses have the discipline-specific theoretical foundation and instruments to advocate for and measure their power.

Without power the profession will be unable to challenge ongoing barriers that prohibit nurses' abilities to autonomously provide access to high-quality, patient-centered, affordable care to decrease health inequities. The capability of nursing to collectively embrace their political power at the institutional, community, and national levels is essential. Nursing has been consistently identified as being the highest rated profession in terms of honesty and ethics (Gallup, 2020), while Americans rate their congressman and legislators as having the least honesty and ethical standards. When it comes to public trust in various groups trying to improve the US health care system, Americans generally do not trust any interest major groups, except for nurses (The Commonwealth Fund, 2019). Those who support hierarchal relations are typically those with power (Sidanius & Pratto, 1999). If nurses are disadvantaged in terms of their political power, they need to assemble to collectively challenge the status quo.

POLITICAL POWER

Political power or capital has been defined as the variety of economic, social, and cultural resources available to individuals and groups to affect organizational decisions, actions, and outcomes (Ocasio, 2002). The nursing literature has scant mention of the importance of political power and instead discusses power at the individual, intrapersonal, or institutional levels. This is significant since there are more than three times as many RNs in the United States as physicians, with more than 3.8 million registered nurses (RNs) nationwide

(American Association of Colleges of Nursing [AACN], 2008; Rosseter, 2018). Medicine has historically been perceived as more powerful than nursing (Manojlovich, 2007), and their power has resulted from strategic planning and deliberate actions. These steps included moving into powerful positions in government and creating a strong political voice, while also concentrating on regulation and limiting licensure for other health professions (Nancarrow & Borthwick, 2005).

Nurses have a unique opportunity to unify in efforts to impact health care inequities and disparities that currently plague the American health care system; however, they must understand the political process and how they as individuals can participate. Nurses have historically been apolitical (Des Jardin, 2001) and oblivious to the power they possess (Pelc, 2009). The profession's ongoing values of altruism and caring are associated with nursing's lack of power (Baer, 2009; Bassett, 2002; Cook, & Cullen, 2003). In order to increase political activism, nurse educators need to prepare graduates with the skills required to lead others and develop policy.

Nursing Education and Political Power

The AACN Essentials documents (AACN, 2008, 2011) call for nurses to achieve 12 health policy competencies at the baccalaureate level. However, there are few faculty qualified to teach policy in many schools and some faculty reportedly do not appreciate the importance of policy as it relates to nursing practice and research (Boswell et al., 2005; Des Jardin, 2001; Heiman et al., 2016). This gap in nursing education has been addressed by researchers who incorporated political perspectives within a public health nursing curriculum. Student feedback suggested the course influenced students' values of the political process and increased their knowledge of public policy, the legislative process, teamwork, and organizational skills (Byrd et al., 2004). Service learning has also been utilized to teach baccalaureate students health policy. Course evaluations suggested the experiences were valuable in helping students learn social justice, determinants of health, and the policy process (O'Brien-Larivée, 2011). Recently, recommendations have been made to stage policy education within nursing by tailoring content in undergraduate and graduate courses to prepare students to participate in health policy development. At a bare minimum, future nurses need to be provided with an introduction to how health policy is drafted along

with the opportunity to meet local political leaders to learn how to serve their communities on local school boards and city councils. Novice nurses would greatly benefit from learning how their colleagues have shaped important legislation influencing nursing practice, including mandatory patient/staff ratios (Spetz et al., 2008), mandatory nursing overtime, and mandated staffing committees (ANA, 2015).

Group/Team Power

The strategic contingencies theory of power (Hickson et al., 1971) hypothesized that organizations consisted of interdependent subunits, thus shifting the emphasis of power from individuals to groups (Friend & Sieloff, 2018). The concept of group power is essential to nurses who practice in teams regardless of their setting. Team power has been defined as the ability of teams to control resources to enable the influence of others (Greer et al., 2011). However, this definition is based upon providing or withholding resources or punishments (French & Raven, 1959). In contrast, Sieloff defined group power as the group's ability to achieve goals, rejecting the paternalistic view of power as depending upon either the environment or other individuals within that environment rather than on the efforts of the work team (Sieloff & Friend, 2015). Group power has profound impact on the social realities of nursing, which has repeatedly been referred to as oppressed.

Powerlessness/Oppression

Nursing has been described as powerless and unable to control its own destiny (D'Antonio et al., 2010). Powerless implies being unable to exercise your capacities to produce the goals you are capable of (Sieloff, 2004; Abood, 2007). The profession has often also been referred to as oppressed. According to Webster, oppression is "the unjust or cruel exercise of authority or power; or a sense of being weighed down in body or mind" (Merriam-Webster, n.d.). Frye (1983) described oppression as living one's life shaped by barriers that restrict or penalize motion. The nursing profession, historically restrained by the barriers of hospital bureaucracy, physicians, and senior nurse authority, may be compared to this analogy (Friend, 2013). Oppressed or powerless nurses were first described by Roberts (1983) who affirmed that submissive, passive-aggressive behaviors in nursing develop in response to domineering practices of physicians and hospital administrators.

The nursing literature is replete with manuscripts describing negative nursing interactions characterized as incivility, horizontal and lateral violence, and nurse bullying in academic and clinical environments (Baltimore, 2006; Clark, 2008; Roberts, 2015; Trossman, 2014). Regardless of the label for these behaviors, these actions are consistently associated with increased burnout and turnover intentions, and decreased job satisfaction and commitment (Smith et al., 2010; Laschinger et al., 2009). Of note, these toxic nursing behaviors are not limited to the United States but have also been reported worldwide (Flateau-Lux & Gravel, 2014; Losa Iglesias & Becerro de Bengoa Vellajo, 2012a; Nixon, 2014). A review of the literature proposes these nursing actions are the result of a cycle where behaviors are tolerated and repeated, suggesting that noxious nursing practices are learned from one generation and passed on to another (Hutchinson & Jackson, 2013). What is less clear is how to break the cycle of oppressed behaviors in order to support a unified, powerful profession that can impact individual, community and global health outcomes.

Empowerment

Empowerment, like power, is complex and has multiple perspectives, including structural, psychological, and group. Rappaport (1987) suggested that the ability to identify the absence of empowerment was easier than actually defining the concept. Historically, empowerment gained momentum during the civil right struggles and, unlike power, is consistently considered positive and is either an outcome or process (Friend & Sieloff, 2018). Empowerment has also been described at the individual, organizational, and community levels.

Empowerment was first described within the nursing literature at a time of hospital down-sizing, a nursing shortage, and initiation of quality improvement projects (Bartunek & Spreitzer, 2006). Nursing empowerment was initially described in terms of individual nurses empowering their patients until Rodwell (1996) reported that nurses cannot empower patients and only people can empower themselves. Rao (2012) later defined nurse empowerment as a state in which an individual nurse has assumed control over their practice, enabling them to successfully fulfill professional nursing responsibilities within an organization. Of note, much of the nursing research related to nursing empowerment has been conducted using theoretical frameworks other than nursing, including the social-structural and psychological theories of empowerment.

Empowerment Theories

The social-structural empowerment theory (Kanter, 1977; 1993) focused on how social, political, and organizational forces create powerlessness. Kanter (1977) defined power as the capacity to mobilize resources to accomplish work and believed that workers become empowered by their work environments, not as a result of their personal predisposition. According to Kanter, empowerment is influenced by the degree of formal and informal power an individual has within an organization. Kanter's perspective emphasizes changing organizational policies and practices that support top-down control systems, where power is held by few (Friend, 2013). The concept of psychological empowerment, first described by Conger and Kanungo (1988), suggested empowerment involves more than sharing power. Thomas and Velthouse (1990) expanded upon Conger and Kanungo (1988) by conceptualizing psychological empowerment as intrinsic task motivation consisting of four dimensions: meaning, competence, self-determination, and impact. Spreitzer (1996) built upon Thomas and Velthouse and confirmed that psychological empowerment consisted of four dimensions including meaning, competence, self-determination, and impact. An additional description of power espouses a poststructuralist approach based on the work of Foucault (1980) who believed power is not fixed but instead changes based on context and induces pleasure. Bradbury-Jones et al. (2008) suggested this poststructuralist perspective should be used by nurses to "consider hierarchical observation, normalizing judgment, the examination and knowledge/power relationships in order to illuminate taken-for-granted areas of nursing practice" (p. 264). However, they also asserted that this approach can be used by other disciplines other than nursing. Since nursing is a unique profession, nursing empowerment is best examined using discipline-specific theories and frameworks including Sieloff's nursing theory of group empowerment within organizations (Sieloff & Bularzik, 2011).

Nursing Theory and Empowerment

Sieloff utilized the strategic contingencies theory of power (Hickson et al., 1971) to provide conceptual guidance to understand nursing's lack of power within organizations (Sieloff, 2007). The strategic contingencies theory of power (Hickson et al., 1971) hypothesized that organizations consist of interdependent subunits and that there is a distribution of power in the division of labor, thus shifting the emphasis of power from persons to groups. Three concepts are included within the theory: (1) centrality, (2) coping with uncertainty, and (3) substitutability (Hickson et al., 1971). The centrality of a subunit is the degree to which its activities are interlinked into the system. Centrality refers to working in a central part of the organization giving one a critical role and bargaining power. Uncertainty is defined as "lack of information about future events so that alternatives and their outcomes are unpredictable" (Hickson et al., 1971, p. 5). Substitutability is defined as the ability of the organization to obtain alternative performance for the activities of a subunit. Power comes from the ability to cope with uncertainty, substitutability, and centrality.

Sieloff reconceptualized the concepts of organizational power to address the human context of nursing (Sieloff, 1995). Centrality, coping with uncertainty, and substitutability were relabeled as position, controlling the effects of environmental forces, and role, respectively. In addition, Sieloff (1995) added resources as a fourth source of power. According to Sieloff, these four variables contribute to a group's empowerment capacity. To explain why some groups are not empowered despite empowerment capacity, four variables associated with group empowerment were identified through observations and labeled based on the results of a factor analysis of instrument data (Sieloff, 1995). The variables were (1) communication competency, (2) goal/outcome competency, (3) nurse leaders' empowerment competency, and (4) empowerment perspective (Friend, 2013). The theory has been refined and an associated instrument developed, the Sieloff King Assessment of Work Team/Group Empowerment within Organizations (SKAWGEO) (Friend & Sieloff, 2018).

Gaps in knowledge. Past research has attempted to examine the relationship between work team/group empowerment and nursing-sensitive patient outcomes and safety (Sieloff, 2010). However, due to a lack of the availability of consistent data, this relationship has yet to be studied. It is critical to establish whether a relationship exists between work team/group empowerment and the achievement of safe and quality care as the identification of a relationship between work team/group empowerment and safe, quality nursing care may provide a foundation for future interventional research designed to identify processes to increase cost effective quality nursing care.

Furthermore, past research has identified that work team/group empowerment is a unique construct that exists within all nursing work settings. However, it is not known which factors have the most effect on improving a work team's/group's overall empowerment. If this knowledge could be identified, strategies could be selected using the most effective, yet least expensive, approaches. Rather than using non-nursing theories to develop knowledge to effect nursing work environments, the use of a nursing-theory based perspective and reliable and valid instrument may generate sufficient knowledge to change workplace practices both now and in the future. Regardless of the definition, power is an essential concept because power differentials in health care settings are universal.

The perspective that nurses wait for empowerment to occur as a result of something or someone else has supported the patriarchal view of empowerment and the perception that nurses are oppressed. There is a current need to focus on empowerment at the group or work team level as a strategy to transform nursing education, practice, and research. If, as the nursing literature suggests, factors associated with nursing's oppressed group behavior continue to include lack of empowerment, authoritative leadership, oppression, learned helplessness (Lewis, 2006), negative nursing unit culture and toxic work environment (Freshwater, 2000; Hamlin, 2000), suppressed anger and gender issues (Rowell, 2005), and low self-esteem (Longo & Sherman, 2007), empowered nursing teams are desperately needed.

AUTHORITY AND INFLUENCE

Definitions

Authority and influence are two major content dimensions of power identified in classic theory. Barnard (1938, p. 161) defined authority as "the character of a communication (order) in a formal organization by virtue of which it is accepted by a contributor to or 'member' of the organization as governing the action he contributes." Weber's (1968) work is considered the most influential related to authority. He defined three types of authority: traditional, rational-legal, and charismatic authority. Weber defined traditional authority as resulting from customs and traditions passed from one generation to the next. Rational-legal authority was born from laws, rules, and power with a legitimate office. Charismatic authority is the result of personal abilities to inspire. Authority generally refers to those who have expertise (theoretical authorities) or practical authorities who have particular positions in an organization or social system (Wendt, 2018).

Influence has been defined as the capacity to impact agendas and outcomes and to bring other people on board (Heath, 1988). Influence is associated with leadership as a way to request a behavior that encourages followers to act (Gardner & Avolio, 1998), and the ability to influence others has been described as the most important determinant of managerial effectiveness (Yukl, 1989). Influence then is the attempt to affect or control the behaviors of others (Bierstadt, 1950; Pfeffer, 1992). Beauchamp and Childress (1994) stated that persuasion is one of three categories of influence and includes convincing someone to believe in something through the merit of reasons by another person.

Typically, influence is considered as something that flows downhill from powerholders to subordinates (Oc et al., 2019). However, followers may also use influence tactics upwardly, impacting organizational effectiveness (Goldrick et al., 1994). There have been three conceptualizations of authority and influence: (1) some authors equate these terms, (2) others tend to equate power with influence and assert that authority is a special case of power, and (3) still others view authority and influence as distinctly different dimensions of power. Several points of contrast are summarized in Table 10.1.

Influence Tactics

Nurse Managers (NMs) confront multiple challenges as they are often charged with fiscal, quality, and human resource responsibilities (Bradley & Moore, 2019). Managers operate at the nexus between the nurse and central decision authority levels. Thus they influence the flow and implementation of resources and support. Most of the research on influence has been conducted within the psychology, business, and organizational frameworks. Kipnis et al. (1980) were among the first to investigate the influence behavior of managers. Content analysis led to the identification of 370 different forms of influence behavior, which were condensed into 14 categories. Subsequently, factor analysis brought about the following eight forms of influence behavior:

1. Assertiveness means expressing one's own position to another without inhibiting the rights of others.
2. Ingratiation means trying to make the other person feel important, giving praise or sympathizing. Ingratiation is attempting to advance oneself by trying to make another person feel important.

TABLE 10.1   Authority and Influence Contrasted

Authority	Influence
Authority is the static, structural aspect of power in organizations.	Influence is the dynamic, tactical element.
Authority is the formal aspect of power.	Influence is the informal aspect.
Authority refers to the formally sanctioned right to make decisions.	Influence is not sanctioned by the organization and is therefore not a matter of organizational rights.
Authority implies involuntary submission by subordinates.	Influence implies voluntary submission and does not necessarily entail a superior–subordinate relationship.
Authority flows downward, and it is unidirectional.	Influence is multidirectional and can flow upward, downward, or horizontally.
The source of authority is solely structural.	The source of influence may be personal characteristics, expertise, or opportunity.
Authority is circumscribed.	The domain, scope, and legitimacy of influence are typically ambiguous.

3. Rationality means using logical and rational arguments, providing pertinent information, presenting reasons, and laying out an idea in a logical, structured way.
4. Sanctions are threats. Positive sanctions, or rewards, are addressed within motivation mechanisms.
5. Exchange means that to persuade, an exchange is offered; this is sometimes called "scratching each other's back."
6. Upward appeal means going to a higher authority. It is the childhood threat of "if you don't play by my rules, I am going to go tell Mom." Upward appeal simply means taking the appeal to a higher authority to arbitrate.
7. Blocking means deliberately keeping others from getting their way, threatening to stop working with them, ignoring them, not being friendly, or simply

attempting to make sure others cannot accomplish their aims. This may take the form of bullying.

8. Coalitions are the result of a group of people getting together to speak or negotiate as one voice.

Influence behaviors translate into power strategies. In their three-nation study of managerial influence styles, Kipnis et al. (1984) identified the most to least popular strategies (Table 10.2). Yukl and Falbe (1991) continued the work of Kipnis et al. (1980). They developed the Influence Behavior Questionnaire (IBQ), an instrument to measure the influence behavior of managers. In later studies, the IBQ was developed further, and psychometric tests were performed (Yukl et al., 1992, 1993, 2008). The resulting 11 tactics cover a wide range of influence behavior relevant for managerial effectiveness or, in a broader sense, for getting things done in an organization. Influence tactics are identified in Table 10.3. Research

TABLE 10.2 Most to Least Managerial Influence Strategies Used in All Countries

Strategy Popularity	Managers Influencing Superiors	Managers Influencing Subordinates
Most popular	Reason	Reason
↑	Coalition	Assertiveness
	Friendliness	Friendliness
	Bargaining	Evaluation
	Assertiveness	Bargaining
↓	Higher authority	Higher authority
Least popular	Sanction	

Modified from Kipnis, D., Schmidt, S.M., Swaffin-Smith, C., & Wilkinson, I. (1984). Patterns of managerial influence: Shotgun managers, tacticians, and bystanders. *Organizational Dynamics, 12*(3), 58–67.

TABLE 10.3 Definitions of Influence Tactics

Tactic	Definition
Rational persuasion	The agent uses logical arguments and factual evidence to show that a proposal or request is feasible and relevant for important task objectives.
Inspiration appeals	The agent appeals to the target's values and ideals or seeks to arouse the target's emotions to gain commitment for a request or proposal.
Consultation	The agent asks the target to suggest improvements or help plan an activity or change for which the target's support is desired.
Ingratiation	The agent uses praise and flattery before or during an attempt to influence the target to carry out a request or support a proposal.
Personal appeals	The agent asks the target to carry out a request or support a proposal out of friendship or asks for a personal favor.
Exchange	The agent offers something the target person wants or offers to reciprocate at a later time if the target complies with the request.
Coalition tactics	The agent enlists the aid of, or uses the support of, others to influence the target to do something.
Legitimating tactics	The agent seeks to establish the legitimacy of a request or verify that he or she has the authority to make it.
Pressure	The agent uses demands, threats, frequent checking, or persistent reminders to influence the target to do something.
Collaboration	The agent offers to provide assistance or necessary resources if the target will carry out a request or approve a proposed change.
Apprising	The agent explains how carrying out a request or supporting a proposal will benefit the target personally or help to advance the target's career.

From Yukl, G., Seifert, C.F., & Chavez, C. (2008). Validation of the extended Influence Behavior Questionnaire. *The Leadership Quarterly, 19*(5), 609–621.

utilizing the IBQ suggests that university administrative employees most often used rational persuasion while influencing their superiors (Ghalazi et al., 2012). Nursing research utilizing a modified IBQ suggested that professional practice leaders most frequently used consultation (mean = 4.4, standard deviation [SD] = 0.71) and rational persuasion (mean = 4.3, SD = 0.67), followed by moderate use of inspirational appeal (mean = 3.8, SD = 0.89), legitimizing (mean = 3.8, SD = 0.82), and collaboration (mean = 3.9, SD = 0.72), whereas coalition (mean = 3.0, SD = 0.80) was described as being used occasionally with the manager group (Lankshear et al., 2013). The authors concluded their results were consistent with existing research in that rational persuasion and consultation were often used when trying to influence superiors (Yukl et al., 1993).

Nursing Influence

Historically, nursing influence has focused on how to promote change and outcomes as opposed to how it is acquired and best used (Shilliam et al., 2018). However, the nursing literature currently describes efforts to enhance and to quantify nursing influence. The Adams Influence Model (AIM), originally developed in 2003 to gain an understanding of nurse executive influence, describes the attributes, factors, and processes of influence relating specifically to nurse leaders (Adams & Natarajan, 2016). The original model was based upon French and Raven (1959) and Kipnis and Schmidt (1988) and has since been adapted using three nursing conceptual models, including Neuman's Theory of Health as Expanding Consciousness, Roy's Adaption Model and King's Interacting System Framework and Theory of Goal Attainment.

The current version of the AIM presents an open system model involving a two-person dyad of the influence agent and the influence target. Within the AIM Version V, "there are significant areas of overlap between Barrett's and Sieloff's definitions of power and concepts presented in the AIM, since all three emphasize the role of relationships and intentionality in nurse leaders' efforts to shape the care environment and effect change" (Adams & Natarajan, 2016, p. E 50) (Fig. 10.1). Iteration V of the AIM was evaluated using secondary data analysis resulting in a revised list of influence factors and attributes. The AIM addresses three issues for nursing as identified by King (1964), including the need to further define the nurse leader's practice domain, to identify a standardized, professional language for nurse leaders, and to articulate a theoretical basis for nurse leaders' practice (Adams & Natarajan, 2016). The AIM was recently used to develop an instrument, the Leadership Influence Self-Assessment (LISA©) to help nurse leaders assess and enhance their influence capacity. Factor analysis of the 145-item instrument supports validity and reliability of the tool (Shilliam et al., 2018).

LEADERSHIP AND MANAGEMENT IMPLICATIONS

According to Yukl, "leadership is the process of influencing others to understand and agree about what needs to be done and how it can be done effectively, and the process of facilitating individual and collective efforts to accomplish the shared objectives" (2010, p. 8). Nurses require expertise regarding politics, policy and power to become effective leaders. In order to do this, they must embrace influence and learn to deliver messages that appeal to a wide variety of stakeholders including politicians, policymakers, the media, and the public (Salvage et al., 2019). Dynamic, complex health care organizations require nurse leaders who have the competencies to collaborate across hierarchical boundaries and to influence others towards performance improvement (Dougall et al., 2018). By collaborating across boundaries, nurses can initiate and sustain change from within.

CONFLICT

There are many interpretations of conflict within the literature. **Conflict** is a process that begins when one party perceives that another party has negatively affected, or is about to negatively affect, something that the first party cares about (Robbins, 1998). Marquis and Huston (2012) defined conflict as the consequences of experienced or perceived variations in common goals, values, ideas, attitudes, beliefs, feelings, or actions.

The consequences of unresolved or dysfunctional conflict "hinder organizational performance" (Kreitner & Kinicki, 2010, p. 375). Estimates suggest that US employees spend 2.8 hours per week dealing with unnecessary conflict, corresponding to approximately $359 billion in paid hours and 385 million working days each year (CPP Global Human Capital Report, 2008; Dunford et al., 2020). Conflict between health

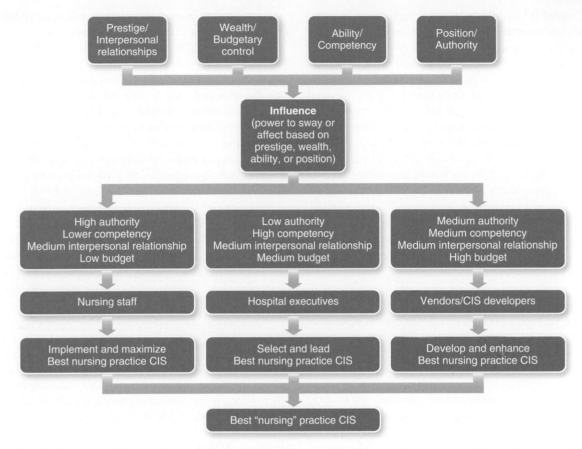

Fig. 10.1 Adams Influence Model, iteration 1. Note: CIS is clinical information systems. (From: Adams, J., & Natarajan, S. (2016). Understanding influence within the context of nursing: Development of the Adams influence model using practice, research, and theory. *Advances in Nursing Science*, 39(3):E40–E56, Figure 1).

care professionals has been associated with decreased providers' attention to patient care, employee satisfaction and morale, and increased turnover (Rosenstein & O'Daniel, 2005). The most damaging outcome of conflict is dysfunctional organizational culture, which stifles change, innovation, and organizational effectiveness. Sentinel events, defined as patient safety events that result in death, permanent harm, or severe temporary harm, have been associated with hospital leadership that fails to establish cultures of safety in hospitals (Smetzer et al., 2010). Conflict resulting in disruptive behaviors in hospitals prompted The Joint Commission (2017), the agency that provides hospital accreditation, to develop a new leadership standard that addressed intimidating behaviors in its elements of performance. Specifically, the standard mandates Chief Executive Officers (CEOs)

to advance trust within the organization by adopting and modeling appropriate behaviors and championing efforts to eradicate intimidating behaviors.

Conflict in nursing has been associated with job dissatisfaction. Nurses have also reported that their managers and nursing colleagues are the most common source of conflict (Bishop, 2004; Lawrence & Callan, 2006; Warner, 2001). Conflict has been reported by 53% of nurses as common (Dewitty et al., 2009) and as contributing to practice errors (Rowe & Sherlock 2005). Unresolved conflict may have negative impacts on organizations, individuals, and patient outcomes (Johansen, 2012; McKibben, 2017). Interpersonal conflicts can lead to nurse attrition and thereby contribute to increasing nurse shortages (Almost et al., 2010; Brinkert, 2010).

Conflict is not inherently undesirable, and, in some situations, a certain amount of conflict is needed as it can improve the quality of decision-making, stimulate involvement in discussion, and build group cohesion (Henry, 2009). What is required is to make a distinction between poorly managed conflicts and properly managed ones. Ideally, conflicts are resolved at the lowest organizational level possible to avoid higher levels of management (Costantino & Merchant, 1996) suggesting nurses need to appreciate how to address conflict at the individual level. However, nurses receive very little training in conflict management but are extensively trained in therapeutic communication (Northam, 2009). Conflict management should be viewed less from a perspective that aims to solve conflict and more towards the idea to manage conflict in a constructive way to enhance group outcomes (Bagshaw & Lepp, 2005; Leksell et al., 2015; Rahim, 2002).

DEFINITIONS

There is no universally accepted definition of conflict (Patton, 2014), although the construct has been studied for a long time. Scholars view the lack of consensus as a major obstacle to progress within the field because research results cannot be generalized from one study to another (Mikkelsen & Clegg, 2018). **Conflict** is defined as a situation where the concerns of two people appear to be incompatible (Thomas & Kilmann, 1974). Conceptual analysis suggested that conflict is a multidimensional construct with both detrimental and beneficial effects (Almost, 2006). The source of conflicts in nursing can be categorized in terms of the degree to which individual characteristics, interpersonal factors, and organizational factors affect working relationships. (Almost, 2006).

Organizational conflict is defined as the struggle over scarce organizational resources. Values, goals, roles, money, or structural elements may be the specific locus of the struggle for scarce organizational resources. For example, two parties may be in opposition because of perceived differences in goals, a struggle over budget allocations, or interference in goal attainment. This opposition prevents cooperation (Deutsch, 1973). **Workplace conflict** emerges when one party—be it an individual or a group of individuals—perceives its goals, values, or opinions being thwarted by an interdependent counterpart (Pondy, 1967; Thomas, 1992; Wall & Callister, 1995). These conflicts may result from scarce resources, such as time, responsibilities, status, or budgets or they

may involve different political preferences, or religious convictions or a combination of issues (De Dreu & Gelfand, 2007; Deutsch, 1973; Druckman, 1994; Kelley & Thibaut, 1969; Rapoport, 1960). **Task-related conflicts** are about the way the team is doing its job, including the pros and cons of certain task approaches (Jehn, 1994). Task conflict is often viewed as healthy because it stimulates discussions and prevents premature consensus, leading to enhanced work-team effectiveness and performance (De Dreu & Beersma, 2005). **Relationship conflicts** are about people, their values, political convictions, or religious preference (Jehn, 1994, 1995; Simons & Peterson, 2000). Relationship conflict leads to biased information-processing and rigid stances, which negatively affect decision-making (de Wit et al., 2013). **Process conflict** involves incompatibilities in views about how the work should be accomplished (e.g., distribution of workload, order of tasks to be completed) (Jehn, 1997).

CONFLICT MANAGEMENT

There has been a decrease in the negative connotation of conflict to include a more positive view where conflict is seen as an inevitable phenomenon that can have beneficial effects and lead to personal, as well as organizational, growth (Almost, 2006; Alper et al., 2000; Brinkert, 2010; Slabbert, 2004). Conflict is functional, or constructive, when it improves the quality of decisions, stimulates creativity and innovation, encourages interest and curiosity, provides a medium through which problems can be aired and tensions released, and fosters an environment of self-evaluation and change (Box 10.2). In contrast, dysfunctional or destructive outcomes

---

BOX 10.2   Effects of Conflict

Constructive Effects
- Improves decision quality
- Stimulates creativity
- Encourages interest
- Provides a forum to release tension
- Fosters change

Destructive Effects
- Constricts communication
- Decreases cohesiveness
- Explodes into fighting
- Hinders performance

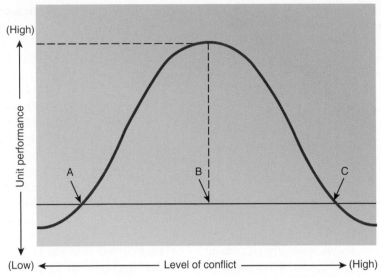

Fig. 10.2 Conflict and unit performance. (Modified from Brown, L.D. [1983]. *Managing conflict at organizational interfaces*. Reading, MA: Addison-Wesley Publishing.)

include a degrading of communication, reduction in group cohesiveness, and subordination of group goals to the primacy of infighting among members. Extremely high or low levels of conflict hinder performance. An optimal level is high enough to prevent stagnation and stimulates creativity, releases tension, and initiates change. However, it is not so high as to be disruptive or counterproductive (Brown, 1983) (Fig. 10.2).

LEVELS OF CONFLICT

Thomas (1992) identified two broad types of conflict. The first refers to incompatible response tendencies within an individual, which Rahim and Bonoma (1979) referred to as intrapersonal conflict (Fig. 10.3). Intrapersonal conflict means discord, tension, or stress inside—or internal to—an individual that results from unmet needs, expectations, or goals. Intrapersonal conflict is conflict that generates from within an individual (Rahim, 1983). It is often manifested as a conflict over two competing roles. For example, a parent with a sick child who has to go to work faces a conflict: the need to take care of the sick child against the need to make a living. A nursing example occurs when the nurse determines that a patient needs teaching or counseling, but the organization's assignment system is set up in a

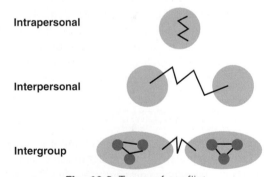

Fig. 10.3 Types of conflict.

way that does not provide an adequate amount of time. When other priorities compete, an internal or intrapersonal conflict of roles exists.

The second use refers to conflicts that occur between different individuals, groups, organizations, or other social units. Rahim and Bonoma (1979) identified these as interpersonal conflict, a category that includes intragroup conflict, intergroup conflict, and interorganizational conflict. Interpersonal means conflict emerging between two or more people, such as between two nurses, a doctor and a nurse, or a nurse manager and a staff nurse. In this case, two people have a disagreement, conflict, or clash. Either their values or styles do not match or there is a misunderstanding or miscommunication between them. Interpersonal conflict can be viewed as happening between two individuals or among individuals within a group. When it specifically involves multiple individuals within a group, interpersonal conflict is called intragroup conflict, which refers to disagreements or differences among the members of a group or its subgroups about goals, functions, or activities of the group.

Intergroup conflict refers to disagreements or differences between the members of two or more groups or their representatives over authority, territory, and resources. Interorganizational conflict occurs across organizations (Rahim & Bonoma, 1979). It is conflict occurring between two distinct groups of people. For example, physicians and nurses may disagree about role functions and activities, or lay midwives may seek to perform home deliveries without being prepared as licensed nurse midwives. Intergroup conflict may also arise during decision-making about the use of postoperative life-sustaining treatment in the intensive care unit due to their perceptions of professional roles and responsibilities (Pecanac & Schwarze, 2018). Sometimes the conflict arises between departments or units as groups. For example, hospital nurses might find themselves in conflict with central purchasing if supplies are provided that do not meet nursing needs or are defective.

CONFLICT MANAGEMENT

Conflict management is used within the organization when facing disagreement or conflict to achieve organizational goals like effectiveness and efficiency. According to De Dreu et al. (2001), conflict management is the intention of a person's actions tailored with their conflict experiences. Follett (1940) identified three main

ways of dealing with conflict: domination, compromise, and integration; and two other ways of handling conflict in organizations: avoidance and suppression. Blake and Mouton (1964) later created a framework for classifying approaches for handling interpersonal conflicts into five activities: (1) forcing, (2) withdrawing, (3) smoothing, (4) compromising, and (5) problem-solving. Rahim and Magner (1995) identified five ways of handling conflict: integrating (cooperation among the parties to reach a solution mutually acceptable), obliging (reducing differences and trying to satisfy the other party), dominating (solution-oriented win–lose or behavior forced to win the position), avoiding (behavioral withdraw or escape), and compromising (both parties give and accept or adjust to each other).

Thomas and Kilmann (1974) developed a model of conflict management based on assertive behavior (the desire to satisfy yourself) and cooperative behavior (the desire to satisfy the other party). They identified five strategies involved with conflict resolution including: competing, collaborating, avoiding, accommodating, and compromising. Competing strategy is characterized by the urge to maximize benefits to the individual, but it is a loss for others. Compromising includes not taking sides and involves making concessions towards the resolution of the conflict. Avoiding involves escape from the conflict. Accommodating behaviors involve sacrificing self-interest for satisfying the needs of others. Models including five management strategies have been most widely utilized in the literature (Kristanto, 2017).

Pondy (1967), Filley (1975), and Thomas and Schmidt (1976) described conflict dynamics across a temporal sequence of stages or phases. These models provide significant insight into understanding the nature of conflict phenomena (Table 10.4). These models are similar in that all indicate that conflict follows a

TABLE 10.4 **Comparison of Four Process Models of Conflict**			
Pondy (1967)	**Filley (1975)**	**Thomas (1976)**	**Robbins & Judge (2016)**
1. Latent (antecedent conditions)	1. Antecedent conditions	1. Frustration	1. Potential opposition
2. Perception and feeling	2. Perceived conflict	2. Conceptualization	2. Cognition and personalization
3. Behavior manifestation (manifest)	3. Felt conflict	3. Behavior	3. Intentions
4. Aftermath	4. Manifest behavior	4. Others' reactions (interaction)	4. Behavior
	5. Resolution or suppression	5. Outcome	5. Functional or dysfunctional outcomes
	6. Conflict aftermath		

predictable course. However, they differ in the number of identifiable stages or elements in a particular pattern. The following elements exist in all the models:

- Causes, identified as conditions, that occur before the conflict
- Core processes, including the perception that conflict exists, followed by some kind of affective state or emotional response
- Conflict behaviors, including a variety of behaviors from very subtle to violent
- Effect that includes outcomes such as resolution or aftermath consequences

Cause, Core Process, Effect

Wall and Callister (1995) described a generic model of conflict. As with any social process, there are causes and a core process that have effects. These effects in turn have an impact on the original cause. This conflict cycle takes place within a context (environment), and the cycle flows through numerous iterations. Wall and Callister (1995) indicated that the model is a general one that displays how the major pieces in the conflict puzzle fit together. The value of this model is that concepts from all other models may be subsumed under the major concepts of this generic model. In addition,

the simplicity of the model facilitates the discussion of conflict according to cause, core process, and effect. Fig. 10.4 uses Wall and Callister's model as a beginning and incorporates the work of Boynton (2012), Patton (2014), and Robbins and Judge (2016). A recent meta-analysis of the literature to identify and synthesize key triggers and impact of healthcare conflicts identified three gaps in the research literature including: (1) lack of holistic approaches to understanding the multi-layered factors involving healthcare conflicts, (2) few studies associating resource depletion and low psychological capital with conflict triggers, and (3) the need to understand the role of psychological safety in healthcare power hierarchy (Kim, 2017, p. 3).

Causes of Conflict

According to Wall and Callister (1995), conditions that occur before conflict is identified are causes. Patton (2014) identified some causes of conflict as personality differences, value differences, blurred job boundaries, battle for limited resources, constraints on the decision-making process, communication, departmental competition, unmet expectations for co-workers, and the complexity of organizations. Additional causes of conflict include lack of clarity with expectations or

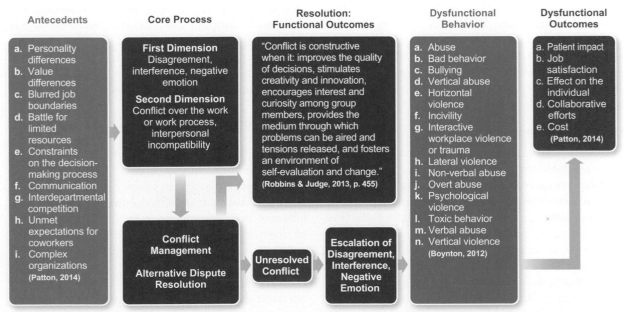

Fig. 10.4 Conceptual framework: antecedents, core process, and functional and dysfunctional outcomes of intragroup conflict.

guidelines, poor communication, lack of clear jurisdiction, personality differences, conflicts of interest, and changes within the organization (Umiker, 1999).

A recent longitudinal study to explore health care professionals' experiences of conflicts and their characteristics identified six sources of conflict: relationships, patient-related tasks, other tasks, team processes, structural processes, and social representations (Bochatay et al., 2017). The authors suggested that disagreements on patient care tended to be the primary trigger of conflict, whereas sources related to communication contributed to conflict escalation without directly triggering conflict.

Moore's Circle of Conflict Model (Moore & Kordick, 2006) included five sources of conflict: (1) data based, (2) interest based, (3) structural based, (4) relationship based, and (5) value based. Data-based conflict occurs when important information is withheld, late, error ridden, irrelevant, or poorly interpreted to the patient or family. Interest-based conflicts occur when a health facility's protocols, processes, or policies frustrate patients' or their loved ones' goals or objectives. Relationship conflicts may not involve important interests, yet they evoke strong reactions. An example of relationship conflict includes poor bedside manner. Structural conflicts arise from the health care system's essential makeup and culture. At the organizational level, structural conflicts involve resource allocations, status differences, role assignments, spatial and organizational relationships, and rules and regulations. Values-based conflicts involve most deeply held beliefs and moral systems that fuel conflicts which are often edgy, "angry," emotional, unforgiving, and disruptive to good care; they are also strongly linked to staff burnout and turnover (Nelson, 2012).

The Core Process of Conflict

Although conflict has been defined in many ways, disagreement, interference, and negative emotion are thought to underlie conflict situations (Barki & Hartwick, 2001). Disagreement, interference, and negative emotion can be viewed as reflecting cognitive, behavioral, and affective manifestations of interpersonal conflict. Disagreement is the most commonly discussed and assessed cognition in the literature. Although a number of different behaviors have been associated with and may be typical of conflict, they do not always indicate the existence of conflict. Conflict exists when the behavior of one party interferes with or opposes another party's attainment of its own interests, objectives, or goals. Several affective states have been associated with conflict. However, it is the negative emotions such as fear, anger, anxiety, and frustration that have been used to characterize conflict. Barki and Hartwick (2001) proposed that interpersonal conflict exists only when disagreement, interference, and negative emotion are present in the situation.

In Barki and Hartwick 2004, conducted a comprehensive review of the literature, and two dimensions of conflict were identified. The first dimension identifies disagreement, interference, and negative emotion as three properties generally associated with a conflict situation. The second dimension identifies relationship and task content or task process as two targets of interpersonal conflict encountered in organizational settings. Conflict management and alternative dispute resolution (ADR) are also components of the core process of conflict.

Effects of Conflict

Patton (2014) noted that conflict has an impact on job satisfaction, individuals, collaborative efforts, and organizational costs. However, the most serious effect is the negative impact on patients. Positive functional outcomes of conflict include increased group performance, improved quality of decisions, stimulation of creativity and innovation, encouragement of interest and curiosity, provision of a medium for problem-solving, and creation of an environment for self-evaluation and changes. In contrast, dysfunctional outcomes include development of discontent, reduced group effectiveness, disrupted communication, reduced group cohesiveness, and infighting among group members, which then overrides the focus on group goals (Robbins & Judge, 2016).

BULLYING AND DISRUPTIVE BEHAVIOR

Interestingly, many authors addressed the negative impact of unresolved conflict, but few have addressed the escalation of conflict to dysfunctional behavior. Disruptive behavior is defined differently but includes behavior that can negatively impact labor relations, effectiveness of communication, information transfer, and the care process and its outcomes (Rosenstein et al., 2002). Disruptive Behavior in Healthcare Work is a theoretical construct made from the combination of several attributes that represent a spectrum of behaviors ranging from incivility to physical and/or sexual violence (Oliveira et al., 2016, p. 695). After a meta-analysis,

Oliveira and colleagues promulgated the following definition: "any inappropriate behavior, confrontation or conflict—ranging from verbal abuse (abusive, intimidating, disrespectful, or threatening behavior) to physical or sexual harassment—which can negatively impact labor relations, effectiveness of communication, information transfer, and the care process and its outcomes." Disruptive behaviors have been classified as including primarily psychological violence, followed by incivility, and physical or sexual violence. There are an increasing number of professionals in hospital organizations whose behavior includes intimidation and hostility, reflected in poor communication and reduced information transfer endangering patient safety (Walrath et al., 2013).

Precursors of disruptive behavior include intrapersonal, organizational, and interpersonal antecedents. Consequences of disruptive behavior primarily affect the worker/health team followed by the patient and the health care organization (Oliveira et al., 2016). Disruptive behavior in the workplace is shown to have significant negative effects on individuals and on patient care and safety, and it can undermine the organization itself (Small et al., 2015). Consequences for workers and the health care team were most often cited, including burnout and decreased morale. Disruptive behaviors were also associated with decreased job satisfaction of nurses and their decisions to leave the profession (Rosenstein & O'Daniel, 2005). Of note, many nurses who reported disruptive behaviors often did not report or comment about them to their peer or manager (Oliveira et al., 2016). The authors also identified three themes of disruptive behavior: incivility, psychological aggression, and violence (Walrath et al., 2010). Given that disruptive behaviors can result in compromised patient safety and costs to the organization and physical violence, nurses need to understand how to address the antecedents of these behaviors and have the difficult conversations to address them head on. Likewise, hospital leaders must strive to decrease the organizational antecedents of disruptive behaviors, including high workload pressure, volume, and number of patients, in addition to unsolved systemic problems (Oliveira et al., 2016.)

Prevention of conflict would be ideal; however, the multiple antecedents and diverse nature of hospital environments preclude preventing conflict. The use of Conflict Management Interviews (CMIs) has gained popularity in health care settings. CMIs are private in-person meetings between two individuals to confront and resolve emerging conflict (Cummings & Worley, 2015). In CMIs, communication and feedback are exchanged in both directions between the supervisor and subordinate as opposed to the top-down method with traditional performance appraisal-related meetings (Dunford et al., 2020). A recent study evaluated a major preventive conflict management initiative in a US health care system in the eastern United States over an 8-year period. The initiative consisted of training and enabling employees and supervisors to conduct CMIs (Boss 1983; Whetten & Cameron, 2016) with one another throughout the health system. The authors used a combination of survey and administrative data and analyzed using ordinary least squares (OLS) and fixed effects panel regression models to test how line managers' participation in CMIs with their employees affected formal grievances, their employees' perceptions of department culture, and actual retention. Study findings suggested that high quality CMIs are associated with a lower likelihood of formal grievances, significantly more perceptions of participative department culture, and lower turnover rates (Dunford et al., 2020).

CONFLICT SCALES

Three conflict inventories are available to measure conflict. The Rahim Organizational Conflict Inventory-I (Rahim, 1983) is designed to measure three dimensions of conflict: intrapersonal, intragroup, and intergroup. The Perceived Conflict Scale (Gardner, 1992) contains four subscales of conflict: intrapersonal, interpersonal, intergroup/other departments, and intergroup/support services. This scale is designed to measure conflict in nursing. Cox (2014) developed a new intragroup conflict scale based on Barki and Hartwick's two dimensions. The scale consists of six subscales: (1) interference over the task, (2) negative emotion over the task, (3) negative emotion and interference related to interpersonal incompatibilities, (4) disagreement over the task process, (5) disagreement over the task, and (6) disagreement related to interpersonal incompatibilities.

CONFLICT MANAGEMENT AND ALTERNATIVE DISPUTE RESOLUTION

Although conflict management and conflict resolution are often used interchangeably, there are differences in the terms (Rahim, 2010). Conflict management involves the control, but not resolution, of a long-term or deep-rooted conflict. In contrast, conflict resolution involves eliminating all forms of conflict. Negotiation, mediation, and arbitration are often referred to in discussions of conflict resolution. These terms are also included under the umbrella of ADR. ADR consists of several forms of conflict resolution that are used to avoid going to court (Brubaker et al., 2014).

Conflict Management Styles

Although other labels have been used for conflict management styles, those identified by Thomas and Schmidt in 1976 are the most frequently cited. The author labeled the five conflict management styles as accommodating, avoiding, collaborating, competing, and compromising.

- **Accommodating** results when one party seeks to appease an opponent; that party is willing to be self-sacrificing.
- **Avoiding** emerges when a person recognizes that a conflict exists and wants to withdraw from it or suppress it.
- **Collaborating** ensues when the parties to conflict each desire to fully satisfy the concerns of all parties. The intention is to solve the problem by clarifying differences rather than by accommodating.
- **Competing** occurs when one person seeks to satisfy his or her own interests regardless of the impact on the other parties to the conflict.
- **Compromising** may develop when each party to the conflict seeks to give up something and sharing occurs, with the result of a compromised outcome. There is no clear winner or loser, and the solution provides incomplete satisfaction of both parties' concerns (Robbins & Judge, 2016).

Shargh et al. (2013) indicated that each of the conflict management styles can be used for different situations. The challenge is for nurses to know when to use each style. Thomas (1976) identified situations for the appropriate use of each conflict management style (see Table 10.5).

Conflict Competence

Conflict competence is the ability to develop and use cognitive, emotional, and behavioral skills that enhance productive outcomes of conflict while reducing the likelihood of escalation or harm (Runde & Flanagan, 2010). An essential skill associated with this competency includes being able to have difficult or crucial conversations. A crucial conversation is defined as "a discussion between two or more people where (1) the stakes are high, (2) opinions vary, and (3) emotions run strong (Patterson et al., 2005). In addition to the ability to hold crucial conversations, one must also be able to confront someone about their behavior face to face (Patterson et al., 2005).

Carefronting

Sometimes conflict between two individuals can be managed by carefronting, which is defined as "a method of communication that entails caring enough about one's self, one's goals, and others to confront courageously in a self-asserting, responsible manner" (Kuperschmidt, 2008, p. 12). Issues are the focus of the interaction. Individuals speak for themselves but in a way that decreases defensiveness and allows another person to hear the message. "I" messages are used; "you" messages are avoided.

Studies of Conflict Management in Nursing

Historically, nursing experienced intrapersonal conflict because of role confusion (Benne & Bennis, 1959). They identified four sources of role confusion for nursing, including institutional expectations, expectations from other nurses including peers and supervisors, professional associations, and the nurse's own self expectations. They summarized role conflicts as involving (1) frustration between their image of "real" nursing and the functions they assume in actual work situations, (2) the nurse–doctor relationship as often a tension area, and (3) promotion for the nurse all too frequently being a conflict between a desire for higher status and a psychological need to give bedside care. Of note, they identified that many of these role conflicts were related to continuing and accelerated change in the health field, stating that change has become the law of contemporary organizational life. Through their research they identified three patterns that nurses use to address conflict: (1) the nurse may lose interest in the job or forsake the effort to find satisfaction in it, (2) the nurse rationalizes away the conflicting demands by calling the schools of nursing and the professional associations "impractical," "theoretical," and "disoriented to the realities of nursing" (Benne & Bennis, 1959, p. 383), and (3) the nurse may formally or informally organize with others to resist the demands of the institution where they work, including a slowdown of efforts and watering down of orders in the execution of them.

TABLE 10.5   Use of Conflict Management Styles According to Situation

Conflict Management Style	Situation
Collaborating	When both sets of concerns are too important to be compromised When objective is to learn To merge insights from people with different perspectives To gain commitment by incorporating concerns into a consensus To work through feelings that have interfered with a relationship
Accommodating	To allow a better position to be heard and to show reasonableness When issues are more important to others than yourself To build social credit for later issues To minimize loss when you are outmatched and losing When harmony and stability are especially important To allow subordinates to develop by learning from mistakes
Competing	When quick, decisive action is vital On important issues where unpopular actions need implementing On issues vital to organization and when you know you are right Against people who take advantage of non-competitive behavior
Avoiding	When an issue is trivial, or more important issues are pressing When you see no chance of satisfying your concerns To let people "cool down" and regain perspective Gathering information supersedes the immediate decision When others can resolve the conflict more effectively
Compromising	When goals are important but not worth potential disruption of more assertive modes When equal power opponents are committed to mutually exclusive goals To find temporary settlements of complex issues To arrive at expedient solutions under time pressure

Adapted from Thomas, K.W. (1977). Toward multidimensional values in teaching: The example of conflict behaviors. *Academy of Management Review, 2*(3), p. 487.

Nursing conflict has been examined widely since then, with older studies finding that avoiding and compromising were the most frequently used conflict handling intentions in nursing. For example, Sportsman and Hamilton (2007) conducted a study to determine prevalent conflict management styles chosen by students in nursing and to contrast these styles with those chosen by students in allied health professions. The associations among the level of professional health care education and the style chosen were also determined. A convenience sample of 126 university students completed the Thomas-Kilmann Conflict Mode Instrument (TKI). The difference was not significant between the prevalent conflict management styles chosen by graduate and undergraduate nursing students and those in allied health. Some of the students were already licensed in their discipline; others had not yet taken a licensing examination. Licensure and educational level were not associated with choice of styles. Women and men had similar preferences. The prevalent style for nursing students was compromise, followed by avoidance. The prevalent style for allied health students was avoidance, followed by compromise and accommodation. Compared with the TKI norms, slightly more than one-half of all participants chose two or more conflict management styles—commonly avoidance and accommodation—at the 75th percentile or above. Only 9.8% of the participants chose collaboration at that level.

Professional nurses in Madrid, Spain, who worked in either a university setting, or a clinical care setting were surveyed to identify conflict resolution styles based on TKI (Thomas & Kilmann, 1974). The styles most frequently used by nurses overall were compromising (27.7%) and competing (26.2%), followed by avoiding

(23.1%) and accommodating (18.5%). Very few participants (4.6%) were assessed as using a collaborating approach (Losa Iglesias & Becerro de Bengoa Vallejo, 2012b). The authors suggested that these results confirm previous findings (Shell, 2001; Valentine, 1995). They concluded that the inclination toward compromise may reflect the powerlessness associated with some nursing positions.

CONFLICT RESOLUTION

Conflict resolution involves eliminating all forms of conflict. Negotiation, mediation, and arbitration are often referred to in discussions of conflict resolution. These terms are also included under the umbrella of ADR. According to Knickle et al. (2012) the resolution continuum includes negotiation, mediation, arbitration, and litigation as a spectrum of third-party dispute resolution.

Negotiation: Negotiation can be used by individuals to come to an agreement or in third-party negotiations such as ADR. Negotiation is the major process used in any ADR technique. It is the process whereby two or more parties come to an agreement. There are no official rules for the negotiation process. Robbins and Judge (2016) described negotiation as a five-step process: (1) preparation and planning, (2) definition of ground rules, (3) clarification and justification, (4) bargaining and problem-solving, and (5) closure and implementation.

Principled negotiation: Principled negotiation is an approach proposed by Fisher et al. (1991), who urged negotiators to use the following five fundamental principles to negotiate effectively with each other instead of against each other:
1. Separate the people from the problem.
2. Focus on interests, not positions.
3. Invent options for mutual gain.
4. Insist on using objective criteria.
5. Know your BATNA (Best Alternative to Negotiated Agreement).

The authors were also the first to coin the acronym BATNA. This term essentially describes the need to conceive of creating and developing backup plans when all else fails. Invariably, not even the best intentions to find agreement will necessarily come to fruition.

Conciliation: A conciliator is like a third friend who might attempt to intercede in an argument between two other friends. Conciliators attempt to diffuse the negative emotions that are often involved in the conflict, and they strive to establish more effective communications between the parties. They attempt to understand each party's point of view as a basis for common ground. The conciliator might also meet with managers and co-workers who are involved in order to have greater insight into the conflict situation (Brubaker et al., 2014).

Mediation: Mediation is often used when the parties have tried to negotiate on their own, but the negotiation has not been successful. The mediator is a process expert and acts as a neutral third party. Although the mediator controls the process, the parties control the outcome. The mediator's job is to listen to the evidence, assist the parties to understand each other's viewpoint regarding the controversy, and then facilitate the negotiation of a voluntary resolution to the conflict situation (Brubaker et al., 2014).

Arbitration: Arbitration also involves the use of a neutral third party, which may be an individual or panel. The arbitrator(s) make the decision for the parties in conflict. Arbitration may be binding or non-binding (Brubaker et al., 2014).

There are several advantages of ADR. It is usually faster and less costly than litigation. Everyone in the conflict situation has the opportunity to explain their perceptions of the situation. ADR is more flexible and responsive to the individual needs of the people involved, and it is less formal than litigation. Because of the parties' involvement in the process, greater commitment results, and the parties may be more compliant. Confidentiality is maintained as well as the relationship, which is especially important if the relationship will continue.

Face Negotiation Theory

Face negotiation is the focus of a theory developed by Ting-Toomey to describe and explain differences in responses to conflict based on cultural backgrounds (Ting-Toomey, 1988; Ting-Toomey & Kurogi, 1998). This theory draws on the idea that face is a metaphor for our public identity, or self-image, and is an important element of social situations throughout the world. The theory suggested that face influences conflict behavior because in any conflict individual parties have to consider protecting self-interest and/or honoring or attacking another person's conflict goals (Ting-Toomey & Kurogi, 1998). Specifically, face refers to a claimed sense of favorable social self-worth that people want others to have of them (Ting-Toomey & Kurogi, 1998). In the theory, facework refers to a set of communicative behaviors that people use to regulate their social dignity. All individuals want others to see them in a certain way, even though they may not be consciously aware of this desire.

Ting-Toomey (1988) originally considered face negotiation theory as a way to explain differences in conflict communication styles stemming from cultural preferences for individualism versus collectivism. She proposed that those in cultures best described as collectivistic would be more likely to seek to uphold "other-face," whereas those in individualistic cultures would more likely seek to uphold "self-face."

Face negotiation theory builds on the five-style dual-concern framework developed by Rahim (1983, 2002) and is based on the degree to which a person is concerned with self-interest, as well as with the interests of others. The five styles are problem-solving (also called integrating, collaborating, or cooperating), forcing (also called competing or dominating), avoiding (also called suppressing or withdrawing), yielding (also called obliging, accommodating, or smoothing), and compromising (Putnam & Poole, 1987; Rahim, 2010). The theory posits that collectivistic cultures favor the avoiding, yielding, and compromising styles; in contrast, individualistic cultures reputedly favor forcing and problem-solving styles (Ting-Toomey, 1988).

In 1998, the face negotiation theory was revised, and the dimension of self-construal (self-image) was discussed in terms of the independent and interdependent self, or the degree to which people conceive of themselves as relatively autonomous from or connected to others (Ting-Toomey & Kurogi, 1998). The revised theory posits that the degree to which people see themselves as autonomous (independent; self-face) or connected to others (interdependent; other face) is a better predictor of conflict interaction than their cultural or ethnic background. Ting-Toomey and Kurogi (1998) also added the concept of power to the theory to explain communicative differences based on the cultural dimension of power distance. In low power-distance cultures, differences in treatment based on status are less accepted. On the other hand, in high power-distance cultures, differences in treatment based on status are more accepted. The authors proposed that individuals of different status levels in low power-distance cultures are more likely to use the forcing style to resolve conflict, whereas in high power-distance cultures, those in lower status roles may use styles such as yielding.

Two cross-cultural empirical tests of the revised face negotiation theory supported much of the theory (Oetzel & Ting-Toomey, 2003; Oetzel et al., 2001). The 2001 study involved a cross-cultural comparison of four national cultures (Oetzel et al., 2001). In the 2003 study of face negotiation theory, Oetzel and Ting-Toomey tested the underlying assumption that face mediates the relationship between cultural or individual-level variables and conflict styles. The findings provide supportive evidence of the face negotiation theory, especially that face concerns provide a mediating link between cultural values and conflict behavior. The authors also suggested that these findings are particularly significant given the relatively large sample size across four national cultures.

Results of the studies indicated that nursing administrators need to be more attuned to face issues in the conflict dialogue process. The findings of Oetzel and Ting-Toomey (2003) demonstrated that display of other-face concern, which is maintaining the poise or pride of the other person and being sensitive to the other person's self-worth, can lead to a collaborative, win–win integrative approach or an avoiding approach. In contrast, individuals who are more concerned with maintaining self-pride or self-image during a conflict episode would devote effort to defending their conflict position to the neglect of other-face validation issue. Face negotiation theory has been applied to physician communication in the operating room (Kirschbaum, 2012). Study findings suggested (1) the theory and instrument can be utilized for health communication research, (2) face-negotiation theory can be expanded beyond traditional intercultural communication boundaries, and (3) theoretically-based communication structures applied in a medical context could help explain physician miscommunication in the operating room to assist future design of communication training programs for operating-room physicians (p. 292).

Conflict Resolution Outcomes

Whatever conflict resolution style is used, the individual needs to be aware of the outcome that results from the strategy selected. The outcomes of conflict are what actually happens as a result of the conflict management process. The three ways in which conflicts resolve are (1) win–lose, (2) lose–lose, and (3) win–win (Filley, 1975) (Box 10.3). Filley (1975) described the win–win resolution as the optimum conflict management. Win–lose and lose–lose resolutions also occur, but effective managers should seek win–win resolutions. Win–win strategies focus on problem-solving.

BOX 10.3   Conflict Resolution Outcomes

Win–Lose
One party exerts dominance.

Lose–Lose
Neither side wins.

Win–Win
An attempt is made to meet the needs of both parties simultaneously.

Data from Filley, A.C. (1975). *Interpersonal conflict resolution.* Glenview, IL: Scott, Foresman; Filley, A., House, R., & Kerr, S. (1976). *Managerial process and organizational behavior.* Glenview, IL: Scott, Foresman.

Conflict Resolution Inventories

Several instruments have been developed to measure conflict-handling styles. In the Organizational Conflict Inventory-II, Rahim (1983) divided the handling of interpersonal conflict into the two dimensions of concern for self and concern for others—both in high and low degrees—to form a grid. Rahim then adapted Blake and Mouton's (1964) five types of handling interpersonal conflict (forcing, withdrawing, smoothing, compromising, and problem-solving) into five styles of handling interpersonal conflict (avoiding, obliging, compromising, integrating, and dominating). The inventory measures the five identified styles.

Thomas and Kilmann (1974) also developed a style assessment and diagnosis inventory, called the TKI. Their grid uses dimensions of assertiveness and cooperativeness on high to low degrees. The five styles are avoiding, accommodating, compromising, competing, and collaborating. This model blends a description of an individual's behavior on assertiveness and cooperativeness dimensions in situations in which the concerns of two people appear to be incompatible. The behaviors of individuals are thought to be a function of both personal predispositions and situational contingencies. Avoiding is low on both assertiveness and cooperativeness; collaborating is high on both aspects. Competing is high on assertiveness and low on cooperativeness; accommodating is low on assertiveness and high on cooperativeness. Compromising is in the middle.

LEADERSHIP AND MANAGEMENT IMPLICATIONS

Organizational Conflict

Thomas and Schmidt (1976) identified a "big picture" structural model of conflict that examines four factors that seem to influence the way conflict is handled in organizations: behavioral predispositions of individuals, social pressure in the environment, the organization's incentive structure, and rules and procedures. Different levels of power exist as a result of bureaucratic hierarchy and the resultant position power.

Organizational conflict is a form of interpersonal conflict that is generated from aspects of the institution, such as the style of management, rules, procedures, and communication channels. Conflicts that arise when an individual's needs and goals cannot be met within the system are generally organizational. Conflict may be necessary to groups and organizations. Conflict serves to unify and bind together a group by setting boundaries and strengthening a group's identity. Conflict may help stabilize a group by serving as a test of opposing interests within the group. Conflict may help integrate a group by distributing power. Thus conflict may be necessary for the growth of a group and its members and serves to stimulate creativity, innovation, and change.

Organizational leadership sets a tone for conflict and conflict management. This occurs because leaders and managers model behaviors of positive or negative conflict management and choose when and how to intervene in conflict situations. Choice of intervention style and timing of conflict management are functions of the individuals' behavioral predispositions and environmental pressure coupled with the organization's reward structure and coordination and control methods.

Specifically related to organizational conflict and the focus on groups in organizations, Pondy (1967) identified three strategies to use when attempting to resolve organizational conflicts by using bargaining; rules, procedures, and administrative control; and a systems integrator. Bargaining might be useful when a conflict exists over scarce monetary resources. The administrative control approach might be helpful when clarification of role boundaries is needed, such as disagreements over delegation by RNs. The systems integrator approach might be appropriate in a matrix structure or where there is a need to coordinate personnel in vertical and horizontal organizational structures.

Ellis and Abbott (2011) recommended avoiding the seven Cs as ground rules before approaching conflict:

Commanding by way of telling people how to behave

Comparing the person or situation to other people and situations

Condemning individuals

Challenging behavior and condescension

Contradictory or Confusing actions may lead to uncertainty and frustration

Johansen (2012) identified strategies for NMs to use to resolve conflict. The strategies are also useful for all nurses:

- Recognize conflict early. Recognizing the early warning signs of conflict is the first step toward resolution. Pay attention to body language and be cognizant of the moods of the staff.
- Be proactive. Address the issue of concern at an early stage. Avoiding the conflict may cause frustration and escalate the problem.
- Actively listen. Focus attention on the speaker. Try to understand, interpret, and evaluate what is being said. The ability to listen actively can improve interpersonal relationships, reduce conflicts, foster understanding, and improve cooperation.
- Remain calm. Keep responses under control and emotions in check. Do not react to volatile comments. Calmness will help set the tone for the parties involved.
- Define the problem. Clearly identify and define the problem. A clear understanding of the issues will help minimize miscommunication and facilitate resolution.
- Seek a solution. Manage the conflict in a way that successfully meets the goal of reaching an acceptable solution for both parties.

The goal of conflict resolution is to create a win–win situation for all. Although it is not realistic to think that every conflict can be resolved in such an ideal fashion, a win–win solution is a worthy goal requiring hard work, creativity, and sound strategy.

CURRENT ISSUES AND TRENDS

There are numerous trends and issues in the continually changing health care environment that have an impact on nursing and health care organizations related to power and conflict. The availability of nursing theories that conceptualize power and group power as a positive resource are essential to advancing discipline-specific knowledge to help nurses identify how to obtain and use power to achieve goals. Nursing theorists strove to understand nursing as a practice from theoretical points of view that moved beyond a task orientation and served to demarcate distinctive boundaries for nursing as a practice and a realm of knowledge (Meleis, 2018; Walker & Avant, 2019). Walker suggested that the "gifts" of nursing theorists including Orlando, Johnson, Roy, and Orem, are as relevant today as they were in the 60s and 70s and are "are worthy of rediscovery and reformulation as nursing navigates present-day challenges" (Walker, 2020, p. 2).

The one constant in health care is change and by using nursing theory and adopting instruments developed using conceptual frameworks of nursing, the profession will be able to address these changes in discipline specific ways. Issues with health care access, quality, and costs of care will continue to be addressed by nursing leaders who must develop conflict competency, in addition to core competencies including knowledge of health systems, health technology, and policy development. Nurses have been and will continue to be essential to reducing medication errors, reducing infection rates, and ensuring safe transitions of care from hospital to home.

Perhaps the most important reason for nurses to stay at the forefront of technological advances is that medical errors are the third leading cause of death in the United States (Makary & Daniel, 2016). Medical errors are defined by the IOM (1999) as the failure of a planned action to be completed as intended or the use of a wrong plan to achieve an aim. James (2013) referred to medical errors as preventable adverse events and separated the errors into these categories: (1) errors of commission, (2) errors of omission, (3) errors of communication, (4) errors of context, and (5) diagnostic errors. Ehteshami et al. (2013) indicated that a variety of technologies reduce medical errors, especially medication errors, and prevent them in the health care system. Nurses are at the forefront of implementing information technology and use their expertise power throughout the process.

Healthcare information technology (HIT) has been widely adopted with four goals including to (1) inform clinical practice, (2) interconnect clinicians, (3) personalize care, and (4) improve population health (Thompson, & Brailer, 2004). Electronic health records

(EHRs) are an example of technology that increases the effectiveness of health care and reduces medical errors through reminders, alerts, and internal intelligent capabilities. EHRs directly or indirectly improved patient safety by minimizing medicals errors, improving documentation of data, enhancing the completeness of data, and improving the sustainability of data (Tubaishat, 2017). By improving interpersonal communication and collaboration, EHRs may also help decrease intragroup and intergroup conflict and litigation.

Participation in High-Level Decision-Making

Nurses need to participate in high-level decision-making in order to influence patient care and the nursing profession. Power needs to be leveraged and conflict managed. The Robert Wood Johnson Foundation's (RWJF, 2018) Future of Nursing Campaign for Action advocated for a nurse in every boardroom. Thew (2016) suggested that if nurses are interested in entering the boardroom, they need to (1) find an organization in which they are interested, (2) know their own strengths, (3) express interest, and (4) not allow time constraints to interfere with participation in the boardroom.

Stalter and Arms (2016) described six competencies needed by nurses who are serving on boards and/or policy committees so that they can contribute in a productive manner. These competencies include a professional commitment to serving on a governing board; knowledge about board types, bylaws, and job descriptions; an understanding of standard business protocols, board member roles, and voting processes; a willingness to use principles for managing and leading effective and efficient board meetings; an appreciation for the ethical and legal processes for conducting meetings; and the ability to employ strategies for maintaining control during intense/uncivil situations.

Building a Personal Power Base

Huston (2008) emphasized the importance of building a personal power base and proposed 11 strategies that can be used by both NMs and staff to establish a personal power base. These are demonstrating expertise possibly through certification, identifying positive role models and seeking mentoring relationships, networking and coalition building, maintaining freedom of maneuverability, being aware of self, staying focused on goals, choosing battles carefully, demonstrating willingness to take risks, giving up some ego, working hard and being a team player, and finally, taking care of oneself. The author concluded that building a personal power base will take time, but the outcome is the ability to achieve personal and professional goals and is therefore well worth the effort.

Political Action

With 3.8 million RNs in the nation, the nursing profession should be a tremendous force in political and public policy debates. This is an area for nurses to unite and use their power to improve patient care. Nurses have great potential to contribute to the development of health policy through political action, and their involvement in health policy development ensures that health care is safe, of a high quality, accessible and affordable. Knowledge, skills, and abilities in understanding, using, and managing power and conflict are crucial to nursing in both personal and professional arenas.

◢ RESEARCH NOTE

Source
Kang, S. W., Lee, S., & Choi, S. B. (2017). The impact of nursing leader's behavioral integrity and intragroup relationship conflict on staff nurses' intention to remain. *JONA: The Journal of Nursing Administration, 47*(5), 294–300.

Purpose
This study tested a multilevel model examining the effect of nursing leaders' (NL) behavioral integrity and intragroup relationship conflict on staff nurses' intent to remain.

Discussion
This study was the first to examine the impact of the NL behavioral integrity on hospital nurses' intention to remain. In addition, the effect of unit-level intragroup relationship conflict on hospital nurses was examined. The study was framed methodologically using the Social Exchange perspective, which proposed both leaders and followers enter into reciprocal relationships to maximize their benefits. The theory suggests that a NL's behavior integrity causes staff nurses to perceive them as trustworthy and believe that they have the best interests of

RESEARCH NOTE—cont'd

staff nurses in mind, because of the congruence between their words and actions. In contrast, when a nursing unit is subjected to a high level of intragroup relationship conflict, the quality of social exchange between staff nurses is often poor, and it is important that they maintain good social exchange with the NL. Therefore, in nursing units with a high level of intragroup relationship conflict, the impact of the NLs' behavioral integrity on staff nurses' intention to remain is stronger relative to that in units without this conflict.

Sample and design. The survey participants were RNs working at a large public hospital in South Korea. Surveys were distributed to RNs from 34 nursing units, and English survey items were translated into Korean. Of 552 RNs, 480 returned completed questionnaires (response rate, 87%). Measures of the NLs' behavioral integrity and staff nurses' intention to remain were used as individual-level variables, and intragroup relationship conflicts were aggregated to a unit level as specified in a hypothesized research model.

Data analysis. The model was tested using a multilevel technique (i.e., hierarchical linear modelling) to examine the relationships between individual- and unit-level variables simultaneously. The program 28 STATA Data Analysis and Statistical Software 12.1 (StataCorp, College Station, TX) was used in the analysis.

Results. Nursing leaders' behavioral integrity was positively related to nurses' intention to remain ($b = 0.34$, $P < .001$). In addition, job stress and individual perceptions of intragroup relationship conflict exerted a negatively significant effect on staff nurses' intention to remain ($b = -0.22$ [$P < .001$] and $b = -0.12$ [$P < .05$], respectively).

The simple slope analysis indicated that the coefficient for the relationship between the NLs' behavioral integrity and staff nurses intention to remain differed significantly from zero when the level of intragroup relationship conflict was either low ($b = 0.23$, $P < .01$) or high ($b = 0.48$, $P < .001$).

Discussion. The main implication of the study is that it presented a specific means of enhancing staff nurses' intention to remain. Another implication of the study was that NLs should care about intragroup relationship conflict in the workplace. The experience of relationship conflict with other nurses could intensify staff nurses' intention to resign. Specifically, workplace bullying or nurse–nurse interpersonal conflict can cause problems, and NLs need to disseminate the anti-bullying message through nursing units and provide group activities to foster teamwork to decrease interpersonal conflict between staff nurses.

Application to Practice

This study presents a practical solution to this issue in that the impact of the NLs' behavioral integrity on staff nurses' intention to remain is stronger in units where levels of intragroup relationship conflict are high relative to those where levels are low. Staff nurses working in an unfriendly workplace often engage in social exchanges with the NL they trust, instead of their co-workers, and try hard to maintain high-quality social exchange with the NL. In this circumstance, the impact of the NL on staff nurses can be intensified. Therefore NLs assigned to nursing units with a high level of intragroup relationship conflict should endeavor to maintain their behavioral integrity to promote staff nurses' intention to remain.

CASE STUDY

A new nurse manager, 2 years post-graduation from a large baccalaureate program, is experiencing increased unit conflict among her staff, presumably due to ongoing increased patient acuity and the recent resignations of two senior nurses. The unit had previously enjoyed a healthy work environment with a stable team, but morale is low and unit nurses are considering transferring to another unit or choosing to work at the larger local hospital with Magnet status. The nurse manager has never received conflict management training, has limited experience dealing with conflict, and tends to utilize avoidance when confronted. She has promised her nurses that she is working to improve morale and has worked many additional shifts to help the staff. However, when staff come to the manager for help and to discuss their issues with one another, the nurse manager has little feedback and tells them "to work it out among themselves." The nurse manager has asked hospital leadership to provide formal staff development to help nurse mangers deal with staff conflict and believes that the training would be beneficial not only for new nurse mangers, but also for experienced managers who may have never thought about nor analyzed their conflict management or leadership styles. When she reaches out to several of the more senior nurse managers, they report that their units are doing well and they do not feel additional training would be

Continued

CASE STUDY—cont'd

helpful, but instead would simply add additional workload to their overburdened schedules. The Chief Nursing Officer (CNO) has stated she is reluctant to offer the training due to financial constraints and has requested that the nurse mangers collectively identify evidenced-based support for the additional education with documentation that the associated expense would benefit the organization. The CNO has been with the organization for 20 years and is widely respected for her clinical expertise.

1. What is the relationship between intragroup conflict and nursing intent to leave?
2. What examples of behavioral integrity are demonstrated by the nurse manager? What is she doing well and how could she improve?

3. If the nurse manager is unable to resolve the unit conflict, what are the possible consequences to patient care?
4. How can the nurse manager convince the other managers that this training would be helpful to the organization?
5. What resources could the nurse manager use to convince the CNO that this training would be helpful?
6. In lieu of the additional staff development, what could the nurse managers do to ensure a healthy work environment within their hospital?

CRITICAL THINKING EXERCISE

Mary is a registered nurse who graduated 2 years ago from a Bachelor of Science in Nursing (BSN) program. She has worked on a very busy unit and in a short period of time has established herself as a natural leader. She loves the unit that she works on and intends to stay with the organization. She has been invited by her chief nursing executive to become the nurse manager for a unit with an ongoing history of nurse turnover and intragroup conflict. Mary has never served in a management position but would like to accept the offer. She has aspirations to become a nursing manager and during her undergraduate education was required to attend interprofessional conflict management training during senior year. Mary also participated in a capstone project where she facilitated an anti-bullying campaign with her preceptor on a busy medical surgical unit. While deliberating about whether to accept the position, she met with the Chief Nursing Officer (CNO) and asked her impressions about issues with the previous nurse manager for recommendations to help turn the unit around. She asked the CNO about the unit. They suggested the previous manger had become burned out and typically

avoided staff when they demonstrated bullying behaviors or approached her for advice about how to deal with conflict. She increasingly refused to help her staff to provide direct patient care and instead stayed in her office most of the day except to attend mandatory meetings. The CNO also indicated that when first hired, the nurse manger had been outstanding, but as the conflict within her unit grew, she became distant.

1. What is significant about Mary's undergraduate training in relation to the nurse manager opportunity?
2. What information did the CNO share with Mary about the previous nurse manger that may be helpful?
3. If Mary accepts the new position, what should she do *first* to demonstrate behavioral integrity to her staff?
4. What could the CNO have done to prevent burnout of the previous nurse manager and to assist with improving morale on the unit?
5. What should CNOs understand about the relationship between intragroup conflict and nurse turnover?
6. Why is behavioral integrity important for NMs to demonstrate as related to staff turnover and patient outcomes?

REFERENCES

Abood, S. (2007). Influencing health care in the legislative arena. *OJIN: The Online Journal of Issues in Nursing, 12*(1), 2.

Adams, J. M., & Natarajan, S. (2016). Understanding influence within the context of nursing. *Advances in Nursing Science, 39*(3), E40–E56.

Alexander, R. K., & Diefenbeck, C. (2020). Challenging stereotypes: A glimpse into nursing's difficulty recruiting African Americans. *Journal of Professional Nursing, 36*(1), 15–22.

Alligood, M. R., & Tomey, A. M. (2010). *Nursing theorists and their work* (7th ed.). Maryland Heights, MO: Mosby.

Almost, J. (2006). Conflict within nursing work environments: concept analysis. *Journal of Advanced Nursing, 53*(4), 444–453.

Almost, J., Doran, D. M., McGillis Hall, L., & Spence Laschinger, H. K. (2010). Antecedents and consequences of intra-group conflict among nurses. *Journal of Nursing Management, 18*(8), 981–992.

Alper, S., Tjosvold, D., & Law, K. S. (2000). Conflict management, efficacy, and performance in self-managing work teams. *Personnel Psychology, 53*(3), 625–642.

American Association of Colleges of Nursing (AACN). (2008). *The essentials of baccalaureate education for professional nursing practice.* Washington, DC: AACN. http://www.aacn.nche.edu/education-resources/BaccEssentials08.pdf.

American Association of Colleges of Nursing (AACN). (2011). *The essentials of master's education in nursing.* http://www.aacn.nche.edu/education-resources/MastersEssentials11.pdf.

American Nurses Association (ANA). (2015). Optimal nurse staffing to improve quality of care and patient outcomes: Executive summary [White paper]. https://cdn.ymaws.com/www.anamass.org/resource/resmgr/docs/NurseStaffingWhitePaper.pdf.

Baer, E. D. (2009). "Do trained nurses… work for love, or do they work for money?" nursing and altruism in the twenty-first century. *Nursing History Review, 17*, 28–46.

Bagshaw, D., & Lepp, M. (2005). Ethical considerations in drama and conflict resolution research in Swedish and Australian schools. *Conflict Resolution Quarterly, 22*(3), 381–396.

Baltimore, J. J. (2006). *Nurse collegiality: Fact or fiction? Nursing Management, 37*(5), 28–36.

Barki, H., & Hartwick, J. (2001). Interpersonal conflict and its management in information system development. *MIS Quarterly, 25*(2), 195–228.

Barki, H., & Hartwick, J. (2004). Conceptualizing the construct of interpersonal conflict. *International Journal of Conflict Management, 15*(3), 216–244.

Barnard, C. I. (1938). *The functions of the executive.* 7th printing. Cambridge, MA: Harvard University Press.

Barrett, E. A. M. (1989). A nursing theory of power for nursing practice: Derivation from Rogers' paradigm. In J. Riehl (Ed.). *Conceptual models for nursing practice* (3rd ed.) (pp. 207–217). Norwalk, CT: Appleton & Lange.

Barrett, E. A. M. (2010). Power as knowing participation in change: What's new and what's next. *Nursing Science Quarterly, 23*(1), 47–54.

Barrett, E. A. M. (2017). Again, what is nursing science? *Nursing Science Quarterly, 30*(2), 129–133.

Bartunek, J. M., & Spreitzer, G. M. (2006). The interdisciplinary career of a popular construct used in management: Empowerment in the late 20th century. *Journal of Management Inquiry, 15*(3), 255–273.

Bassett, C. (2002). Nurses' perceptions of care and caring. *International Journal of Nursing Practice, 8*(1), 8–15.

Beauchamp, T. L., & Childress, J. F. (1994). Principles of biomedical ethics (4th ed.). New York: Oxford University Press.

Benne, K. D., & Bennis, W. (1959). Role confusion and conflict in nursing: The role of the professional nurse. *The American Journal of Nursing, 59*(2), 196–198.

Bierstadt, R. (1950). An analysis of social power. *American Sociological Review, 15*, 730–738.

Bishop, S. R. (2004). *Nurses and conflict: Workplace experiences.* Dissertation, University of Victoria (Canada).

Blake, R. R., & Mouton, J. S. (1964). *The managerial grid.* Gulf Publishing.

Bochatay, N., Bajwa, N. M., Cullati, S., Muller-Juge, V., Blondon, K. S., Perron, N. J., et al. (2017). A multilevel analysis of professional conflicts in health care teams: Insight for future training. *Academic Medicine, 92*(11S), S84–S92.

Boss, R. W. (1983). Team building and the problem of regression: The personal management interview as an intervention. *Journal of Applied Behavioral Science, 19*(1), 67–83.

Boswell, C., Cannon, S., & Miller, J. (2005). Nurses' political involvement: responsibility versus privilege. *Journal of Professional Nursing, 21*(1), 5–8.

Bourdieu, P. (1985). The social space and the genesis of groups. *Information (International Social Science Council), 24*(2), 195–220.

Boynton, B. (2012). *Disruptive behavior, bullying, & incivility: A glossary of violence in healthcare workplaces.* https://www.confidentvoices.com/2012/04/04/disruptive-behavior-bullying-incivility-workplace-abuse-a-glossary-of-violence/.

Bradbury-Jones, C., Sambrook, S., & Irvine, F. (2008). Power and empowerment in nursing: a fourth theoretical approach. *Journal of Advanced Nursing, 62*(2), 258–266.

Bradley, J. M., & Moore, L. W. (2019). The perceptions of professional leadership coaches regarding the roles and challenges of nurse managers. *The Journal of Nursing Administration, 49*(2), 105–109.

Brinkert, R. (2010). A literature review of conflict communication causes, costs, benefits and interventions in nursing. *Journal of Nursing Management, 18*(2), 145–156.

Brody, A. A., Farley, J. E., Gillespie, G. L., Hickman, R., Hodges, E. A., Lyder, C., et al. (2017). Diversity dynamics: The experience of male Robert Wood Johnson Foundation nurse faculty scholars. *Nursing Outlook, 65*(3), 278–288.

Brown, L. D. (1983). *Managing conflict at organizational interfaces*. Reading, MA: Addison Wesley Publishing Company.

Brubaker, D., Noble, C., Fincher, R., Park, S. K. Y., & Press, S. (2014). Conflict resolution in the workplace: What will the future bring? *Conflict Resolution Quarterly, 31*(4), 357–386.

Butts, J. B., Rich, K. L., & Fawcett, J. (2012). The future of nursing: How important is discipline-specific knowledge? A conversation with Jacqueline Fawcett. *Nursing Science Quarterly, 25*(2), 151–154.

Byrd, M. E., Costello, J., Shelton, C. R., Thomas, P. A., & Petrarca, D. (2004). An active learning experience in health policy for baccalaureate nursing students. *Public Health Nursing, 21*(5), 501–506.

Catalano, J. T. (2019). *Nursing now: Today's issues, tomorrows trends*. F.A. Davis.

Chinn, P. L., & Falk-Rafael, A. (2015). Peace and power: A theory of emancipatory group process. *Journal of Nursing Scholarship, 47*(1), 62–69.

Chinn, P. L., & Kramer, M. K. (1995). *Theory and nursing a systematic approach*. Mosby.

Clark, C. M. (2008). Faculty and student assessment of and experience with incivility in nursing education. *Journal of Nursing Education, 47*(10), 458–465.

Cohen, L. B. (1992). Power and change in health care: Challenge for nursing. *Journal of Nursing Education, 31*(3), 113–116.

Conger, J. A., & Kanungo, R. N. (1988). The empowerment process: Integrating theory and practice. *Academy of Management Review, 13*(3), 471–482.

Cook, P. R., & Cullen, J. A. (2003). CARING as an imperative for nursing education. *Nursing Education Perspectives, 24*(4), 192–197.

Costantino, C. A., & Merchant, C. S. (1996). *Designing conflict management systems: A guide to creating productive and healthy organizations*. San Francisco: Jossey-Bass.

Cox, K. B. (2014). The new Intragroup Conflict Scale: Testing and psychometric properties. *Journal of Nursing Measurement, 22*(1), 59–76.

Cummings, T. G., & Worley, C. G. (2015). *Organization development and change* (10th ed.). Stamford, CT: Cengage.

D'Antonio, P., Connolly, C., Wall, B. M., Whelan, J. C., & Fairman, J. (2010). Histories of nursing: The power and the possibilities. *Nursing Outlook, 58*(4), 207–213.

De Dreu, C. K., Evers, A., Beersma, B., Kluwer, E. S., & Nauta, A. (2001). A theory-based measure of conflict management strategies in the workplace. *Journal of Organizational Behavior: The International Journal of Industrial, Occupational and Organizational Psychology and Behavior, 22*(6), 645–668.

De Dreu, C. K., & Beersma, B. (2005). Conflict in organizations: Beyond effectiveness and performance. *European Journal of Work and Organizational Psychology, 14*(2), 105–117.

De Dreu, C. K. W., & Gelfand, M. J. (2007). Conflict in the workplace: Sources, dynamics, and functions across multiple levels of analysis. In C. K. W. De Dreu, & M. J. Gelfand (Eds.), *The psychology of conflict and conflict management in organizations*. New York: Lawrence Erlbaum.

Des Jardin, K. E. (2001). Political involvement in nursing—Education and empowerment. *AORN Journal, 74*(4), 467–475.

de Wit, F. R., Jehn, K. A., & Scheepers, D. (2013). Task conflict, information processing, and decision-making: The damaging effect of relationship conflict. *Organizational Behavior and Human Decision Processes, 122*(2), 177–189.

Deutsch, M. (1973). *The resolution of conflict: Constructive and destructive processes*. New Haven: Yale University Press.

Dewitty, V. P., Osborne, J. W., Friesen, M. A., & Rosenkranz, A. (2009). Workforce conflict: What's the problem? *Nursing Management, 40*(5), 31–33, 37.

DiCicco-Bloom, B., Frederickson, K., O'Malley, D., Shaw, E. Crossan, J.C. & Looney, J. A. (2007). Developing a model of social capital: Relationships in primary care. *Advances in Nursing Science, 30*(3), E13–E24.

Dougall, D., Lewis, M., & Ross, S. (2018). *Transformational change in health and care. Reports from the field*. London: The King's Fund.

Druckman, D. (1994). Determinants of compromising behaviour in negotiation: A meta-analysis. *Journal of Conflict Resolution, 38*(3), 507–556.

Dunford, B. B., Mumford, K. J., Boss, R. W., Boss, A. D., & Boss, D. S. (2020). Integrated conflict management systems pay off with lower levels of formal grievances and lower turnover rates. *ILR Review, 73*(2), 528–551.

Ehteshami, A., Rezaei1, P., Tavakoli, N., & Kasaei, M. (2013). The role of health information technology in reducing preventable medical errors and improving patient safety. *International Journal of Health System and Disaster Management, 1*(4), 195–199.

Ellis, P., & Abbott, J. (2011). Strategies for managing conflict within the team. *British Journal of Cardiac Nursing, 7*(3), 138–140.

Fawcett, J. (1999). The state of nursing science: hallmarks of the 20th and 21st centuries. *Nursing Science Quarterly, 12*(4), 311–315.

Filley, A. C. (1975). *Interpersonal conflict resolution*. Glenview, IL: Scott, Foresman.

Filley, A., House, R., & Kerr, S. (1976). *Managerial process and organizational behavior*. Glenview, IL: Scott, Foresman.

Fisher, R., Ury, W., & Patton, B. (1991). *Getting to yes: Negotiating agreement without giving* (2nd ed.). New York: Penguin Group.

Fiske, S. T. (2010). Interpersonal stratification: Status, power, and subordination. In S. T. Fiske, D. T. Gilbert, & G. Lindzey (Eds.) (5th ed.), *Handbook of social psychology* (pp. 941–982). Hoboken, NJ: John Wiley & Sons Inc.

Flateau-Lux, L. R., & Gravel, T. (2014). Put a stop to bullying new nurses. *Home Healthcare Now, 32*(4), 225–229.

Follett, M. P. (1940). Constructive conflict. In H. C. Metcalf & L. Urwick (Eds.), *Dynamic administration: The collected papers of Mary Parker Follett* (pp. 30–49). New York and London: Harper.

Foucault, M. (1980). *Power/knowledge: Selected interviews and other writings, 1972–1977.* New York: Vintage.

French, J., & Raven, B. (1959). The bases of social power. In D. Cartwright (Ed.), *Studies in social power* (pp. 150–167). Ann Arbor, MI: University of Michigan, Institute for Social Research.

Freshwater, D. (2000). Crosscurrents: Against cultural narration in nursing. *Journal of Advanced Nursing, 32*(2), 481–484.

Friend, M. L. (2013). *Group empowerment capacity and capability in schools of nursing* (Doctoral dissertation). Retrieved from ProQuest Dissertations & Theses. (Order No. 3577616).

Friend, M. L., & Sieloff, C. L. (2018). Empowerment in nursing literature: An update and look to the future. *Nursing Science Quarterly, 31*(4), 355–361.

Frye, M. (1983). *The politics of reality: Essays in feminist theory.* Trumansburg, NY: Crossing Press.

Future of Nursing. (n.d.). *Campaign for action: Campaign progress—dashboard indicators.* Center to Champion Nursing in America. http://campaignforaction.org/dashboard.

Gallup. (2020). *Nurses continue to rate highest in honesty, ethics.* Gallup. https://news.gallup.com/poll/274673/nurses-continue-rate-highest-honesty-ethics.aspx.

Gardner, D. L. (1992). Conflict and retention of new graduate nurses. *Western Journal of Nursing Research, 14*(1), 76–85.

Gardner, W. L., & Avolio, B. J. (1998). The charismatic relationship: A dramaturgical perspective. *Academy of Management Review, 23*(1), 32–58.

Ghazali, M., Hashim, R., & Ismail, N. M. (2012, April). Gender and influence tactics among university administrative employees. In *2012 IEEE Business, Engineering & Industrial Applications Colloquium (BEIAC)* (pp. 237–240), IEEE.

Goldrick, B., Leclair, J., & Larson, E. (1994). Intraorganizational influence in the health care setting: A study of strategies preferred by head nurses and infection control practitioners. *American Journal of Infection Control, 22*(1), 6–11.

Greer, L. L., Caruso, H. M., & Jehn, K. A. (2011). The bigger they are, the harder they fall: Linking team power, team conflict, and performance. *Organizational Behavior and Human Decision Processes, 116*(1), 116–128.

Hamlin, L. (2000). Horizontal violence in the operating room. *British Journal of Perioperative Nursing (United Kingdom), 10*(1), 34–42.

Heath, R. L. (Ed.). (1988). *Strategic issues management: How organizations influence and respond to public interests and policies.* Thousand Oaks, CA: Jossey-Bass.

Heiman, H. J., Smith, L. L., McKool, M., Mitchell, D. N., & Roth, C. (2016). Health policy training: A review of the literature. *International Journal of Environmental Research and Public Health, 13*(1), ijerph13010020.

Henry, O. (2009). Organizational conflict and its effects on organizational performance. *Research Journal of Business Management, 2*(1), 16–24.

Hickson, D. J., Hinings, C. R., Lee, C. A., Schneck, R. E., & Pennings, J. M. (1971). A strategic contingencies theory of intraorganizational power. *Administrative Science Quarterly, 16*(2), 216–229.

Huntington, A. D., & Gilmour, J. A. (2001). Re-thinking representations, re-writing nursing texts: possibilities through feminist and Foucauldian thought. *Journal of Advanced Nursing, 35*(6), 902–908.

Huston, C. (2008). Preparing nurse leaders for 2020. *Journal of Nursing Management, 16*(8), 905–911.

Hutchinson, M., & Jackson, D. (2013). Hostile clinician behaviours in the nursing work environment and implications for patient care: A mixed-methods systematic review. *BMC Nursing, 12*(1), 25.

Institute of Medicine (IOM). (1999). *To err is human: Building a safer health system.* Washington, DC: National Academies Press.

Institute of Medicine (IOM). (2011). *The future of nursing: Leading change, advancing health.* Committee on the Robert Wood Johnson Foundation Initiative on the Future of Nursing. Washington, DC: National Academies Press. https://www.nap.edu/read/12956/chapter/1#v.

James, J. T. (2013). A new, evidence-based estimate of patient harms associated with hospital care. *Journal of Patient Safety, 9*(3), 122–128.

Jehn, K. (1994). Enhancing effectiveness: An investigation of advantages and disadvantages of value-based intragroup conflict. *International Journal of Conflict Management, 5*, 223–238.

Jehn, K. A. (1995). A multi-method examination of the benefits and detriments of intragroup conflict. *Administrative Science Quarterly, 40*, 256–282.

Jehn, K. A. (1997). A qualitative analysis of conflict types and dimensions in organizational groups. *Administrative Science Quarterly, 42*(3), 530–557.

Johansen, M. L. (2012). Keeping the peace: Conflict management strategies for nurse managers. *Nursing Management, 43*(2), 50–54.

Kang, S. W., Lee, S., & Choi, S. B. (2017). The impact of nursing leader's behavioral integrity and intragroup relationship conflict on staff nurses' intention to remain. *JONA: The Journal of Nursing Administration, 47*(5), 294–300.

Kanter, R. M. (1977). *Men and women of the corporation*. New York: Basic Books.

Kanter, R. M. (1993). *Men and women of the corporation* (2nd ed.). New York: Basic Books.

Kelley, H. H., & Thibaut, J. (1969). Group problem solving. In G. Lindzey & E. Aronson (Eds.), *The handbook of social psychology* (2nd ed.). Reading, MA: Addison-Wesley.

Kim, S. (2017). A new focus in healthcare conflict research. *Journal of Community and Public Health Nursing, 3*(4), 1–2.

King, I. M. (1964). Nursing theory—Problems and prospect. *Nursing Science, 2*(5), 394–403.

King, I. M. (1981). *A theory for nursing: systems, concepts, process*. New York: Wiley & Sons.

King, I. M. (1992). King's theory of goal attainment. *Nursing Science Quarterly, 5*(1), 19–26.

Kipnis, D., & Schmidt, S. M. (1988). Upward-influence styles: Relationship with performance evaluations, salary, and stress. *Administrative Science Quarterly, 33*, 528–542.

Kipnis, D., Schmidt, S. M., Swaffin-Smith, C., & Wilkinson, I. (1984). Patterns of managerial influence: Shotgun managers, tacticians, and bystanders. *Organizational Dynamics, 12*(3), 58–67.

Kipnis, D., Schmidt, S. M., & Wilkinson, I. F. (1980). Intraorganizational influence tactics: Explorations in getting one's way. *Journal of Applied Psychology, 65*(4), 440–452.

Kirschbaum, K. (2012). Physician communication in the operating room: Expanding application of face-negotiation theory to the health communication context. *Health Communication, 27*(3), 292–301.

Knickle, K., McNaughton, N., & Downar, J. (2012). Beyond winning: Mediation, conflict resolution, and non-rational sources of conflict in the ICU. *Critical Care, 16*, 308. https://doi.org/10.1186/cc11141.

Kreitner, R., & Kinicki, A. (2010). *Organizational behavior* (9th ed.). Boston: McGraw-Hill Higher Education.

Kristanto, H. (2017). Demographic characteristics and conflict management strategies. *International Journal of Economic Perspectives, 11*(4), 566–580.

Kupperschmidt, B. R. (2008). Conflicts at work? Try care fronting. *Journal of Christian Nursing, 25*(1), 10–17.

Lankshear, S., Kerr, M. S., Laschinger, H. K. S., & Wong, C. A. (2013). Professional practice leadership roles: the role of organizational power and personal influence in creating a professional practice environment for nurses. *Health Care Management Review, 38*(4), 349–360.

Laschinger, H. K. S., Read, E., Wilk, P., & Finegan, J. (2014). The influence of nursing unit empowerment and social capital on unit effectiveness and nurse perceptions of patient care quality. *JONA: The Journal of Nursing Administration, 44*(6), 347–352.

Lauder, W., Reel, S., Farmer, J., & Griggs, H. (2006). Social capital, rural nursing and rural nursing theory. *Nursing Inquiry, 13*(1), 73–79.

Lawrence, S., & Callan, V. J. (2006). *Interpersonal conflict and support mobilization: Nurses' experience of coping in the workplace*. Paper at Annual Meeting of the Academy of Management. Glassboro, NJ: June 2006. https://www.researchgate.net/publication/29462063_Interpersonal_conflict_and_support_mobilisation_Nurses'_experience_of_coping_in_the_workplace.

Leksell, J., Gardulf, A., Nilsson, J., & Lepp, M. (2015). Self-reported conflict management competence among nursing students on the point of graduating and registered nurses with professional experience. *Journal of Nursing Education and Practice, 5*(8), 82–89.

Lewis, M. A. (2006). Nurse bullying: organizational considerations in the maintenance and perpetration of health care bullying cultures. *Journal of Nursing Management, 14*(1), 52–58.

Longo, J., & Sherman, R. (2007). Leveling horizontal violence. *Nursing Management, 38*(3), 34–37.

Losa Iglesias, M. E., & Becerro de Bengoa Vallejo, R. (2012a). Prevalence of bullying at work and its association with self-esteem scores in a Spanish nurse sample. *Contemporary Nurse, 42*(1), 2–10.

Losa Iglesias, M. E., & Becerro de Bengoa Vallejo, R. (2012b). Conflict resolution styles in the nursing profession. *Contemporary Nurse, 43*(1), 73–80.

Makary, M. A., & Daniel, M. (2016). Medical error—the third leading cause of death in the US. *British Medical Journal, 353*, i2139.

Mannix, J., Wilkes, L., & Daly, J. (2013). Attributes of clinical leadership in contemporary nursing: An integrative review. *Contemporary Nurse, 45*(1), 10–21.

Manojlovich, M. (2007). Power and empowerment in nursing: Looking backward to inform the future. *Online Journal of Issues in Nursing, 12*(1), 2.

Marquis, B. L., & Huston, C. J. (2012). *Leadership and management tools for the new nurse: A case study approach*. Philadelphia: Lippincott Williams & Wilkins.

McKibben, L. (2017). Conflict management: Importance and implications. *British Journal of Nursing, 26*(2), 100–103.

Meleis, A. I. (2018). *Theoretical nursing: Development and progress* (6th ed.). Philadelphia, PA: Wolters Kluwer.

Merriam-Webster. (n.d.). *Oppression*. https://www.merriam-webster.com/dictionary/oppression.

Mikkelsen, E. N., & Clegg, S. (2018). Unpacking the meaning of conflict in organizational conflict research. *Negotiation and Conflict Management Research, 11*(3), 185–203.

Moore, J. B., & Kordick, M. F. (2006). Sources of conflict between families and health care professionals. *Journal of Pediatric Oncology Nursing, 23*(2), 82–91.

Nahapiet, J., & Ghoshal, S. (1998). Social capital, intellectual capital, and the organizational advantage. *Academy of Management Review, 23*(2), 242–266.

Nancarrow, S. A., & Borthwick, A. M. (2005). Dynamic professional boundaries in the healthcare workforce. *Sociology of Health & Illness, 27*, 897–919. https://doi.org/10.1111/j.1467-9566.2005.00463.x.

National Academies of Sciences, Engineering, and Medicine (was the IOM). (2016). *Assessing progress on the Institute of Medicine Report The Future of Nursing.* Washington, DC: National Academies Press.

Nelson, H. W. (2012). Dysfunctional health service conflict: Causes and accelerants. *The Health Care Manager, 31*(2), 178–191.

Nixon, J. (2014). Looking at the culture of nursing through fresh eyes. *Kai Tiaki: Nursing New Zealand, 20*(1), 26–27.

Northam, S. (2009). Conflict in the workplace: Part 1. *AJN The American Journal of Nursing, 109*(6), 70–73.

Oakes, L. S., Townley, B., & Cooper, D. J. (1998). Business planning as pedagogy: Language and control in a changing institutional field. *Administrative Science Quarterly, 42*(3), 257–292.

O'Brien-Larivée, C. (2011). A service-learning experience to teach baccalaureate nursing students about health policy. *Journal of Nursing Education, 50*(6), 332–336.

Oc, B., Bashshur, M. R., & Moore, C. (2019). Head above the parapet: How minority subordinates influence group outcomes and the consequences they face for doing so. *Journal of Applied Psychology, 104*(7), 929.

Ocasio, W. (2002). Organizational power and dependence. In J. Baum (Ed.), *Companion to organizations* (pp. 363–385). Malden, MA: Blackwell.

Ocasio, W., Pozner, J. E., & Milner, D. (2020). Varieties of political capital and power in organizations: A review and integrative framework. *Academy of Management Annals, 14*(1), 303–338.

Oetzel, J. G., & Ting-Toomey, S. (2003). Face concerns in interpersonal conflict: A cross-cultural empirical test of the face negotiation theory. *Communication Research, 30*(6), 599–624.

Oetzel, J., Ting-Toomey, S., Masumoto, T., Yokochi, Y., Pan, X., Takai, J., et al. (2001). Face and facework in conflict: A cross-cultural comparison of China, Germany, Japan, and the United States. *Communication Monographs, 68*(3), 235–258.

Oliveira, R. M., Silva, L. M. S. D., Guedes, M. V. C., Oliveira, A. C. D. S., Sánchez, R. G., & Torres, R. A. M. (2016). Analyzing the concept of disruptive behavior in healthcare work: An integrative review. *Revista da Escola de Enfermagem da USP, 50*(4), 695–704.

Patterson, K., Grenny, J., McMillan, R., & Switzler, A. (2005). *Crucial confrontations: Tools for resolving broken promises, violated expectations, and bad behavior.* New York: McGraw-Hill.

Patton, C. M. (2014). Conflict in health care: A literature review. *The Internet Journal of Healthcare Administration, 9*(1), 1–11.

Paynton, S. T. (2009). The informal power of nurses for promoting patient care. *OJIN: The Online Journal of Issues in Nursing, 14*(1). http://ojin.nursingworld.org/MainMenuCategories/ANAMarketplace/ANAPeriodicals/OJIN/TableofContents/Vol142009/No1Jan09/ArticlePreviousTopic/InformalPowerofNurses.html.

Pecanac, K. E., & Schwarze, M. L. (2018). Conflict in the intensive care unit: Nursing advocacy and surgical agency. *Nursing Ethics, 25*(1), 69–79.

Pelc, K. (2009). The political power of nurses: power to influence, power to change. *AAACN Viewpoint, 31*(6), 1.

Pfeffer, J. (1992). Understanding power in organizations. *California Management Review, 34*(2), 29–50.

Pondy, L. R. (1967). Organizational conflict: Concepts and models. *Administrative Science Quarterly, 12*(2), 296–320.

Putnam, L. L., & Poole, M. S. (1987). Conflict and negotiation. In F. M. Jablin, L. L. Putnam, K. Roberts, & L. W. Porter (Eds.), *Handbook of organizational communication* (pp. 549–599). Newbury Park, CA: Sage.

Rahim, M. A. (1983). *Rahim organizational conflict inventories: Experimental edition: Professional manual.* Palo Alto, CA: Consulting Psychologists Press.

Rahim, M. A. (2002). Toward a theory of managing organizational conflict. *International Journal of Conflict Management, 13*(3), 206–235.

Rahim, M. A. (2010). *Managing conflict in organizations* (4th ed.). Piscataway, NJ: Transaction Publishers.

Rahim, M. A., & Bonoma, T. V. (1979). Managing organizational conflict: A model for diagnosis and intervention. *Psychological Reports, 44*(3), 1323–1344.

Rahim, M. A., & Magner, N. R. (1995). Confirmatory factor analysis of the styles of handling interpersonal conflict: First-order factor model and its invariance across groups. *Journal of Applied Psychology, 80*(1), 122.

Rao, A. (2012). The contemporary construction of nurse empowerment. *Journal of Nursing Scholarship, 44*(4), 396–402.

Rapoport, A. (1960). *Fights, games, and debates.* Ann Arbor: University of Michigan Press.

Rappaport, J. (1987). Terms of empowerment/exemplars of prevention: Toward a theory for community psychology. *American Journal of Community Psychology, 15*(2), 121–148.

Raven, B. H. (1965). Social influence and power. In I. D. Steiner, & M. Fishbein (Eds.), *Current studies in social psychology* (pp. 371–382). New York: Holt, Rinehart, Winston.

Read, E. A. (2014). Workplace social capital in nursing: an evolutionary concept analysis. *Journal of Advanced Nursing, 70*(5), 997–1007.

Robbins, S. P. (1998). *Organizational behaviour.* (8th ed.). Englewood Cliffs, NJ: Prentice Hall.

Robbins, S. P., & Judge, T. A. (2016). *Organizational behavior* (17th ed.). Upper Saddle River, NJ: Prentice Hall Publishing.

Robert Wood Johnson Foundation (RWJF). (2018). *Nurses and nursing. Future of nursing: Campaign for action.* https://www.rwjf.org/en/our-focus-areas/topics/nurses-and-nursing.html.

Roberts, S. J. (1983). Oppressed group behavior: Implications for nursing. *Advances in Nursing Science, 5*(4), 21–30.

Roberts, S. J. (2015). Lateral violence in nursing: A review of the past three decades. *Nursing Science Quarterly, 28*(1), 36–41.

Rodwell, C. M. (1996). An analysis of the concept of empowerment. *Journal of Advanced Nursing, 23*(2), 305–313.

Rogers, M. E. (1970). *An introduction to the theoretical basis of nursing.* Philadelphia: F. A. Davis.

Rogers, M. E. (1990). Nursing: Science of unitary, irreducible, human beings: Update 1990. In E. A. M. Barrett (Ed.), *Visions of Rogers' science-based nursing* (pp. 5–11). New York: National League for Nursing.

Rosenstein, A. H., & O'Daniel, M. (2005). Disruptive behavior & clinical outcomes: Perceptions of nurses & physicians: Nurses, physicians, and administrators say that clinicians' disruptive behavior has negative effects on clinical outcomes. *Nursing Management, 36*(1), 18–28.

Rosenstein, A. H., Russell, H., & Lauve, R. (2002). Disruptive physician behavior contributes to nursing shortage: Study links bad behavior by doctors to nurses leaving the profession. *Physician Executive, 28*(6), 8–11.

Rosseter, R. (2018). *Nursing faculty shortage fact sheet.* American Association of Colleges of Nursing. https://www.aacnnursing.org/News-Information/Fact-Sheets/Nursing-Fact-Sheet.

Rowe, M. M., & Sherlock, H. (2005). Stress and verbal abuse in nursing: Do burned out nurses eat their young? *Journal of Nursing Management, 13*(3), 242–248.

Rowell, P. A. (2005). Being a "target" at work: Or William Tell and how the apple felt. *JONA: The Journal of Nursing Administration, 35*(9), 377–379.

Runde, C., & Flanagan, T. (2010). *Developing your conflict competence: A hands-on guide for leaders, managers, facilitators and teams.* San Francisco, CA: Jossey-Bass.

Salancik, G. R., & Pfeffer, J. (1977). Who gets power—and how they hold on to it: A strategic-contingency model of power. *Organizational Dynamics, 5*(3), 3–21.

Salvage, J., Montayre, J., & Gunn, M. (2019). Being effective at the top table: developing nurses' policy leadership competencies. *International Nursing Review, 4*, 449. https://doi.org/10.1111/inr.12567.

Shargh, F. S., Soufi, M., & Dadashi, M. A. (2013). Conflict management and negotiation. *International Research Journal of Applied and Basic Sciences, 5*(5), 538–543.

Shell, R. (2001). Perceived barriers to teaching for critical thinking by BSN nursing faculty. *Nursing Education Perspectives, 22*(6), 286–291.

Shillam, C. R., Adams, J. M., Bryant, D. C., Deupree, J. P., Miyamoto, S., & Gregas, M. (2018). Development of the leadership influence self-assessment (LISA©) instrument. *Nursing Outlook, 66*(2), 130–137.

Sidanius, J., & Pratto, F. (1999). *Social dominance: An intergroup theory of social hierarchy and oppression.* New York: Cambridge University Press.

Sieloff, C. L. (1995). Development of a theory of departmental power. In M. Frey & C. L. Sieloff (Eds.), *Advancing King's systems framework and theory of goal attainment* (pp. 46–65). SAGE Publications.

Sieloff, C. L. (2003). Measuring nursing power within organizations. *Journal of Nursing Scholarship 35*(2), 183–187.

Sieloff, C. L. (2004). Leadership behaviors that foster nursing group power. *Journal of Nursing Management, 12*(4), 246–251.

Sieloff, C. L. (2007). The theory of group power within organizations—Evolving conceptualization within King's conceptual system. In C. L. Sieloff & M. A. Frey (Eds.), *Middle range theory development: Using King's conceptual system* (pp. 196–214). New York: Springer Publishing Company.

Sieloff, C. L. (2010). Improving the work environment through the use of research instruments: An example. *Nursing Administration Quarterly, 34*(1), 56–60.

Sieloff, C. L. (2012). *Theory of group empowerment within organizations.* https://sites.google.com/site/theoryofnursinggrouppower.

Sieloff, C. L., & Bularzik, A. M. (2011). Group power through the lens of the 21st century and beyond: Further validation of the Sieloff-King Assessment of Group Power within Organizations. *Journal of Nursing Management, 19*(8), 1020–1027.

Sieloff, C. L., & Friend, M. L. (2015, November 9–10). *A global resource for Nurses: Work team empowerment.* Poster session presented at Sigma Theta Tau International Conference. Las Vegas, NV.

Simons, T. L., & Peterson, R. S. (2000). Task conflict and relationship conflict in top management teams: The pivotal role of intragroup trust. *Journal of Applied Psychology, 85*, 102–111.

Slabbert, A. D. (2004). Conflict management styles in traditional organisations. *The Social Science Journal, 41*(1), 83–92.

Small, C. R., Porterfield, S., & Gordon, G. (2015). Disruptive behavior within the workplace. *Applied Nursing Research, 28*(2), 67–71.

Smetzer, J., Baker, C., Byrne, F. D., & Cohen, M. R. (2010). Shaping systems for better behavioural choices: lessons learned from a fatal medication error. *The Joint Commission Journal on Quality and Patient Safety, 36*(4), 152–AP2.

Smith, L. M., Andrusyszyn, M. A., & Spence Laschinger, H. K. (2010). Effects of workplace incivility and empowerment on newly-graduated nurses' organizational commitment. *Journal of Nursing Management, 18*(8), 1004–1015.

Spence Laschinger, H. K., Leiter, M., Day, A., & Gilin, D. (2009). Workplace empowerment, incivility, and burnout: Impact on staff nurse recruitment and retention outcomes. *Journal of Nursing Management, 17*(3), 302–311.

Spetz, J., Donaldson, N., Aydin, C., & Brown, D. S. (2008). How many nurses per patient? Measurements of nurse staffing in health services research. *Health Services Research, 43*(5p1), 1674–1692.

Sportsman, S., & Hamilton, P. (2007). Conflict management styles in the health professions. *Journal of Professional Nursing, 23*(3), 157–166.

Spreitzer, G. M. (1996). Social structural characteristics of psychological empowerment. *Academy of Management Journal, 39*, 483–504.

Stalter, A. M., & Arms, D. (2016). Serving on organizational boards: What nurses need to know. *Online Journal of Issues in Nursing, 21*(2). https://ojin.nursingworld.org/MainMenuCategories/ANAMarketplace/ANAPeriodicals/OJIN/TableofContents/Vol-21-2016/No2-May-2016/Articles-Previous-Topics/Serving-on-Organizational-Boards.html.

The Commonwealth Fund/The New York Times/Harvard T.H Chan School of Public Health. (2019). *Americans' values and beliefs about national health insurance reform.* https://cdn1.sph.harvard.edu/wp-content/uploads/sites/94/2019/10/CMWF-NYT-Harvard_Final-Report_Oct2019.pdf.

The Joint Commission. (2017). Sentinel Event Alert 57. *Leadership committed to safety.* The Joint Commission. https://www.jointcommission.org/-/media/tjc/documents/resources/patient-safety-topics/sentinel-event/sea_57_safety_culture_leadership_0317pdf.pdf.

Thew, J. (2016). *4 strategies for nurses who want to enter the boardroom.* HealthLeadersMedia. https://www.healthleadersmedia.com/nursing/4-strategies-nurses-who-want-enter-boardroom.

Thomas, K. W. (1976). Conflict and conflict management. In M. D. Dunnette (Ed.), *The handbook of industrial and organizational psychology* (pp. 889–935). Chicago, IL: Rand McNally.

Thomas, K. W. (1977). Toward multidimensional values in teaching: The example of conflict behaviors. *Academy of Management Review, 2*(3), 487.

Thomas, K. W. (1992). Conflict and negotiation processes in organizations. In M. D. Dunnette, & L. M. Hough (Eds.), *The handbook of industrial and organizational psychology* (2nd ed., Vol. 3. pp. 651–717). Palo Alto, CA: Consulting Psychologists Press.

Thomas, K. W., & Kilmann, R. H. (1974). *Thomas-Kilmann conflict mode instrument.* Tuxedo, NY: Xicom.

Thomas, K. W., & Schmidt, W. H. (1976). A survey of managerial interests with respect to conflict. *Academy of Management Journal, 19*(2), 315–318.

Thomas, K. W., & Velthouse, B. A. (1990). Cognitive elements of empowerment: An "interpretive" model of intrinsic task motivation. *Academy of Management Review, 15*(4), 666–681.

Thompson, T. G., & Brailer, D. J. (2004). *The decade of health information technology: delivering consumer-centric and information-rich health care.* Washington, DC: US Department of Health and Human Services.

Ting-Toomey, S. (1988). Intercultural conflict styles: A face negotiation theory. In Y. Y. Kim & W. Gudykunst (Eds.), *Theories in intercultural communication* (pp. 213–235). Newbury Park, CA: Sage.

Ting-Toomey, S., & Kurogi, A. (1998). Facework competence in intercultural conflict: An updated face-negotiation theory. *International Journal of Intercultural Relations, 22*(2), 187–225.

Trossman, S. (2014). Healthy work environment toward civility. ANA, nurses promote strategies to prevent disruptive behaviors. *The Oklahoma Nurse, 59*(2), 6.

Tubaishat, A. (2017). Evaluation of electronic health record implementation in hospitals. *CIN: Computers, Informatics, Nursing, 35*(7), 364–372.

Turkel, M. C., Fawcett, J., Amankwaa, L., Clarke, P. N., Dee, V., Eustace, R., et al. (2018). Thoughts about nursing curricula: Dark clouds and bright lights. *Nursing Science Quarterly, 31*(2), 185–189.

Umiker, W. (1999). Principles of workforce stability. *Health Care Manager, 18*(2), 58–64.

Valentine, P. E. (1995). Management of conflict: Do nurses/women handle it differently? *Journal of Advanced Nursing, 22*(1), 142–149.

Walker, L. O. (2020). Gifts of wise women: A reflection on enduring ideas in nursing that transcend time. *Nursing Outlook.* https://doi-org.libdata.lib.ua.edu/10.1016/j.outlook.2020.01.004.

Walker, L. O., & Avant, K. C. (2019). *Strategies for theory construction in nursing* (6th ed.). New York: Pearson.

Wall, J. A., & Callister, R. R. (1995). Conflict and its management. *Journal of Management, 21*(3), 515–558.

Walrath, J. M., Dang, D., & Nyberg, D. (2010). Hospital RNs' experiences with disruptive behavior: A qualitative study. *Journal of Nursing Care Quality, 25*(2), 105–116.

Walrath, J. M., Dang, D., & Nyberg, D. (2013). An organizational assessment of disruptive clinician behavior: Findings and implications. *Journal of Nursing Care Quality, 28*(2), 110–121.

Warner, I. J. (2001). Nurses' perceptions of workplace conflict: Implications for retention and recruitment. MA dissertation, Royal Roads University, Canada. Retrieved from Dissertations & Theses: Full Text. (Publication No. AAT MQ62041).

Weber, M. (1968). *Economy and society: An outline of interpretive sociology* (Vol 3). New York: Bedminster Press.

Wendt, F. (2018). *Authority*. Hoboken, NJ: John Wiley & Sons.

Whetten, D. A., & Cameron, K. S. (2016). *Developing management skills* (9th ed.). Boston: Prentice Hall.

Yukl, G. (1989). Managerial leadership: A review of theory and research. *Journal of Management, 15*(2), 251–289.

Yukl, G. (2010). *Leadership in organizations* (7th ed.). Upper Saddle River, NJ: Prentice Hall.

Yukl, G. (2013). *Leadership in Organizations* (9th ed.). Harlow, UK: Pearson Education Limited.

Yukl, G., & Falbe, C. M. (1991). Importance of different power sources in downward and lateral relations. *Journal of Applied Psychology, 76*(3), 416–423.

Yukl, G., Falbe, C. M., & Youn, J. Y. (1993). Patterns of influence behavior for managers. *Group & Organization Management, 18*(1), 5–28.

Yukl, G., Lepsinger, R., & Lucia, T. (1992). Preliminary report on development and validation of the Influence Behavior Questionnaire. In K. E. Clar, M. B. Cla, & D. P. Campbell (Eds.), *The impact of leadership* (pp. 417–427). Greensboro, NC: Center for Creative Leadership.

Yukl, G., Seifert, C. F., & Chavez, C. (2008). Validation of the extended Influence Behavior Questionnaire. *The Leadership Quarterly, 19*(5), 609–621.

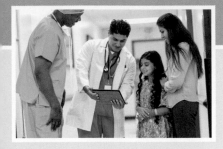

11

Workplace Diversity and Inclusion

Kupiri Piri Ackerman-Barger

 http://evolve.elsevier.com/Huber/leadership

Health care values include service to others, quality care, and justice. However, a paradox in health care occurs when values fall short of outcomes. In response to this, nursing organizations are prioritizing workforce diversity as an essential approach to promoting health equity (American Association of Colleges of Nursing [AACN], 2019; Campaign for Action, 2019; National League for Nursing [NLN], 2016). This chapter guides nurses through definitions needed to understand the value of workplace diversity as well as strategies for creating and maintaining workplace diversity and inclusion.

DEFINITIONS

A long existing and pernicious issue in health care is health disparities. **Health disparities** can be defined as "a particular type of health difference that is closely linked with social, economic, and/or environmental disadvantage. Health disparities adversely affect groups of people who have systematically experienced greater obstacles to health based on their racial or ethnic group; religion; socioeconomic status; gender; age; mental health; cognitive, sensory, or physical disability; sexual orientation or gender identity; geographic location; or other characteristics historically linked to discrimination or exclusion" (Healthy People 2020, 2020). Health equity "means that everyone has a fair and just opportunity to be as healthy as possible. This requires removing obstacles to health such as poverty, discrimination, and their consequences, including powerlessness and lack of access to good jobs with fair pay, quality education and housing, safe environments, and health care" (Braveman et al., 2017, p. 2). The term **health equity** encompasses health disparities

data, but also includes a purposeful focus on actions and solutions to mitigate health disparities.

Diversity in its broadest sense refers to the condition of having or being composed of different elements (Merriam-Webster, 2020). In terms of racial/ethnic diversity a student or patient cannot be diverse as an individual but may add diversity to an otherwise homogeneous group of people. A group of people who are all black or all Hispanic are not necessarily a diverse group of people. A racially/ethnically diverse group of people would have representation from multiple groups. Nursing has historically and continues to be comprised of primarily white females: a homogeneous group of people who create policies and procedures, define nursing theories, create nursing school curricula, and decide what and how topics will be researched. This creates a problem on several levels. One is that perspectives of white women are overrepresented while perspectives of other groups are underrepresented. Another issue is the lack of **cognitive diversity**, which refers to differences in information, knowledge, representations, mental models, and heuristics to better outcomes on specific tasks such as problem-solving, predicting, and innovating (Page, 2017). In other words, when groups of health care providers who think differently, who have different perspectives, and who hold varied world views come together, there is an increased likelihood that some of the complex health issues such as health disparities can be solved. It is imperative that nurses do not oversimplify the value of workforce diversity by reducing it to **compositional diversity (identity diversity)** or by looking at demographics as the sole indicator for diversity. Neither one should be a proxy for the other, rather to

209

truly leverage the value of diversity, representation, and inclusion of the many social identities that exist such as race/ethnicity, gender identity and sexual orientation, political viewpoints, socio-economic status, diversability as well as the many ways these identities can intersect are needed.

Inclusion is the binding force for diversity and the foundation for the kind of teamwork and collaboration that is necessary for health care providers to provide quality care. It is the process by which individuals view themselves as active members of the workplace, where their background, insights, and contributions are valued as part of the creativity and productivity of the organization (Ackerman-Barger et al., 2016).

Intersectionality: Crenshaw (1989) developed a framework called "intersectionality" designed explore how the overlapping and interdependent forms of social stratification (such as race/ethnicity, gender, gender identity, sexual orientation, socio-economic status, and diversability) shape the experiences of individuals. Intersectionality is an important framework to help nurses provide patient-centered care and avoid stereotyping and anchoring biases. The concept of intersectionality also suggests that it is difficult to assess someone's "culture" based on assumptions, stereotypes, or generalizations about culture. It is important to engage with patients, families, and communities authentically and with **cultural humility** (see discussion below).

Representation refers to the degree to which the nursing workforce accurately reflects the patient demographic. This can be analyzed from a national, state or regional perspective. There are several groups that are underrepresented in nursing. The percentage of black/African American patients was 22.16% and Hispanic/Latino was 36.27 in 2018 (Health Resources and Service Administration, 2018). However, according to Smiley et al. (2018) only 6.2% of the nursing workforce is black/African American, and 5.3% is Hispanic/Latino. Men compose nearly half the patient population but only 9.1% of the nursing workforce. Each of these groups are *underrepresented in nursing.*

Cultural competence: Leininger is one of the first nurse scholars to advocate the importance of culture in the profession of nursing. Leininger (2006) stated that culture was one of the broadest, most comprehensive, holistic, and universal features of humans and that it must be understood in order to provide care to clients. Leininger emphasized the interdependence of the

concepts of culture and care, and developed The Culture Care Theory. Leininger's work set the stage for the concept of cultural competence.

A widely used definition of cultural competence describes a set of congruent behaviors, attitudes, and policies that come together in a system, agency, or among professionals and enables that system, agency, or those professionals to work effectively in cross-cultural situations (Cross et al., 1989; Isaacs & Benjamin, 1991). AACN (2008) defined cultural competence as "the attitudes, knowledge and skills necessary for providing quality care to diverse populations" (p. 1). Campinha-Bacote (2007) created a conceptual framework for cultural competence that included the following components: cultural desire, cultural awareness, cultural knowledge, cultural skill, and cultural encounters. **Cultural desire** is when the health care provider is motivated to become engaged in becoming culturally competent because they want to not because they have to. She stated the concepts of love and caring, the capacity to sacrifice biases, a commitment to social justice, and humility are central to cultural desire. **Cultural awareness** "is the deliberate self-examination and in-depth exploration of our personal biases, stereotypes, prejudices and assumptions that we hold about individuals who are different from us" (p. 27). Cultural awareness helps the health care provider avoid cultural imposition. Cultural imposition was defined by Purnell and Paulenka (2003) as the intrusive application of the majority group's cultural view upon others. **Cultural knowledge** is the process of actively seeking knowledge about culturally diverse groups. **Cultural skill** refers to the ability of the health care provider to collect culturally relevant data about patients and to conduct culturally based physical assessments. **Cultural encounter** is the process of engaging in direct contact with culturally diverse groups to understand more about those groups. Campinha-Bacote (2007) warned that interacting with three or four people from a particular group does not make the health care provider an expert on that group.

The term cultural competence has been controversial. The criticism about this term is the implication that an individual can take a class or classes and become competent. Competence suggests a state of arrival that allows us to relinquish accountability for actively engaging in lifelong learning about others. If individuals view themselves as competent in understanding the myriad of cultures and intersections of cultures, identities, or roles that an individual inhabits, they are prone to stereotyping and likely to miss critical nuances. Fundamentally, the idea of cultural competence is not a set of functions or skills that are applied in certain situations but a way of being in the world. Cultural competence comes from recognizing one's own biases and taking the time to understand others in the context of their worldview. Davidhizar et al. (1998) warned against using a "cookbook" approach for assessing cultural and ethnic differences. Cultural knowledge should serve as a framework for inquiry rather than a strategy to generalize ethnic groups, which can lead to stereotyping.

Cultural humility is a term that first appeared in the health professions literature in 1998 in an article written by Tervalon and Murray-Garcia (1998). It provides a lens for how to learn about other people and other cultures. Cultural humility is rooted in the idea that one can never be competent in a culture other than one's own, but that we continue to grow and learn about others throughout our lives. Cultural humility has three tenets: (1) a lifelong commitment to self-evaluation, self-critique and growth; (2) a recognition of the existence of power differentials, to understand how they shift and to level them during interactions; and (3) a partnership with communities and groups who advocate for others by having them serving as experts on their own respective communities (Tervalon & Murray-Garcia, 1998).

Structural and institutional inequities are those factors that are largely responsible for historical inequities and perpetuate them into current inequities. The weight of structures and institutions is far more powerful than individual intent. This means that unless there are intentional and active efforts to reverse inequities, the status quo will remain unchanged. A health professions workforce armed with structural competencies has the potential to move the dial toward health equity. Hansen and Metzel (2016) stated that the notion of structural competency suggests that many health disparities are the consequence of downstream decisions about larger structural contexts, including health care and food delivery systems, zoning laws, local politics, urban and rural infrastructures, structural racisms, or even the very definitions of illness and health. **Structural competencies** are therefore necessary to identify upstream causes of health inequities. They "direct clinical training and healthcare systems to intervene at the level of social structures, institutions and policies that must be altered

to improve population health and promote health equity" (Hansen & Metzel, 2016, p. 180).

BACKGROUND

Statistics show that the racial/ethnic profile of nurses, who are predominantly white and female, does not reflect the general patient population. Nurses from non-white backgrounds represent 19.2% of the nursing population, whereas 80.8% of the nursing population is white/Caucasian (Smiley et al., 2018). In contrast, according to the National Health Center Data, the total number of non-white patients based on race/ethnicity in 2019 was 62.99% (Health Resources and Services Administration, 2019), indicating a wide gap in racial/ethnic representation of the patient population compared with nursing (Table 11.1).

There are many benefits to having a nursing workforce that reflects the patient population. First is the concept of racial concordance (also known as racial match), which indicates that patients are more comfortable and satisfied with nurses (and other health care providers) who speak their language and understand their culture. This care symmetry can increase the likelihood that patients and families will seek medical care and follow through with treatments. Second, diverse perspectives can provide a greater number of innovations and solutions to health care challenges because differing

TABLE 11.1 Racial Ethnicity of Nurses Compared With Patients

	% Nurses by Race Ethnicity	% Patients by Race Ethnicity
White	**80.8**	**40.99**
Black/African American	6.2	21.69
Asian	7.5	4.22
Hispanic	5.3	36.84
American Indian/Native Alaskan	0.4	1.45
Two or more races	2.6	3.45
Non-white totals	**19.2**	**62.99**

Source: Health Resources and Services Administration (HRSA). (2019). *Total patients by age and race/ethnicity from 2016 to 2018.* US Department of Health and Human Services, National Health Center Data. https://bphc.hrsa.gov/uds/data-center.aspx; Smiley et al., 2018).

experiences, ideas, and ways of thinking lead to better problem-solving. Third, increasing workforce diversity can make it much easier to recruit and retain minority nurses.

CREATING DIVERSITY AND INCLUSION IN THE WORKPLACE

Effective leaders will seek a diversity of people and ideas knowing that they will then have a wide selection of options from which to choose in order to solve problems. However, when teams represent a diversity of backgrounds, communication and interaction can be more challenging than when individuals are from the same culture. We tend to be attracted to people who are more like us than different from us (a concept known as *homophily*). In fact, those who are different from us can make us feel uncomfortable or even anxious. Yet fostering comfort with the unfamiliar and promoting inclusion must be a standard that is upheld consistently for an organization to benefit from diversity. Nurse managers who supervise diverse teams need to be aware of how cultural difference and backgrounds can affect interactions and communications between the health care team and with patients. To reduce miscommunications across diverse groups and to improve patient satisfaction, health care practitioners need to have skills. Communicating across cultures can take effort and is a skill that needs to be developed and nurtured over time because in the health care field, miscommunications can be fatal.

Another important concept that nurse managers need to be aware of when leading teams is that each of us carry biases, whether unconscious or not, that have the potential to hamper communication, negatively impact interactions and relationships, and ultimately impede quality patient care. Unconscious (or implicit) bias refers to beliefs and prejudices that reside outside of our awareness. There are many ways that these can manifest. Ross (2014) outlined multiple types of unconscious bias.

Selection attention (intentional blindness) is a mental process through which we selectively see some things but not others. We select what information to retain and what to discard. We tend to discard information that complicates our individual views of the world (Ross 2014). The notion of the existence of racism in current times is difficult for many white people to acknowledge. Dovidio et al. (2017) discussed the concept of aversive racism, which describes individuals who

hold egalitarian values but maintain racial implicit bias. Because of the cognitive dissonance related to having one's values and beliefs in conflict, selection attention can be a helpful tool in avoiding painful realities. For example, an individual may say, "I don't think racism exists anymore. I have never seen it." Closely related to selection bias is **confirmation bias,** which is a tendency to gather information or respond to a circumstance in a way that confirms an already established belief or idea. **Commitment confirmation** supports selection attention and confirmation bias. It is when our minds become attached to particular points of view, even when they are wrong, and can lead to a form of confidence bias or self-motivated reasoning. This is an over attachment to being right rather than a genuine seeking of the truth.

Diagnosis bias is the propensity to label people, ideas, or things based on our initial opinions or first impressions (Ross, 2014). For example, if you believe that women and black people are prone to exaggerating their pain or discomfort, as a provider, you might be less likely to believe women or black people or black women, in particular, about their pain. This may account for the chronic disparities in pain management that exist for people of color. Another example is the account of an otherwise healthy black woman who died shortly after giving birth. In 2018 Charles Johnson shared the story of his wife, who had many signs of hemorrhaging after the delivery of their baby, but whose care was delayed because, as her husband described, she was not considered a priority. When asked whether he thought this incident was related to her being black, he responded, "The very fact that we have to ask that question is a problem." (This video can be found on YouTube in the video titled, "Charles Johnson shares the tragic story of his wife Kira's death hours after giving birth.")

Pattern recognition is the tendency to sort and identify information based on prior experience or habit. Stereotyping is an example of pattern recognition (Ross, 2014). This shortcut is common among health care providers. "If you have seen one drug-seeker, you have seen them all" is typical pattern recognition bias. We remember the patient who complained of back pain and was treated generously with opioids only to discover that he did not really have back pain, but rather was addicted to pain killers. Now, every time someone complains of back pain, we think we recognize a pattern and are determined not to be tricked again. However, we are not always correct in pattern recognition. And when we are wrong, we risk undertreating patients who are indeed experiencing excruciating pain.

Value attribution is the inclination to imbue a person or thing with certain qualities based on initial perceived value (Ross, 2014). Although nurses are highly educated and skilled health care providers, many nurses have experienced a time when they explained a procedure or condition to a patient or family only to have them respond with doubt or skepticism. However, when the physician explained the exact same information, the patient and family believed the physician. This is related to a perception that the information provided by the physician is more credible and therefore more valuable. Nurses internalize value attribution in favor of a physician's decision-making at the cost of their own. An example of this is when nurses do not question or clarify physician's orders and simply follow them because "the doctor said." This is disempowering at best and can have catastrophic consequences for patients.

Anchoring bias is a tendency to rely too heavily on one trait or piece of information when making decisions (Ross, 2014). Members of the transgender community often experience anchoring bias when health care providers are too focused on their gender identity rather than their reason for entering the health care system. For example, a common story from transgender patients is that they have endured a genital exam even when they have come in for a cough or respiratory issue. In other words, they receive an exam for a respiratory issue although cisgender people rarely have this exam when they present with the same symptoms.

Group think is a function of accepted patterns of bias that have become part of the organizational culture. When people respond to questions with "This is how we have always done it," they exemplify group think. When health care providers prioritize group membership over independent thought, they tend to conform to unit norms rather than think differently or question the status quo. Ross (2014) stated that this kind of bias is one of the greatest deterrents to true diversity of thought.

LEADERSHIP AND MANAGEMENT IMPLICATIONS

Valuing and Leveraging Diversity

Health care services in the United States are arguably unnecessarily complex and inefficient, with often disappointing outcomes. Further, the state of health care leaves many consumers of health and health care providers frustrated and powerless. How, then, can we change health care and health care organizations to meet the health care needs of the United States? The answer is certainly not simple, but there are ways to begin. Ross (2011) stated, "Organizations across every part of the economic spectrum—hospitals, corporations, schools, religious institutions, banks, utility companies, law offices, architectural firms, government agencies, and nonprofits and charities—all share a common link. They are bound together in the acknowledgement that the way to a new future cannot be found by using the old models of limited leadership and participation. It can only be discovered by constructing a new way of *being with each other* in organizations" (p. 15). Page (2017), who used logic models to explain the value of diversity, stated, "Complexity increases in a problem's dimensionality and interdependencies. On complex tasks, no single person's repertoire will be sufficient, so teams will be needed, and those teams need to be diverse" (p. 68). Page argued that it is cognitive diversity that increases problem-solving and innovation and that identity diversity is the source of cognitive diversity. The following outlines some aspects of diversity and how they can be beneficial to health care. This is not intended to be an exhaustive list, rather an illustrative list.

Racial and Ethnic Minority Employees

The concept of race is often understood as a biological or genetic difference between groups of people. Our historical medical knowledge has often sought to differentiate individuals based on a construct of race and to even ascertain from a scientific perspective the inferiority and superiority of groups of people. However, science has not been able to make this association. The National Human Genome Research Institute (n.d.) stated, "Race is a fluid concept used to group people according to various factors including, ancestral background and social identity. Race is also used to group people that share a set of visible characteristics, such as skin color and facial features. Though these visible traits are influenced by genes, the vast majority of genetic variation exists within racial groups and not between them. Race is an ideology and for this reason, many scientists believe that race should be more accurately described as a social construct and not a biological one." Yudell et al. (2016, p. 564) stated, "In the wake of the sequencing of the human genome in the early 2000s, genome pioneer and social scientists alike called for an end to the use of race as a variable in genetic research." The concept of race is a social construct rather than a biological construct. Racism therefore describes something that we do to each other, not what we are. Disparities based on race that exist across institutions indicate that racism still exists and influences the access to resources and availability to opportunities for individuals in the United States.

One of the ways to ameliorate racial disparities in health care is to diversify the health care workforce by hiring, retaining, and promoting more individuals of color. In the hiring process, nurse leaders must be attentive to mitigating bias in individuals on hiring committees and bias that might be embedded into hiring processes. In order to retain nurses of color, nurse leaders need to acknowledge that nurses of color are often dealing with burdens that their white counterparts are not, such as discrimination and racial microaggressions. Acts of discrimination can be a patient stating they do not want a nurse of color caring for them. Racial microaggressions describes interactions, whether intentional or not, that convey negative messages about specific groups of people, in subtle but powerful ways (Sue, 2007; Sue et al., 2019). Examples of microaggressions are, "You were only hired to increase diversity in our department" (this implies that the individual of color was somehow less qualified for the job and should not have been hired). These interactions can be extremely taxing and tend to wear on nurses of color. Nurses of color are also notably absent in leadership positions, often overlooked and passed up for promotion. To foster diversity and representation in nursing there will need to be active steps taken to move the dial forward. This means that acknowledging the problem and stating values will not be enough. Neither will good intentions. It means that organizations need to take active steps to set the tone for valuing diversity and requiring inclusion excellence, creating and adhering to policies that protect from workplace discrimination, and establishing transparent career ladders that provide equal opportunities for professional growth.

LGBT (Lesbian, Gay, Bisexual, and Transgender) Employees

Minority stress, a concept coined by Meyer (2003), describes the excess stress individuals from stigmatized social groups experience as a result of their social position and often as a member of a minority group. This term highlights how stigma, prejudice, and discrimination create a hostile and stressful social environment that causes mental health problems. The model describes stress processes, including the experience of prejudice events, expectations of rejection, hiding and concealing, internalized homophobia, and ameliorative coping processes. Some health disparities that exist for LGBT individuals that may be the result of minority stress include higher rates of depression and anxiety, higher rates of smoking and substance abuse, higher rates of obesity (Institute of Medicine [IOM], 2011; Medley et al., 2016; Meyer, 2003; National LGBT Health Education Center 2016). Some of the most staggering suicide attempt rates are among transgender individuals. McNeil et al. (2017) conducted a systematic literature review to summarize the evidence concerning factors that correlate with suicide ideation and attempts in transgender populations. They found suicide attempt rates that ranged from 37% to 83% in the general transgender population. Toomey et al. (2018) found that suicide rates for transgender youth were as high as 50.8%. Additional health factors are higher rates of HIV (human immunodeficiency virus) and STI (sexually transmitted infection) transmission for men, and lower rates of mammography and Pap smear screening for women (National LGBT Health Education Center, 2016). One way to mitigate these health disparities in LGBT populations is care given by openly LGBT health care providers and staff.

National LGBT Health Education Center (2015) recommended several strategies for recruiting and retaining LGBT employees, such as commitment statements to LGBT employees from boards and senior management, sponsoring LGBT employee resource groups, attending LGBT job fairs, advertising positions in LGBT publications, ensuring that health benefits plans include same-sex partners, and having health benefits cover the health needs of transgender employees, including transition-related expenses. They further recommended that all employees receive training on culturally affirming care for LGBT people and have policies that reflect the needs of LGBT people. Individuals can promote inclusive workplace environments for LGBT co-workers by recognizing the tendency to make gender-binary assumptions about others. Respect for LGBT individuals can be shown by asking for their preferred pronouns. Many organizations recommend that when you introduce yourself, you state your name and your preferred gender pronouns, which opens the door for the person you are speaking with to reciprocate. For example, "Hello, my name is XXX and my preferred gender pronouns are she/her. What is your name and what are your preferred gender pronouns?" Leveraging allyship means that you use your social privilege to advocate for LBGT inclusive work environments, policies, and training.

Divers-ability

Workplace diversity focuses on inclusiveness beyond race and LGBT. It also applies to being inclusive of persons with hearing, vision, mobility, and other challenges. There are many differing abilities that have often been called "disabilities." The term divers-ability reframes how we think about abilities and provides an opportunity to value the perspectives that people with divers-abilities bring to the workplace. For example, consider an employee who is hard of hearing and reminds speakers to use the microphone during a forum. A co-worker states "my voice is loud, I don't need to use a microphone." The employee who is hard of hearing explains that although using a raised voice may work for people who have normal hearing, for those who are hard of hearing the pitch of raised voice is often difficult to hear. She also explains that many people who are hard of hearing feel uncomfortable having to request a microphone. That department then adopted a custom of using a microphone when speaking to large groups as a standard practice. It is also served as a reminder that shouting to communicate with patients who are hard of hearing is not effective.

Under the ADA, employment discrimination is prohibited regarding qualified individuals with disabilities. This 180 PART III Communication and Relationship Building applies to persons who have impairments; these must substantially limit major life activities such as seeing, hearing, speaking, walking, breathing, performing manual tasks, learning, caring for oneself, and working. An individual with epilepsy, paralysis, HIV infection, AIDS, a substantial hearing or visual impairment, mental retardation, cancer, mental illness, or a specific learning disability is covered (US Equal Employment Opportunity Commission, n.d.).

Politics

Navigating political differences at work can be challenging and doing so poorly can quickly lead to conflict.

However, when viewed through a lens of cognitive diversity, political differences, whether Democratic/Republican, liberal/conservative, or even rural/urban, can be a way of deepening the collective understanding of topic areas and problem-solving in such a way to meet health needs for the broadest possible groups of people. Although it may not be wise to debate politics at work, it is important to listen to and value differing viewpoints.

Language Diversity

Culturally and linguistically appropriate health care and services are broadly defined as care and services that are respectful of and responsive to the cultural and linguistic needs of all individuals. These are increasingly seen as essential to reducing disparities and improving health care quality. The National Standards for Culturally and Linguistically Appropriate Services in Health and Health Care (the National CLAS Standards) were originally developed in 2000 by the US Department of Health and Human Services Office of Minority Health (OMH) (2013) and then enhanced in 2010. They were intended to advance health equity, improve quality, and help eliminate health care disparities by providing a blueprint for individuals and health and health care organizations to implement culturally and linguistically appropriate services. The original National CLAS Standards provided guidance on cultural and linguistic competency, with the ultimate goal of reducing racial and ethnic health care disparities. The HHS Office of Minority Health undertook the National CLAS Standards Enhancement Initiative from 2010 to 2012 to recognize the nation's increasing diversity, reflect the tremendous growth in the fields of cultural and linguistic competency over the past decade, and ensure relevance with new national policies and legislation, such as the Affordable Care Act. A compendium titled *National Standards for Culturally and Linguistically Appropriate Services in Health and Health Care* (US Department of Health and Human Services, 2016) is a comprehensive view of the 15 standards and recommendations for implementing and maintaining culturally and linguistically appropriate services.

Nurses encounter patients who do not speak or understand the English language well. Patients who are limited English proficient (LEP) are likely to require the services of an interpreter. This person should be a neutral outsider instead of a family member, especially in the case of a bilingual child of the patient, except in extreme emergencies. Robust and readily available policies and procedures are needed to guide health care personnel in the use of interpreter services. Knowledge about the major ethnic and cultural groups in the patient population is a key aspect of success. Health care interpreters can be trained bilingual staff, on-staff interpreters, contract interpreters, telephone interpreters, and trained volunteers. Some people, however, should **not** serve as health care interpreters: patients' family and friends, children under 18 years old, health care personnel not involved in direct care, other patients or visitors, and untrained volunteers.

Communication style

reflects social, cultural, and family structures and varies among groups of people. Anthropologists Hall and Hall (1990) introduced the concept of 'low-context' and 'high-context' communication styles. Low-context people tend to communicate with the purpose of exchanging information directly and clearly, separating personal and professional relationships, and one situation from another. Low-context individuals feel less need to be subtle and worry less about how their communication will be received by others (Ward et al., 2016). Although a low-context style can be efficient and direct it can also be reductionist, narrow, and lacking in sensitivity. High-context communicators tend to focus more on relationship building and connecting ideas or situations, giving meaning to a broader or more contextual whole. High-context communicators tend to be more conflict avoidant and deferential to those perceived as having a higher position in the social hierarchy. Low-context communicators are more likely to speak up and share their views in work settings than high-context communicators (Ward et al., 2016). In terms of culture, Western societies like the United States tend to be low context and Eastern cultures like Japan tend to be high context (Hall & Hall, 1990; Ward et al., 2016). In health care, physicians might be considered largely low context and nurses high context.

Neither communication style should be considered more valuable than the other. Rather, both are essential to any team and exemplify how cognitive diversity can enhance problem-solving. Physicians specialize in specific systems and are trained in minute detail about the inner workings of that system. This knowledge is essential for diagnosing and providing medical interventions. Consider, however, nurses who are trained to understand how individuals, families, and communities experience illness and to create care plans that ensure

patients can and will follow through with medical interventions. These approaches represent interdependent ways of thinking and addressing illness that, viewed as a whole, can produce better outcomes.

Generational Diversity

A growing challenge in nursing leadership for both nurses in practice and for nurse managers is the management of generational workforce diversity. Sociologists categorize generational groups into cohorts, called *generational markers*. These cohorts are members of a generation who are linked through shared life experiences in their formative years. Phillips (2016) stated that it is important to appreciate and embrace these differences and outlined some of the general descriptions of each generation.

Baby boomer nurses (1946–1964). Baby boomers, the second largest generational group, currently occupy many of the leadership positions, including those in health care organizations. Having been influenced by the Vietnam War, Watergate, and the Civil Rights movement they have questioned traditional authority structures, blurred gender roles, and made vigorous attempts to push systems toward their ideas of perfection. They grew up thinking they could ignore or break rules and still be successful. Consequently, financial security is a central issue for this generation, and many boomers will work past the age of retirement. In the workplace they tend to be loyal, team-oriented, and appreciative of promotions and monetary gains. Their preference is for a more participative and less authoritarian workplace (Hendricks & Cope, 2013; Phillips, 2016). The impending retirement of large numbers of baby boomer nurses is predicted to create further nurse and nurse faculty shortages.

Generation X nurses (1965–1980). People from Generation X (Gen X) grew up in a time of rapid social, economic, and technological change. Many were latchkey children who watched their parents work long hours (Phillips, 2016). Although they tend be averse to authority like baby boomers, they tend to seek work–life balance. Gen X nurses learned to set limits and manage their own time. They are self-directed, do not feel obligated to work in teams, and practice very comfortably by themselves. Gen X nurses desire facts rather than emotions. They believe quality of life is important, and they are self-reliant and resourceful (Phillips, 2016).

Millennial nurses (1981–1996). As the largest group in US history, millennial workers are the most demographically diverse generation. The common marker of their developmental years is technology. These workers have astonishing multitasking skills. They also tend to have a positive outlook and a desire to improve the world. People from older generations tend to believe that millennials are shallow on basic skills; but because they grew up with computers, they can create solutions that other generations could not have imagined. Technology guides their every move. They are problem-solvers who grew up in a flourishing economy. Millennials matured in a world in which shortcuts, manipulation of rules, and situational ethics seem to have reigned. They got the message somehow that the final word is not the final word. They do not live to work; they work to live. Thus they have a different set of expectations about the world of work. Phillips (2016) noted that millennial nurses, like Gen X nurses, strive for work–life balance, and prefer flexible work shifts and job portability. Millennial nurses also tend to have a great sense of morality and civic duty.

Generation Z nurses (1997–2012). The newest cohort just entering the workforce is called Generation Z (Gen Z). Projections about the overarching influences for Gen Z are speculative. They are the most racially and ethnically diverse adult generation. Most members of Gen Z have no memory of the 9/11 terrorist attack. Donald Trump would be the first US president most Gen Z's know as they turn 18. The political environment in 2020 may influence the attitudes and engagement of Gen Z. Technology and the internet explosion are generation-shaping elements, with the rapid way people communicate and interact, including social media and an "always-on" technology environment that has produced dramatic shifts in behaviors, attitudes, and youth lifestyles (Dimock, 2019).

Like any demographic group, people from different generations have their own cultural perspectives and social expectations. These can cause workplace conflict. However, there is great potential for cross-generational growth and support as each generation has experienced its own set difficulties and has developed its own strengths. Barry (2014) suggested that by acknowledging the strengths of each generation there is the potential for effective mentoring, reducing work-place conflict, and diversification of the nursing workforce.

It is acceptable to take a sincere interest in a co-worker's or patient's background or culture. However, many Americans are afraid to ask people about their culture or background because they worry, "I don't want to offend anyone." The challenge with this thinking is that if nurses do not ask about people's differences, then the only option is to make assumptions. It is far more likely that others will be offended by people making assumptions than asking them directly about differences in their behavior or beliefs. In fact, asking other people directly about their culture can often help build rapport and a much deeper working relationship than simply talking about the weather or current events. Exploring and assessing the individual's preferences can bring to light the impact of culture on health care needs. Their culture could have an impact on their views about health issues such as health care, diet, and lifestyle. When people do not ask others about their cultural differences, those unasked questions can create a kind of "cultural static" that can keep the nurse from hearing a co-worker or patient clearly. This is a part of patient assessment and is also important for fostering co-worker relationships. Nurses can miss important facts that would enlighten care delivery and healthy work environments. However, it is important to note that is not an obligation for individuals to teach you about their culture.

Generational differences can be seen as both a challenge and an opportunity (Douglas & Gray, 2020). This is because of the acceleration of change and radical shifts in technology and information processing. There can be more than four generations working together in the workplace. Part of the complexity is whether or not the individuals grew up immersed in technology. Despite all of this, a highly qualified nurse workforce is desperately needed. A holistic perspective that considers generational differences along with universal human characteristics will aid in creating a foundation that sustains nursing through the path ahead (Douglas & Gray, 2020).

CURRENT ISSUES AND TRENDS

Strategies for Creating and Maintaining Workplace Diversity

The Pipeline

An important step in increasing nursing workforce diversity is looking at the long-term pipeline. The American Association of Colleges of Nursing (2019) and National League for Nursing (2016) outlined steps they are taking to increase nursing workforce diversity, including recruiting and retaining students from diverse backgrounds. A significant portion of nursing student education occurs in the practice setting. This means that hospitals, clinics, nursing homes, and other practice settings can contribute to workforce diversity by ensuring that students from underrepresented backgrounds feel welcomed, included, and valued during their clinical experiences. Ackerman-Barger et al. (2020) found that students of color experienced racial microaggressions from preceptors during their clinical rotations. Organizations can take steps to promote inclusion by having strong mission and vision statements related to diversity, inclusion and health equity; staff who exemplify and uphold the mission statement; and by having staff nurses and nursing leaders who reflect the characteristics of the general population.

Outreach and Recruitment

Advertisements for positions need to include inclusive language, organizational diversity, and inclusion statements. Increased recruiting efforts from historically black colleges and universities, Hispanic serving institutions, and Native American communities can help. Targeting the networks of underrepresented groups like minority nursing organizations and LGBT groups like Gay and the Lesbian Medical Association (GLMA), which has a nursing branch, can increase diversity. Using connections to personally reach out to potential candidates is also a helpful strategy.

Hiring

Organizations need to develop hiring committees with diverse compositions. Individuals who serve on hiring committees should undergo unconscious bias training. This training can include how to account for bias that may be present in letters of recommendation. Further, prior to reviewing applications the committee needs to discuss the qualification criteria for candidates and processes that will be followed during the hiring process. A discussion about the value that diversity brings to the organization and to patient care should be central in conversations about hiring. Be flexible in reviewing resumes and tend toward inclusion versus exclusion when deciding upon which applicants to invite for interview. Recognize that some applicants, often women and individuals from collectivist cultures, may not include or may minimize their accomplishments as opposed to those from individualist cultures who may be more comfortable with self-promotion. Include diversity, inclusion, and health equity themed questions to ask candidates during the interview. An iterative appraisal process of hiring procedures should occur periodically to ensure that biased processes have not become embedded into hiring procedures. Things to ask during periodic appraisals are: how does the pool of people hired compare with the list of who to interview and who applied for the position? Are applicants from underrepresented groups held to different standards than well-represented groups? If there was a high percentage of underrepresented groups who did not make it to the interview or hiring pool, why did this occur?

Retention and Promotion

Organizations are better served when they invest in long-term employees. There are cost savings and valuable institutional memory that is retained when turnover rates are reduced. Women and employees of color have historically and are currently paid less and are promoted less compared with their male and white counterparts. This is true in nursing as well. A first step is to consistently offer competitive and transparent hiring packages. Note that not all individuals have the same comfort with, or knowledge about, how to negotiate. For example, men and women tend to negotiate differently, in ways that leave women at a disadvantage. There are cross-cultural differences as well. In the United States, Canada, Western Europe, and a few other countries, people only negotiate the most expensive purchases like cars and houses, whereas they will pay exactly what is asked on almost everything else. In countries and regions such as Mexico, Asia, India, South America, and the Philippines, negotiation is a daily expectation (Lewis, 2017). Suggestions for equitable negotiations are as follows:

- Provide education to business office staff, individuals serving on hiring committees, and managers about how negotiating styles can vary based on gender, culture, and individual background.
- Create a fair, transparent hiring process. Organizations who 'low-ball' their new employees on hiring may pay a much bigger price later in turnover when disgruntled employees leave the organization.

RESEARCH NOTE

Source
O'Connor, M.R., Barrington, W.E., Buchanan, D.T., Bustillos, D., Eagen-Torkko, M., Kalkbrenner, A., et al. (2019). Short-term outcomes of a diversity, equity, and inclusion institute for nursing faculty. *Journal of Nursing Education*, *58*(11), 633–640.

Purpose
The purpose of this study was to develop faculty knowledge and effectiveness in addressing diversity, equity, and inclusion (DEI) topics in teaching. Specific objectives were to provide school of nursing faculty with the knowledge and skills they need to create truly inclusive learning environments, facilitate crucial conversations on racism and other-ism, and incorporate DEI topics through all curricula. To this end, the researchers offered a 3-day DEI Institute that included content experts, exercises on how to facilitate conversations on racism and other-isms led by social justice facilitators, and active learning opportunities such as individual self-reflection and small and large group discussions.

Discussion
This study found that the DEI Institute resulted in overwhelmingly positive increases in satisfaction and impact and statistically significant increases in DEI-related teaching self-efficacy post institute. These results suggest that workshops such as these show promise as interventions to create more inclusive learning environments. The researchers noted that significant institutional support from both the university and school of nursing were needed for the success of their DEI Institute. They discussed the importance of allowing participants to self-select into the workshop because of the evidence showing that mandatory DEI workshops may have the opposite effect than intended. Finally, they highlighted that a singular event or approach is not adequate to create inclusive learning environments, rather institutions need multiple resources and activities and ongoing trainings and discussions to make an impact.

Application to Practice
Training and skills are needed to achieve diversity, equity, and inclusion. An important place to start this process is in schools of nursing where future nurses can have DEI modeled for them and bring these skills to clinical practice. Although this study focused on nursing academic settings, it highlights the value and impact DEI training can have on participants, which could be applicable in multiple workplace settings.

CASE STUDY

Carol, a black nurse, has been assigned to care for a patient. When she walks into the patient's room and introduces herself, the patient responds, "I don't want you to be my nurse. I need a nurse who is not a (insert racial epithet)." A co-worker observed this interaction and called the nurse manager. The nurse manager comes to the floor.

1. Describe the impact this interaction could have had on Carol.
2. What would support for her look like?
3. Describe the impact this interaction could have had on other members of the unit who belong to marginalized groups.
4. What would support for them look like?
5. Describe the impact that not addressing this issue could have on unit as a whole.
6. What response should be made to the patient?
7. Imagine this same scenario but the nurse is a white male instead of a black female. What would be similar and/or different about the response?

CRITICAL THINKING EXERCISE

With the ever-increasing use of social media in our society, health care is grappling with new issues. Platforms like LinkedIn, Facebook, and Instagram have been helpful in recruiting nurses and can be a mechanism for providing news and education. However, there have also been challenges related to social media in the form of posts made with images of patients in clinical environments and complaints about co-workers and/or hospitals. A nurse manager is preparing a staff development workshop about the positive and negative aspects of social media platforms currently in health care.

1. What differing generational perspectives should the nurse manager anticipate when developing this training? In what ways might millennial nurses view social media differently than baby boomers?

2. What facilitation strategies could the nurse manager use to ensure all participants feel included and valued during the social media workshop?

3. Describe some activities the nurse manager can use to build community and create meaningful and productive dialogue among participants during the social media workshop.

REFERENCES

Ackerman-Barger, K., Boatright, D., Gonzalez-Colaso, R., Orozco, R., & Latimore, D. (2020). Seeking inclusion excellence: Understanding microaggressions experienced by underrepresented medical and nursing students. *Academic Medicine, 95*(5), 758–763. https://doi.org/10.1097/ACM.0000000000003077.

Ackerman-Barger, K., Valderama-Wallace, C., Latimore, D., & Drake, C. (2016). Understanding health professions students' self-perceptions of stereotype threat Susceptibility. *Journal of Best Practices in Health Professions Diversity, 9*(2), 1232–1246.

American Association of Colleges of Nursing (AACN). (2008). *Cultural competency in baccalaureate nursing education.* https://www.aacnnursing.org/Portals/42/AcademicNursing/CurriculumGuidelines/Cultural-Competency-Bacc-Edu.pdf.

American Association of Colleges of Nursing (AACN). (2019). *Enhancing diversity in the nursing workforce.* https://www.aacnnursing.org/Portals/42/News/Factsheets/Enhancing-Diversity-Factsheet.pdf.

Barry, M. (2014). Creating a practice environment that supports multigenerational workforce collaboration. *American Nurse, 46*(1), 13.

Braveman, P., Arkin, E., Orleans, T., Proctor, D., & Plough, A. (2017). *What is health equity? and what difference does a definition make?* Princeton, NJ: The Robert Wood Johnson Foundation: National Collaborating Centre for Determinants of Health.

Campaign for Action: Center to Champion Nursing in America. (2019). *The importance of diversity in nursing.* https://campaignforaction.org/the-importance-of-diversity-in-nursing/.

Campinha-Bacote, J. (2007). *The process of cultural competence in the delivery of healthcare services: The journey continues.* Cincinnati, OH: Transcultural C.A.R.E. Associates.

Crenshaw, K. (1989). Demarginalizing the intersection of race and sex: A Black feminist critique of antidiscrimination doctrine, feminist theory and antiracist politics. *The University of Chicago Legal Forum, 140*(1989), 139–167.

Cross, T., Bazron, B., Dennis, K., & Isaacs, M. (1989). *Towards a culturally competent system of care: A monograph on effective services for minority children who are severely emotionally disturbed (volume I).* Washington, DC: Georgetown University Child Development Center.

Davidhizar, R., Dowd, S. B., & Giger, J. N. (1998). Educating the culturally diverse nursing student. *Nurse Educator, 23*(2), 38–42.

Dimock, M. (2019). *Defining generations: Where Millennials end and Generation Z begins.* Pew Research Center. January 17. https://www.pewresearch.org/fact-tank/2019/01/17/where-millennials-end-and-generation-z-begins/.

Douglas, K., & Gray, S. (2020). Generational complexities present new challenges for nurse leaders. *Nurse Leader, 18*(2), 126–129.

Dovidio, J. F., Gaertner, S. L., & Pearson, A. R. (2017). Aversive racism and contemporary bias. In C. G. Sibley & F. K. Barlow (Eds.), *The Cambridge handbook of the psychology of prejudice* (pp. 267–294). Cambridge, UK: Cambridge University Press.

Hall, E. T., & Hall, M. R. (1990). *Understanding cultural differences.* Boston: Intercultural Press.

Hansen, H., & Metzl, J. M. (2016). Structural competency in the U.S. healthcare crisis: Putting social and policy interventions into clinical practice. *Bioethical Inquiry, 13*, 179–183.

Health Resources and Services Administration (HRSA). (2018). *Total patients by age and race/ethnicity from 2016 to 2018.* US Department of Health and Human Services, 2018 National Health Center Data. https://bphc.hrsa.gov/uds/datacenter.aspx.

Healthy People 2020. (2020). *Disparities.* https://www.healthypeople.gov/2020/about/foundation-health-measures/Disparities.

Hendricks, J. M., & Cope, V. C. (2013). Generational diversity: What nurse managers need to know. *Journal of Advanced Nursing, 69*(3), 717–725.

Isaacs, M., & Benjamin, M. (1991). *Towards a culturally competent system of care. Programs which utilize culturally competent principles (volume II).* Washington, DC: Georgetown University Child Development Center.

Institute of Medicine (IOM). (2011). *The health of Lesbian, Gay, Bisexual, and Transgender people: Building a foundation for better understanding.* Washington, DC: National Academies Press.

Leininger, M. M. (2006). Culture care diversity and universality theory and evolution of the ethnonursing method. In M. M. Leininger & M. R. McFarland (Eds.), *Culture care diversity and universality: A worldwide nursing theory* (2nd ed) (pp. 1–41): Sudbury, MA: Jones and Bartlett.

Lewis, B. (2017). *Negotiation tactics: How to haggle like your life depends on it.* https://www.fluentin3months.com/negotiation-tactics/.

McNeil, J., Ellis, S. J., & Eccles, F. J. R. (2017). Suicide in trans populations: A systematic review of prevalence and correlates. *Psychology of Sexual Orientation and Gender Diversity, 4*(3), 341–353. https://doi.org/10.1037/sgd0000235.

Medley, G., Lipari, R. N., Bose, J., Cribb, D. S., Kroutil, L. A., & McHenry, G. (2016). *Sexual orientation and estimates of adult substance use and mental health: Results from the 2015 National Survey on Drug Use and Health.* Substance Abuse and Mental Health Services Administration. https://www.samhsa.gov/data/sites/default/files/NSDUH-SexualOrientation-2015/NSDUH-SexualOrientation-2015/NSDUH-SexualOrientation-2015.pdf.

Merriam-Webster. (2020). *Diversity.* https://www.merriam-webster.com/dictionary/diversity.

Meyer, I. H. (2003). Prejudice, social stress, and mental health in Lesbian, Gay, and Bisexual populations: Conceptual issues and research evidence. *Psychological Bulletin, 129*(5), 674–697.

National Human Genome Research Institute. (n.d.). *Race.* https://www.genome.gov/genetics-glossary/Race.

National League for Nursing (NLN). (2016). *Achieving diversity and meaningful inclusion in nursing education: A living document from the National League for Nursing.* http://www.nln.org/docs/default-source/about/vision-statement-achieving-diversity.pdf?sfvrsn=2.

National LGBT Health Education Center. (2015). *10 things: Creating inclusive health care environments for LGBT people.* https://www.lgbthealtheducation.org/wp-content/uploads/Ten-Things-Brief-Final-WEB.pdf.

National LGBT Health Education Center. (2016). *Understanding the health needs of LGBT people.* https://www.lgbthealtheducation.org/publication/understanding-health-needs-lgbt-people/.

Page, S. (2017). *The Diversity bonus: How great teams pay in the knowledge economy.* Princeton, NJ: Princeton University Press.

Phillips, M. (2016). Embracing the multigenerational nursing team. *MEDSURG Nursing, 25*(3), 197–200.

Purnell, L. D., & Paulenka, B. J. (2003). *Transcultural health care: A culturally competent approach* (2nd ed). Philadelphia, PA: F.A. Davis.

Ross, H. (2011). *Reinventing diversity: Transforming organizational community to strengthen people, purpose, and performance.* Lanham, MD: Rowman & Littlefield.

Ross, H. (2014). *Everyday bias: Identifying and navigating unconscious judgments in our daily lives.* Lanham, MD: Rowman & Littlefield.

Smiley, R. A., Lauer, P., Bienemy, C., Berg, J. G., Shireman, E., Reneau, K. A., et al. (2018). The 2017 national nursing workforce survey. *Journal of Nursing Regulation, 9*(3), S1–S88.

Sue, D. W., Capodilupo, C. M., Torino, G. C., et al. (2007). Racial microaggressions in everyday life: Implications for clinical practice. *American Psychologist, 62*(4), 271–286. https://doi.org/10.1037/0003-066X.62.4.271.

Sue, D. W., Alsaidi, S., Awad, M. N., Glaeser, E., Calle, C. Z., & Mendez, N. (2019). Disarming racial microaggressions: Microintervention strategies for targets, white allies, and bystanders. *American Psychologist, 74*(1), 128–142.

Tervalon, M., & Murray-Garcia, J. (1998). Cultural humility versus cultural competence: A critical distinction in defining physician training outcomes in multicultural education. *Journal of the Healthcare Poor and Underserved, 9*(2), 117–123.

Toomey, R. B., Syvertsen, A. K., & Shramko, M. (2018). Transgender adolescent suicide behavior. *Pediatrics, 142*(4), 1–8.

US Department of Health and Human Services, Office of Minority Health (OMH). (2013). *National standards for CLAS in health and health care: A blueprint for advancing and sustaining CLAS policy and practice.* https://thinkculturalhealth.hhs.gov/pdfs/EnhancedCLASStandardsBlueprint.pdf.

US Department of Health and Human Services, Office of Minority Health (OMH). (2016). *National standards for culturally and linguistically appropriate services in health and health care: Compendium of state-sponsored national CLAS standards implementation activities.* U.S. Department of Health and Human Services. https://thinkculturalhealth.hhs.gov/pdfs/CLASCompendium.pdf.

US Equal Employment Opportunity Commission. (n.d.). *Americans with Disabilities Act: Questions and answers.* https://search.ada.gov/search?query=Americans+with+Disabilities+Act%3A+Questions+and+ans&search=go&sort=date%3AD%3AL%3Ad1&output=xml_no_dtd&ie=iso-8859-1&oe=UTF-8&client=default_frontend&proxystylesheet=default_frontend&affiliate=justice-ada.

Ward, A.-K., Ravlin, E. C., Klaas, B. S., Ployhart, R. E., & Buchan, N. R. (2016). When do high-context communicators speak up? Exploring contextual communication orientation and employee voice. *Journal of Applied Psychology, 101*(10), 1498–1511.

Yudell, M., Roberts, D., DeSalle, R., & Tishkoff, S. (2016). Taking race out of human genetics. *Science, 351*(6273), 564–565.

12

Organizational Structure

Christopher J. Louis

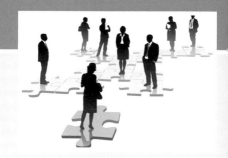

(e) http://evolve.elsevier.com/Huber/leadership

Organizations are essentially social structures that rely on human activity. An organization meaningfully coordinates group activity toward a shared goal because collective efforts are often necessary to manage large-scale work processes and outcomes efficiently and effectively. Many types of organizations are necessary in order to deliver nursing and health care services to diverse populations across sectors and geography. In health care, obvious organizational goals might be safety and quality of care, cost reduction, and increased efficiency. Yet the challenges and consequences of system fragmentation and care coordination continue to plague the US health care system (Louis et al., 2019). Understanding organizational structure helps nurses be more effective and efficient in their work lives.

Whether as employees or as independent practitioners, nurses work for or interact with organizations. How nurses' roles interface with the structure of the organization influences the accomplishment of organizational goals. Research examples throughout this chapter highlight associations between the organizational structures in which nurses work and clinical, nurse, and organizational outcomes.

DEFINITIONS

Structure refers to the arrangement of the parts within a larger whole. In Donabedian's (1980) classic quality framework of structure, process, and outcomes, structure affects process, which affects outcomes. **Organizations** are entities that contain groupings that consolidate smaller elements into a larger, systematized whole. **Organizational social structure** is defined as the

ways in which work is divided and coordinated among members and the resulting network of relationships, roles, and work groups (e.g., units, departments). The social structure of an organization influences the flow of information, resources, and power among its members.

BACKGROUND

Organizational Theory

Organizations are complex and dynamic. Yet for nurses to function as effective health care workers, an understanding of organizations is essential. There are many ways to understand organizations, and each understanding reflects different assumptions and tensions regarding the nature and dynamics of organizations. The history of organizational theory has been shaped by multiple disciplines, including management, engineering, psychology, sociology, and anthropology, and by study over a long period of time. Although this has created a rich and varied understanding of organizations, the field of organization theory contains a variety of approaches to and assumptions about the phenomenon of "organization." Objectivism, subjectivism, and postmodernism reflect three broad perspectives regarding the nature of reality and the nature of knowledge with respect to the concept of "organization" (Hatch & Cunliffe, 2013). These perspectives are reviewed briefly with attention to the meanings of social structure, management, and power.

Objective Perspective

The objective (also called modern) perspective centers interest on causal explanation that entails describing the antecedents and results of a particular phenomenon (Hatch & Cunliffe, 2013). When approached as an objective entity, an organization exists as an external reality, independent of its social actors. Organizations are viewed as logical and predictable objects with identifiable and scientifically measurable characteristics (e.g., size) that can be predicted, observed, or manipulated (Hatch & Cunliffe, 2013). The purpose is to uncover laws that enhance the generalizability of knowledge. Organizational structure is a consequence of both the division of and the coordination of labor, which results in a formal set of interrelated and interdependent roles and work groups. Management determines the formal relationships and standardizes the behaviors of individuals and groups in order to align organizational functioning with internal demands (e.g., technology) and external demands (e.g., market conditions, regulatory standards) (Reed, 1992). Typically, power is conceptualized as a resource to be allocated among roles and groups. Modernist theories related to bureaucracy and systems—as well as the schools of scientific management and human relations—have focused on improvements to efficiency, motivation, and performance in the achievement of collective goals (Reed, 1992). These theoretical approaches, which focus on the *formal* aspects of organizations, are examined in detail in this chapter.

Subjective Perspective

In contrast to objectivism, a symbolic or subjective approach to the phenomenon of organization asserts that an organization cannot exist independent of its social actors. The organization is a social reality that can be known only through human experience, relationships, and shared meanings and symbols (Hatch & Cunliffe, 2013). Because knowledge is considered to be relative, open to interpretation, and context dependent, the purpose of inquiries is to uncover collective meanings and understandings that resonate with the experiences of those involved (Hatch & Cunliffe, 2013). Social structure therefore arises from and is continuously transformed through social interaction, which is played out against a backdrop of formal rules and material resources directed by management (Reed, 1992). Power is reflected in the struggle between social actors who proactively and self-consciously shape organizational arrangements and secure scarce resources to serve their interests (Hatch & Cunliffe, 2013; Reed, 1992).

The subjective perspective focuses on the *informal* aspects of organization and on the freedom of individuals to make choices and to influence organizational life. Symbolic–interpretive theorists are interested in "how the everyday practices of organizational members construct the very patterns of organizing that guide their actions" (Hatch & Cunliffe, 2013, p. 113). Examples of daily social practices include routines (e.g., clinical protocols), interactions, and communities of practice. For example, instead of viewing routines as mechanisms to standardize the behavior of individuals (i.e., an objective approach), a subjective approach might examine the changing nature or pattern of routines as members selectively modify, adapt, and retain practices in response to varying conditions and evidence-based practice. In a community of practice, learning occurs through voluntary social interaction whereby clinicians who are committed to a common interest self-organize informally to build ongoing relationships, partake in joint activities, and share resources (Wenger, 2008). An example in nursing would be an informal group of staff nurses who routinely have lunch together and who come to rely on this activity as a source of knowledge related to patient care in terms of problem-solving, information exchange, and networking.

Postmodern Perspective

Departing from the polarization between objectivism (or modernism) and subjectivism (symbolism), the postmodern view offers critique and appreciation by challenging the meanings and interpretations associated with the concept of organization. The basic premise is that the world is known through language. Because language is continually reconstructed and context dependent, knowledge is essentially a power play (Hatch & Cunliffe, 2013). Notions of order and structure are the subject of scrutiny, and organizations may be thought of as chaotic entities characterized by conflicts and misunderstandings (Reed, 1992). Managerial practices and structures within organizations are seen to legitimize the interests of those in power. Even classic organization theorists such as Weber (1978) cautioned that bureaucracies were essentially domination structures that shape the form and purpose of social action through a system of rational rules and norms. Those who control bureaucracies therefore exert significant power over social action. For example, occurrences of sexual harassment can be either ignored or aggressively sanctioned as consistent with organizational values and norms. Thus the postmodern organization is understood both as an arena in which power struggles between dominant and subordinate groups play out and as a text to be rewritten to free its members from exploitative and controlling influences (Hatch & Cunliffe, 2013; Reed, 1992).

Postmodernists challenge the assumption that social structure results from the division and coordination of work among roles and groups. Clegg (1990) suggested that excessive fragmentation of work results in a disjointed and confusing experience for workers who become dependent on more powerful members in the hierarchy to make sense of workflow and goals. To counter this excess control over member actions, he proposed the idea of **differentiation**, whereby people self-manage and coordinate their own activities. Other examples of postmodern approaches to organization include feminist critiques of bureaucracies (e.g., Eisenstein, 1995) and anti-administration theory (Farmer, 1997). Each perspective contributes to stretching the thinking about how organizations are structured and function.

KEY THEORIES OF ORGANIZATIONS AS SOCIAL SYSTEMS

In the field of organizational design, the organization is most commonly approached as a social system from the objective perspective. Different theories within this tradition have contributed to understanding organizational social structure over an extensive period of study. However, these theories have also been critiqued for rationalizing social action, for favoring efficiency and productivity over other values (e.g., equity, justice), and for adopting an elitist view of management (e.g., O'Connor, 1999).

Bureaucratic Theory

Although often criticized for its oppressive qualities and administrative burden, the concept of bureaucracy may be better understood when placed within a historical context. Theorist Max Weber (1864–1920) was a German lawyer, professor, and political activist who noted the push of industrialism toward mass production and technical efficiency (Prins, 2000). Weber sought to explain from a historical perspective how the bureaucratic structure of large organizations differed from and improved on other forms of societal functioning (e.g.,

feudalism). He viewed bureaucracy as a social leveling mechanism founded on impartial and merit-based selection (i.e., legal authority), rather than a social ordering determined by kinship (i.e., traditional authority) or personality (i.e., charismatic authority) (Weber, 1978). However, Weber warned of the potential dehumanizing effects of bureaucracies that emphasized purely economic results (i.e., formal rationality) at the expense of other important social values such as social justice and equality (i.e., substantive rationality) (Weber, 1978). Weber's descriptions of authority and rationality are foundational concepts in the study of organizations. His interpretation of hierarchy and its relevance to health care organizations are explored later in the chapter.

Scientific Management School

Arising from the experiences and ideas of business leaders and engineers in manufacturing industries, the scientific management school sought to determine the single best way to structure an organization. A well-known theorist in this field is Frederick W. Taylor (1856–1915), an engineer who authored *The Principles of Scientific Management* in 1914 (Prins, 2000). Along with colleagues, Taylor's vision was to improve labor relations and the low industrial standards that plagued the American manufacturing industry by the application of technical solutions (e.g., time and motion studies) (Prins, 2000). The goal was to enhance organizational performance in a milieu of improved cooperation between management and labor by matching the work performed with the worker's skills and with economic incentives. However, the experiments and engineering techniques associated with this approach were ultimately criticized for reducing the worker to a mere input in the production process (Prins, 2000). The application of scientific principles to improve the task performance and productivity of workers reflected a bottom-up approach to organizational design (Scott, 1992). In nursing, efforts to redesign nursing jobs, such as by using nurse practitioners or to measure nursing workload, often rely on this tradition.

Classical Management Theory

In contrast, classical theorists such as Fayol, Urwick, and Gulick evolved a top-down approach to organizational design. Based on experience as company executives, they identified principles of administration and management functions that could be applied in the design of organizations. Key concepts such as differentiation, coordination, the scalar principle, centralization, formalization, specialization, and span of control became central to the study of organizational structure. These concepts, which describe the *formal* aspects of an organization's social structure and their application to health care organizations, are examined in relation to nursing later in the chapter.

Human Relations School

Theorists in the human relations school emphasized the *informal*, rather than *formal*, aspects of organization social structure. The disciplines of industrial psychology and industrial relations founded this approach, which now persists as the field of organizational behavior (O'Connor, 1999). The social and psychological needs and relationships of workers and groups were thought to be important to work productivity. Improved cooperation between management and workers was proposed to enhance performance and reduce industrial strife (O'Connor, 1999). The famous Hawthorne experiments were influential in this school of thought. Initial interpretations of the Hawthorne experiments suggested that psychological factors influenced worker motivation because improved worker productivity was observed when researchers gave special attention to workers, regardless of changes to physical surroundings (Scott, 1992). Concepts such as job enlargement and job rotation were promoted to offset the alienation workers experienced because of excessive **formalization** and division of work processes (Scott, 1992). Formalization is the extent to which the organization uses explicit rules, procedures, job descriptions, and communications to prescribe roles and role interactions, govern activities, and standardize behaviors (Hatch & Cunliffe, 2013).

Streams of study included leadership behavior, small group dynamics, participative decision-making, morale, motivation, and other worker characteristics and behaviors (Scott, 1992). In nursing, this school of thought is reflected in efforts to meet the professional development needs of nurses, enhance nurse autonomy and empowerment, and involve nurses in decision-making processes to improve organizational functioning.

Open System Theory

Open system theory emphasizes the dynamic interaction and interdependence of the organization with its external environment and its internal subsystems. Meyer and O'Brien-Pallas (2010) conceptualized the health care organization as an open system characterized by energy transformation, a dynamic steady state, negative entropy, event cycles, negative feedback, differentiation, integration and coordination, and equifinality. *Inputs* (i.e., characteristics of care recipients, nurses, resources), *throughputs* (the delivery of nursing services arising from the nature of the work, structures, and work conditions), and *outputs* (i.e., clinical, human resource, and organizational outcomes) were theorized to interact dynamically to influence the global work demands placed on nursing work groups at the point of care in production subsystems.

Contingency theory is a subset of open system theory positing that there is no single right way to structure an organization. Effective organizational performance depends on the fit between the structure and multiple contingency factors such as technology, size, and strategy. Mark et al. (1996) applied contingency theory to the evaluation of nursing care delivery system outcomes. The basic premise was that to perform effectively and produce quality outcomes, an organization must structure and adapt its nursing units to complement the environment and technology.

Technology is a core concept in contingency theory and refers to the work performed. Technology can be examined in terms of task uncertainty (i.e., repetitive nature of the task), diversity (i.e., number of different components), and interdependence (i.e., degree to which work processes are interrelated) (Scott, 1992). Highly repetitive and distinct tasks are amenable to mass production technologies (e.g., manufacturing industry). In contrast, highly uncertain and interdependent tasks require discretion, improvisation, and more intense coordination structures across team-driven networks. The work performed by health care professionals such as nurses is often considered to be highly uncertain, diverse, interdependent, and reliant on group coordination. For example, in a study of hospital care for persons with joint replacements, the use of teams with high levels of shared knowledge and goals and mutual respect positively influenced patient-assessed quality of care despite shortened lengths of stay (Gittell, 2004). In this study, task uncertainty was intensified by time constraints (i.e., shorter lengths of stay), task diversity was reflected by the multidisciplinary roles, task interdependence resulted as multidisciplinary work was performed concurrently, and the coordination device was teamwork.

Newer Organizational Theories

In this section, two newer organizational theories that have been applied in health care—including **complexity theory** (see Chapter 1), which suggests that organizations are complex adaptive systems, and **network theory**—are briefly reviewed. Complexity science arose out of the field of physical sciences in the latter half of the twentieth century. It has also provided new perspectives to reconsider both natural and human systems. The theory carries specific assumptions about systems characterized by nonlinearity and feedback loops (Hatch & Cunliffe, 2013; McDaniel et al., 2013). Complexity science is concerned with complex systems and problems that are constantly changing, multidimensional, and unpredictable, comprising interconnected diverse elements and relationships. Concepts such as chaos, self-organization, and complex adaptive systems (CAS) have been used to understand both irregular aspects of nature and provide frameworks to explore regularities that arise in complex systems. A hallmark of these ideas is the existence of nonlinearities in systems, which means that the behavior of the system is more than the sum of the behaviors of individual components (McDaniel et al., 2013).

The notion that organizations, and specifically health care systems, can be viewed as CAS has been proposed by organizational researchers (Hatch & Cunliffe, 2013; McDaniel et al., 2013). This perspective has been applied to current issues in today's health care organizations with the goal of finding new ways to understand the roles of individuals and groups (*agents*) and their effects on health care delivery processes. For example, CAS are *nonlinear and dynamic* and do not essentially reach stable equilibrium states. As a result, system behaviors may appear to be unplanned or chaotic (Rouse, 2008). As agents operate in the system, gain experience, or learn and change their behaviors, the overall system behavior naturally changes over time. This change or adaptation and learning tend to result in *self-organization* and these organizational behavior patterns can be viewed as evolving rather than being planned or constructed into the system. However, these emergent behaviors may range from valuable advances to unfortunate errors. In CAS, there is *no single point(s) of control*, and, as a result, the behaviors of CAS can usually be more easily influenced than controlled. That is, hierarchy plays a less significant role as knowledge, expertise, and decision-making are more distributed across organizational members than invested in authorities at the top of the organization. Leaders using the principles of complexity theory engage in influencing, collaborating, and relational activities rather than aiming for control of others and the future (McDaniel et al., 2013).

Theories of networks are also applied to organizational structure. Social network analysis, which builds on a system view of organizations, examines and interprets the structures and patterns of the formal and informal relationships among members of the organization (Tichy et al., 1979). A recent review of the literature by Bae et al. (2015) focused on health care provider social network analysis found that relationships among care providers were primarily built upon personal characteristics, practice settings and patient type (e.g., disease-oriented). This study also found that social networks affected some patient outcomes, care coordination approaches, and the utilization of health information systems (Bae et al., 2015). **Social capital** is another concept that has been identified in studies using social network theory and refers to resources produced by and rooted in social relationships. The concept is founded on the idea that the relationships among people in the workplace are resources that in turn can provide access to other resources through social exchange (Hatch & Cunliffe, 2013). The concept has been identified by health care leaders as an important resource that is instrumental to the success of health care organizations (Read, 2014) and that leadership in health care organizations was associated with increasing attention to social capital over time (Strömgren et al., 2017). It is receiving current attention in nursing research because greater knowledge about nurses' relationships at work may provide new insights into the creation of healthier work environments that promote positive outcomes for nurses, patients, and health care organizations.

KEY ORGANIZATIONAL DESIGN CONCEPTS

The structure of an organization can be described as the overall way work is divided into tasks and roles, grouped into subunits, and coordinated across an organization. Leaders need to address key elements when they design an organizational structure: division of labor (specialization), departmentalization, differentiation, hierarchy (chain of command), span of control, coordination (integration), centralization and decentralization, standardization, and formalization. In Table 12.1 each of

TABLE 12.1	**Dimensions of Organizational Design**	
Dimension	**Definition or Measure**	**Examples in Health Care and Nursing**
Centralization and decentralization	The degree to which decision-making is concentrated at a single point in the organization versus the degree to which decisions are made by lower-level employees	Centralized or tall organization with several layers of management above the direct care unit level (e.g., unit coordinator, manager, director, vice president, chief executive officer [CEO]) versus flat organization with one layer (vice president) between unit manager and CEO
Coordination or integration	The coordination of activities through accountability, rules, and procedures, liaison roles, committees, task forces, cross-functional teams, or direct communication	Bed management specialist role who links across hospital units to manage access and efficient use of available beds, or a quality improvement team that works across patient care programs to improve a particular aspect of patient care such as infection rates, or inter-professional rounds on patient care units
Departmentalization	The basis by which jobs are grouped	Jobs may be grouped by function (e.g., the human resources department), or by product or service/program (e.g., cardiac surgery, palliative care)
Differentiation	The process of dividing the work in an organization. *Vertical* differentiation is shown in the number of levels in the hierarchy, and *horizontal* differentiation is shown in the number of departments or divisions across an entire organization	*Vertical* includes several levels from care units to departments or programs/service lines to divisions, and *horizontal* refers to number of units or departments at the same level across the organization
Division of labor (or specialization)	The degree to which work activities/tasks in an organization are divided into separate jobs	Large acute care hospitals with several levels of nursing care roles, such as patient care assistants, registered nurses, specialty nurses, advanced practice nurses, etc.
Formalization	The degree to which jobs within the organization are standardized and employee behavior is guided by rules and procedures	Formal job descriptions, certification and educational requirements for each role, standards of practice, clinical protocols, care guidelines, written procedures for various treatments, union contractual agreements
Hierarchy (or chain of command)	The structure of authority in an organization The chain of command is an unbroken line of authority that extends from the top of the organization to the lowest level and clarifies who reports to whom	CEO at the top has several vice presidents (e.g., patient care divisions, human resources, finance, etc.) who in turn have directors who in turn have unit managers who may have staff nurses and other professionals reporting to them
Size	Number of employees in the organization	Health system of multiple organizations with 2000 employees versus small rural hospital with 100 employees
Span of control	The number of subordinates a manager can efficiently and effectively direct	A nurse manager of an intensive care unit with 100 direct reports of nurses and charge nurses versus a manager of a small outpatient clinic with 20 direct reports of nurses plus support personnel
Standardization	The extent to which standard procedures govern the organization's functions and activities rather than using individual judgment	Mission and vision statements, organizational policies and procedures, clearly defined communication channels, or supervisory roles and functions

Adapted from: Hatch, M.J., & Cunliffe, A.L. (2013). *Organization theory: Modern, symbolic, and postmodern perspectives* (3rd ed.), p. 95. Oxford, UK: Oxford University Press.

these elements is presented, with definitions and examples, and the following sections describe them.

Division and Coordination of Labor

A formal organization that employs people to achieve predetermined goals divides the work among its members by assigning tasks and delegating responsibilities to positions and work units. Structure is a byproduct of the basic need to divide the labor into the specific tasks to be performed and a consequent need to coordinate these tasks to accomplish the activity or goal. The division (or differentiation) of work by occupation or by function is a form of **specialization**. As occupations and functions multiply in number, an organization increases in complexity and **size**. Size is a quantitative measure of personnel, physical capacity, volume of inputs or outputs, or discretionary resources of an organization.

The advantages of specialization include improved work performance and a critical mass of experts (Charnes & Tewksbury, 1993). In health care, specialist roles have emerged to address the increasing complexities of care and technology. Within nursing, specialist roles have also evolved to address particular areas of nursing practice and include advanced practice roles such as clinical nurse educators, nurse practitioners, and nurse anesthetists.

Organizations may also **differentiate** work units by function (also called **departmentalization**) to serve distinct client populations. For instance, rather than a single, general intensive care unit, an organization may establish several intensive care units by medical specialty (e.g., cardiovascular, neurosurgical, neonatal) or grouped into a "service line," such as palliative care or cardiac care programs. At the work group level, nursing care delivery models (e.g., team, primary, or total nursing care models) reflect different ways of dividing and coordinating the work among a team of nurses caring for clients.

Subdividing work may create breaks or fragmentation in work flow, which can be addressed in organizations by integrating work processes across roles and subunits using coordination devices (Hatch & Cunliffe, 2013). At the work group level, coordination may involve specific roles, standardization (programming), groups, or feedback devices. For example, handoff communication and techniques such as Situation, Background, Assessment, and Recommendation (SBAR) are used to coordinate between units or providers in the delivery of care.

In health care, common programming devices used to control work processes are the following:

- Standardization of worker skills coordinates work indirectly by stipulating the kind of training or education required to perform the work. In nursing, the standardization of worker skills might occur if specific degrees or certifications are required for certain roles such as nurse practitioners or critical care nurses.
- Standardization of work processes coordinates work by prespecifying or programming content before the work is undertaken, such as nurses being required to use clinical protocols or evidence-based best practice guidelines in practice.
- Standardization of work outputs coordinates work through the specification of the results, product, or performance desired or expected and includes the specification of outcome targets such as reduction of nosocomial infection rates.
- Standardization of communication methods coordinates work by providing a uniform structure for information delivery and flow in order to facilitate exchange among those involved in common work processes. In nursing, this might be achieved through electronic health records and relational databases with alerts that allow nurses and other care providers to have direct and simultaneous access to client information in a consistent format.

In addition, feedback mechanisms are used in the transfer of information in an adaptive and reciprocal manner to foster the exchange of information (Gittell, 2002):

- Mutual adjustment coordinates work by using simple informal communication and may occur when one nurse consults another nurse about practice issues, such as how to interpret a policy, or when nurses, physicians, and allied health professionals participate in clinical rounds.
- Direct supervision coordinates work through the use of a supervisor taking responsibility for the instruction and monitoring of the work of others, such as when a nurse supervises the work of assistive personnel.
- Boundary spanning roles coordinate work by managing relationships as well as the bidirectional flow of information and materials across functional divisions. For example, case managers exemplify boundary spanning because these roles manage relationships, exchange information, and negotiate resources with internal and external parties to facilitate care across occupations, services, sectors, funding agencies, and locations.

The types of **coordination** that are used may depend on the degree of stability and predictability of the work situation and the size of the work unit. For instance, acute health care settings are typically characterized as highly uncertain and interdependent work situations in which patient health needs, acuity, and care trajectories are often highly variable and unpredictable. To ensure comprehensive care, nurses coordinate patient care activities with the work of others in a reciprocal manner because the work performed is highly interdependent. As conditions become increasingly uncertain and variable, as in health care, coordination by feedback or specific liaison roles may be used. Improved health care team performance has been associated with both programming and feedback devices because standardized routines may enhance, rather than replace, the interactions among health care providers, particularly in situations of increasing uncertainty (Gittell, 2002). Recent research has shown that improved provider ratings of coordination in inpatient medicine units were linked with an organization's alignment and commitment to high-quality patient care, adequate staffing, resources that support health care professionals to do their jobs, and approaches that promote interactions and communication between nurses and physicians, such as regular multidisciplinary rounding (McIntosh et al., 2014).

At the organizational level, the coordination and division of labor influence the size and degree of organizational centralization and formalization. As organizations grow in size, work units are increasingly subdivided to ensure tasks are accomplished. However, this process slows as organizations become very large, because the gains achieved by subdividing work occur at the expense of the coordination mechanisms necessary to unify system functioning across subunits. In centralized structures, top leaders make all the decisions, and lower-level managers and staff have little decision-making discretion. In a highly formalized job, the individual has minimal discretion over what to do and when and how to do it. Organizational coordination is often measured by the degree of centralization and formalization. Health care organizations tend toward being decentralized and less formalized because professionals are employed to manage highly uncertain work. However, as organizations grow and the work becomes increasingly complex, specialized, and interdependent, there is a pull toward greater centralization and formalization (Hatch & Cunliffe, 2013).

Hierarchy

Hierarchy is the structure of authority in an organization. Authority is equated with the enforcement of regulations, which creates a governing order among the formal social relationships of organizational members (Weber, 1978). Authority is vested in positions, rather than in persons, and creates an impartial mechanism whereby the supraordinate position directs the actions and the norms expected of subordinate positions. Centralization is a multidimensional concept frequently associated with authority and hierarchy and describes the extent to which decision-making authority is concentrated in the top level of the hierarchy (i.e., centralized) versus spread down through the hierarchy (i.e., decentralized). In nursing, shared governance structures signify decentralization. **Hierarchical centralization** can vary according to the decision type.

Corporate strategy is likely to be decided by top executives, whereas procedural work decisions may be decentralized to work units or employees. For instance, a nurse executive could be required to centralize some budgetary decisions, whereas others could be decided at lower levels in the hierarchy. A specific example would be the need to centralize a component of professional development expenditures required by union contracts (e.g., organization-wide funding for nursing certification) in contrast to decisions at the work unit level to possibly fund nurses to attend their specialty conferences (some units do, some do not). Participation is an alternate dimension of centralization that refers to the scope of involvement and influence of organizational members in decision-making. Findings from a study of Belgian hospitals showed that nurses who perceived that their work decisions were tightly controlled by a supervisor (i.e., high hierarchical centralization) and they had little influence on program decisions (i.e., low participative centralization) reported lower job satisfaction (Willem et al., 2007).

In addition, hierarchy creates a reporting structure whereby formal lines of communication, in conjunction with role descriptions, delineate the responsibilities and accountability of each position for work processes and outcomes. Organizational positions are traditionally described in terms of staff and line positions (Hatch & Cunliffe, 2013). Staff positions are outside the direct hierarchical authority chain. These positions provide expertise and knowledge to support the line positions in meeting the organization's goals. The clinical nurse specialist (CNS) who is hired for knowledge development and expert consultation for selected patient groups is an example of a staff position. Line positions are in the direct line of hierarchical authority from top to bottom in an organization and are central to controlling or generating the product or service of the organization. Line positions include vice presidents, directors, managers, and frontline nurses because these positions are authorized either to supervise production processes or to produce the organization's output. In nursing, although frontline nurses are commonly referred to as "staff" nurses, these nurses hold line positions that deliver services to care recipients.

Hierarchy also enables organizations to assign responsibilities based on the complexity and skill requirements of the work and to ensure individual accountability. Responsibility is the obligation to take on and accomplish work and to secure the desired results. A manager assigns or delegates responsibility to a subordinate, and thus responsibility flows down the organizational chain. In accepting the obligation of an assigned task, the staff person is accepting responsibility to accomplish the task, whereas accountability is the liability for task performance and is determined in a retrospective analysis of what occurred. The assignment of responsibility and the granting of authority create accountability. Accountability flows upward or outward, from staff to manager or from provider to client. Reporting relationships are important for creating channels of appeal (Weber, 1978), to ensure employees are held accountable for the work assigned, and to invest managers with the necessary authority to ensure the completion of work. The manager represents the organization at the point of contact with staff, and thus the reporting relationship is also a mechanism by which staff can access organizational resources to identify and solve complex problems. Ideally, managers also apply their leadership skills to reporting relationships to release the energy and talents of people in ways that add value to the work performed. Examples of "value-added" outcomes include improved employee productivity, organizational commitment, and organizational citizenship behaviors.

Organizational Forms

The division and coordination of labor lead to varied organizational forms. As illustrated by the sloping triangles in Fig. 12.1, organizational forms reflect a trade-off between differentiation by function and integration by program. **Differentiation by function** refers to the division of work by occupation. **Integration by program** means the coordination of work around the delivery of particular products or services. Five basic organizational forms can be situated along a differentiation–integration continuum (Charnes & Tewksbury, 1993). Functional and program forms represent extreme examples of differentiation and integration. The matrix form represents the most balanced form. In reality, organizations are not usually found in these pure forms but instead reflect hybrids of the forms described next.

Functional Form

At the extreme left end of the continuum, dividing the work by occupation leads to a functional organization

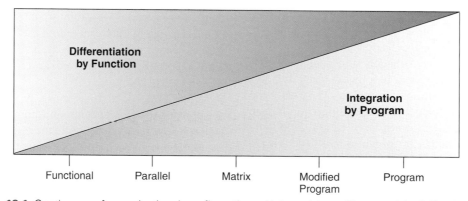

Fig. 12.1 Continuum of organizational configurations. (Adapted from Charnes, M., & Tewksbury, L. [1993]. *Collaborative management in health care: Implementing the integrative organization* [p. 28, Fig. 2.1]. San Francisco, CA: Jossey-Bass. This material is used by permission of John Wiley & Sons.)

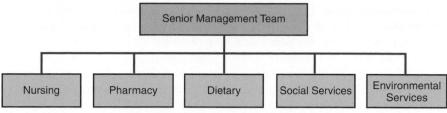

Fig. 12.2 Simplified functional form.

whereby health professions and nonprofessional services are arranged according to the type of work performed. The emphasis is on the human resources inputs to the organization (Fig. 12.2). Examples are nursing, respiratory therapy, admitting, and environmental services. Within each functional department, management develops specific structures, policies, procedures, and human resource practices. In this type of organizational form, professionals report directly to a discipline-specific supervisor (e.g., nurses would report to a nurse manager). Members of a functional group (e.g., nursing) are likely to interact more frequently, develop social relationships, receive supervision and evaluations from within the group, and conform to professional standards (Charnes & Tewksbury, 1993).

By dividing personnel according to the type of work performed, organizations can capitalize on the expertise, experience, efficiency, and professional standards that each discipline offers (Charnes & Tewksbury, 1993). Other benefits include cost reduction through shared resources; enhanced monitoring of cost, performance, and quality; and promotion of professional development, identity, autonomy, advocacy, and career advancement. Disadvantages of the functional form are

its potential to overemphasize professional silos, discourage informal relationships across disciplines, and fragment care delivery (Charnes & Tewksbury, 1993). Coordination of activities becomes challenging because group members have functionally based differences in work goals, cognitive patterns, and status (Gittell, 2004). Because the work of nursing is highly interdependent with other professional and nonprofessional work, nurse leaders in functional forms may use coordination mechanisms and leadership behaviors to span the boundaries between disciplines and facilitate the flow and exchange of information, resources, and work activities. Although prevalent in health care in the 1980s, functional forms have gradually been replaced by program or matrix forms to enhance patient centeredness.

Program Form

At the extreme right end of the continuum, program organizations emphasize integration of the work by consumer, service, or geography (Charnes & Tewksbury, 1993). The emphasis is on the outputs of the organization (Fig. 12.3). In health care, programs may be managed according to consumer health needs (e.g., diabetes, cancer), consumer age (e.g., elderly, neonates, women),

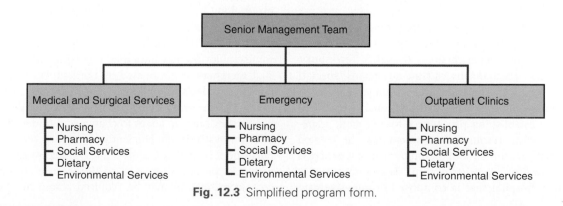

Fig. 12.3 Simplified program form.

services (e.g., addictions, rehabilitation), medical specialty (e.g., neurosciences, endocrinology), or geography (e.g., catchment areas). Although the corporate structure is shared, each program tends to operate as a semiautonomous unit with its own management team composed of medical, administrative, and nursing representatives (Charnes & Tewksbury, 1993). Professionals who work in program organizations may not report to a discipline-specific supervisor.

Program designs can optimize service delivery because local experts with accountability for costs, outcomes, and staffing control resources and can make timely operational decisions (Leatt et al., 1994). Patients can access integrated services from an array of health professionals with specific clinical expertise. With the program form, there is a push toward a multidisciplinary team approach. However, clients who require access to more than one program may find it difficult to coordinate services among different programs. Integration by program occurs at the expense of decreased coordination among programs (Charnes & Tewksbury, 1993). Although organizational relationships with medical staff are enhanced when programs are grouped by medical specialty, health care professionals may be isolated from their colleagues in other programs, and this has been associated with job dissatisfaction and lack of professional development opportunities (Young et al., 2004). For nursing, the concern is that no organization-wide mechanisms would exist to systematically handle professional nursing issues in terms of standards, resources, or professional advocacy. Because each program operates independently, processes and procedures are likely to be duplicated, and programs may compete for resources or develop goals that diverge from the corporate mission (Leatt et al., 1994).

Parallel Form

To address the challenges of purely functional forms, mechanisms in the parallel form assist in coordinating across functional departments (Charnes & Tewksbury, 1993). These mechanisms can include teams, specialists, task forces, liaison roles, and standing committees. For example, rather than each functional department separately establishing procedures to hire staff, a specialized human resource department may be created to deal with recruitment and employment issues across the organization. Another example is a rapid response team in a hospital that is composed of intensive care

physicians and nurses and respiratory therapists. This team assists staff throughout the hospital in detecting and managing imminent patient deterioration and in resuscitating compromised patients. Likewise, in home care, nurses with specialized expertise such as wound care or palliative care might be responsible for referrals across multiple areas. Task forces bring together members from various divisions in an organization to address a concern. For example, developing and implementing critical pathways, evidence-based practices, disease management initiatives, case management projects, or outcomes management efforts generally require an interdisciplinary team of specialists. These types of mechanisms foster collaboration and cross-fertilization of knowledge across divisions and can reinforce consistency in clinical and management practices by standardizing procedures.

Modified Program Form

To offset the fragmentation and isolation of functions in pure program structures, organizations maintain the program structure and develop integrative mechanisms to unify functions and occupations across programs (Charnes & Tewksbury, 1993). For example, a nurse executive could address professional nursing issues related to standards, educational resources, and research activities across the organization. Unlike their counterpart in a functional nursing department who has line authority, a nurse executive in a modified program would not directly control operations, finances, or personnel issues (known as *staff authority*). A nurse executive with staff authority need to use personal influence and leadership skills to effect change.

Matrix Form

In a pure matrix form, people and work are organized along both functional and program dimensions (Charnes & Tewksbury, 1993). Essentially, the program form overlays the functional form (Fig. 12.4). Although some employees may have dual reporting relationships, staff members are evaluated by both supervisors. The budget and decision-making are shared between functional and program divisions. A matrix configuration has the flexibility to adapt to change and to deliver services innovatively and efficiently by drawing on a varied talent pool (Hatch & Cunliffe, 2013). In contrast, innovation in program forms is costly because additional cross-coordination may be required across functional

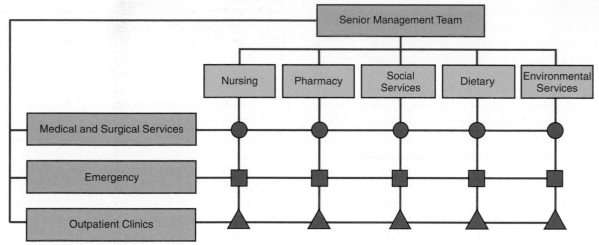

For example, team members for Outpatient Clinics (▲) are drawn from different functions.

Fig. 12.4 Simplified matrix form.

divisions, or specialists may need to be hired for each program. However, true matrix forms are rarely seen and are difficult to maintain because the additional management infrastructure is costly and dual reporting relationships may be ambiguous and lead to conflict (Charnes & Tewksbury, 1993). Success requires well-educated workers who can handle a multifaceted communication and authority web. Nurses in matrix organizations need strong interpersonal and teamwork skills to negotiate these complex environments.

ORGANIZATIONAL CHARTS

Hierarchy reflects the *formal* structure of the organization, which can be identified on an organizational chart. An organizational chart is a visual display of the organization's positions and the intentional relationships among positions. The organizational chart reflects the various positions and the formal relationships between and among the positions and, by extension, the people who are a part of the organization. The organizational chart generally presents the line positions, linked together by solid lines to show the flow of authority. Administrative roles are generally shown in vertical and horizontal dimensions. Staff positions or advisory bodies may be depicted on the chart with dotted lines to show consultative relationships. Organizational charts help with administrative control, policy making and planning, and the evaluation of the organization's

strengths and weaknesses. They clearly depict who reports to whom. Charts are used to orient personnel because relationships and expected patterns of interaction within the formal organization are made clear. For example, an organizational chart of a matrix structure may show dotted lines for the project or interdisciplinary team relationships. Dotted lines mean that a relationship to the position or the group would form for a project. In the process of applying for a job, obtaining the employer's organizational chart will help understand the relative positioning of individuals within the organization and how the organization is structured—or at least how decision makers believe it is structured.

In addition to a *formal* structure, organizations are characterized by an *informal* structure. The *informal* structure is simply the network or pattern of social relationships and friendship circles that are outside the formal structure. It is an interconnected web of relationships that operate in and around the formally designated lines of communication. The *informal* structure does not appear on the *formal* organizational chart.

ORGANIZATIONAL SHAPES

The shape of an organization structure can be described as relatively tall or flat. Several structural factors influence the shape of an organization. The formal reporting relationships among positions ensure the assignment of responsibility, authority, and accountability and result in hierarchical levels. The **span of control** of managers—the number of employees reporting directly to a management position—also influences organizational shape (Meyer, 2008). For instance, when managers on average have fewer direct-report staff, the organizational shape is relatively taller. Another structural factor involves decisions about the number of management layers in the hierarchy (i.e., the **scalar principle**). Increased layers of management help the organization cope with increasing work complexity and extended timelines (Jaques, 1990). A tall organization structure assumes a pyramidal shape with multiple management layers (Fig. 12.5). In contrast, a flat organization structure has minimal management layers (Fig. 12.6). Advantages and disadvantages associated with tall and flat organizational shapes are summarized in Table 12.2. However, a narrow focus on the hierarchical structure of an organization without attention to the people and processes within the organization or the outcomes achieved can be misleading. For instance, factors that can potentially offset the effects

of tall organizations include the competence and leadership of members, the use of merit-based rewards, the effectiveness of reporting relationships, and the sharing of information and authority (Jaques, 1990).

Span of management refers to the number and ordering of management positions and resources relative to other personnel and can be measured at organizational, departmental, managerial, work group, or employee levels (Meyer, 2008). There are many competing arguments about factors influencing the span of management, and decisions about the amount, type, and distribution of nursing management resources within health care organizations are influenced by a multitude of factors at the consumer, nurse, work group, manager, organizational, and regional levels (Meyer, 2008). A key controversy about the span of control of nurse managers relates to supervisory responsibilities. On the one hand, wider spans of control for managers are proposed because nurses and other health care professionals are experts committed to professional codes of ethics and regulated

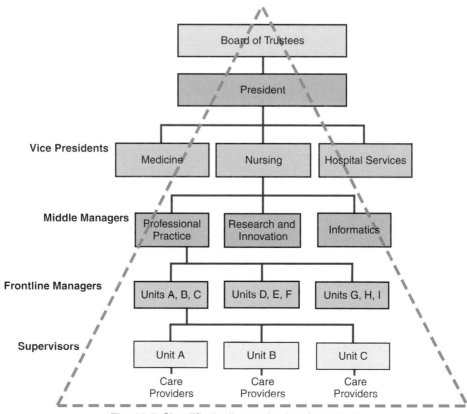

Fig. 12.5 Simplified tall organizational structure.

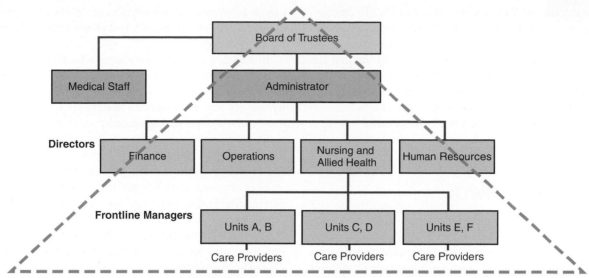

Fig. 12.6 Simplified flat organizational structure.

TABLE 12.2	**Comparison of Flat and Tall Organization Structures**	
	Tall Organization	**Flat Organization**
Advantages	• Increased access to managers and organizational resources • Greater supervisory capability • Layers of skill to deal with varying degrees of work complexity • Layers of accountability for work completion • Layers of responsibility to address short, medium, and long-term issues and planning	• Fewer divisions facilitate streamlining of goals, problem-solving, and resource use • Greater hierarchical decentralization; potential for greater staff autonomy through increased delegation • Greater innovation • Enhanced responsiveness to consumers at point of service • Less cross-coordination required • Less costly management infrastructure
Disadvantages	• More hierarchical centralization; potential to micromanage staff activities • Slowed vertical decision-making and distorted communication • Less innovation • Difficult way-finding for consumers • Greater cross coordination required • Costly management infrastructure	• Decreased access to managers and organizational resources • Decreased supervisory capability • Overextension of managers • Vertical communication delays

Copyright 2012 Raquel M. Meyer. Used with permission. Table based on: Alidina & Funke-Furber, 1988; Jaques, 1990; Pabst, 1993.

standards, therefore requiring less direct supervision (Meier & Bohte, 2003). On the other hand, narrow spans of control are deemed necessary because (1) nurses require managerial support and access to organizational resources and information to coordinate complex work processes to achieve positive outcomes, and (2) the introduction of unlicensed workers into health care settings has required more direct, hands-on supervision to ensure that care standards and organizational expectations are met. This counterargument suggests that the span of control of frontline nurse managers should factor in the needs of staff nurses for their manager's support and supervision. In nursing, relationships between the span of control of frontline managers and manager, nurse, and clinical outcomes have been investigated (Wong et al., 2015).

STRUCTURAL POWER

Within the objective perspective, power has been conceptualized as a resource. Kanter's (1977) classic theory of the structural determinants of behavior in organizations has been investigated in nursing systems (Laschinger, 1996). For Kanter (1977, p. 166), power refers to "the ability to get things done, to mobilize resources." It is not the power to control or dominate others. When power is shared, rather than monopolized, employees are empowered, and the organization is more likely to benefit. More activity can be accomplished by organizational members, and the capacity for effective action is increased. Kanter (1977) described three work empowerment structures: opportunity, power, and proportion. The structure of *opportunity* refers to expectations and future prospects (e.g., opportunities for growth, mobility, job enrichment). The structure of *power* stems from access to information, support, and resources. The structure of *proportion* denotes the social composition of the organization's workforce (e.g., gender, minorities). Empowered work environments are those in which all employees have access to opportunities to learn and grow and to information, support, and resources necessary for the job. Indeed, frontline nurses' job-related or structural empowerment has been linked to positive nurse outcomes, including greater nurse job satisfaction (Cicolini et al., 2014; Wong & Laschinger, 2013), increased organizational commitment (Smith et al., 2010; Yang et al., 2013), feelings of trust and respect in the workplace (Laschinger et al., 2014), lower job and career turnover intentions (Choi et al., 2014; Laschinger & Fida, 2014), and lower burnout and workplace incivility (Laschinger et al., 2013). Nurses who occupy positions at higher levels in the nursing hierarchy reported increasingly greater degrees of empowerment (Laschinger et al., 2012), which may mean that nurses in management positions are likely to perceive greater access to opportunity and power structures than frontline nurses.

In Kanter's (1977) study, effective leaders were seen as both competent and powerful. Sensitivity with subordinates was secondary to having upward credibility within the organization; leaders to whom others listened, who accessed resources, and who produced results within the broader organization were perceived to be effective. Kanter (1977) proposed that effective leadership evolves from both *formal* and *informal* sources of power in the organization. *Formal* power is derived from work that is relevant to pressing organizational issues and that provides opportunities to perform extraordinary and highly visible activities; *informal* power comes from relationships and alliances with people in the organization.

Kanter (1977, p. 168) also theorized that "power begets power." Research indicates that nurses who are managed by empowered leaders are also empowered (Laschinger, 1996). For example, frontline nurses in organizations where chief nurse executives had line authority reported significantly greater global empowerment with respect to resources than their counterparts in organizations where chief nurse executives had staff authority (Matthews et al., 2006). The authors suggested that the *formal* power accessible to nurse executives with line authority enabled them to secure the staffing resources necessary for frontline nurses to provide high quality of care. Magnet hospitals typically consist of flat organizational structures with nursing councils that empower nurses through decentralized decision-making. This structure engages staff nurses in decisions affecting their work, for example, when inter-professional staff work together to redesign workflow. Considered overall, the research suggests that empowerment structures have a positive impact on both nurses and managers and can inform the design of the organizational structures in which nurses work.

LEADERSHIP AND MANAGEMENT IMPLICATIONS

The global and local challenges for nursing within organizations and across systems are numerous. Leaders and managers can influence the structure in which goals are accomplished. In fact, determining the structure is a key responsibility of leaders and managers in planning an organization that is conducive to high-quality nursing care. As environments and technologies evolve, the leadership and management team may need to rethink and redesign the organization and work group structures to better match the changing conditions and achieve the desired outcomes. In nursing, determining the structure is a planning and organizing aspect of the management process that can be informed by evidence and theory from the management field.

Leaders and managers may be involved in revising or changing organizational structures. *Restructuring* means revising or modifying the structure to reshape it or switch to another structural form. Restructuring efforts have typically been geared toward fixing existing operational processes. Lean, decentralized, self-governing organizations that empower first-line caregivers are the preferred structures. To begin anew, processes are analyzed from the point of view of the consumer (patient and family) as well as the requirement to achieve greater cost containment, quality, service, and speed. User-friendly processes, efficiency, and economy are key ideas. Job redesign focuses on who does what tasks and on maximizing flexibility, cross-training, and productivity.

Changes to organization structure afford opportunities to empower nurses. Strategies include maximizing nurses' scope of practice, creating autonomous and visible nursing roles relevant to organizational priorities, and providing more leadership opportunities for nurses at all levels. Fiscal and material resources can also be deployed to empower nurses by facilitating access to knowledge-development opportunities (e.g., courses, conferences) and by providing adequate resources for job completion (e.g., staffing). A decentralized, participative structure can be promoted through coordination mechanisms that involve nurses in shared governance councils and task forces (e.g., related to clinical practice or nurse retention) and in information exchange (e.g., newsletters, open forums, web technologies).

A transparent and participative approach to the development of programming devices to standardize work processes (e.g., clinical protocols, electronic health records) can be used to build shared goals for interdisciplinary teams. Organizations can also deliberately foster informal coordination mechanisms to enhance the relational and functional networks in which work is accomplished (Hatch & Cunliffe, 2013). For example, physical colocation, communal space, communities of practice, rotational job assignments, electronic chat groups, and interdisciplinary training programs can foster spontaneous interactions and relationships across functional, professional, and geographical silos, resulting in knowledge sharing, problem-solving, and innovation.

Hierarchical reporting relationships can be greatly enhanced by transformational leaders who establish trust with nurses by communicating role and behavior expectations, giving constructive performance feedback, and recognizing and rewarding successes (Wong & Laschinger, 2013). When workers fall outside organizational lines of authority (e.g., outsourced services, nursing agencies such as travelers), managers and leaders need skills in negotiating standards and performance outcomes, in resolving problems across organizational boundaries, and in building relationships and shared goals to overcome differing alliances (Porter-O'Grady & Malloch, 2014).

In more highly matrixed organizations, nurse managers and leaders need to network with interdisciplinary stakeholders within and across programs and support services. Success for leaders with line authority requires strong relational skills, credibility, an ability to link resource use to outcomes using a business model, and an in-depth understanding of the needs of clients and staff (Lorenz, 2008). The trends toward increased outsourcing, decreased reliance on traditional inpatient services for revenues, and increased specialization of health services require an entrepreneurial skill set and innovative leadership roles to build business partnerships and alliances and to foster change at the point of service delivery (Porter-O'Grady, 2015). In the context of nurse and manager shortages, organizations need to recruit and deploy management resources in line with objectives by reevaluating the number of management layers and the span of control of individual positions, as well as by developing a nursing leadership succession plan. To be supportive of nursing staff, nurse managers need access to the support and information of senior management and peers, professional development and mentorship, an office that is easily accessible to staff, administrative support, and a strong and shared organizational culture.

Organizational Assessment

Nurse leaders can use organizational assessment to generate data needed for analysis that serves as the foundation for planning and change management as well as to identify the status of quality and safety efforts. Organizational assessments focus on assisting teams, departments, organizations, and systems to better understand the organization as it is and to continuously improve by indicating areas in need of further development. There are a variety of organizational assessments. Some are commercial or not in health care, like the Organizational Assessment (Lusthaus et al., 2002). Some are both in business and industry as well as health care, such as the Malcolm Baldrige National Quality Award (American Society for Quality [ASQ], n.d.), which recognizes US companies that have implemented successful quality management systems. Some focus specifically on the unit, such as the Dartmouth Institute for Health Policy & Clinical Practice's (2010) Microsystems at a Glance and the Institute for Healthcare Improvement's (IHI) (2016) Clinical Microsystem Assessment Tool. In nursing, the Magnet Recognition Program (American Nurses Credentialing Center, n.d.) only focuses on the quality of nursing services and resources for nurses.

CURRENT ISSUES AND TRENDS

During the 1990s, health care systems in many developed countries were subjected to restructuring, decentralization, specialization, and performance management, resulting in the de-layering of management structures in an effort to contain costs and achieve outcomes (Mahon & Young, 2006). Those managers remaining in the system faced expanded roles. Instead of a traditional head nurse position responsible for patient care on a single unit, the role of the nurse manager typically grew to encompass the management of finances, operations, and human resources across multiple clinical areas and services in program management structures with regulated and unregulated multidisciplinary staff.

The twenty-first century has ushered in significant concerns related to the global community and public safety. These issues are intensified by calls for transparency, accountability, and public reporting in the management of health care services, which in turn have increased demands on the internal structures and external boundaries of organizations. In addition, at a societal level, preparedness for disasters, bioterrorism, and pandemics has required health care organizations, communities, and jurisdictions to pool resources and coordinate activities along the external boundaries of organizational structures. Furthermore, large

companies in the business world have been working to eliminate *vertical* and *horizontal* boundaries within and to break down *external* barriers between the company and its customers and suppliers. This **boundaryless** organization seeks to eliminate the hierarchical chain of command, replace departments with empowered teams, and promote learning in order to keep pace with rapid change (Hatch & Cunliffe, 2013). Although achieving a boundaryless state may never be completely actualized, especially in health care organizations, there is evidence of moves to create better integration of care delivery processes across care sectors and organizations within health systems (Edgren & Barnard, 2012).

Attempts to remove vertical boundaries, flatten the hierarchy and implement cross-functional and cross-organizational teams (which include senior executives, middle managers, supervisors, employees, and care recipients), participative decision-making practices, and boundary-spanning leadership practices are being implemented in health care to break down vertical and horizontal boundaries (Shirey & White-Williams, 2015). With wide-ranging changes introduced with the Affordable Care Act (ACA) of 2010 and the Institute for Healthcare Improvement's (IHI's) Triple Aim framework for optimizing health system performance, a focus for organizations is on improving individual patient and family care experiences, increasing the health of populations, reforming primary care, and reducing overall costs. All of these priorities require high levels of system integration and even transformation (Shirey & White-Williams, 2015). One solution has been a rise in the number of health care organizations (hospitals, ambulatory facilities, continuing care homes, and home health) merging not only to achieve economies of scale but as also as a way of better organizing the clinical functions across different sites and locations (Kerfoot & Luquire, 2012; Shirey & White-Williams, 2015). With the emergence of these larger health systems, the role of the system chief nurse executive has increased (Bradley, 2014).

At a global level, increasing shortages of nurses and other health care professionals has engendered a call for developed countries to create self-sufficient and sustainable nursing workforces by increasing domestic supply (Gantz et al., 2012). At the organizational level, employers need to attract and retain nurses through changes to work conditions and structures such as creating full-time positions, re-dividing work to continue to remove non-nursing tasks, supplying adequate staffing and material resources to accomplish the work, and improving work climates that support exemplary professional nursing practice (Gantz et al., 2012). These strategies are necessary to stabilize the nursing workforce within organizations and to ensure that the knowledge, skills, and competence that nurses possess are retained and appropriately deployed in the organization.

Increased awareness and disclosure about medical errors and preventable adverse events have encouraged organizations to address consumer safety through risk reduction and the development of cultures of safety (DiCuccio, 2015). To address safety, new coordination mechanisms and explicit safety standards are based on the science of human factors engineering, which takes a systems approach to understanding and preventing critical incidents (Carayon et al., 2014). A systems approach considers how adverse events occur in relation to management, organization, and regulatory factors such as policies and procedures, information technology, staffing practices, and physical structures. Recall that policies, procedures, and information systems are coordination devices. For instance, safety risks may be reduced when nurses standardize care through the use of evidence-based clinical protocols. Organizations are also compelled to collaborate in the development and sharing of safety innovations. The Center for Quality Improvement and Safety in the United States and the Canadian Patient Safety Institute in Canada are examples of how safety innovations can be widely shared and standardized across organizations.

---

⑤ RESEARCH NOTE

Source
Louis, C. J., Clark, J. R., Gray, B., Brannon, D., & Parker, V. (2019). Service line structure and decision-maker attention in three health systems: Implications for patient-centered care. *Health Care Management Review, 44*(1), 41–56.

Purpose
The aim of this study was to understand the role of service line structure in producing coordinated, patient-centered care.

Description
Prior research has identified a disconnect between the level at which structure is typically examined (the organization level) and where coordination effort actually takes place (e.g., the delivery of services). However, we know little about the role that structure plays in care coordination. In this study, a comparative case study approach was used to understand the role structure played in care coordination efforts at three different health systems. The study specifically investigated the delivery of breast cancer care, the care providers involved, and services provided.

Results
This study found that the three health systems had substantial variation in service line structure. Corresponding variation was also found in terms of where each health system primarily focused in coordinating care. These results draw a clear connection between the organization's structural characteristics and the dominant focus of attention (operational tactics, provider roles and relationships, or patient needs and engagement) at the service line level.

Application to Practice
The structure and design of health care organizations and service lines influences how care providers function and can enable (or hinder) their propensity to collaborate. In each of the organizations in this study, a different dominant focus of attention was found and ultimately influenced the level at which the care providers could put the patient at the center of care processes. Achieving a patient-centered attention may require careful internal planning of service line structure such that inter-departmental barriers are removed and collaborative efforts across provider specialties are prioritized. The alternative is a less desirable, more fragmented orientation where staff and care providers are constantly focusing on operational process workarounds and overcoming barriers to timely, efficient care.

CASE STUDY

Consolidation of Inpatient Services at Two Community Hospitals

Hospital A is the flagship hospital in a two-hospital health system and is located in the suburbs of a major US city. Hospital A is comprised of 240 medical/surgical and telemetry beds and has eight units, each with the maximum capacity of 30 beds. Over the past 12 months the average daily census (ADC) in this hospital is 40% (96 patients), with a peak census of 70% (168 patients). Hospital A also has 20 Intensive Care Unit (ICU) beds and the ADC over the past 12 months was 40% (eight patients), with a peak census of 90% (18 patients).

Hospital B is located 7 miles away from Hospital A and is in a rural location. Hospital B is comprised of 100 medical/surgical and telemetry beds and has five units, each with the maximum capacity of 20 beds. The ADC over the past 12 months is 33% (33 patients), with a peak census of 75% (75 patients). Hospital B also has a six-bed

ICU, and the ADC over the past 12 months is 33% (two patients), with a peak census of 100% (six patients).

Health system leadership has noticed a steady decline in inpatient admissions at their two hospitals over the past 3 years resulting in the current census numbers. The organization has been running at a loss ("in the red") for the past 2 years. Moreover, challenges with patient throughput, care coordination, and timely discharge have plagued the organization for years. The current average length of stay (ALOS) across both hospitals for medical/surgical patients is 5.9 days and ICU patients is 9.8 days. When compared to other local competitors, these ALOS data suggest that they are approximately 10%–20% higher on average.

The current situation is not sustainable. Alternatives for restructuring were reviewed and evaluated. What is the best way to improve the functioning of inpatient services?

▌ CRITICAL THINKING EXERCISE

Nursing leadership been asked to assess the feasibility of consolidating inpatient services across the two hospitals. Hospital A and Hospital B have a long history of serving the communities for decades, so the decisions must be considered carefully. They need your help in understanding the operational, cultural, and political benefits and drawbacks of each option. Financial analysis will be performed by the Finance team at the completion of this operational exercise and is not your responsibility.

1. What elements of organization structure and design must be considered in determining whether consolidation of inpatient services is feasible?

2. Who are the key internal and external stakeholders that would be impacted by a decision to consolidate

inpatient units at the two hospitals? Why must their perspectives be considered?

3. What are the key operational challenges with consolidating the medical/surgical and telemetry units at both hospitals? What about with the intensive care units (ICUs)?

4. What role might improve care coordination, reduced average length of stay (ALOS), or more timely discharge play in your decision to consolidate units? Would consolidation prompt a culture change within the health system?

5. You are the Chief Nursing Officer. What is your recommendation to other health system leadership—do you recommend consolidating the inpatient units or not? Why or why not?

REFERENCES

Alidina, S., & Funke-Furber, J. (1988). First line nurse managers: Optimizing the span of control. *Journal of Nursing Administration, 18*(5), 34–39.

American Nurses Credentialing Center. (n.d.). *Magnet model–Creating a Magnet culture.* https://www.nursingworld.org/organizational-programs/magnet/magnet-model/.

American Society for Quality (ASQ). (n.d.). *Malcolm Baldrige National Quality Award (MBNQA).* http://asq.org/learn-about-quality/malcolm-baldrige-award/overview/overview.html.

Bae, S., Nikolaev, A., Seo, J., & Castner, J. (2015). Health care provider social network analysis: A systematic review. *Nursing Outlook, 63*(5), 566–584.

Bradley, C. (2014). Leading nursing through influence and structure: The system nurse executive role. *Journal of Nursing Administration, 44*(12), 619–621.

Carayon, P., Xie, A., & Kianfar, S. (2014). Human factors and ergonomics as a patient safety practice. *BMJ Quality & Safety, 23*(3), 196–205.

Charnes, M., & Tewksbury, L. (1993). The continuum of organization structures. In *Collaborative management in health care: Implementing the integrative organization.* (pp. 20–43). San Francisco, CA: Jossey-Bass.

Choi, S., Jang, I., Park, S., & Lee, H. (2014). Effects of organizational culture, self-leadership and empowerment on job satisfaction and turnover intention in general hospital nurses. *Journal of Korean Academy of Nursing Administration, 20*(2), 206–214.

Cicolini, G., Comparcini, D., & Simonetti, V. (2014). Workplace empowerment and nurses' job satisfaction: A systematic literature review. *Journal of Nursing Management, 22*(7), 855–871.

Clegg, S. R. (1990). *Modern organizations: Organization studies in the postmodern world.* Sage Publications.

Dartmouth Institute for Health Policy & Clinical Practice. (2010). *Microsystems at a glance.* https://studylib.net/doc/8879258/microsystems-at-a-glance—the-dartmouth-institute—micr...

DiCuccio, M. H. (2015). The relationship between patient safety culture and patient outcomes: A systematic review. *Journal of Patient Safety, 11*(3), 135–142.

Donabedian, A. (1980). *Explorations in quality assessment and monitoring: The definition of quality and approaches to its assessment* (Vol. 1). Ann Arbor, MI: Health Administration Press.

Edgren, L., & Barnard, K. (2012). Complex adaptive systems for management of integrated care. *Leadership in Health Services, 25*(1), 39–51.

Eisenstein, H. (1995). The Australian femocratic experiment: A feminist case for bureaucracy. In M. M. Ferree, & P. Y. Martin (Eds.), *Feminist organizations: Harvest of the new women's movement* (pp. 69–83). Philadelphia, PA: Temple University Press.

Farmer, D. J. (1997). The postmodern turn and the Socratic gadfly. In H. T. Miller, & C. J. Fox (Eds.), *Postmodernism "reality" and public administration* (pp. 105–117). Burke, VA: Chatelaine Press.

Gantz, N. R., Sherman, R., Jasper, M., Choo, C. G., Herrin-Griffith, D., & Harris, K. (2012). Global nurse leader perspectives on health systems and workforce challenges. *Journal of Nursing Management, 20*(4), 433–443.

Gittell, J. H. (2002). Coordinating mechanisms in care provider groups: Relational coordination as a mediator and input uncertainty as a moderator of performance effects. *Management Science, 48*(11), 1408–1426.

Gittell, J. H. (2004). Achieving focus in hospital care: The role of relational coordination. In R. E. Herzlinger (Ed.), *Consumer-driven health care: Implications for providers, payers, and policymakers* (pp. 683–695). San Francisco, CA: Jossey-Bass.

Hatch, M. J., & Cunliffe, A. L. (2013). *Organization theory: Modern, symbolic, and postmodern perspectives* (3rd ed.). Oxford, UK: Oxford University Press.

Institute for Healthcare Improvement (IHI). (2016). *Clinical microsystem assessment tool.* http://www.ihi.org/resources/pages/tools/clinicalmicrosystemassessmenttool.aspx.

Jaques, E. (1990). In praise of hierarchy. *Harvard Business Review, 68*(1), 127–133.

Kanter, R. M. (1977). *Men and women of the corporation.* New York, NY: Basic Books.

Kerfoot, K. M., & Luquire, R. (2012). Alignment of the system's chief nursing officer: Staff or direct line structure? *Nursing Administration Quarterly, 36*(4), 325–331.

Laschinger, H. K. S. (1996). A theoretical approach to studying work empowerment in nursing: A review of studies testing Kanter's theory of structural power in organizations. *Nursing Administration Quarterly, 20*(2), 25–41.

Laschinger, H. K. S., & Fida, R. (2014). A time-lagged analysis of the effect of authentic leadership on workplace bullying, burnout, and occupational turnover intentions. *European Journal of Work and Organizational Psychology, 23*(5), 739–753.

Laschinger, H. K., Wong, C. A., Cummings, G. G., & Grau, A. (2014). Resonant leadership and workplace empowerment: The value of positive organizational cultures in reducing workplace incivility. *Nursing Economics, 32*(1), 5–15, 44.

Laschinger, H. K., Wong, C. A., & Grau, A. (2013). Authentic leadership, empowerment and burnout: A comparison in new graduates and experienced nurses. *Journal of Nursing Management, 21*(3), 541–552.

Laschinger, H. K., Wong, C. A., Grau, A. L., Read, E. A., & Pineau Stam, L. M. (2012). The influence of leadership practices and empowerment on Canadian nurse manager outcomes. *Journal of Nursing Management, 20*(7), 877–888.

Leatt, P., Lemieux-Charles, L., & Aird, C. (1994). Program management: Introduction and overview. In L. Lemieux-Charles, P. Leatt, & C. Aird (Eds.), *Program management and beyond: Management innovations in Ontario hospitals* (pp. 1–10): Ottawa, ON, Canada: Canadian College of Health Service Executives.

Lorenz, H. L. (2008). Service line leadership. *Nurse Leader, 6*(1), 42–43.

Louis, C. J., Clark, J. R., Gray, B., Brannon, D., & Parker, V. (2019). Service line structure and decision-maker attention in three health systems: Implications for patient-centered care. *Health Care Management Review, 44*(1), 41–56.

Lusthaus, C., Adrien, M., Anderson, G., Carden, F., & Montalvan, G. P. (2002). *Organizational assessment: A framework for improving performance.* Inter-American Development Bank/International Development Research Centre. https://www.idrc.ca/sites/default/files/openebooks/998-4/index.html.

Mahon, A., & Young, R. (2006). Health care managers as a critical component of the health care workforce. In C. Dubois, M. McKee, & E. Nolte (Eds.), *Human resources for health in Europe* (pp. 116–139). Berkshire, UK: Open University Press.

Mark, B. A., Sayler, J., & Smith, C. S. (1996). A theoretical model for nursing systems outcomes research. *Nursing Administration Quarterly, 20*(4), 12–27.

Matthews, S., Laschinger, H. K. S., & Johnstone, L. (2006). Staff nurse empowerment in line and staff organizational structures for chief nurse executives. *Journal of Nursing Administration, 6*(11), 526–533.

McDaniel, R. R., Driebe, D., & Lanham, H. J. (2013). Health care organizations as complex systems: New perspectives on design and management. *Advances in Health Care Management, 15*, 3–26.

McIntosh N., Meterko M., Burgess J. F., Jr., Restuccia J. D., Kartha A., Kaboli P., et al. (2014). Organizational predictors of coordination in inpatient medicine. *Health Care Management Review, 39*(4), 279–292.

Meier, K. J., & Bohte, J. (2003). Span of control and public organizations: Implementing Luther Gulick's research design. *Public Administration Review, 63*(1), 61–70.

Meyer, R. M. (2008). Span of management: Concept analysis. *Journal of Advanced Nursing, 63*(1), 104–112.

Meyer, R. M., & O'Brien-Pallas, L. (2010). Nursing Services Delivery Theory: An open system approach. *Journal of Advanced Nursing, 66*(12), 2828–2838.

O'Connor, E. S. (1999). The politics of management thought: A case study of the Harvard Business School and the Human Relations School. *Academy of Management Review, 24*(1), 117–131.

Pabst, M. K. (1993). Span of control on nursing inpatient units. *Nursing Economic$, 11*(2), 87–90.

Porter-O'Grady, T. (2015). Confluence and convergence: Team effectiveness in complex systems. *Nursing Administration Quarterly, 39*(1), 78–83.

Porter-O'Grady, T., & Malloch, K. (2014). *Quantum leadership: Building better partnerships for sustainable health* (4th ed): Burlington, MA: Jones & Bartlett Learning.

Prins, G. (2000). *Testing theories on structure and strategy: An assessment of organizational knowledge.* Delft, The Netherlands: Eburon.

Read, E. A. (2014). Workplace social capital in nursing: An evolutionary concept analysis. *Journal of Advanced Nursing, 70*(5), 997–1007.

Reed, M. I. (1992). *The sociology of organizations: Themes, perspectives and prospects.* New York, NY: Harvester Wheatsheaf.

Rouse, W. B. (2008). Health care as a complex adaptive system: Implications for design and management. *Bridge-Washington-National Academy of Engineering, 38*(1), 17.

Scott, W. R. (1992). *Organizations: Rational, natural, and open systems* (3rd ed.). Englewood Cliffs, NJ: Prentice-Hall.

Shirey, M. R., & White-Williams, C. (2015). Boundary spanning leadership practices for population health. *Journal of Nursing Administration, 45*(9), 411–415.

Smith, L., Andrusyszyn, M. A., & Spence Laschinger, H. K. (2010). Effects of workplace incivility and empowerment on newly-graduated nurses' organizational commitment. *Journal of Nursing Management, 18*(8), 1004–1015.

Strömgren, M., Eriksson, A., Ahlstrom, L., Bergman, D., & Dellve, L. (2017). Leadership quality: A factor important for social capital in healthcare organizations. *Journal of Health Organization and Management, 31*(2), 175–191.

Tichy, N. M., Tushman, M. L., & Fombrun, C. (1979). Social network analysis for organizations. *Academy of Management Review, 4*(4), 507–519.

Weber, M. (1978). *Economy and society: An outline of interpretive sociology.* In E. Fischoff, H. Gerth, A. M. Henderson, F. Kolegar, C. W. Mills, T. Parsons, M. Rheinstein, G. Roth, E. Shils, & C. Wittich, (Eds.). Trans. (Vol. 2): Berkeley, CA: University of California Press.

Wenger, E. (2008). *Communities of practice: A brief introduction.* https://scholarsbank.uoregon.edu/xmlui/bitstream/handle/1794/11736/A%20brief%20introduction%20to%20CoP.pdf.

Willem, A., Buelens, M., & De Jonghe, I. (2007). Impact of organizational structure on nurses' job satisfaction: A questionnaire survey. *International Journal of Nursing Studies, 44*, 1011–1020.

Wong, C. A., & Laschinger, H. K. (2013). Authentic leadership, performance and job satisfaction: The mediating role of empowerment. *Journal of Advanced Nursing, 69*(4), 947–959.

Wong C. A., Elliot-Miller P., Laschinger H. K., Cuddihy M., Meyer R., Keatings M., et al. (2015). Examining the relationships between span of control and manager and unit work outcomes in Ontario academic hospitals. *Journal of Nursing Management, 23*(2), 156–168.

Yang, J., Liu, Y., Huang, C., & Zhu, L. (2013). Impact of empowerment on professional practice environments and organizational commitment among nurses: A structural equation approach. *International Journal of Nursing Practice, 19*(S1), 44–55.

Young, G. J., Charnes, M. P., & Heeren, T. C. (2004). Product line management in professional organizations: An empirical test of competing theoretical perspectives. *Academy of Management Journal, 47*(5), 723–734.

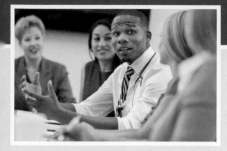

Decentralization and Governance

M. Lindell Joseph, Richard J. Bogue

 http://evolve.elsevier.com/Huber/leadership

The US health care system is constantly adapting in the face of changes in governmental policies, payment mechanisms, population health priorities, local disasters, and to meet the daily challenges of patient care across the continuum of care. Among critical assets for adaptation in health care organizations are innovations that liberate the strengths of nurses, care teams, and the field of nursing. Such adaptations in health systems, hospitals, and clinics include ensuring that the right personnel, with the right training, the best situational understanding, and the authority and flexibility to act are free to meet any given challenge at the needed time. Promptly meeting these complex challenges requires teams composed of staff who feel encouraged to exercise their competencies to their full scope of practice in their respective part of the health system. This decentralization of authority is a core feature of shared governance: having authority for decision-making at the right level in the organization from the local work unit and up the levels of leadership, with ramifications for nursing participation at the level of the governing board.

Participation in shared governance, especially in unit-based councils, is an evidence-based practice that is integral to the Magnet Recognition Program® (https://www.nursingworld.org/organizational-programs/magnet). In a review of 20 articles, it was found that shared governance makes a meaningful difference for nurses. Shared governance promotes autonomy, higher job satisfaction, greater control over nursing practice, better quality and safety outcomes, greater engagement, and an improved work environment (Al-Marri & Kehyayan, 2018). In situations where nurses are dissatisfied and turnover is high, one significant remedy is to institute shared governance using unit-based councils to give nurses a venue

for greater satisfaction and participation. This chapter reviews key definitions, approaches to operationalize decentralization and governance, implications for leadership, and current issues and trends.

DEFINITIONS

Board Governance

A **governing board** is a decision-making body with fiduciary and strategic accountability for an organization's mission and the assets for advancing that mission. Board members provide oversight for corporations, not-for-profits, agencies of government, and other entities by exercising four duties. These four duties are (1) Duty of Fiduciary, acting in the organization's best interests, ensuring that resources are used in a reasonable, appropriate, and legally accountable manner, (2) Duty of Care, making responsible decisions and providing appropriate oversight, (3) Duty of Loyalty, avoiding conflicts of interest or self-interest, and (4) Duty of Obedience, ensuring compliance with applicable laws, rules, and regulations, and to act within the scope of their authority under the organization's articles, bylaws, and applicable laws (American Hospital Association [AHA], 2009). The vision of the Nurses on Boards Coalition (NOBC), for example, is "to build healthier communities in America by increasing nurses' presence on corporate, health-related, and other boards, panels, and commissions" (2020).

Governance is how society or groups within it organize to make decisions or achieve collective action. It is defined as "Establishment of policies, and continuous monitoring of their proper implementation, by the members of the governing body of an organization. It includes the mechanisms required to balance the powers of the members (with the associated accountability), and their primary duty of enhancing the prosperity and viability of the organization" (Business Dictionary.com, 2020a).

Centralization and decentralization

Describe both the degree of hierarchical power distribution for decision-making authority in an organization *and* how power is manifested in the organizational structure, reflected in the locus of decision-making authority. In a highly centralized organization (BusinessDictionary. com, 2020b), the power of planning and decision-making are exclusively in the hands of top management. Decentralization (BusinessDictionary.com, 2020c) means that authority for planning and decision-making are widely distributed throughout the organization.

Structural Empowerment

Structural empowerment refers to organizational structures and procedures that help advance or maintain generally flat, flexible, and decentralized decision-making. In nursing, this means adopting shared governance and/or decentralized decision-making structures and processes that establish and reinforce standards of practice and opportunities for improvements that advance the performance of nurses and others up and down the organization's formal hierarchy (American Nurses Credentialing Center [ANCC], 2019).

Subsidiarity and Decentralization

The phrase "decentralization of authority" and the term subsidiarity both refer to one core feature of organizations aiming to be more effective and better democratized: engaging all members of the team in the journey toward excellence. **Subsidiarity** is the principle that "functions which are performed effectively by subordinate or local organizations belong more properly to them than to a dominant central organization" (Merriam-Webster, 2020); in other terms, decision-making power should be decentralized to the extent possible.

Tsagourias summarized the history of the principle of subsidiarity:

"The origins of the principle of subsidiarity go back to Aristotle, but it is Catholic doctrine that popularized this concept. Subsidiarity was invoked in 1891 by the Catholic Church and has been reaffirmed

since then in different contexts as a principle of social ordering of constituent parts in order to serve and attain the common good" (Tsagourias, 2011, p. 547).

The supranational European Union embedded subsidiarity in its constitution. From the Glossary of summaries in EUR-Lex we learn:

"The principle of subsidiarity is defined in Article 5 of the Treaty on European Union. It aims to ensure that decisions are taken as closely as possible to the citizen and that constant checks are made to verify that action at EU level is justified in light of the possibilities available at national, regional or local level" (EUR-Lex, 2020).

The General Effective Multilevel Theory for Shared Governance (GEMS)

GEMS is a theory-based approach to nursing shared governance. It offers a precise, specific, and systematic approach to enacting, evaluating, and improving shared governance. GEMS guides the implementation of effective shared governance by using both the unit-level work team and the leadership team to improve outcomes at the individual level, unit level, department level, and organizational level (Bogue et al., 2009; Joseph & Bogue, 2016).

BACKGROUND

Approaches Used for Decentralization and Governance
Board Governance

The Institute of Medicine's (IOM, 2011) *The Future of Nursing: Leading Change, Advancing Health* report, challenged nurses to strive for board engagement. The recommendations encouraged nurses to participate in the redesign of care delivery, including by aspiring to board membership (IOM, 2011). Many nurses hold esteemed leadership roles throughout the health care field. However, they often cannot or do not participate at the highest level of organizational leadership—the governing board. An outcome of the report was a Campaign for Action. This campaign resulted in the development of NOBC. The primary mission of the NOBC is to get an additional 10,000 nurses on governing boards by 2020. According to the (NOBC, 2018), the positioning of nurses with diverse knowledge, expertise, and independence on boards has become essential to enable and capture diverse thoughts and contributions. The approaches of decentralization, governance, improvement methods, and innovations enable buy-in, collaborative decision-making, alignment, and sustainability for the reshaping of health care. As of April 11, 2020, there were 7309 nurses on boards (NOBC, 2020). The work of the NOBC will not end until the right nurses are serving on the right boards creating strategic value.

Regardless of nurses' level of education, background, or experience, there is a place on a board, commission, or other leadership entity for every nurse. Nurses are suited to impact board discussions and outcomes. Nurses are accustomed to using critical thinking skills, evidence-based approaches, good listening skills, and to formulate key questions that often result in new thinking, discussions, and outcomes. Each nurse who is appointed to a board brings America one step closer to the collective goal of healthier communities and a healthier nation. The following are strategies for an effective presence when on a board (Joseph & Benson, 2017 a,b,c; 2018; 2019):

1. Show attentiveness by using nonverbal cues that show understanding such as nodding, eye contact, and leaning forward
2. Be gracious by not using ungracious expressions such as "whatever" and reflect on your social skills
3. Use storytelling since it is an effective strategy that helps to build relationships, demonstrate effective communication, and engage others in the issues
4. Be confident by learning from setbacks, failures, and successes
5. Take an ethical stance by striving for the best possible outcomes for the benefit of all and express empathy

Nurses' Role in Health Care

Nursing has its own organizational structure within health care for extremely good reasons. Nurses, in teams, are expected to be persistently and readily at the call to care for patients, 24 hours a day, 7 days a week, all year around in hospitals. Each individual nurse is expected to apply their knowledge and skills of nursing to every moment that a patient needs them. In the performance of their duties, nurses are expected to represent the most flexible and persistently available health care professionals until a need arises that calls for a different configuration of the system. This is not true of physicians, let alone administrators or financial or IT managers, or any of the other roles that might be useful for other specific aspects of patients' needs within the system of health care. At least in inpatient settings, nursing is a unique role that demands effective, nurse-driven teamwork and problem-solving on a constant basis. Nursing, therefore, from top to bottom in the organization, requires its own organizational structure and can perform better using formal, organized, and effective methods for nursing shared governance.

As noted above, subsidiarity drives decision-making to the most local or personal level of a complex organization but also recognizes that certain decisions and actions may be more effective when addressed at the organizational level directly above the most local members. In the case of nursing, if the nursing team working together cannot effectively meet the demands of decision-making and action for a particular issue, that issue should be elevated to the nursing unit. If the unit cannot effectively handle an issue, that issue should be elevated to the department level or, if needed, higher in the organization.

Centralization Versus Decentralization on 4 East and 5 West

Organizations have an identifiable structure that affects decision-making authority and the power that nurses have to control and make improvements in their practice. The higher the degree of decentralization in an organization, the more decision-making is done at the point of activity or "the front line." Institutions organize and structure themselves by defining departmental function and authority to achieve a more coordinated effort. This drives plans and decisions about responsibilities and who reports to whom. The following two scenarios provide a contrast to illustrate the operationalization of centralization and decentralization in an institution:

- In scenario one, Abigail Hutton is the nurse manager in the primary care clinic, a medical nursing unit in General Medical Center. Once a candidate is screened for a position by the human resources department, Nurse Hutton interviews applicants to fill open nursing positions in the clinic. At the conclusion of the interviews, she decides whom to hire and notifies human resources. Although this is a somewhat simplistic example, of note is that the decision-making authority is vested solely in the nurse manager.

- In scenario two, Jordan Jones is the nurse manager of 4 East and 5 West, medical nursing units in City Hospital. With three staff nurse positions vacant, he posts the openings and asks the unit council—made up of nurses and other staff on the unit who have had human resources training on behavioral interviewing—to act as part of the selection committee. Based on the needs of the nursing unit and the availability of nursing applicants who match those criteria, human resource staff screen the files of the applicants. They pass on the applications of those nurses who meet the requirements for the positions to the selection committee, who then schedules interviews with the applicants. Once the selection committee has interviewed the candidates, they decide on the best candidate for each position. The committee's recommendations, along with the rationale for its choices, are relayed to the manager. The manager (1) meets with the candidates and takes into consideration the recommendations by the selection committee, (2) interviews them, and (3) makes the job offers.

In this second scenario, the staff nurses are involved in making a hiring decision that directly affects their work environment. This scenario clearly illustrates a more decentralized organizational philosophy. In such an organization, decision-making authority rests in levels closer to the point of service rather than in the executive levels. Decentralization encourages and facilitates greater innovation, more input, and faster response times because staff who are directly responsible for implementing changes and delivering care are a major part of decision-making at the point of implementation.

Nursing Shared Governance Effectiveness

The principle of subsidiarity—or decentralization—has been applied widely, including as a fundamental precept of models of nursing shared governance even if not worded in these terms. O'May and Buchan (1999) described types of nursing shared governance *based on the level at which councils operate*: the nursing unit, the department, the executive level (coordinating activities of lower-level councils), and system-wide (where representative staff participate through top-level cabinets). In any of these types, the target of shared governance is to guide and improve practice. In 2009, Bogue and colleagues argued for the importance of practice councils at

the unit level, built on the concept of subsidiarity: where the action is. Subsidiarity works because it also illustrates the importance of pushing issues up the organization when that would be more effective. Effectiveness in nursing relies on "supportive nursing group power and the concomitant exercise of power by nursing work units—vertically aligned empowerment" (Bogue et al., 2009, p. 6).

There has been little research evidence available about best practices in establishing shared governance. GEMS theory represents an innovative and evidence-based approach to nursing shared governance that is based on the critical importance of the principle of subsidiarity. GEMS theory guides the implementation of shared governance using leadership strategies both within the unit work team and the leadership team, to improve outcomes for patients, nurses, and the overall organization. Such successes lead to increased understanding of challenges and improved performance in goal attainment (Bogue et al., 2009; Joseph & Bogue, 2016).

There are nine essential competencies required for unit-level work teams or nursing practice councils to become increasingly effective. These nine competencies are grouped into three major categories that reflect increasing levels of competence in goal achievement: team foundations, empowering, and aligning (Fig. 13.1). Team foundations for nursing practice council effectiveness include these competencies: (1) skillful group formation and group tasks, (2) creating group identity and norms, and (3) focusing on driving improvements in nursing practice. The empowering competencies include actively gaining the active support of management. The unit council must take responsibility for gaining the support of local management and do so while helping drive unit practices toward achieving outcomes and enabling excellence in patient safety initiatives. In the aligning competencies phase, the unit council leadership group is conducting highly efficient meetings that are oriented toward identifying, achieving, and regularly demonstrating an ability to identify, design, conduct, and promulgate evidence from their successes in a patient care improvement agenda; in the aligning phase, unit councils are practicing excellence and providing leadership in improving patient outcomes.

A local unit council may be fluid as to membership due to time, reassignments, family considerations, or other reasons. This means two things: (1) there may

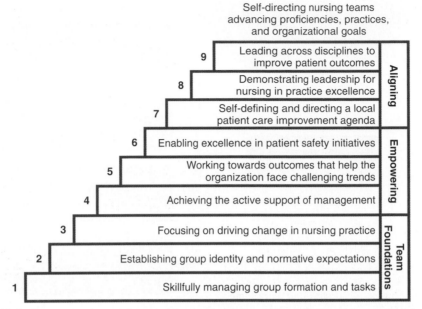

Fig 13.1 Competencies stair-stepping toward becoming self-directing nursing teams. From: Bogue, R. J. & Joseph, M. L. (2011, October 16–19). *A general theory for effective multilevel shared governance: A model for driving change in nursing practice.* International Conference on Communication in Healthcare, Chicago, IL.

be changes in the council membership, and (2) there must be ongoing, but not highly time-consuming, efforts to keep other nurses, nursing assistants, nurse practitioners, physicians, or others on the unit aware of and, ideally, engaged in the unit's progress. When a strong and mutually supportive relationship is developed between the unit manager(s), the nursing practice council, and other personnel who frequent the unit, this structure becomes more natural.

Nursing shared governance effectiveness can be reliably measured on GEMS' nine specific-nursing competencies using the Nursing Practice Council Effectiveness Scale (NPCes). Research has shown that higher NPCes scores were associated with improvements in various measures at the individual level, unit level, departmental level, and organizational level. These improvements included manager support, job satisfaction, self-efficacy, and pressure ulcer rates (Bogue et al., 2009; Joseph & Bogue, 2016).

It is inconceivable that an organization would implement a new shared governance process and expect it to flourish automatically. Ongoing improvement requires *kaizen*, a spirit of continuous improvement and a simple, clear, consistent process. GEMS

theory describes and contains a developmental, iterative process that generates experience in reaching goals, as local councils and nursing units achieve higher levels of self-directed goal attainment. GEMS enables this through time-efficient methods, relying on goals inherent in the unit's aspirations but also an initial GEMS site visit, quick self-assessments twice per year for target setting, feedback reports at all levels, online or telephonic support as needed, and other assistance if desired.

Fig. 13.2 illustrates the overall framework of GEMS theory. The nursing unit work team, engaged by its local leadership and nursing practice council, accelerates progress toward goals by gaining and exercising the competencies shown in Fig. 13.1. The nursing leadership team provides clarity, effective communications, encouragement, and buffering from externalities that might otherwise disrupt progress. These two GEMS inputs from below and above interact in the process of GEMS effective shared governance to adopt and track target outcomes for improvement. These targets should respect the organization's goals and individual goals, as well as goals for the specific unit and for the nursing department.

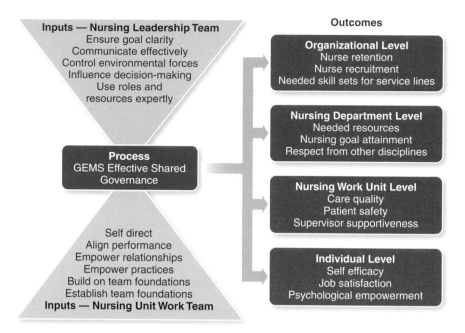

Fig. 13.2 GEMS, general theory for effective multilevel shared governance. From: Bogue, R. J. & Joseph, M. L. (2011, October 16–19). *A general theory for effective multilevel shared governance: A model for driving change in nursing practice.* International Conference on Communication in Healthcare, Chicago, IL.

Organizations Fostering Decentralization and Governance in Health Care

Magnet Hospitals

In the Magnet Recognition Program®, structural empowerment provides organizations with a framework for empowerment and governance (American Nurses Credentialing Center [ANCC], 2019). According to study findings (Spence Laschinger et al., 2003), empowering work conditions and Magnet Hospital characteristics were significantly predictive of nurses' satisfaction with their jobs. McHugh and et al. (2013) found that patients treated in Magnet hospitals had 14% lower odds of mortality and 12% lower odds of failure-to-rescue.

Structural empowerment (SE) is evaluated based on the following criteria (ANCC, 2019, pp. 26–27):

1. Clinical nurses are involved in interprofessional decision-making groups at the organizational level.
2. The health care organization supports nurses' participation in local, regional, national, or international professional organizations.
3. The organization supports nurses' continuous professional development.
4. Nurses participate in professional development activities designed to improve their knowledge, skills, and or practices in the workplace.
5. Professional development activities are designed to improve the professional practice of nursing or patient outcomes, or both.
6. Nursing education opportunities are provided for those interested in a nursing career.
7. The organization provides opportunities to improve nurses' expertise in effectively teaching a patient or family.
8. The organization facilitates the effective transition of registered nurses and advanced practice nurses (APRNs) into the work environment.
9. The organization provides educational activities to improve the nurse's expertise as a preceptor.
10. The organization supports nurses' participation in community health care outreach.
11. Nurses participate in the assessment and prioritization of the health care needs of the community.
12. Nurses are recognized for their contributions in addressing the strategic priorities of the organization.

The Lean Model

The Lean model is another illustration of the centrality of subsidiarity in more effective organizations. Lean has been widely used in health care and owes its existence to Toyota's kaizen quality improvement principles. The kaizen path refers to accelerating the implementation of kaizen (continuous incremental improvement) to processes within the organization (Black & Miller, 2008). Both kaizen and Lean rely upon the core importance of subsidiarity in fostering effective organizations. In both cases, the aim is to achieve continuous improvements that reduce waste and improve outputs. To do this, both models depend on workers at all levels in their various roles to notice problems and propose improvements, keeping in mind that the workers closest to production are also generally those who are furthest from the board, the CEO, and the management at division and department levels. The classic Toyota example is Toyota Principle #5: Build a culture of stopping to fix the problem, to get quality right the first time. This principle means that any worker on a production line can pull the cord to illuminate the location of a production problem and alert support personnel to immediately go to the location, identify, and resolve the problem (Gao & Low, 2014). In health care the same principle applies when workers at all levels, but starting where actual care processes occur, are empowered to ensure high-quality, defect-free health care (Black & Miller, 2008).

The Institute for Health Care Improvement (IHI)

The Institute for Health Care Improvement (IHI) was founded in 1991, but their work began in the late 1980s as part of the National Demonstration Project on Quality Improvement in Health Care. This group was created with the commitment to redesign health care into a system without errors, waste, delay, and unsustainable costs (IHI, 2019). IHI's structure and vision supports Follesdal's (1998) definition of subsidiarity, whereby powers or tasks should rest with the lower-level subunits of that order, and the higher-level central unit would ensure higher comparative efficiency or effectiveness in achieving health care improvement and health. IHI has been an influential force toward a journey of excellence in the United States and has had a rapidly growing influence in such countries as Canada, England, Scotland, Denmark, Sweden, Singapore, Latin America, New Zealand, Ghana, Malawi, South Africa,

and the Middle East. IHI's governance structure is not an organization with walls but more of a movement for collaboration and change. IHI governance is organized around multiple stakeholders such as an Executive Team, Management Team, Board of Directors, Faculty, IHI Senior Fellows, IHI Alumni, IHI Scientific Advisory Group, and anyone who has a passion for improvement of patient care and who wants to profoundly change health and health care for the better. In addition to these groups, IHI uses a grassroots multiforum approach to enable engagement and participation (IHI, 2020). These include:

1. ihi.org
2. IHI Open School
3. Women's Health Initiative (WHI)
4. Conferences, seminars and direct consultations, such as:
   a. National Forum on Quality Improvement in Health Care
   b. International Forum on Quality and Safety in Healthcare
   c. Annual Summit on Improving Patient Care in the Office Practice and in the Community, Face-to-Face seminars and trainings
   d. Virtual Training Programs such as Virtual Expeditions
   e. IHI Open School
   f. the ability to bring IHI staff for consultation
5. Training in improvement skills such as the Breakthrough Series College and Patient safety Executive Development Program
6. Working strategically with IHI with programs such as IHI Leadership Alliance, and Cutting-Edge Innovation

LEADERSHIP AND MANAGEMENT IMPLICATIONS

Although shared governance shifts decision-making away from a health care organization's leader and into the hands of empowered staff, shared governance does not mean that leaders can ignore their responsibility in the decision-making process. Nor does it mean that all decisions are made by nurses. To be effective, leaders must be ready for and accepting of this shift. So too must leaders be prepared to empower staff.

"Staff who experience empowerment feel that they are respected and trusted to be active participants.

Staff who feel empowered also demonstrate a positive image to other healthcare team members, patients and their families, and the public. Nurses who do not feel empowered will not be effective in conveying a positive image, because they will not be able to communicate that nurses are professionals with much to offer. Empowerment that is not clear to staff is just as problematic as no staff empowerment. Empowered teams feel a responsibility for the team's performance and activities, which in turn can improve care and reduce errors" (Finkelman & Kenner, 2016, p. 457).

"An interprofessional approach to Shared Governance must be embedded throughout the organization adopting it, from the clinical decisions at points of service to the strategic priorities placed on interprofessional issues by senior leadership. A cornerstone of this approach to practice may be the inclusion of patients and families as full partners on both care teams and planning groups. Respecting and valuing the knowledge and service of all team members contributes to a trusting, openly communicative, learning environment and positive patient care and practice outcomes" (Swihart & Hess, 2014, p. 87).

An inter-professional approach:

"[O]ften engages patients and families as partners. Keys to successful implementation ... include active participation of all team members contributing to mutually respectful, trusting, collaborative, openly communicative, safe, and effective learning environments of care and practice across disciplines and departments. Interprofessional Shared Governance provides a unique structure for shared decision-making reflective of the current and devolving demands of an increasingly diverse and integrated care delivery system" (Swihart & Hess, 2014, p. 4).

CURRENT ISSUES AND TRENDS

There are four key issues and trends today. These include (1) whether to use the terms shared governance versus profession nursing governance, (2) types of councils, (3) whole system integration, (4) engagement, and (5) the appropriateness of selected measures.

Shared Governance Versus Professional Nursing Governance

A debate exists about using the terms shared governance versus professional nursing governance. Porter-O'Grady (2017) stated that in the early 1980s shared governance was an alternative term used for professional governance because the term professional was not considered as legitimate when applied to nurses. Because nursing has been a predominantly employed work group primarily composed of women, the usual requisites of ownership, control over practice, and membership were rarely applied to nurses.

However, in 1998 Hess published his seminal works on professional governance. Hess defined professional governance as a multidimensional organizational characteristic that encompasses the structure and processes by which professionals direct, control, and regulate goal-oriented efforts of one another. To measure these types of professional governance, he developed and tested the Index of Professional Nursing Governance and the Index of Professional Governance. The latter is a more generic version for nurses, physicians, pharmacists, and allied health professionals (Swihart & Hess, 2018).

Although both Hess and Porter-O'Grady have published on shared governance and professional governance extensively, the evidence-based knowledge for nursing shared governance and professional governance was sparse. In the early 2000s, there was a call for a stronger link between theory and practice so that evaluations can build nursing theory, science, and practice for shared governance (Anthony, 2004). And in 2011, the Institute of Medicine called for nurses to become active in building research knowledge. The seminal theory of GEMS has provided the most progressive evidence to advance nursing practice. GEMS is the only theory for shared governance in the field of nursing (Bogue et al., 2009; Joseph & Bogue, 2016).

Types of Councils

The decision to implement the most appropriate type of shared governance for an organization may be a challenging. In a blog by Lippincott (2019), the authors described three levels of councils. These include unit practice-level councils, hospital-level councils, and themed level councils. In some institutions one, two, or all types may be implemented. The following core types are discussed. (1) **Unit practice councils are** organized and implemented by direct care nurses. This format offers direct care nurses the opportunity to share their opinions, suggest ways to improve the patient care experience, and make decisions regarding process improvements. (2) **Hospital councils are at the meso-system level.** Direct care nurses from many units gather to discuss issues affecting nursing practice and patient care throughout the entire organization. Members of nursing leadership should be present to support staff nurses in their decision-making and act as intermediaries between the staff and upper management. (3) **Themed councils are organized to address** broader issues such as quality and safety, professional development, or the healing environment.

The key in selecting the appropriate type of council is to ensure that councils are not too big so that they limit participant engagement and motivation. Williams noted, "I have observed hospital and themed councils with 60–100 participants but if you read the research on teams, the ideal group size should be based on your purpose. Are these shared governance councils convening to problem solve? How can 60–100 people engage? Secondly, alignment may be absent in many institutions. In many institutions nurses voice that they are usually delegated to by upper management and are sometimes working in a vacuum with minimal influence when alignment is absent" (J. Williams, personal communication, May 17, 2013).

Whole-System Integration

Practice leaders see the benefits of decentralization and the shared governance model extending beyond nurses and all care providers to all employees. "As for the future of Shared Governance, Susan Allen PhD, RN (assistant vice president, Cincinnati Children's Hospital) says it would be ideal to see whole-system integration involving all hospital staff. But will Shared Governance ever be the sole governing system or will there always be a traditional system to manage operations? Shared Governance would have to be highly integrated, says Allen" (Gray, 2013). Clearly, the next steps in this vision are to include patients and the community more deliberatively into the shared governance model. Allen says Cincinnati Children's Hospital has a family advisory council and a teen council that get involved in projects, including reviewing potential educational materials and designing a new learning center (Gray, 2013).

Engagement

Shared governance is the gold standard for engaging nurses in solving problems at the point of care. An ongoing challenge among US employers, including health care systems, is to keep employees engaged. A Gallup poll (2017) indicated that only 33% of employees in the United States report they are "engaged at work," meaning they are committed to their job and feel they are making positive contributions. Fifty-one percent reported they are "not engaged at work," meaning they are not likely to put effort into organizational goals. Sixteen percent are "actively disengaged," described as unhappy, unproductive and likely to spread negativity.

Perhaps improved technology can also make a difference. According to AHA (2016), "almost 30% of clinicians aren't satisfied with technology used by their organization." It will become more and more important for nurses to leverage the power of shared governance to improve practice and help deliver desired outcomes. Nurses need to both structure and participate in shared governance as a routine part of their work life.

Appropriateness of Selected Measures
Nursing Practice Council Effectiveness Scale (NPCes)

NPCes is a valid and reliable index of nursing practice council effectiveness. It measures nine competencies at the practice/unit council level. These competencies include skillfulness, usefulness, effectiveness, supported by management, empowering nurses and nursing, improves patient care, improves patient safety, leads with professional practice issues, and improves professional practice (Bogue et al., 2009). NPCes is used as a self-assessment tool for nursing practice councils, so they can identify their progress across the competencies and craft "lean" plans for improving their competencies as a group as they strive toward leadership.

The GEMS Self-Assessment

The GEMS self-assessment measures shared governance at the team level and leadership level to examine team effectiveness, alignment, and goal attainment. This measure consists of 21 items; initial uses indicate that the GEMS self-assessments are valid and reliable (Joseph & Bogue, 2016).

The Index of Professional Nursing Governance (IPNG)

IPNG is used to identify an organization's place on a continuum of traditional governance, shared governance, and self-governance. Two instruments currently exist: (1) the Index of Professional Nursing Governance, and (2) the Index of Professional Governance (this version evaluates the health care team). This is in multiple languages and may be perceived as lengthy (Swihart, & Hess, 2018).

The Structural Professional Governance Self-Assessment Survey (SPGS-A)

This is a new tool in development. It measures attributes of professional governance. These attributes include accountability, professional obligation, collateral relationships, and effective decision-making (Porter-O'Grady & Clavelle, 2019).

⚑ RESEARCH NOTE

Source

Al-Marri, A.H., & Kehyayan, V. (2018). Nurses' lived experience serving on unit-based councils: A literature review. *Journal of Nursing Education and Practice*, *8*(12), 21–28. https://doi.org/10.5430/jnep.v8n12p21.

Purpose

This literature review examined studies reporting results about nurses' lived experiences on unit-based councils (UBCs) within shared governance (SG) structures. The aims of the review were to describe whether and how UBCs affect decisions about nursing practice, standards of nursing care, nurse work environment, nurses' sense of empowerment, and any other findings.

Discussion

A literature review was designed to identify full texts of English-language empirical studies with results associated with shared governance that were published in peer-reviewed journals between January 2006 and January 2017. Search terms were "shared governance AND nurses' experience OR perspective OR view OR attitude," "shared governance AND healthcare," and "unit-based councils." This search strategy was employed in CINAHL, Academic Search Complete, and Academic Search Elite. Of 120 articles found, 15 were duplicates, 13 were excluded based on the title, 48 were excluded based on the abstract, and 35 were excluded based on full text review. The results are based on 20 articles, representing results from Belgium, Brazil, UK, Jordan, the Kingdom of Saudi Arabia, and the United States.

After extracting all the results associated with UBCs in SG, the study team reviewed general perceptions of UBCs and SG. General perceptions about UBCs in SG included (1) an increased desire for decisional involvement related to more experience in UBCs, and (2) participation in SG at the unit-level (UBCs) increases voice for nursing and for individual nurses, as well as greater voice in interdisciplinary contexts. Hospitals successfully achieving Magnet designation are "known for fostering positive work environments."

The researchers also identified four themes grouping results documented in one or another study. **Theme 1: Leadership and management** results demonstrated that UBCs in SG may promote autonomy among nurses, provide active support for engagement in SG, and increase the chance of offering patient care coverage and compensation for SG effort outside normal schedules, as well as mentoring staff nurses to improve performance and fostering a healthy work environment. **Theme 2: Increased job satisfaction** was composed of findings of higher job satisfaction from SG in UBC participation and greater control over nursing practice; job satisfaction was also positively associated with years of experience in one's current work Findings under **Theme 3: Improved patient care** demonstrated that nurses participating in decisions affecting nursing practice produced better quality and safety outcomes; moreover, quality and safety benefits appeared to increase as engagement in decision-making increased. **Theme 4: Improved work environment** suggests that SG facilities where UBCs enable greater engagement in SG, nurses are more empowered to have control over their own polices, thereby experiencing their work more as managing patient care, being bedside leaders. This demonstrates that nurses gain satisfaction when nurses enjoy greater active decision-making at the point of care. In general, older nurses and more experienced nurses both tend to be more satisfied and more active in shared governance.

Application to Practice

The findings from the studies in this review suggest that SG participation specifically in UBCs makes a meaningful difference. Where nurses cannot participate in SG at the level of UBCs, nurses are more likely to be confused about expectations for their roles in SG and/or perceive that SG does not make a difference. Participation in SG at the unit level tends to generate a different set of expectations that are associated with greater work satisfaction and more active engagement in improving performance

RESEARCH NOTE—cont'd

for patient experience and patient care quality. These findings offer a recommendation that hospitals and health systems can achieve greater performance and higher nurse satisfaction by investing in the establishment and maintenance of unit-level councils for nursing shared governance.

NEXT-GENERATION NCLEX® EXAMINATION-STYLE CASE STUDY

After one year of employment on 3 South, nurse Maria was invited to join the unit's Shared Governance Council Committee (SGCC). Maria has listened to her fellow nurses complain about not being listened to or valued, and the unit's nurse turnover rate is climbing. Morale is low. She is thrilled that this will be a venue to communicate ways to mitigate the increasing turnover and to communicate her peer's perceptions of being powerless and not having a voice. However, it is important that the SGCC operate as an effective structure. At the first meeting, Maria decided to observe and gain trust with the group versus voicing her concerns. After the meeting, Maria made an appointment with the chairperson (Elyssa) to discuss her observations about how the SGCC operates. Elyssa was open to her feedback.

Choose the most likely options to complete the question below.

Question
Which actions, observed while on the committee, indicate that the Shared Governance Council is demonstrating effectiveness? **Select all that apply.**
1. The council meetings are skillful
2. The council enables leadership
3. The information discussed is useful
4. The committee goals are supported by management
5. The council members are empowered to act
6. The council is improving patient safety
7. The council is improving nursing practice

CRITICAL THINKING EXERCISE

Kimani Joseph is a member of the unit-level SG council. A group of nurses approach him because the nurse manager has locked up all personal protective equipment (PPE) and is dolling them out sparingly. Nurses are afraid for personal safety; lately staff have been absent from work, and the unit's staff satisfaction scores are decreasing. Kimani is concerned about the complaints; he has observed them himself.

1. What are the areas of concern in this scenario?
2. Using the General Effective Multilevel Theory for Shared Governance, which competencies would be essential for the nursing team to execute?
3. With shared governance in mind, what should Kimani do? What would you do?

REFERENCES

Al-Marri, A. H., & Kehyayan, V. (2018). Nurses' lived experience serving on unit-based councils: A literature review. *Journal of Nursing Education and Practice, 8*(12), 21–28.

American Nurses Credentialing Center (ANCC). (2019). *Magnet recognition program: Application manual.* Silver Spring, MD: American Nurses Credentialing Center.

American Hospital Association (AHA). (2009). *The guide to good governance for hospital boards.* https://trustees. aha.org/sites/default/files/trustees/09-guide-to-good-governance.pdf.

American Hospital Association (AHA). (2016). *2016 American Hospital Association environmental scan.* http://www.hhnmag.com/articles/3199-american-hospital-association-environmental-scan.

Anthony, M. K. (2004). Shared governance models: the theory, practice, and evidence. *Online Journal of Issues in Nursing, 9*(1), 7.

Black, J., & Miller, D. (2008). *The Toyota way to healthcare excellence: increase efficiency and improve quality with Lean*: Chicago, IL: Health Administration Press. https://www.amazon.com/Toyota-Way-Healthcare-Excellence-Efficiency/dp/1567932932.

Bogue, R. J., Joseph, M. L., & Sieloff, C. L. (2009). Shared governance as vertical alignment of nursing group power and nurse practice council effectiveness. *Journal of Nursing Management, 17*(1), 4–14. https://doi.org/10.1111/j.1365-2834.2008.00954.x.

Bogue, R. J., & Joseph, M. L. (2011, October 16–19). *A general theory for effective multilevel shared governance: A model for driving change in nursing practice*, International Conference on Communication in Healthcare, Chicago, IL.

BusinessDictionary.com. (2020a). *Governance*. http://www.businessdictionary.com/definition/governance.html.

BusinessDictionary.com. (2020b). *Centralization*. http://www.businessdictionary.com/definition/centralization.html.

BusinessDictionary.com. (2020c). *Decentralization*. http://www.businessdictionary.com/definition/decentralization.html.

EUR-Lex. (2020). *EUR-Lex: Access to European Common Law*: Publications Office of the European Union. https://eur-lex.europa.eu/homepage.html.

Follesdal, A. (1998). Survey article: Subsidiarity. *The Journal of Political Philosophy, 6*(2), 190–218. https://philpapers.org/rec/ANDSAS.

Finkelman, A., & Kenner, C. (2016). *Professional nursing concepts*. Sudbury, MA: Jones & Bartlett Learning.

Gallup Inc. (2017). *State of the American workplace*. https://www.gallup.com/workplace/238085/state-american-workplace-report-2017.aspx.

Gao, S., & Low, S. P. (2014). The Toyota Way model: an alternative framework for lean construction. *Total Quality Management, 25*(6), 664–682. https://doi.org/10.1080/14783363.2013.820022.

Gray, B. B. (2013). *Taking control through shared governance*. https://www.nurse.com/blog/2013/02/18/taking-control-through-shared-governance-2/.

Hess, R. (1998). Measuring nursing governance. *Nursing Research, 47*(1), 35–42.

Institute for Healthcare Improvement (IHI). (2019). *Improving health and health care worldwide*. http://www.ihi.org/.

Institute for Healthcare Improvement (IHI). (2020). *About us*. http://www.ihi.org/about/Pages/History.aspx.

Institute of Medicine (IOM). (2011). *The future of nursing: Leading change, advancing health*. Washington, DC: The National Academies Press.

Joseph, M. L., & Benson, L. (2017a, May 30). Confidence and truthfulness. *Building a Healthier America Blog*. https://www.nursingcenter.com/ncblog/may-2017/confidence-and-truthfulness.

Joseph, M. L., & Benson, L. (2017b, September 18). Take an ethical stance! *Building a Healthier America Blog*. https://www.nursingcenter.com/ncblog/september-2017/take-an-ethical-stance.

Joseph, M. L., & Benson, L. (2017c, December 15). Influence and storytelling. *Building a Healthier America Blog*. https://www.nursingcenter.com/ncblog/december-2017/influence-with-storytelling.

Joseph, M. L., & Benson, L. (2018, June 12). The art of being gracious. *Building a Healthier America Blog*. http://lippincottsolutions.lww.com/blog.entry.html/2018/06/12/building_a_healthier-1F2z.html.

Joseph, M. L., & Benson, L. (2019, May 30). Nurses on Boards: 5 ways to show attentiveness while serving on a board. *Building a Healthier America Blog*. http://lippincottsolutions.lww.com/blog.entry.html/2019/05/30/nurses_on_boards5-8vKF.html.

Joseph, M. L., & Bogue, R. J. (2016). A theory-based approach to nursing shared governance. *Nursing Outlook, 64*(4), 339–351. PMID: 27005400. https://doi.org/10.1016/j.outlook.2016.01.004.

Lippincott. (2019, February 27). *How shared governance in nursing works*. http://lippincottsolutions.lww.com/blog.entry.html/2019/02/27/how_shared_governanc-oiGj.html.

McHugh, M. D., Kelly, L. A., Smith, H. L., Wu, E. S., Vanak, J. M., & Aiken, L. H. (2013). Lower mortality in Magnet hospitals. *Medical Care, 51*(5), 382–388. http://www.ncbi.nlm.nih.gov/pubmed/23047129.

Merriam-Webster. (2020). *Subsidiarity*. https://www.merriam-webster.com/dictionary/subsidiarity.

Nurses on Boards Coalition (NOBC). (2018). *Resources*. https://www.nursesonboardscoalition.org/resources/.

Nurses on Boards Coalition (NOBC). (2020). About. https://www.nursesonboardscoalition.org/about/.

O'May, F., & Buchan, J. (1999). Shared governance: a literature review. *International Journal of Nursing Studies, 36*(4), 281–300.

Porter-O'Grady, T. (2017). A response to the question of professional governance versus shared governance. *Journal of Nursing Administration, 47*(2), 67–71.

Porter-O'Grady, T., & Clavelle, J. (2019). The structural framework for nursing professional governance. *Nurse Leader, 18*(2), 181–189.

Laschinger, Spence, H. K., Almost, J., & Tucr-Hodes, D. (2003). Workplace empowerment and Magnet Hospital characteristics: Making the link. *Journal of Nursing Administration, 33*(7/8), 410–422.

Swihart, D., & Hess, R. (2014). *Shared governance. A practical approach to transforming interprofessional healthcare* (3rd ed): Danvers, MA: HCPro.

Swihart, D., & Hess, R. (2018). *Shared governance. A practical approach to transforming interprofessional healthcare* (4th ed): Danvers, MA: HCPro.

Tsagourias, N. (2011). Security Council Legislation, Article 2(7) of the UN Charter, and the principle of subsidiarity. *Leiden Journal of International Law, 24*(3), 539–559. https://www.cambridge.org/core/journals/leiden-journal-of-international-law/article/security-council-legislation-article-27-of-the-un-charter-and-the-principle-of-subsidiarity/B68B4E6DBDED98406FAA814DA80481FD.

14

Strategic Management

Cole Edmonson

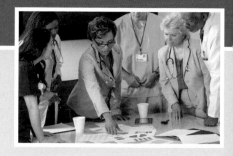

ⓔ http://evolve.elsevier.com/Huber/leadership

Thinking and acting strategically are crucial for nurses to be proactive in a complex, fast-changing, rapid-cycle environment. Arising from the business field, strategic management has made its way into health care leadership, including nursing. The leadership role of nurses has become an area of increasing focus since the Institute of Medicine (IOM, now called the National Academies of Sciences, Engineering, and Medicine, Health and Medicine Division), in its 2010 *Future of Nursing* report, called for increased leadership development and participation in leadership among nurses. Evaluation of progress toward the *Future of Nursing* goals indicates that although leadership development opportunities have been created since the release of the IOM report, insufficient data exist to determine progress toward nurses serving on "executive management teams and other key leadership positions" (National Academies of Sciences, Engineering, and Medicine [NAM], 2015). Leadership development and participation continues to be an area of focus for nursing as the profession strives to fulfill the IOM goals.

In order to be effective leaders, nurses need to gain competence in a variety of areas. The American Organization for Nursing Leadership (AONL), formerly the American Organization of Nurse Executives (AONE), divided these competencies into five broad categories: communication and relationship management, knowledge of the health care environment, leadership, professionalism, and business skills and principles (AONL, 2015). One key area of business skills includes strategic management. Competencies that align with strategic management consist of several processes, including organizational assessment,

planning, management of implementation, and evaluation. The American College of Healthcare Executives (ACHE) also provides a competency assessment tool that offers health care leaders an opportunity to conduct a self-evaluation of key competencies necessary for strategic leadership (ACHE, 2020).

In alignment with the competencies developed by AONL (2015), strategic management involves conducting an environmental scan, knowing the competition, establishing goals, setting targets, developing an action plan, implementing the plan, and evaluating success (Management Study Guide, 2020; Pearce & Robinson, 2012). This approach has long been used in business to ensure a competitive advantage over similar enterprises. Issues in the health care industry, including the Hospital Consumer Assessment of Healthcare Providers and Systems (HCAHPS) and the Hospital Value-Based Purchasing Program, among others, require health care organizations to function as businesses to obtain and maintain a competitive advantage. In the last 10 years, health systems are challenged with meeting the Institute for Healthcare Improvement's (IHI) Quadruple AIM (Sikka et al., 2015) that consists of improving care to the individual, optimizing health outcomes, and lowering overall cost while improving the work environment in health care. Bowles et al. (2018) described the importance of nurse leaders' roles and actions in accomplishing IHI's quadruple aims. The success of a health care enterprise depends on competitive advantages of how well it does something compared with similar efforts and how well it is able to continuously achieve superior performance. Those enterprises that do not do so fail to remain viable for long. Lasater et al. (2016) reported that hospitals known for their excellence in nursing also perform better on value-based purchasing outcomes.

Strategic management involves strategic planning and implementation. It provides a "blueprint" for operating a business, establishing a competitive position, ensuring customer satisfaction, and reaching strategic objectives or goals. Although most strategic planning occurs at the "macro" level (i.e., the executive levels of the health care institution), its implementation typically becomes the responsibility of the "micro" level, such as the nursing division, department, or unit and even the individual nurse. As a result, success depends on the engagement of the entire workforce (Jasper & Crossan, 2012). Fortunately, strategic management prepares nurses to adapt to the current health care environment and helps them achieve their goals, whether related to the workplace or to the profession.

DEFINITIONS

A review of literature by Jasper and Crossan (2012) determined that strategic management is a multifaceted concept that is difficult to define. These authors embraced the definition of strategic management offered by Nag et al. (2007, p. 944), which asserted that "strategic management deals with the major intended and emergent initiatives taken by general managers… involving utilization of resources, to enhance the performance of firms in their external environments." This definition encompasses the five characteristics of strategic management found by Jasper and Crossan (2012):

- Engagement of the entire workforce in organizational leadership
- Alignment with the external environment
- Future orientation
- Use of change management strategies to achieve performance goals
- Facilitation of decision-making with well-communicated decisions

The concept of strategic management includes strategic planning and strategy implementation (Management Study Guide, 2020). Additional terms associated with an organization's use of strategy include *organizational mission and vision, core values, core purpose, strategy, tactics, strategic plan, objectives,* and *stakeholders.* The **organizational mission and vision** collectively is a guiding framework that describes the organization's purpose and future direction (Society for Human Resource Management [SHRM], 2018). **Core values** define the characteristics or beliefs that underlie the organization's activities. The core purpose is the reason the organization is in business. **Strategy** is a competitive move or business approach designed to produce a successful outcome. **Tactics** are operational choices for action that are made to implement a strategy. A **strategic plan** is a document that specifies a plan for actualizing the mission. A strategic plan may also involve a *business plan* or an *action plan* (either as part of the strategic plan or as an adjunct to it) that consists of the who, what, by when, where, and in general terms, the costs involved in implementing the activities identified as objectives in the strategic plan. Weston (2020, p. 54) defined **strategic planning** as "a thoughtful, systematic process of determining a direction and course of actions for achieving a desirable envisioned future." **Objectives** are defined as the targets an organization wants to achieve. These can be financial or performance based with short-range or long-range targets. Finally, **stakeholders** are individuals, groups, or another institution with a financial interest in—or who are affected by—what happens with the organization (BusinessDictionary, 2020).

BACKGROUND

Strategic Planning Process

Strategic management generally begins with a strategic planning process, triggered by recognition of the need for an organization to establish its competitive position in the marketplace or to address some other perceived need (e.g., seeking Magnet Recognition from the American Nurses Credentialing Center's Magnet Recognition Program®, [2017], applying to become a Certified Comprehensive Stroke Center through The Joint Commission [2020], or simply establishing future directions). These are questions to be answered in the strategic planning process: Where are we currently? Where do we want to go? How will we get there? What differentiates us from other organizations?

The components of the nursing process—assessment, planning, implementation, and evaluation—are similar to those employed in strategic management. Although a variety of strategic planning frameworks

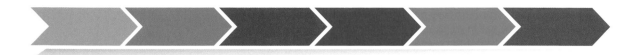

Fig. 14.1 Strategic planning process.

exist, they include the following six components, as shown in Fig. 14.1:

- Creating strategic mission and vision
- Assessing the environment
- Setting objectives
- Developing strategies to achieve the objectives
- Planning for implementation
- Planning for evaluation

The strategic plan provides a framework for strategic management, considering both external and internal environmental factors. Although the strategic planning process may appear to be sequential, it may be iterative as each stage illuminates new ideas for consideration.

Creating Mission and Vision Statements

The first step of the strategic planning process is to formulate or review and update as needed the organization's mission and vision in alignment with the organization's core purpose and values. The mission delineates what the organization does, while the vision articulates the preferred future state of the organization (SHRM, 2018). This step requires a determination of what the organization is, what business it is in and for whom, and where the business seeks to be in the future. The documentation of the mission and vision serves to communicate both purpose and direction to all stakeholders.

The mission and vision are informed by the core values of the organization. The core values held by an organization are those values that are held regardless of whether circumstances—either internal or external—change. They provide a standard for decision-making processes (SHRM, 2018). These core values are so embodied in the culture of the organization that even if they were seen as a liability, they would not be abandoned. Core values do not change even if the industry in which the organization operates changes. Thus, in health care, the organization that has as its core values quality care, patient safety, integrity, and social responsibility would retain those core values despite internal changes (e.g., changes in chief executive officers [CEOs]) or external changes (e.g., reimbursement, the nursing shortage).

The organization's core purpose is the reason the organization exists. The mission defines what the organization does, and the core purpose delineates why (Jones, 2018). The core purpose, like the core values, is relatively unchanging. It provides direction to the organization and contributes to the articulation and implementation of its mission.

In the strategic planning process, the following questions can help develop or revise vision and mission statements:

- What business are we in now?
- What business do we want to be in?
- What do our customers expect of us now?
- What will the customers' expectations be in the future?
- Who are our customers now?
- Who will our customers be in the future?
- Who are our current stakeholders (other than customers)?
- How will those stakeholders change in the future? What about their expectations?
- Who are our primary competitors currently?
- Who will our competitors be in the future?
- What about partners, now and in the future?
- What will the effect of technology be?
- What are the available and the needed resources, both human and financial?
- What is happening in the environment both internally and externally, now and in the future, that may affect us?

In many cases, the core values and the core purpose of the organization may have been defined previously, but if not, planners engaged in the strategic planning process should develop them using questions such as the following:

- What are the values on which we base our work?
- How central or essential are these to the organization?
- Would these values be supported if circumstances changed, or if the industry in which we currently operate changes?

The core purpose can be defined and refined by asking, "Why are we in business?" As a result, the initial response, "We are in the business of health care," may be further refined to "We want to contribute to the community in which we exist." Thus asking "why" may result in the core purpose of providing needed health care services to the community in which the organization is located. Sinek (2009) referred to the "why" in his book *Start with Why* as the core reason that individuals commit to a purpose, profession, or organization, which he later expounded on as an organization's "just cause" and, in his third book, *The Infinite Game* (2019), as the reason that individuals continue to engage in an organization and profession.

Responses to these questions by the principals involved in an organization (e.g., executive management, supervisory staff, department heads) shape an organization's mission, vision, strategic plan, and, as a result, its strategic management. However, involving individuals at all levels of the organization (e.g., staff nurses, clerical workers) in addition to those at the top of the hierarchy ensures a variety of perspectives and more buy-in to the final product. Such inclusion also engages all levels of staff in helping make the vision a reality. When everyone involved in an institution shares the same vision, individuals know where the organization is going and can be instrumental in helping it get there through their daily activities. As the old saying goes, "If you don't know where you're going, then any path will take you there." Conversely, if all of the individuals in the institution know the mission and vision, they are more likely to take the same path. Thus, although it is tempting to skip the mission, vision, and values review, sound strategic planning is premised on a firm linkage to them so that the plan then makes sense and flows out from this core.

Assessing the Environment

A key component of the strategic planning process is to assess the environment. This assessment, called environmental scanning, consists of analyzing both internal and external environmental factors. A SWOT analysis is often used in the environmental assessment and reviews four key areas: strengths, weaknesses, opportunities, and threats (Centers for Disease Control & Prevention, 2015). A grid such as the one seen in Table 14.1 is often used for documenting the SWOT analysis. In

TABLE 14.1 SWOT Analysis Template

Internal factors	Strengths	Weaknesses
External factors	Opportunities	Threats

this approach, strengths and weaknesses internal to the organization are identified. These strengths and weaknesses are generally related to resources, programs, and operations in key areas of the organization, examples of which are the following:

- *Operations:* efficiency, capacity, processes
- *Management:* systems, expertise, resources
- *Products:* quality, features, prices
- *Finances:* resources, performance

Once identified, these components are analyzed for the purpose of drafting a picture of the critical features of the organization, its achievements and failures, and its good points and bad points.

The external components are described as opportunities and threats, and they are identified in the same manner as the internal factors. Opportunities and threats may include changes in industry, marketplace, economy, political climate, technology, and competition.

Once identified, these strengths, weaknesses, opportunities, and threats must be analyzed for their impact on the organization. Next, priorities are established for the critical issues so that strategies are based on the priority issues. For example, a change in the market for the organization's services may be a threat but a low priority, so the organization determines it is not essential to target resources (e.g., human, financial) to deal with the threat when a higher priority is to take advantage of an opportunity involving technology. The SWOT analysis often leads to strategies in which the organization determines to build on **s**trengths, resolve or minimize **w**eaknesses, seize **o**pportunities, and avoid **t**hreats.

The strategies identified through the SWOT analysis help shape the strategic plan on which strategic management is based. The more carefully the analysis is conducted, the more reliable the strategic plan. A plan based on faulty assumptions or careless analysis does not serve the organization well and indeed may lead eventually to its demise.

There are a variety of methods used to analyze and craft a strategic plan. Besides the SWOT analysis, the SOAR (**s**trengths, **o**pportunities, **a**spirations, and **r**esults) planning model has been used in nursing to encourage innovation (Wadsworth et al., 2016). SOAR is a more positive alternative to the more traditional SWOT, places greater emphasis on the organization's future, and encourages employee involvement.

In addition to a SWOT or SOAR analysis of the current environment, individuals engaged in the strategic planning process must project the future. The assessment of future environmental impact takes the form of assumptions. These assumptions encompass the sociodemographic, political, economic, and technological aspects of the external environment. Of course, these assumptions are merely best guesses, because it is impossible to predict the future with certainty.

Setting Objectives

Once the organization's mission and vision have been established and the environmental assessment conducted, the next step in strategic planning is to develop the ways and means to achieve the vision. Strategic goals and objectives are crafted in this step. These objectives generally define the "who," "what," and "where" of the strategies to be implemented. Clearly defined objectives allow individuals to recognize where the organization wants to go and how much time it will take to get there. Absence of strategic objectives results in individuals trying to move in too many directions without a coordinated plan or not moving at all because of confusion about the organization's direction.

Strategic objectives provide a way of converting the rather abstract mission and vision of an organization into concrete terms. These are targets of performance that when taken together will achieve the mission and vision. Objectives also offer a way of measuring progress toward achieving the organization's mission and vision. These objectives generally are written to reflect not what *is* but what *should be*—activities that encourage the individuals implementing them to be creative, stretch beyond their current limits, and challenge themselves to improve their performance. These objectives must be achievable, however, lest individuals lose faith that they can accomplish them. If the strategic objectives are challenging but achievable, they prevent employees of an institution from becoming complacent or settling for the status quo.

Objectives may be written in terms of financial outcomes that relate to improvements in an organization's fiscal health and result in a stronger position for the institution in the industry. For example, a hospital may set a financial objective to decrease expenses by a specific percentage each year. This objective may be accomplished through tactics to decrease length of stay or prevent hospital-acquired conditions such as pressure ulcers (HAPU) or ventilator-associated pneumonia (VAP). In addition, the organization may have objectives to enhance their position as a health care provider or employer of choice. These objectives may relate to obtaining high scores on publicly reported data such as HCAHPS or achieving quality recognition such as Magnet designation.

Developing Implementation Strategies

Objectives are the targeted results and outcomes, and strategies are actions taken to achieve those outcomes. The strategies must be aligned with the organizational culture. In addition, they must be realistic, planned, and intentional, yet flexible enough to respond to unanticipated events.

In the strategic management process, tactics need to be developed with patient safety and quality care as the guiding force (Jasper & Crossan, 2012). Operational strategies need to be evidence based and engage employees at all levels of the organization. Because of this, individuals who develop implementation strategies need to be cognizant of the organizational culture and the impact of changes on those who are tasked with carrying out the plans. As Jasper and Crossan (2012, p. 843) stated, "[I]f we accept that part of the organization's culture is a sense of agreement among staff as to what constitutes the best way forward in any given situation then acknowledgment of those values and beliefs when formulating strategy will be key to successful implementation."

Plans that engage employees are realistic. The need for realistic yet flexible plans is emphasized by the American Nurses Association's (ANA, 2018) Leadership Institute Competency Model. This model identifies the leadership competency of strategic planning as the ability to "translates his or her vision into realistic business strategies" (ANA, 2018, p. 9). Behaviors that demonstrate this competency include:

- Adjusting plans as needed based on circumstances
- Developing plans with consideration for organization-wide needs
- Formulating realistic tactical plans that align with organizational strategies

- Creating contingency plans
- Balancing "long-term goals with immediate organizational needs" (ANA, 2018, p. 9)

This ability to rapidly adapt to changing environmental influences is referred to as *strategic agility* (Kotter, 2014; Shirey, 2015). Kotter maintains that organizations that are not able to shift their operational focus quickly are at risk in an environment of ever-increasing change. Strategic agility has become a key to organizational success. A flexible implementation plan helps an organization remain strong enough to withstand competition, overcome obstacles, and achieve peak performance. The organization's strategy needs to be flexible to respond appropriately to the following:

- Evolving needs and preferences of customers and stakeholders
- Advances in technology
- Changes in political climate and regulatory requirements
- New opportunities
- New entrants/disrupters in the market
- Economic variability
- Altered market conditions
- Disasters and crises

Planning for Implementation

Once the strategies have been delineated, the next step in the strategic planning process is planning for implementation. Implementation involves trying out the activities in a way that determines how best to close the gap between how things are done and what it takes to achieve the strategy. For example, given an objective related to improvement of the financial bottom line, the first step is to determine current cost and then compare it with desired cost to decide what needs to be changed to reach the desired lower cost.

If strategies are to be effective, they must be implemented proficiently, efficiently, and in a timely manner. For this to occur, the organization must attend to its capabilities, the reward structure, available support systems, and the organizational culture. For example, if employees are not rewarded in ways that are meaningful to them, they are unlikely to initiate or maintain efforts to implement the strategy. If the organizational culture does not support innovation or risk taking, or if the prevailing attitude is "if it's not broken, don't fix it," then efforts to improve performance or outcomes may be doomed. Support systems such as education,

policies, and procedures must be developed to support the implementation plan.

Implementing strategy is closely linked to an organization's operations; it involves managing, budgeting, motivating, changing culture, supervising, and leading. Strategic planning and implementation are managerial processes that accomplish the following:

- Demonstrate leadership in implementation of the strategy
- Develop accountability structures
- Reward those who carry out the strategy successfully
- Allocate necessary resources to activities critical to the strategy
- Formulate policies and procedures that support the identified strategy
- Initiate continuous quality improvement activities
- Develop and reward best practices
- Maintain a culture that supports the strategy

Effective implementation is more likely when an action plan is developed with input from the individuals who are responsible for implementing the strategic plan. The action plan should include a priority order for achieving the strategic objectives or outcomes, the determination of who (individual or group) is responsible for achieving these objectives, an indication of available or necessary financial support, and a timetable outlining when achievement of the objectives can be expected. If the strategic objective is long term or complex, it may also be advisable to include interim activities and time frames so that progress can be evaluated.

Planning for Evaluation

The final step in the strategic planning process is developing the evaluation design. Planning for evaluation is imperative to ensure that systems and measurements are in place to determine whether the strategic plan has been achieved. During the strategic planning process, measures of success are delineated, responsible individuals are identified, and frequency of evaluation and reporting of these measures is determined. If these progress reports reveal that the measures of success are not being achieved, further evaluation—such as environmental scanning with additional SWOT analysis—may be indicated.

Strategic plan progress reports may appear in a variety of formats from a simple narrative to use of complex strategic management software. Whatever format is used, it should clearly indicate the organization's progress toward its strategic goals.

ELEMENTS OF A STRATEGIC PLAN

Strategic planning results in a written document called the strategic plan. This document may be written by the individuals involved in the strategic planning process or by the individual who facilitated the process (e.g., consultant). Strategic plan documents generally contain the following sections:

- **Executive summary:** A two- to three-page synopsis of the plan, written in language understandable by all potential readers.
- **Background**: A description of the institution, its history, and current state, including its accomplishments, as well as the situation that prompted the strategic planning process.
- **Mission, vision, and values:** A description of the philosophy of the organization.
- **Goals and strategies:** A list of the target objectives and the strategies identified to ensure achievement of the objectives.
- **Appendices:** All additional documentation related to the strategic planning process to provide the background information used by the strategic planners to arrive at the final plan.

Appendix materials may include the annual reports of the institution, SWOT analysis results, financial information, environmental scan results, staffing information, and current and projected programs and services. Other materials may be included as desired. Caution should be exercised, however, to not include confidential data that should not be viewed by individuals outside of the organization.

The strategic plan should be disseminated widely throughout the institution. However, the document does not need to be reproduced in its entirety for everyone in the institution. A decision needs to be made about which parts of the strategic plan are appropriate for the individuals who will receive them. Some may need the entire plan, others may need only the executive summary, and still others may need only the goals and strategies.

In any case, the strategic plan should be communicated to stakeholders: board members, management, and staff. Copies should be included in orientation programs for new employees. The institution's vision and mission—including the core values—should be displayed in public areas (e.g., waiting rooms, cafeteria), as well as in areas reserved for employees. The core values can be listed on employee identification badges and printed in all marketing materials for the organization. The strategic plan tenets should be incorporated into all of the institution's policies and procedures.

Copies of the plan may also be provided to trade or professional organizations with which the institution is associated. The public relations or community outreach department in the institution can use the strategic plan as the basis for a media campaign to educate the community and other stakeholders and audiences about the institution's vision and mission. Patients may be provided with a condensed summary of the strategic plan on admission, particularly those sections related to their care. Patients should be informed of the institution's core values as well.

IMPLEMENTATION OF THE STRATEGIC PLAN

At this point, strategic management often fails. Strategic plans are developed and then allowed to languish as the necessary commitment to implementation is not realized. Strategy projects are said to fail in the range of 50%–90% of the time (Weston, 2020). This may be due to lack of a well-executable plan or lack of follow-through. Often competing priorities impede implementation of the plan. Executives and staff in health care organizations have numerous responsibilities, and implementing strategic objectives adds another burden to an already overwhelming workload. To overcome this obstacle, the strategic plan needs to be integrated into the organization's daily activities. Everyone needs to be committed to implementing the strategic plan, from the leaders to the staff at all levels and in all departments. Focusing on the strategic plan and its meaning to the viability and future of the institution is imperative.

An operational plan is key to maintaining focus on implementation of the strategic plan. The operational plan breaks the strategic plan into manageable components with defined tactics, particularly for those individuals who were not directly involved in crafting the strategic plan. During implementation, the operational plan needs to become a living document that is constantly referenced, consulted, and discussed. The operational plan should be reviewed and updated at regular intervals. Actions that have been completed or those that do not move the organization toward achievement of its goals should be deleted, and new actions based on existing environmental conditions should be added. It may also be necessary to readjust the timeline for completion of some activities in response to external or internal factors that affect the ability to accomplish the desired activities.

Ensuring that the operational plan remains at the forefront of daily activities—whether in an institution as a whole, a department, or a unit—often requires a "champion." This champion is an individual who is passionate and committed to the implementation process and who can inspire others. Often a champion appears as the strategic planning process unfolds; generally, this individual contributes freely, is engaged in the work groups, and expresses interest in the process. Champions can be selected as well, but those who volunteer are usually more enthusiastic about the work than those who are "drafted." Leaders often consider not only formal champions, but also informal champions who have influence in the area of the operational plan in order to increase the chance for success.

LEADERSHIP AND MANAGEMENT IMPLICATIONS

Strategic management is useful for nursing leaders and managers because it can be used to analyze the environment for opportunities and threats; to set measurable, achievable goals and strategies; and to help determine the future of the nursing department or unit. There are two predominant schools of thought today related to strategic planning at the enterprise, facility, department, and unit level. First is the opportunity to develop strategic plans for each of the levels, to align them, and then deploy. Second is the idea that the only one strategic plan should be developed at the highest organizational level, meaning a health system would develop a strategic plan at the enterprise level and the remainder of the plans would then be operational plans to support the overarching strategic plan. Regardless of the approach, strategic plans need to cascade and align to link and relate to the organization's overall mission, vision, and values. Success in strategic planning and implementing the operational plan will position nursing well, and more importantly this is critical to the success of the organization. The process provides an opportunity for nursing to shine, because the similarities between the nursing process and the strategic

planning process allow nurses to shortcut the learning curve and begin to move forward with the implementation phase while others may still be grappling with the planning process. Nursing skills and abilities make it relatively easy to plan strategically, and nurses, as 24-hour workers, can approach implementation as an ongoing, continuous, and seamless process. Nurses' involvement with continuous quality improvement and performance improvement systems provides a basis for participation in strategic planning that is systematic and thorough.

Implementation of the organization's strategic plan can be useful in unifying staff on a nursing unit or in a department. Collaboration and cooperation among staff generally are required to accomplish strategic objectives. Working together to accomplish a strategic objective keeps staff engaged. Involvement in decisions that ultimately will affect them is essential and often results in positive spin-offs; for example, staff members feel a sense of ownership in the process and pride in their accomplishments.

CURRENT ISSUES AND TRENDS

Many current issues and trends affect the strategic management process in health care organizations and nursing. These trends include a focus on the Institute for Health care Improvement's (IHI) Quadruple Aim, the effect of the Patient Protection and Affordable Care Act (ACA), and continued attention to the goals of the IOM's *Future of Nursing* report.

First proposed in 2008, the Triple Aim established by the IHI includes goals related to population health, improving the patient experience, and decreasing per capita cost (IHI, 2016; Whittington et al., 2015). The Triple Aim transformed to become the Quadruple Aim, with the fourth aim being that of improving work environments and the experience of health care workers (Sikka et al., 2015). The IHI posited that these goals can strengthen other health care reform measures such as accountable care organizations (ACOs), bundled payments, avoidance of penalties for preventable events such as hospital readmissions or hospital-acquired infections, and the conservation of human capital in health care. Strategic management in health care organizations requires attention to these goals in order to maintain optimal reimbursement and remain financially viable.

Tenets of the original Triple Aim were incorporated in the ACA, another trend that affects strategic management in health care organizations. Provisions of the ACA, which was implemented in 2010, continue to evolve (Rand Health Care, 2017). Overall, the ACA has resulted in fewer uninsured individuals but has also affected hospital and provider reimbursement. As the ACA's mandates continue to be phased into practice, health care organizations must strategically manage their impact on overall operations.

Finally, the continued focus on the IOM's (2010) *Future of Nursing* goals drives the strategic goals of health care organizations and nursing practice. Elimination of barriers to practicing at the full scope of practice, advancing educational preparation of nurses, creating diversity in the nursing workforce, leading change to promote health, and improving collection of nursing workforce data all require continued effort (NAM, 2015). However, the shifting health care environment requires more inter-professional collaboration and mandates that organizations and nursing professionals engage with a broad base of stakeholders to promote the Quadruple Aim targets of population health, patient satisfaction, and decreased costs of health care while also improving the care giver's experience.

CONCLUSION

Strategic planning is not reserved for activities such as seeking recognition through the ANCC Magnet Recognition Program® or for ameliorating workforce issues in a particular institution. Any business venture benefits from having a strategic plan. The plan provides for assessment of the environment, including current and future opportunities, and identification of specific, measurable, realistic ways of taking advantage of those opportunities. Most importantly, perhaps, the strategic plan answers the question, "What business are we in?" Clearly defining a mission and vision helps a nursing unit or department focus its efforts on its core business.

Strategic planning and strategic management are necessary components of business in today's competitive and highly unstable health care environment. Strategic planning is a process similar to the nursing process, with defined and specific steps to be taken to ensure that a comprehensive and thorough process occurs. Strategic management involves implementation of the strategic plan to ensure that the organization is responsive to changes in its environment as well as to internal events.

Strategic planning and strategic management are not reserved exclusively for organizations. Individuals such as nurses can use these techniques to determine their own direction and establish objectives to ensure that they meet the goals they have set for themselves. Nurses in all areas of practice and in all employment settings can use the principles of strategic planning to explore programs, projects, and services and to advance their careers. Nurses who are involved in any aspect of an institution's strategic planning efforts should incorporate those activities into a personal portfolio (Cope & Murray, 2018) and use those activities to reflect their competence and expertise as well as their own professional development.

⚡ RESEARCH NOTE

Source

Alvarez-Maldonado, P., Reding-Bernal, A., Hernandez-Solis, A., & Cicero-Sabido, R. (2019). Impact of strategic planning, organizational culture imprint and care bundles to reduce adverse events in the ICU. *International Journal for Quality in Health Care, 31*(6), 480–484.

Purpose

To evaluate the impact of a multi-faceted program on quality outcomes and adverse events in a respiratory intensive care unit (ICU) in a large tertiary care setting using a cross-sectional secondary analysis design.

Discussion

Adverse events in hospital settings contribute to significant morbidity and mortality and are responsible for approximately 400,000 deaths per year in hospitalized patients. The authors undertook the project with the primary goal of reducing the number of nosocomial infections related to mechanical ventilation and central venous catheters.

The team implemented a multi-pronged program based upon three "Es" from the Michigan Keystone organizational change model: Engage (strategic planning and organizational culture imprint), Educate (training and practice), and Execute (implementation of care bundles). The project leadership team then conducted strategic planning sessions and completed a SWOT analysis prior to implementing the project based on the three Es framework. Some of the threats identified included work overload, resistance to change and a lack of commitment to the organization's mission and vision. As part of the organizational culture aspect of project implementation, key messages emphasized the importance of "belonging to the organization," also known as wearing the institution's t-shirt. The educational presentations centered on the organization's strong foundation and focus on the roles and value of all health care team members' contributions to care and implementation of specific care bundles aimed at reducing ventilator- and central venous catheter-associated infections.

As a result of the project, infections related to central venous catheters and mechanical ventilators were reduced by 40% per 1000 patient catheter or ventilator days. As a secondary finding in the analysis, the authors also monitored other adverse events and observed reductions in some of those patient outcomes as well, including accidental extubation, pneumothorax, endotracheal tube changes, and atelectasis. They observed an 18% reduction in ICU death rates.

Application to Practice

Current health care environments are filled with complexity. As organizations face ever-increasing demands to achieve quality clinical and financial outcomes, traditional linear approaches often no longer prove effective in solving problems or attaining desired goals and objectives. Interprofessional health care team members each bring unique knowledge, competencies and skill sets that bring value to care delivery and patient outcomes.

Strategic planning is the foundation of any organization, department, unit, and team initiative and involves bringing interprofessional teams together to conduct SWOT analyses, set goals, and plan, implement, and evaluate the project. Aligning processes with organization mission, vision, and values and engaging interprofessional team members and key stakeholders throughout the project is vital to success.

CASE STUDY

The Chief Nursing Officer (CNO) in a large urban health care facility approached the Chair of the organization's shared governance council (SGC) about engaging the council in a project to improve patient satisfaction scores. The senior leaders had implemented various strategies to improve the "patient experience" without successfully achieving health system targets. Senior executives and leaders were concerned about the impact of these patient outcomes on Centers for Medicare & Medicaid Services reimbursement and the organization's financial outcomes.

Since the SGC chair was working with council leadership to plan council activities and set goals for the coming year, she agreed that this initiative was certainly an important area of focus that impacted the majority of clinical areas represented by council members. The Chair also believed that council members' involvement and engagement in this work could have significant impact on patient, unit, and organization outcomes.

Once the CNO and SGC Chair set expectations and planned an approach, the CNO attended the January SGC meeting to present an overview of the organization's mission, vision, and values; a synopsis of strategies implemented and recent annual patient satisfaction outcome results. Following the formal presentation, the CNO hosted an open forum and question and answer session with council members regarding the patient experience.

Following the initial SGC meeting, the SGC Chair then worked with a task force of leaders and interprofessional team members to set goals, develop a timeline, and formalize the project overview and presented the information to the entire SGC membership at the next meeting. Following the task force presentation, the SGC Chair and task force members facilitated work group sessions with all SGC members present. Members were divided into small groups to complete their assigned tasks for the meeting.

CRITICAL THINKING EXERCISE

Pursuant to the Shared Governance Council's "patient experience" improvement project, the Chair charged the council members with homework assignments that included meeting with their managers and unit council leaders to present the project information and expectations. Each council member, in collaboration with their unit leaders, would identify and implement at least two interventions aimed at improving patients' experiences on their units.

As council members returned to their units and clinical areas to partner with their managers to complete their assignments and lead these efforts, each member engaged their interprofessional team members in finding the best evidence-based interventions that their disciplines could implement to improve patient satisfaction scores.

1. Which team members have the greatest impact on patients' satisfaction with their hospital experiences, and how can they be involved?

2. Once the team develops a plan for improving these patient experience outcomes, what elements of strategic planning, implementation, and evaluation will lead to accomplishing the best team, patient and unit outcomes?

3. What measures can team members use to periodically evaluate outcomes?

REFERENCES

Alvarez-Maldonado, P., Reding-Bernal, A., Hernandez-Solis, A., & Cicero-Sabido, R. (2019). Impact of strategic planning, organizational culture imprint and care bundles to reduce adverse events in the ICU. *International Journal for Quality in Health Care, 31*(6), 480–484.

American College of Healthcare Executives (ACHE). (2020). *ACHE healthcare executive 2020 competencies assessment tool.* https://www.ache.org/-/media/ache/career-resource-center/competencies_booklet.pdf.

American Nurses Association (ANA). (2018). *ANA leadership competency model.* https://www.nursingworld.org/~4a0a2e/globalassets/docs/ce/177626-ana-leadership-booklet-new-final.pdf.

American Nurses Credentialing Center (ANCC). (2017). *Magnet® application manual* 2019: Silver Spring, MD.: American Nurses Credentialing Center.

American Organization of Nurse Executives (AONE)/ American Organization for Nursing Leadership (AONL). (2015). *AONE nurse executive competencies*: Chicago, IL: AONE. https://www.aonl.org/sites/default/files/aone/nec.pdf.

Bowles, J. R., Adams, J. M., Batcheller, J., Zimmermann, D., & Pappas, S. (2018). The role of the nurse leader in advancing the quadruple aim. *Nurse Leader, 16*(4), 244–248. https://doi.org/10.1016/j.mnl.2018.05.011.

BusinessDictionary. (2020). *Stakeholder.* http://www.businessdictionary.com/definition/stakeholder.html.

Centers for Disease Control & Prevention (CDC). (2015). Do a SWOT analysis. In *Communities of practice resource kit.* https://www.cdc.gov/phcommunities/resourcekit/evaluate/swot_analysis.html.

Cope, V., & Murray, M. (2018). Use of professional portfolios in nursing. *Nursing Standard, 32*(30), 55–63.

Institute for Healthcare Improvement (IHI). (2016). *IHI triple aim initiative: Better care for individuals, better care for populations, and lower per capita costs.* http://www.ihi.org/Engage/Initiatives/TripleAim/Pages/default.aspx.

Institute of Medicine (IOM. (2010). *The future of nursing: Leading change, advancing health.* https://www.nap.edu/read/12956/chapter/1.

Jasper, M., & Crossan, F. (2012). What is strategic management. *Journal of Nursing Management, 20*(7), 838–846.

Jones, B. (2018). Mission versus purpose: What's the difference? Talking point. *Disney Institute Blog.* https://www.disneyinstitute.com/blog/mission-versus-purpose-whats-the-difference/.

Kotter, J. P. (2014). *Building strategic agility for a faster moving world.* Cambridge, MA: Harvard Business Press Books.

Lasater, K. B., Germack, H. D., Small, D. S., & McHugh, M. D. (2016). Hospitals known for nursing excellence perform better on Value Based Purchasing measures. *Policy & Politics & Nursing Practice, 17*(4), 177–186.

Guidc, Management Study (2020). *Strategic management—meaning and important concepts.* https://www.managementstudyguide.com/strategic-management.htm.

Nag, R., Hambrick, B. C., & Chen, M.-J. (2007). What is strategic management, really? Inductive derivation of a consensus definition of the field. *Strategic Management Journal, 28*, 935–955.

National Academies of Sciences, Engineering, and Medicine (NAM). (2015). *Assessing progress on the Institute of Medicine Report The Future of Nursing.* Washington, DC: The National Academies Press.

Pearce, J. A., & Robinson, R. (2012). *Strategic management* (13th ed.). New York, NY: McGraw-Hill/Irwin.

Rand Health Care. (2017). *The future of U.S. health care: Replace or revise the Affordable Care Act?* https://www.rand.org/health-care/key-topics/health-policy/in-depth.html.

Shirey, M. R. (2015). Strategic agility for nursing leadership. *Journal of Nursing Administration, 45*(6), 305–308.

Sikka, R., Morath, J. M., & Leape, L. (2015). The quadruple aim: Care, health, cost and meaning in work. *BMJ Quality & Safety, 24*(10), 608–610. https://doi.org/10.1136/bmjqs-2015-004160.

Sinek, S. (2009). *Start with why: How great leaders inspire everyone to take action.* New York: Portfolio.

Sinek, S. (2019). *The infinite game.* New York: Portfolio.

Society for Human Resource Management (SHRM). (2018). *Mission & vision statements: What is the difference between mission, vision and value statements?* https://www.shrm.org/resourcesandtools/tools-and-samples/hr-qa/pages/isthereadifferencebetweenacompany%E2%80%99smission,visionandvaluestatements.aspx.

The Joint Commission. (2020). *Stroke certification.* https://www.jointcommission.org/en/accreditation-and-certification/certification/certifications-by-setting/hospital-certifications/stroke-certification/.

Wadsworth, B., Felton, F., & Linus, R. (2016). SOARing into strategic planning: Engaging nurses to achieve significant outcomes. *Nursing Administration Quarterly, 40*(4), 299–306.

Weston, M. J. (2020). Strategic planning in an age of uncertainty: Creating clarity in uncertain times. *Nurse Leader, 18*(1), 54–58.

Whittington, J. W., Nolan, K., Lewis, N., & Torres, T. (2015). Pursuing the Triple Aim: The first 7 years. *Milbank Quarterly, 93*(2), 263–300. http://www.milbank.org/uploads/documents/featured-articles/pdf/Milbank_Quarterly_Vol-93_No-_2_Pursuing_the_Triple_Aim_The_First_7_Years.pdf.

15

Professional Practice Models

Joy Parchment

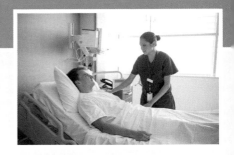

(e) http://evolve.elsevier.com/Huber/leadership

Health care organizations continue to evolve with rapid speed to deliver safe, quality care that meets the needs of patients. Fueling this change is the adoption of the Centers for Medicare & Medicaid Services' (CMS) incentive programs that penalize or reward health care organizations for high quality value rather than the volume of services performed (CMS, 2019; Lasater et al., 2016). The achievement of patient outcomes that demonstrate the delivery of safe, high quality patient care requires organizations to match the caring side of the health care business with available and/or limited resources. The practice of nursing requires nurses to serve as patient advocates, to integrate the best evidence into the delivery of patient care, and to improve the health of individuals (American Nurses Association, 2015). Nurses, intricately linked to the delivery of patient care, are challenged to transform health care with innovative care models that result in positive, sustainable, valued-added benefits to patients, providers, and organizations.

Over 20 years ago, researchers identified nursing sensitive indicators (NSIs) or elements of patient care that nurses directly influence (Heslop & Lu, 2014). In addition to NSIs, the publicly reported patient's perception of care survey known as Hospital Consumer Assessment of Healthcare Providers and Systems (HCAHPS), is used by CMS and other accrediting bodies to determine clinical quality outcomes of patient care or high-quality value that is tied back to hospital reimbursements. Patient's perception of care or patient satisfaction, an outcome measure for all hospitals, includes the ability of nurses to identify and mitigate the inherent suffering that patients experience

when receiving care (Dempsey et al., 2014) (Box 15.1). However, the ability to attain high quality outcomes depends on the organization's approach to matching human and material resources, patient characteristics, and health care needs to professional practice and care delivery models.

DEFINITIONS

The terms *professional practice model* and *care delivery model*, though used interchangeably in practice settings, are quite different. A **professional practice model (PPM** as defined by the American Nurses Credentialing Center (ANCC) is "a schematic depiction of a system, theory, or phenomenon that depicts how nurses practice, collaborate, communicate, and develop professionally to provide the highest-quality care for those served by the organization" (ANCC, 2017, p. 158). This visual representation serves as the foundational guide for how nurses' practice provides meaning for nurses and defines the structure and processes that enable nurses to achieve exemplary outcomes while practicing at top of license (Glassman, 2016; Stallings-Welden & Shirey, 2015).

Core elements of a PPM include a theoretical framework, nursing values or beliefs, leadership, care delivery model, collaborative relationships, autonomous decision-making, environment, research and innovation integration, and development and recognition (Duffy, 2016; Slayter et al., 2016). Organizations that utilize a PPM will typically include it on their website, in organizational documents, and in their nursing annual report.

BOX 15.1   Nursing Sensitive Indicators and Patient Satisfaction Outcomes

Nursing Sensitive Indicators
Structure
- Nursing hours per patient day
- Nursing turnover rate
- Registered nurse (RN) education/certification
- Staff or skill mix

Process
- Pediatric pain assessment and intervention, reassessment

Process and Outcome
- Patient falls
- Patient falls with injury
- Pressure injury (community, hospital, unit acquired)
- RN Survey (job satisfaction, practice environment)

Outcome
- Adverse outcomes of care: wrong site, side, patient, procedure, implant
- Antibiotic stewardship
- Delay in treatment

- Nosocomial infections (catheter-associated urinary tract infection [CAUTI]; central line-associated bloodstream infection [CLABSI]; clostridium difficile [CDIFF]; methi-cillin-resistant staphylococcus aureus [MRSA]; venous thromboembolism [VTE]
- Peripheral intravenous infiltration (PIV)
- Psychiatric physical/sexual assaults
- Pressure injuries, device related, hospital acquired

Patient Satisfaction
Outcome
- Patient engagement or patient-centered care
- Patient education
- Care coordination
- Safety
- Service recovery
- Courtesy and respect
- Responsiveness
- Pain
- Careful listening

(National Database for Nursing Quality Indicators, n.d.; Press Ganey, 2020; Centers for Medicare & Medicaid Services, 2020).

A **care delivery model (CDM** is integrated with the PPM and defines the operational mechanism for organizing care, the skill set needed to provide care, the setting for the care, and what the intended outcome could be for patients and families (ANCC, 2017). Inherent in all CDMs is the authority of the nurse to make informed clinical decisions, the accountability process for decision-making that maximizes quality and safety of nursing care, and the collaborative approach used with other members of the interdisciplinary team (ANCC, 2017). Several types of CDMs are noted in the literature. The two most prominent are total patient care and team nursing. In total patient care, one registered nurse (RN) is responsible for the total care of a patient or groups of patients. With team nursing, a team consisting of care providers with varying skill mix will care for groups of patients throughout their shift (Havaei et al., 2016).

BACKGROUND

Professional practice models were first described in the literature in the 1980s to articulate exemplary nursing practice, nurses' control over the delivery of care, and the practice environment; all core components of Magnet® organizations (ANCC, 2017). Nursing literature chronicles the influence of the work environment on nursing practice and identifies a strong correlation between work environments, safety, and the delivery of quality patient care (Olds et al., 2017). Executive leaders are responsible for designing strategies to create innovative work environments that support the practice of nurses. Given the complexity of nursing practice and the myriad of factors that influence patient, team, and organizational outcomes, nurse leaders need to actively collaborate with clinical nurses to determine the most effective models that can achieve quality outcomes (Wharton et al., 2016; Winslow et al., 2019). If these decisions are made only by executive nurse leaders, exemplary outcomes are less likely to occur.

The conceptual framework by Donabedian (1988) is frequently used to identify structures and processes that promote positive outcomes (S-P-O), and these concepts are causally linked. Structures support the care delivery process and focus on how the delivery of care is organized, the skill mix of the team, and the available number of care providers (ANCC, 2017).

Processes consist of two categories: clinical and inter-personal processes, such as collaborative teamwork, patient–provider communications, cultural sensitivity of care, and patient education. Outcomes answer the "so what" and are organized into three domains to include: patients, nurses, and the organization (ANCC, 2017; Donabedian, 1988).

PROFESSIONAL PRACTICE MODELS

An important predictor of RN job satisfaction is the presence of a PPM. Job satisfaction is directly associated with nurse turnover, which is a significant human resource challenge for nurse leaders (Sabei et al., 2020). Professional practice models consist of structures, processes, and values that support nurses' control over practice, enhance job satisfaction, and decision-making (Basol et al., 2015). Yet, the Magnet Recognition Program®, the highest recognition for nursing practice and known for being associated with organizations' success at attracting and retaining nurses, is credited with bringing to the forefront the PPM. Of the five components of the Magnet model, one component focuses on exemplary professional practice and the enculturation of the PPM into the practice environment (ANCC, 2017; Basol et al., 2015). Though many core elements of PPMs exist, seven major elements will be discussed: theoretical framework, leadership, autonomy and collaborative relationships, practice environment, development and recognition, research and innovation, and the CDM.

Theoretical Framework

PPMs are often grounded within a nursing or organizational theoretical framework, such as Kolcaba's comfort theory, Koloroutis' (2004) relationship-based care theory, systems theory; or PPMs are based on an established nursing concept like professional (shared) governance or Benner's novice to expert model (Cordo & Hill-Rodriguez, 2017; Kolcaba et al., 2006; Slayter et al., 2016). Nurse-driven PPMs prosper when nurse leaders at all levels support nursing professional practice. Evidence of professional practice support includes active professional (shared) governance councils and resources to engage and empower nurses in their practice (Cordo & Hill-Rodriguez, 2017; Glassman, 2016).

A strong link between the PPM, the vision, mission statements, and core values of the organization are vital to ensure adoption of the PPM. Also, alignment of nursing values with organizational values supports a culture of excellence throughout the organization (Slayter et al., 2016). Mission, vision, values, and philosophy also are fundamental to strategic planning. These foundational elements for PPMs will be briefly reviewed here.

Mission Statements

The purpose or goal of an organization is expressed by its *mission statement*. For health care organizations their sole existence is to deliver patient care. Publicly posted mission statements communicate to key stakeholders, the public, and employees the organization's purpose and identity. Mission statements provide information and support an organization's public relations. For management at all levels of an organization, the mission statement acts as a blueprint or foundational guide for developing specific measurable objectives and actions (Alegre et al., 2018).

Measurable *objectives and actions* associated with the mission statement explicitly represent what the organization is trying to do, and these initiatives keep an organization on track by providing guidelines and indicators for measuring present performance. Lack of goal alignment across an organization can trigger conflict and slow progress toward goal completion (Alegre et al., 2018). Nurse leaders are responsible for ensuring their unit, department, service line goals, and performance measures are in alignment with the organization's mission. A common source of conflict related to goal achievement within the complex health care environment is resource allocation, such as nurse staffing. However, an important leadership responsibility is to ensure that stakeholders agree with the mission statement and goals and support their enactment.

Vision Statements

Vision statements are often confused with mission statements. The difference is vision statements focus on the future direction of the organization and are crafted to describe the most desirable state at some future point in time. Vision statements are meant to be an inspirational tool for organizational leadership to reenergize and motivate stakeholders to ensure the fulfillment of the vision. Fully deployed vision statements have demonstrated a positive correlation with financial and growth performance metrics (Gulati et al., 2016).

Values Statements

Core *values* are strongly held beliefs and priorities that guide organizational decision-making. Values do not change but are anchors or fundamental beliefs that are constant and relate to the mission and vision of the organization. Values create the culture of the organization and drive the behaviors of team members. Furthermore, personally held values need to demonstrate congruency with organizational values because value congruency can predict compliance, autonomous practice, and conformity with organizational norms (Eva et al., 2017).

Philosophy

A statement of *philosophy* is defined as an explanation of the systems of beliefs, values, or ethics that determine how the mission and vision will be achieved. The philosophy is abstract; it describes an ideal state and gives direction to achieving the purpose. Philosophy statements typically begin with "we believe" and could be stated in any of the following ways:

- We believe everyone has a right to the highest quality of care.
- We believe we have an obligation to render quality care at a cost-effective price.
- We believe that any person who presents for care should receive care, regardless of his or her ability to pay.

The philosophy has implications for the role of the nurse. If an organization's stated mission includes patient care, education, and research utilization, then the expectation will be for nurses to embrace all aspects of the mission. Nurses develop new knowledge, integrate the best evidence into their practice to ensure exemplary patient outcomes, and participate in educating patients and nursing colleagues. For example, a correlation study of approximately 500 clinical nurses identified a positive significant relationship between the ethical climate of the organization, the level of support given to nurses, and turnover intentions (Abou Hashish, 2017). Nurse leaders, therefore, need to identify misaligned values, address possible sources of ethical conflict, and put strategies in place to decrease ethical conflicts before nurses take action and leave the organization.

Leadership

A key element identified in PPMs is the assumption that all nurses regardless of position are leaders. Leadership for organizational leaders includes setting the vision to ensure alignment with organizational values and strategies; ensuring that nurses have an equal voice at nursing and interprofessional decision-making groups, committees, forums, and councils; and empowering nurses to lead (Slayter et al., 2016). To ensure a professional practice environment of ownership, empowerment and engagement by nurses, some organizations have implemented professional (shared) governance structures at the unit, hospital, and or system levels. This structure has decreased the organizational bureaucratic layers found in most health care organizations and enabled relationship building leadership styles to flourish (Clavelle et al., 2016).

Autonomy and Collaborative Relationships

The practice of nursing is governed by nurses, and this grants nurses the authority to practice within identified scope and standards of practice to benefit patients, families, and communities. Nurses are given the self-governing right to define, credential, and evaluate nursing practice to promote health, protect patients/clients, and prevent illness and injury (Fowler, 2017). To accomplish these directives, nurses are granted the authority by their respective board of nursing to make autonomous decisions and/or to engage various collaborative health care providers to ensure the delivery of appropriate care to patients. Thus, collaborative relationships and/or partnerships built on trust involve effective communication techniques to not only engage patients with their care, but also to facilitate effective relationships between other interdisciplinary providers.

Practice Environment

The practice environment is a driver for nurse satisfaction, burnout, intent to leave, and patient mortality (Cicolini et al., 2014; Olds et al., 2017). Positive practice environments, also known as **healthy work environments,** are often found in Magnet designated organizations (Box 15.2). Magnet hospitals are known for their exemplary nursing care, transformative leadership,

---

BOX 15.2   Organizational Structures for Healthy Work Environment

- Effective leaders at all levels of the organization
- Professional development opportunities
- Staffing structures that consider nurse competencies, patient needs, and teamwork
- Interdisciplinary collaboration
- Empowered, shared decision-making
- Patient-centered culture/culture of safety
- Quality improvement infrastructure, evidence-based practice
- Visible acknowledgment of nursing's unique, valued contributions (e.g., professional practice model, vision/mission/philosophy statements)

(ANCC, 2017; AACN, 2005).

---

low turnover, and superior patient outcomes, such as higher patient care experiences and lower infection, mortality and morbidity rates over non-Magnet hospitals (Lasater et al., 2016; Park et al., 2016; Stimpfel et al., 2016). To achieve these outcomes, Magnet hospitals have structures and processes that support nursing professional practice (ANCC, 2017; Stimpfel et al., 2016). These structures and processes are differentiating factors for nurse satisfaction and quality patient outcomes. Most Magnet-like characteristics are easy to adapt to different work contexts. Characteristics such as involving nurses in practice decisions, providing resources for ongoing development, and utilizing a relationship building leadership style are demonstrated to have a dramatic impact on the environment where nurses practice.

Development and Recognition

Health care is constantly changing. What was current 2 years ago is perhaps now outdated. This never-ending evolution of health care practices and standards requires nurses to have a growth mindset, to pursue professional **development** activities to ensure the safety of patients, and to expand their professional knowledge and competence. Ulep (2018) suggested key strategies to retain millennial nurses included the availability of professional development resources, career advancement pathways or opportunities, and real-time coaching from their nurse leader. Strategies like intentional mentoring, the use of various conversations that help nurses understand

that they make a difference in their practice, and the establishment of early accomplishments can build long-term loyalty with millennial nurses (Ulep, 2018).

Recognition of nurses is positively linked to job satisfaction and retention of nurses (Tang & Hudson, 2019; Ulep, 2018). To ensure a healthy practice environment, the American Association of Critical-Care Nurses (AACN, 2005) included meaningful recognition as an important strategy. Meaningful recognition consists of communicating the value that the nurse brings to the delivery of patient care, identifying exemplary nursing care, and celebrating their accomplishments and milestones. Though there are numerous ways that nurses can be recognized, many organizations utilize the DAISY Award™ (https://www.daisy-foundation.org/daisy-award), an international award program that has grown in notoriety and is described as continuing the legacy of thanks to ensure that nurses understand how critical their role is for the health of nations (Barnes et al., 2016).

Research and Innovation

The utilization of new knowledge and innovative strategies into the practice environment is critical to meet the evolving needs of patients and healthcare. **Research** is defined as "the systematic inquiry that uses disciplined methods to answer specific questions or solve problems. The goal of research is to develop, refine, and expand knowledge" (Polit & Beck, 2017, p. 3). Though the translation of research into the practice environment is slow, the improvement of patient outcomes cannot be undervalued. All completed research studies should be disseminated, but not all research can be adopted into practice because research needs to be evaluated for quality and relevancy to the population at hand (Curtis et al., 2017).

Innovation is described as the utilization of creative or problem-solving techniques that result in a widely adopted strategy, product, or service to fill a need in a way that is new, different, or was non-existent before. Innovations will typically consist of quality improvement or cost effective or efficiency measures that impact the practice environment (Kaya et al., 2016). When integrated together these two concepts of research and innovation focus on what is possible and what is needed. The innovation can be studied to prove a theory, assess feasibility across different populations, or to ensure generalizability. Innovations can also serve as solutions to issues in the current practice environment. Innovation can include new CDMs, new leadership styles, and or new processes that drive change and redefine the practice environment (Weberg, 2009).

STRUCTURES AND PROCESSES THAT SUPPORT CARE DELIVERY MODELS

The appropriate CDM is the one that maximizes existing resources while meeting organizational goals and objectives, specifically the mission of the organization. However, to ensure the effective delivery of patient care, structures and processes such as policies, procedures, and clinical protocols are part of the tools that allow nurses to practice accountably.

Policies and Procedures

Policies and procedures are two functional elements or written rules of an organization that are extensions of the mission statements. Together they determine the requirements of the unit, department, service line, or organization. Policies and procedures provide order and stability so that the unit functions in a coordinated manner within the larger structure of nursing and the health care organization. Standard *operating policies and procedures* integrate behaviors of team members to prevent random chaos and maintain order, function, structure, and most of all decision-making (Amadei, 2016).

Policies

A **policy** serves as a formal guideline that directs action for thinking about and solving recurring problems related to practice and or the objectives of the organization. Throughout the practice arena, specific instances exist when team members are not clear about who is supposed to do something, the circumstances that an action should occur, or what should be done about unusual circumstances (Amadei, 2016). Policies, therefore, clarify actions, direct decision-making, and serve as guides to increase the likelihood of consistency with decisions and actions. Though broad limits are available with policies, there could be some modifications made for unique circumstances.

Written policies are *formal* and general in nature to cover all team members. Unwritten policies are *informal* and are established by patterns of decisions and interpretation of observed behaviors. For instance, an unwritten policy of an organization is the expectation

---

> ### BOX 15.3 **Policies**
> - Serve as guides
> - Help coordinate plans
> - Control performance
> - Increase consistency of action
> - Should be written
> - Usually are general in nature
> - Refer to all employees

that all individuals will receive compassionate care. However, this expectation may not be written as a policy. Yet, by decisions and disciplinary actions that occur, a team member can infer there is a policy that will be enforced even though it is not written (Box 15.3).

Some general nursing areas require the formulation of policies. These include areas where there is confusion about the locus of responsibility and where lack of guidance might result in the neglect, malpractice, or "malperformance" of an act necessary for the patient. Unambiguous policies are necessary for medication error reporting, the protection of patients' or families' rights, and matters of human resource management and personnel welfare. Conflicts arise when a lack of explicit criteria to inform decisions and actions exists (Amadei, 2016).

Procedures

Procedures are descriptions of step-by-step directions, methods for actions to take in common situations, and serve as a ready reference for all personnel. **Procedures** require the best evidence and should be written in enough detail to provide the information required by all persons engaging in the activity. This means procedures will have a statement of purpose, identify who is to perform the activity and include the steps necessary along with a list of supplies and equipment needed for the activity (Box 15.4).

> ### BOX 15.4 **Procedures**
> - Provide step-by-step methods
> - Are written in detail
> - Provide guidelines for commonly occurring events
> - Provide a ready reference
> - Guide performance of an activity
> - Should include the following:
>   - A statement of purpose
>   - Identification of who performs activity
>   - Steps in the procedure
>   - A list of supplies and equipment needed

The similarities between policies and procedures are that both are a means for accomplishing objectives and are necessary for the smooth functioning of any work group, department, or organization. The difference between a policy and a procedure is that a policy is a directive that must be followed, for example, the use of restraints. A procedure provides direction, such as evidence-based steps to perform a urinary catheterization. There are legal implications to the application of policies and procedures. For instance, the nurse may be held liable for failing to follow written policies and procedures. Thus, it is important for nurses to be informed about policies and procedures governing practice in an organization. In addition, both policies and procedures need regular and periodic review (Amadei, 2016).

Clinical Protocols

Clinical protocols fall under the umbrella term of *structured care methodologies* (SCMs). SCMs are interdisciplinary tools that identify best practices, facilitate standardization of care, and provide a mechanism to track variances, quality, and outcomes (Cole & Houston, 1999). *Clinical or critical pathways, evidenced-based algorithms, clinical protocols, standards of care, order sets,* and *clinical practice guidelines* are all types of SCMs. However, the gold standard for clinical protocols is the use of best evidence to reduce practice variation in a patient outcome focused environment.

A *clinical pathway* is a written plan that identifies key, critical, or predictable incidents that must occur at set times to achieve patient outcomes within an appropriate length of stay in a hospital setting. As a pathway, it is a tracking system for the timing of treatments and interventions, health outcomes, complications, activity, and teaching/learning (Pound et al., 2017). Pathways are also considered a method of quality improvement to assist health care providers with clinical process innovation (Pound et al., 2017).

CARE DELIVERY MODELS

A variety of patient CDMs exist. The redesign of a CDM is influenced by fiscal responsibility, accountability to the consumer, available resources, and quality and safety considerations. Although all models have their advantages and disadvantages, there is no one right way to structure patient care. Quite often, aspects of older or traditional, models are incorporated into new delivery

models. Therefore, it is important to understand the variety of models available. They may be old, traditional, new, evolving, and/or innovative. With the proliferation of numerous health care provider roles, expedited care processes, and increased patient acuity and needs, pure nursing models that flourished in less complex environments have yielded to collaborative practice and interdisciplinary approaches. Understanding the historical perspective helps nurses to better analyze options for current practice.

Traditional Nursing Care Delivery Models

Historians mark the emergence of modern nursing from the time of Florence Nightingale's work in the Crimea. Nightingale (1860) believed that nursing care of patients included spiritual well-being as well as their environment. Over the past century, the evolution of nursing models of care has resulted from the impact of economic, social, and political agendas. There are five traditional nursing models of care: (1) private duty, (2) functional, (3) team, (4) primary, and (5) case management. Of those, functional, team, primary, and case management were and are currently associated with hospital nursing practice. Private duty and case management were associated with public health, home health, and community health but have been adapted to the inpatient setting. Private duty, later called *case* or *case management*, was the original way nursing care was delivered; it later became the foundation for public health nursing and community service delivery (Muir, 2019; Whelan, 2012).

Private Duty Nursing

Private duty nursing is sometimes called *case nursing*, because it is based on the case method where each patient is a case. Another term for private duty nursing is total patient care. There are two ways of thinking about *total patient care*. One approach is holistic care of the total patient, including mind, body, and spirit. Another approach is functionally based, where a nurse assumes total care for one patient. Private duty nursing is the oldest care model in the United States. Between 1890 and 1929, graduate nurses in the United States served as private duty nurses, caring for patients in their homes (Muir, 2019; Whelan, 2012). Nurses did the cooking, cleaning, bathing of wounds, and organizing of the household functions, basically functioning as a home manager. A form of hospital case nursing evolved between 1900 and the 1930s. When the Great Depression hit, most families were too poor to afford private duty nurses and so nurses were without jobs. Hospitals then began to employ graduate nurses. As the graduate nurses who had been doing private duty moved into the hospital, the desire was to retain the type of care model to which they had become accustomed. Private duty was transplanted into hospital settings for as long as nurses were paid by patients. When nurses became employees of hospitals, the kind of care that private duty allowed was not possible within the organizational structure of hospital staff nursing (Muir, 2019; Whelan, 2012).

The advantages of private duty nursing were one-to-one care, the ability to foster close nurse–patient relationships, and attainment of a high degree of autonomy. The disadvantages were the high cost and low efficiency associated with this model. With the shift to hospital-based care, nurses' job security was questionable (Whelan, 2012).

Two main variations on the basic pattern of private duty nursing developed within hospitals: group nursing and total patient care.

Group nursing was a care model proposed in the 1930s by Geister, then the executive director of the American Nurses Association (ANA). Defined as nursing group practice, the idea of group nursing in hospitals was similar to divisional private duty in which several patients shared a private nurse. The plan was to reorganize private duty from individual to group practice both inside and outside the hospital. The intention was to link a group practice registry of private duty nurses to a community's public health nursing service, but after political pressure the plan died. Hospitals also experimented with a group nursing care modality, described as being halfway between a private duty arrangement and graduate nurse hospital staff nursing. Under this plan, patients were grouped together in a special unit where several patients shared a private nurse. Thus, three nurses could do 8-hour shifts for two patients instead of four nurses being needed for 12-hour shifts. The hospital paid the nurses' wages but charged the patients directly as a surcharge on the hospital bill. The advantages included shorter hours for nurses, order and regularity in hospital staffing, steady employment for nurses, slightly cheaper rates for patients, and responsibility for the total care of several patients for the nurse. Nurses had the autonomy and care delivery method of private duty without its isolation and uncertainty. Nurses were

members of the hospital's staff, yet their time was specifically allocated only to a set number of patients who paid for this service directly. However, economic and political pressures for more efficiency, productivity, and service cut off the adoption of this system in hospitals (Baas, 1992; Muir, 2019; Reverby, 1987). There is a striking parallel between group nursing and how physicians are organized to practice medicine in today's health care environment.

Total patient care initially occurred in intensive care, hospice care, and home health care. The term total patient care has come to mean the assignment of each patient to a nurse who plans and delivers care during a work shift. With this model, continuity of care can be compromised as patients are allocated by shift, rather than allocated based on admission date to discharge (King et al., 2015).

Functional Nursing

Functional nursing emerged as a care model in the 1940s. With this model, the division of labor is assigned according to specific tasks and technical aspects of the job, such as medication administration and taking vital signs. Under functional nursing, the nurse identifies the tasks to be done for a shift. The work is divided and assigned to nursing and support personnel, such as care assistants.

From the late 1800s through the end of World War II, functional nursing was the norm in US hospitals. In the early 1900s, business and industry concepts of "scientific management" emphasized efficiency. The efficiency was gained by breaking down a work process into its component task steps and then analyzing and timing the steps, establishing standards, and determining the best way to perform each task. Thus, managerial control over the planning and execution of work could be established. Functional nursing was developed as a result of this concern for task analysis and proper division of the nursing workload. With this model, there could be a "temperature nurse," a "medication nurse," a nurse for the right side of the hall, and a nurse for the left side of the hall (Tiedeman, 2004). This model enabled hospitals to improve service efficiency and control labor costs by requiring fewer RNs. Another advantage of this model was clear division of labor. Over time, with the increased complexity of patient care needs, the functional model has become less favored due to the fragmentation of care and patient exposure to multiple care providers.

The focus on tasks diminishes nurses' critical thinking and the patient-centered approach of care delivery (Tiedeman, 2004).

Team Nursing

Team nursing is a care model that uses a group of care providers led by a knowledgeable nurse to achieve a common goal. This model utilizes a delivery approach that provides care to a group of patients by coordinating a team of RNs, licensed practical nurses, and care assistants under the supervision of one RN, called the *team leader*. Team nursing developed in the early 1950s in response to a shortage of RNs and in reaction to the dissatisfaction with functional nursing (Fairbrother et al., 2015; King et al., 2015).

Team nursing is designed to make use of each member's capabilities to meet the nursing needs of their group of patients. When making team assignments, the nurse leader considers the scope of practice, knowledge, and expertise of each team member and gives each team member their own patient assignments. This model requires effective team leadership, collaboration, frequent communication, and the expectation that team members will assist and support each other as needed. A benefit of an effective team is that team members provide extra surveillance for patients and give greater support for novice nurses (Dickerson & Latina, 2017). Blurring of the scope of practice along with educational preparation, critical thinking skills, and knowledge application are significant challenges for team nursing models (Martin & Weeres, 2016). Nursing literature suggests teams with a greater proportion of RNs or richer skill mix have better patient outcomes (Halm, 2019). A national study of nurses across 41 hospitals in the United States identified higher levels of collaboration between nurses, physicians, and their leaders had a strong impact on the quality of care given to patients and increased reports of the job satisfaction of nurses (Ma et al., 2015).

Primary Nursing

Primary nursing began in the 1960s by Manthey to overcome the discontent with functional and team nursing's emphasis on tasks and discrete functions that directed nurses' attention away from the holistic care of the patient. This matched a societal trend toward accountability, as well as nursing's rising level of professionalism. In this model, the primary nurse has 24-hour-per-day accountability for the patient's plan of care from admission to discharge. Associate nurses oversee patient care delivery when the primary nurse is not on shift and are expected to follow the primary nurse's plan of care. This model enhances continuity of care; maximizes RN utilization of professional competencies, such as critical thinking, collaboration, and teaching; and philosophically complements holistic, patient-centered care. Although this model is favored by RNs and patients due to its relational nature, it takes time and energy investment to have 24-hour accountability (Wessel & Manthey, 2015). However, Manthey (2002) believed that the implementation of primary nursing would be a vehicle to return nursing to its true professional role.

Fernandez et al. (2012) completed a systematic review of the literature to evaluate nursing models of care delivery, specifically team and primary nursing, on nurse and patient outcomes. This research team identified sparse differences with respect to quality of communication among staff, nurse job satisfaction, absenteeism rates, and role clarity, while the impact on patient outcomes was ambiguous. Team nursing was associated with significantly decreased medication errors, fewer adverse events involving intravenous management, and lower pain scores for patients, although there were no differences for patient fall rates. Overall, the researchers concluded that team nursing is often preferred when there are staff with less experience or skill level on a unit. In another systematic review, Mattila et al. (2014), revealed that the primary nursing model was less costly than a team nursing model and nurses on primary nursing units reported higher quality care delivery than nurses on team nursing units. Also, the Mattila team identified that primary nursing could have a higher impact in the maternity setting, as continuity of care was enhanced. Mothers reported less breast discomfort and engaged more effectively in breastfeeding. Dal Molin et al. (2018) assessed the relationship between nursing sensitive staff, and organizational outcomes and the effectiveness of primary nursing using a before and after research methodology. After the implementation of primary nursing, patient satisfaction with the care they received improved, and nursing sensitive outcomes such as urinary catheter infections, falls, and pressure injuries (ulcers) decreased.

Case Management

Case management as a nursing model of care evolved in the late 1980s, as both a process (a provider intervention), a CDM, and as a method to manage care. The Case Management Society of America (CMSA), a multidisciplinary organization is the professional organization representing the practice of case managers. The CMSA defined case management as "a collaborative process of assessment, planning, facilitation, care coordination, evaluation, and advocacy for options and services to meet an individual's and family's comprehensive health needs through communication and available resources to promote quality, cost-effective outcomes" (CMSA, 2017). **Care coordination,** an integral role of case managers, is the facilitation of resources, integration of providers to achieve the longitudinal plan for the best patient outcomes (Swan et al., 2019).

Case management and care coordination have been the CDMs used for years by public health and community health nurses, although case management can occur in any health sector (acute care, community), extend across the health care continuum, or be linked to a population focus, such as school nursing (Maughan et al., 2018). In the face of strong economic external forces, acute care hospitals turned to case management to help reduce provider practice variation and to ensure the appropriateness of care. The risk with case management models is that communication and coordination infrastructures, along with standardized practice guidelines, may not be available or integrated for effectiveness of care (Joo & Huber, 2018).

Case management has components of health services delivery, coordination, and monitoring, through which multiple service needs of patients are met. Hospital-based acute care nursing case management focuses on an entire episode of illness, crossing all settings in which the patient receives care. Care is directed by a case manager, who is not always a nurse, and can be unit or population focused (Joo & Huber, 2018). A longitudinal study to determine the effectiveness of a 12-month nursing case management intervention on the functioning of the family, stress of the mother, and outcomes of children with attention deficit hyperactivity disorder found improvement in the functioning of the family and behaviors of the child. Though there was not a statistically significant outcome with the mother's stress level between the intervention and the control group, this study determined that the nursing care management intervention promoted communication, empowered families to take ownership of their care, and strengthened the connection between providers (Churchill et al., 2018). Other research demonstrated that the use of RN case managers within the care delivery system can improve adherence to care treatments resulting in better patient outcomes (Mattei da Silva et al., 2020).

EVOLVING MODELS

Changes to the health care, economic, social, and political environments will continue to have a strong impact on the creation of **traditional and evolving** CDMs. Coupled with these transforming changes is the retirement of baby boomers, the delivery of care across the care continuum, and exploding technological advancements. The seminal and replicated work of Aiken and colleagues (Aiken et al., 2011, 2013, 2017) contributes a body of evidence that richer RN-specific skill mix reduces patient mortality. However, many of the resulting structures for patient care are skill mix models or mixed models that partner RNs with a variety of "extenders" or multi-skilled workers. Even though care teams consist of members with various skills, when redesigning the CDM, the professional practice standards of nursing and the Code of Ethics for Nurses are key drivers to frame any model.

Patient-and-Family-Centered Care

For more than 50 years, **patient-and-family-centered care (PFCC)** has been in the health care literature. However, during the 1980s the Institute for Patient-and-Family-Centered Care (IPFCC, n.d.) partnered with researchers to develop care principles, and they pushed these principles into the health care arena through the revolutionary book *Through the patient's eyes* (Gerteis et al., 1993). PFFC is care that is organized around the patient and family. Providers partner, support, connect, and communicate with patients and families to identify and satisfy their needs and cultural preferences (Institute for Patient-and-Family-Centered Care, n.d.) and to treat symptoms and prevent suffering (Press Ganey, 2014). When the Institute of Medicine (IOM, 2001), now called the National Academies of Sciences, Engineering, and Medicine, Health and Medicine Division, included PFCC as one of its major goals for twenty-first century

---

BOX 15.5   The Eight Dimensions of Patient-Family-Centered Care

1. Respect for patient preferences, values, needs
2. Information, education, communication
3. Coordination, integration of services
4. Emotional support
5. Physical comfort
6. Family/close other involvement
7. Continuity, safe transitions between care settings (e.g., hospital to home; hospital to long-term care)
8. Access to care and services

From Institute of Medicine (IOM). (2001) *Crossing the quality chasm: A new health system for the 21st century.* Washington, DC: National Academies Press.

---

health care improvement, many health care organizations utilized the framework for their CDM (Box 15.5). Foundational to PFCC is nurses' ability to connect with the patient, their determination of patient preferences, their provision of realistic care options, and their assistance with making care decisions based on patient values versus provider values (Ortiz, 2018). Organizing care around the patient is not a new practice for nurses as many nursing theorists did formulate their theories using the patient as a major focus, resulting in patient-centered care becoming a core component of nursing.

PFCC has been studied for its relationship to patient satisfaction. The framework of Compassionate Connected Care inherent in PFCC consists of domains that are linked to clinical excellence and other concepts that identify preventive measures to mitigate the suffering of patients and increase their overall perception of care. The use of this framework provides nurse leaders with the tools to evaluate their patient satisfaction data for the purpose of reducing patient suffering (Dempsey et al., 2014).

A randomized control trial to measure the effectiveness of patient-centered care on the patient's experience after a cardiac event supported the benefits of PFCC on the satisfaction of patients across the care continuum. Approximately 200 patients were randomized to either a standard cardiac care group or person-centered care group. Results demonstrated an increase in the communication between the care provider, the patient and family, increased involvement in decision-making, and improvement in documentation for those who were

randomized to the patient care group (Wolf et al., 2019), suggesting a relationship between patient satisfaction with care and the use of a PFCC model of care.

Transitional Care Model

In the United States and other countries, many older citizens suffer from multiple chronic conditions that involve the interactions of physical, cognitive, and emotional health problems. Due to multiple comorbidities, these individuals have frequent care transitions (e.g., from home to hospital to assisted living) that involve many health care providers in different settings. To promote safe passage of senior patients between the various care continuum providers, the *transitional care model* (**TCM**) emerged as a nurse-led, team-based CDM for chronically ill older adults. The transitional care nurse (TCN) leader is typically an advanced practice, master's prepared nurse with population-specific clinical expertise. Three National Institute of Nursing Research funded randomized controlled trials using TCM have demonstrated improved quality of care outcomes and cost savings. Some notable outcomes are reduced numbers of unnecessary hospital readmissions and enhanced patient satisfaction (Naylor et al., 2018).

Patient-Centered Medical Home

A related CDM is the *patient-centered medical home* (**PCMH**). The PCMH was originally designed by the American Academy of Pediatrics to care for children with special needs with the goal of refocusing patient care from the hospital to the primary care setting. The current model has expanded to include care across the life span (Prokop et al., 2017). Approximately 25% of primary care patients have one or more chronic physical and psychiatric disorders, such as diabetes, heart disease, and psychological disorders, which can often impair the patients' capacity to manage their own care or the care of others. The use of the PCMH with this population is to decrease unnecessary primary care/specialty care visits and hospitalizations and to improve self-care management with diet, exercise, and medication adherence. The PCMH uses a nurse (i.e., care manager) to promote education and decision-making with treatment adjustments (e.g., medication management) and to track outcomes associated with the disorders. The nurse care manager connects weekly with a consultant and updates the PCMH primary care provider as needed. Nurse care managers are tasked with monitoring patients to ensure no one "falls through the cracks." After implementation of a PCMH, researchers identified improved care coordination and a reduction in hospital and emergency services admissions (Prokop et al., 2017).

INNOVATIVE MODELS

The complexity of health care delivery necessitates the use of dynamic and innovative models to ensure patient outcomes are met. The IOM's (2001) report *Crossing the quality chasm: a new health system for the 21st century* described the need for sweeping change and redesign of patient CDMs to foster innovation and improve the delivery of care. As defined by Asurakkody and Shin (2018) the term "innovative" describes an idea or product that has been reframed, something that is new and different from the original idea. Many of the innovative models have as their core component one of traditional CDMs that were previously discussed.

Virtual Nursing

In the 1870s with the invention of the telegraph, telehealth or telemedicine was first introduced into the health care environment. Since those early beginnings, the use of technology to integrate care continues to expand into urban and rural health care organizations to increase access for patients to health care services. The **virtual nursing CDM** is defined as the utilization of telecommunication technologies remotely to perform patient-centered surveillance evaluations, care interventions, and interpretation of data for the promotion of the patient's health and wellbeing. Virtual nursing is a care delivery mode that allows patients access to health care services in a financially responsible manner (American Academy of Ambulatory Care Nursing [AAACN], 2018). Over 19 years ago, the AAACN published the first telenursing scope and standards of practice for telehealth nursing. These standards outline six core roles for virtual nurses to embody: (1) patient education, (2) mentoring and education of teams, (3) surveillance of patient quality and safety using "real-time," (4) admission, (5) discharge activities, and (6) physician rounding (AAACN, 2018). The virtual nurse (VN) demonstrates competencies at the proficient and/or expert level for complex patients and has a strong acumen to lead teams, along with being technologically competent. Virtual nursing can occur in a variety of practice settings to include the home, clinics, long-term care, correctional facilities, hospitals, and essentially any setting where nursing care is needed (Cloyd & Thompson, 2020). Utilizing telephonic and video technology with high resolution, two-way audio and video communication to perform care, the VN serves as the clinical expert to support decision-making among all other members of the care delivery team (Schuelke et al., 2019).

One health care system implemented a virtually integrated care^SM (VIC) team model on two medical-surgical units at two separate hospitals. VN coverage was provided for only 12 hours per day, 5 days per week. Over a period of 2½ years after implementation of the new delivery model, both hospitals observed an increase in their patient satisfaction, teamwork between departments, emergency department throughput, length of stay, discharge times, and financial metrics. Education and mentoring of clinical nurses' efforts uncovered numerous anecdotal examples of conversations with nurses that resulted in the identification of care gaps and assistance with new procedures. This tailored mentoring became a recruitment tool for nurses coming into the unit (Denney & Evans, 2017; Schuelke et al., 2019).

Artificial Intelligence, Machine Learning, and Robotics

The use of artificial intelligence, machine learning, and robotics in the delivery of patient care are innovative technologies that are rapidly disrupting how nurses practice. Health care organizations are charged with achieving positive outcomes yet must attain these outcomes within financial margins that challenge their viability. Innovative technologies are poised to assist organizations to meet health care disruption by reducing the burden of less-value added tasks and increasing data processing, and medical information transfer for effective decision-making (American Hospital Association, 2019). Less value-added nursing activities, now completed by nurses, increases their workload and takes time away from patients; incorporating innovative technologies into the care delivery system could give time back to nurses.

Artificial intelligence (AI) is defined as a collection of technologies, that can learn, teach, perceive, and mimic the thought process of humans (Davenport & Kalakota, 2019; Robert, 2019). Many consumers have already embraced the use of various devices that recognize voice patterns to help achieve various mundane tasks in the home. In health care, the use of AI could be utilized to rank various types of data, provide applicable treatment options for care providers, and deploy a virtual assistant for nurses (Robert, 2019). **Machine learning (ML)** describes the practice of creating and utilizing algorithms to separate data, learn, and then make predictive decisions (Clipper et al., 2018). An example of ML is the use of a risk assessment tool to identify patients at risk for sepsis. Using prescribed algorithms, data are calculated in real time from medical record entries, such as nursing assessments and laboratory values. A predictive index score is then generated and based on the risk score, a prediction for patient safety risk is identified (Robert, 2019). **Robotics** describes the design, construction, and operation of robots through the integration of science and technology. As defined, robots are "re-programmable, physically embodied, intelligent and mobile systems, that can act autonomously or be teleoperated in an environment where the robot has the ability to sense" (Olaronke et al., 2017, p. 44).

A robotics company based in Austin, Texas, designed a robot to assist nurses with various mundane "hunting and gathering" tasks. The social intelligence features of the robot, Moxi, includes blinking eyes, soft curved edges, a neutral voice, and a moving head. Moxi has a robotic arm, can move through the hallways, and sense obstacles. Due to the AI integration, Moxi can learn various behavior patterns and has predictive abilities that allow for coordination of supplies with the patient's plan of care (Schwab, 2019; Stuart, 2019). During the successful beta trials of Moxi at several hospitals in Texas, team members and patients learned to appreciate the capabilities of this robot; essentially Moxi decreased the workload of nurses and other care providers (Schwab, 2019).

LEADERSHIP AND MANAGEMENT IMPLICATIONS

Fundamentally, a CDM is the way patients' needs are matched to health care resources to achieve positive clinical outcomes. Through many complex relationships, the CDM influences the quality of nursing care provided and its cost. Though multiple nursing CDMs have been developed, evidence suggests evolutionary changes are underway. Traditionally, care delivery was provided within a pure nursing framework. Over time, nursing care delivery methods were adapted to better fit external forces and the balance of the needs of patients and the needs of employing organizations. With these changes came variations in modes of delivery (e.g., team nursing, total patient care), skill mix, staffing levels, and nurse roles and accountabilities. The delivery of nursing care has become more complex as integration with other provider disciplines became essential to meet the patients' needs throughout the entire continuum of care. Future trends point to greater integration and inter-professional team collaboration models as health care reform drives changes within the health care industry.

Though the repeal, replace, or change of the Affordable Care Act (ACA) was not completed, the ACA mandates continue to alter the way health care is delivered (Vogenberg & Santilli, 2018). The Health and Medicine Division (HMD), formerly IOM, *Future of nursing report* (2010), is inclusive of the ACA's health care vision of accessible, equitable, and affordable care with a key feature being new CDMs. The themes of integration and coordination of care, addressing needs in a comprehensive manner with patients as key partners, and providing services efficiently continue to predominate and trigger a radical shift in the delivery of health care toward primary health care (Vogenberg & Santilli, 2018). Reimbursement structures and other incentives to health care providers are triggering new models and offering leadership opportunities for nurses (Porter-O'Grady, 2019).

Nursing leaders and managers need to have a broad vision to facilitate the design of CDMs that meet the objectives of cost containment, patient satisfaction, quality, and safety outcomes over the course of the care cycle. Nursing leaders are in the perfect position to lead the changes essential in care delivery redesign. Nursing, as a major percentage of the health care labor force, needs to be able to demonstrate its effectiveness in producing financial as well as clinical outcomes. The challenge to prove "value" will continue.

Mentoring staff to participate in the creation of new care delivery methods is an aspect of effective leadership. Many factors, including the environmental context, influence successful implementation of new models, and nurses need to be engaged in these quality improvement initiatives. Evidence demonstrates that professional practice models, particularly their valuing of nursing and their professional (shared) governance structures and processes, are critical to nurse satisfaction and retention. Furthermore, there is evidence that CDMs, a component of professional practice models, are associated with nurse, patient, and organizational outcomes. Nurses and nurse leaders, therefore, need to be visible and engaged when planning patient care delivery strategies at all levels of the organization. The challenge of nurse leaders is to balance risk taking and adoption of innovations with the practical necessity to be systematic, evaluative, and realistic. To assist nurse leaders with designing and adopting innovative CDMs, the American Organization for Nursing Leadership (AONL) developed a *Guiding principles for the role of the nurse in future patient care delivery* toolkit (2010). These principles outline five assumptions to guide nurse leaders: (1) use a systems approach with all disciplines involved in process and outcome models, (2) recognize that accountable care organizations will influence health care reform provisions to impact differing care delivery venues, (3) be mindful that an increasingly informed public will drive changes in care delivery based on safety concerns and outcomes, (4) remember that as health leaders gain knowledge of funding sources, they will strategically deploy funds to achieve desired outcomes, and (5) joint education of inter-professionals will become the norm to ensure shared knowledge and practice. Today these assumptions are still significant, with some assumptions emerging or peaking in health care environments.

CURRENT ISSUES AND TRENDS

The challenges for patient care in the future are massive. The work environment of the nurse is dramatically different. Cost containment and demands for quality and safety outcomes will continue to drive CDM redesign. The Donabedian S-P-O framework can be used to plan

and test model structures and processes associated with safe quality care delivery outcomes.

Clearly, forces and pressures outside of professional nursing influence care models. What is not known is which model is the best CDM for each patient care setting, and there is limited research evidence to support specific inpatient and ambulatory nursing care models (Fernandez et al., 2012). Nurses are urged to examine their patient populations, understand and embrace the business aspects of health care, and remain vigilant in analyzing emerging economic and clinical trends in order to be active participants in the creation of future patient CDMs.

A final trend worth noting is the shift toward the integration of digital tools in the practice setting, big data management, and the use of evidence to make practice decisions. With this digital integration, practice changes will be time driven and fluid. Speed of implementation of new treatment processes into practice will become the new norm and a definer of value, quality, and effectiveness of care provided to patients (Porter-O'Grady, 2019). Nurses play a critical role in facilitating this transition by encouraging knowledge exchange, shared problem-solving, and the creation and reinforcement of patient-and-family-centered goals. Nurses are exceptionally skilled at building informal and formal relationships across levels, permitting more rapid coordination, practice integration, and more effective communication. The heightened awareness of the social determinants of health on communities will continue to propel nurses to improve access, identify, connect, and implement health care resources to ensure the sustainable health of individuals and communities. Nurse leaders, therefore, are important influencers for leading CDM redesign and developing innovations.

◢ RESEARCH NOTE

Source

Havaei, F., MacPhee, M., & Dahinten, V. (2016). The effect of nursing care delivery models on quality and safety outcomes of care: A cross-sectional survey study of medical-surgical nurses. *Journal of Advanced Nursing, 75*(10), 2144–2155.

Purpose

Havaei et al. (2016) used an exploratory cross-sectional correlational methodology to study the effects of two delivery

care modes (total patient care and team nursing), and skill mix on the quality of nursing care and adverse patient outcomes. Using secondary data from a larger study, this team examined four aspects: (1) the mode of delivery of nursing care on quality of nursing care and patient outcomes, (2) skill mix on quality of nursing care and patient outcomes, (3) the moderating effect of nursing delivery model of care between workload on quality nursing care and patient outcomes, and (4) the moderating effect of skill mix between workload on quality nursing care and patient outcomes.

Continued

RESEARCH NOTE—cont'd

Sample

The Havaei team surveyed 416 clinical nurses whose practice was in acute care medical and or surgical settings across hospitals in British Columbia, Canada. A power analysis identified a sample size of 226 individuals would garner a small effect size for the multiple regression analysis that would be used.

Study Variables

The *mode of delivery of nursing care* was measured using one item that asked nurses to describe how care was delivered on their unit during their shift. Clinical nurses were asked to select either total patient care (one nurse caring for the patient) or team nursing (different care providers caring for groups of patients at one time). *Skill mix* was measured by one item that asked clinical nurses to determine the number and type of nurse that gave nursing care to patients on their unit during their shift. Types of care providers included: registered nurses (RNs), registered practical nurses (RPNs), licensed practical nurse (LPNs), and unlicensed individuals (nursing assistants [NAs]). Based on these skill mix types, the research team further categorized skill mix into skill mix with all RNs and NAs and skill mix with RNs, LPNs, and NAs.

Workload factors included staffing levels inclusive of the number of nurses available to care for the specified number of patients on the unit, acuity level (not acute or very acute), and whether the patient was completely dependent or completely independent. *Work environment factors* were measured using the 28-item Practice Environment Scale-Nursing Work Index (PES-NWI), an instrument validated by Lake (2002).

Patient outcome variables focused on nurse reported quality of care, total number of nursing tasks left undone, and the frequency of adverse events of nurse sensitive measures that included medication errors, urinary tract infections, and patient falls with injuries.

Discussion

Key findings of the study were clinical nurses practicing in a team-based mode of care delivery reported a higher number of tasks left undone when compared with reports from clinical nurses practicing in a total patient care mode of delivery. Clinical nurses in a skill mix team model that included LPNs reported greater occurrences of patient adverse events when compared to a skill mix without LPNs. When the patient acuity level was very acute, clinical nurses in a team-based model reported increased numbers of adverse patient events when compared to clinical nurses in a total patient care model. Work environment factors, such as foundations of nursing care delivery and the availability of resources were linked to patient adverse events.

This study used a cross-sectional correlational design; therefore, findings only demonstrate a relationship between the study variables, rather than causation, and are not generalizable to other study populations. Though study findings are correlational, they are supported by other research where richer skill mix is associated with improved patient outcomes. Work environment factors, along with the mode of care delivery and skill mix impacted adverse patient outcomes. These findings are also supported by other research that documents the relationship between the work environment of nurses, patient outcomes, and staffing (Griffiths et al., 2019; Stalpers et al., 2015; Twigg et al., 2019). With the impetus for health care organizations to attain high quality metrics, all contributory factors that impact quality and safety must evaluated and embraced by all nurses.

Application to Practice

Nurse leaders need to utilize research evidence to deliberately structure and advocate for the adoption of innovative nursing care delivery models and practice environments that drive exemplary patient care.

CASE STUDY

Overview

Ceremony Medical Center (CMC), an 814-bed teaching hospital utilizes Kolcaba's theory of comfort as a framework for their nursing professional practice model (PPM). The values of the organization are quality, safety, teamwork, and service and though listed on CMC documents are not evident in the PPM nor do nurses "live" the organizational values. Total patient care is the care delivery

model (CDM) for all areas. However, RNs of different experience levels have responsibilities for a group of seven to eight patients on four of the medical and surgical units, three to four patients on the four-step-down units, and one to two patients on the three-intensive care units. A nurse manager has 24/7 responsibility for two 36 bed units which serves a mixed population of patients with cardiac, renal, pulmonary, neurological, and

CASE STUDY—cont'd

gastrointestinal diagnoses. Assistant nurse managers are accountable for daily operations and, due to low staffing, must frequently have a patient assignment consisting of one to two patients. Novice nurses, those with less than 15 months of nursing experience, account for 48% of the team. The Registered nurse (RN) voluntary turnover rate for both units continues to climb above 25%. Certified nursing assistants (CNAs) are occasionally assigned to a nurse but are more likely given secretarial tasks to complete. Though responsibilities of the CNA include basic custodial care of patients, they also function as patient safety attendants and are assigned to serve as sitters for Baker Act patients or those patients at high risk for falls.

Complaints from patients and physicians are numerous and cite unsafe nursing care practices, poor transitions to and from various levels of care, and a general lack of responsiveness for the care needs of patients. Reporting of significant incidents and "near misses" have increased, with two incidents resulting in a nurse reporting the medical center to the accrediting agency for endangering the lives of patients. This prompted the accrediting agency to place the medical center on conditional accreditation. These findings trigger the service line nursing director to conduct a comprehensive assessment to ascertain the root cause.

Assessment and Findings

The assessment of the nursing director identified that the professional practice model that guides nursing practice is not fully embraced; this results in disjointed delivery of care. Timely and complete nursing assessments and reassessments, along with evidence of nursing care planning, were not identified in the electronic medical record. Consequently, nurses are unable to speak to the patient's diagnosis and medical plan of care. Novice nurses are challenged with critical thinking and effective decision-making yet can perform some care activities with limited knowledge. Though the policy of CMC requires nurses to begin discharge planning on admission to the unit, discharge education typically will not start until a discharge order is received from the physician; this frequently delays a timely discharge from CMC. Multiple caregivers perform patient care activities. However, communication of the plan of care at shift change is deficient due to a lack of continuity, numerous nurse callouts, poor problem identification, and incomplete coordination and prioritization of care activities. Inter-professional communication, specifically between physicians and nurses, is sporadic and inadequate. Nurses rarely use communication tools such

as situation, background, assessment and recommendation (SBAR) and handoff reports to standardize and share critical information. Nurses are not comfortable with delegation of tasks to CNAs and frequently assume non-nursing functions rather than communicate the patient's care needs to their CNAs. Dedicated preceptors and learning professionals to support the knowledge, skills, and attitudes of novice nurses for the purpose of growing them into competent practitioners is inadequate.

Nursing quality data indicates high rates of catheter associated urinary tract infections (CAUTI), patient falls with injury, central-line associated bloodstream infections (CLABSI), physical assaults by patients on nurses, and delays in treatment. Patient satisfaction scores continue their downward trajectory and have never attained the intended 85th percentile benchmark in over 15 months. The most recent results of the NDNQI RN survey revealed poor teamwork across units, low marks for quality of care, and insufficient staffing and resources that support top of license practice.

Professional Practice Model Enculturation and Care Delivery Redesign

To meet the care needs of patients by "living" the organizational values of quality, safety, teamwork, and service, the nursing director and the vice president of nursing agreed that the PPM needed further enculturation, while a re-design of how care is delivered was also warranted. The nursing director initiated a redesign process by forming a team consisting of RNs, CNAs, and other inter-disciplinary care providers from the two 36 bed medicine units. Using the model for improvement framework, the team clarified the goal of the project, identified changes that can demonstrate improvement, and outlined specific success metrics. Provider focus groups, a focused literature review, discussions with patient representatives, and an assessment of CDMs from other hospitals rounded out the assessment process. Team meetings were used to align nursing practice to the components of the PPM, to brief everyone about planned changes, and to listen for consensus and any new ideas.

Given the spatial layout of the two medicine units, modular nursing was the best option. A form of team nursing, modular nursing allows the clustering of similar patients, grants exposure to, and increases learning about specific patient populations that are cared for within a structural module or pod. Complexity of needed services, patient acuity, and diagnosis are used to further group patients who are admitted to each pod. Based

Continued

CASE STUDY—cont'd

on preference, members of the care team are assigned permanently to a unit but understand that rotation to the sister unit is available after a trial period of 6 months. Each pod consists of 18 patients, an experienced nurse who is partnered with a novice or agency nurse, and one or two CNAs. Shift report is taken by all members of the modular care team. This practice facilitates communication and continuity of care if one team member is off the unit or is not scheduled the next day. Daily inter-disciplinary care planning rounds facilitated by nurses, are established for each pod. The evidence-based practices of bedside shift report, hourly rounding, and focused assessments are instituted to improve monitoring and surveillance of rapidly changing patient conditions.

To increase skills performance, a new CNA level is established, and competency assessments evaluated in the simulation lab. Members of the unit's professional (shared) governance council determined the most valued CNA skills to reduce the non-nursing tasks that nurses perform. Team-building workshops to facilitate understanding of delegation responsibilities and roles were given to both RNs and CNAs. Staffing levels were refined to ensure the assistant nurse manager is free of a patient assignment. This change facilitates communication between physicians, nurses, and other members of the care team, ensures the availability of resource, and establishes effective staffing levels.

Evaluation

Process and outcome indicators that measure quality, safety, patient satisfaction, RN satisfaction, and financial metrics were established and displayed in a dashboard.

Clinical outcomes must follow successful implementation of processes. Therefore, the quality improvement project team made the decision to measure process indicators for 6 months, then quality indicators at 6 months, 1 year, 18 months, and 2 years post implementation.

Fast Forward: The End of the First Year

Nurses understand the components of the professional practice model and integrate the components into their practice. Nursing satisfaction, specifically intent to stay and perceptions of quality care delivery, improved. Nursing practice activities of assessment of psychosocial and clinical needs, evaluation of care treatments, documentation, delegation of non-nursing tasks, patient education, coordination of care, and safe transition to the next care setting are consistently identified in the electronic medical record. Agency usage is almost non-existent and novice nurse attrition is reduced by 10%. Patient satisfaction scores such as pain management, discharge preparation, and responsiveness to the care needs of patients demonstrated improvement by 24 percentage points. The number of patient falls with injury are significantly reduced, while patient assaults and delays in treatment are rare occurrences. Incidence of CAUTIs continues its downward trend, although metrics have not yet attained benchmark.

Conclusions

By using the model as an improvement framework, collaborative and deliberate planning with all stakeholders, and implementation and evaluation of adopted strategies, the enculturation of the PPM along with the redesign of the CDM was successfully achieved.

CRITICAL THINKING EXERCISE

After a 5-month search, your organization brought on a new chief nursing officer (CNO). Within 10 months of hire, all nurse leaders were part of a strategic alignment process with the CNO which resulted in clearly defined outcomes for each nurse leader. Though the PPM incorporates the theory of relationship-based care, the virtual CDM continues to interrupt workflow, exceed costs associated with the level of care, and hinder patient and family interactions. You are the nurse manager for a 72-bed orthopedic unit and your CNO has requested that you use the S-P-O Donabedian framework to determine what structures and processes need to be in place within your work environment to support exemplary VIC

for your patients. To determine your outcomes or goals, you perform patient/family and team surveys to establish preferences and needs. Major care preferences for patients and families include real-time communication with the health care team, assistance with physical needs, and a clear understanding of the roles and responsibilities of the virtual care team. For the virtual care team, their desires centered around technical challenges, resistance to the new model, and interruption of their workflow.

1. What evidence-based structures are necessary to meet your VIC goals or outcomes?
2. What evidence-based processes are necessary to meet your VIC goals or outcomes?

3. Koloroutis' (2004) relationship-based care is a theoretical framework that some Magnet hospitals use for their nursing professional practice model. What Magnet-like characteristics can you use to change the culture of your work environment to become more relationship-based?

Hint: Consider using a matrix or table such as:

Structures	Processes	Desired Outcomes

REFERENCES

Abou Hashish, E. (2017). Relationship between ethical work climate and nurses' perception of organizational support, commitment, job satisfaction and turnover intent. *Nursing Ethics, 24*(2), 151–166.

Aiken, L., Cimiotti, J., Sloane, D., Smith, H., Flynn, L., & Neff, D. (2011). Effects of nurse staffing and nurse education on patient deaths in hospitals with different nurse work environments. *Medical Care, 49*(12), 1047–1053.

Aiken, L., Sloane, D., Bruyneel, L., Van den Heede, K., Sermeus, W., & Consortium, R. (2013). Nurses' reports of working conditions and hospital quality of care in 12 countries in Europe. *International Journal of Nursing Studies, 50*(2), 143–153.

Aiken L., Sloane D., Griffiths P., Rafferty A., Bruyneel L., McHugh M., et al. (2017). Nursing skill mix in European hospitals: Cross-sectional study of the association with mortality, patient ratings, and quality of care. *BMJ Quality & Safety, 26*(7), 559–568.

Alegre, I., Berbegal-Mirabent, J., Guerrero, A., & Mas-Machuca, M. (2018). The real mission of the mission statement: A systematic review of the literature. *Journal of Management & Organization, 24*(4), 456–473.

Sabei, Al, S. Labrague, L., Miner Ross, A., Albashayreh, A., Al Masroori, F., & Al Hashmi, N. (2020). Nursing work environment, turnover intention, job burnout, and quality of care: The moderating role of job satisfaction. *Journal of Nursing Scholarship, 52*(1), 95–104.

Amadei, L. (2016). Why policies and procedures matter. *Risk Management, 63*(9), 12–13.

American Academy of Ambulatory Care Nursing (AAACN). (2018). *Scope and standards of practice for professional telehealth nursing* (6th ed.). Pitman, NJ. AAACN.

American Association of Critical-Care Nurses, (AACN) (2005). AACN standards for establishing and sustaining healthy work environments: A journey to excellence. *American Journal of Critical Care*, (14(3), 187–197).

American Hospital Association (AHA). (2019. *AI and care delivery: Emerging opportunities for artificial intelligence to transform how care is delivered.* https://www.aha.org/system/files/media/file/2019/11/Market_Insights_AI_Care_Delivery.pdf.

American Nurses Association (ANA). (2015). *Nursing scope and standards of practice,* (3rd ed.). Silver Springs, MD. Nursebooks.

American Nurses Credentialing Center (ANCC). (2017). *2019 Magnet® application manual.* Silver Springs, MD. ANCC.

American Organization for Nursing Leadership (AONL). (2010). *Toolkit for patient care delivery.* https://www.aonl.org/toolkit-future-care-delivery.

Asurakkody, T., & Shin, S. (2018). Innovative behavior in nursing context: A concept analysis. *Asian Nursing Research, 12*(4), 237–244.

Baas, L. (1992). An analysis of the writings of Janet Geister and Mary Roberts regarding the problems of private duty nursing. *Journal of Professional Nursing, 8*(3), 176–183.

Barnes, B., Barnes, M., & Sweeney, C. (2016). Putting the "meaning" in meaningful recognition of nurses: The DAISY award. *Journal of Nursing Administration, 46*(10), 508–512.

Basol, R., Hilleren-Listerud, A., & Chmielewski, L. (2015). Developing, implementing, and evaluating a professional practice model. *Journal of Nursing Administration, 45*(1), 43–49.

Case Management Society of America (CSMA). (2017). Little Rock, AR. *What is a case manager?* https://www.cmsa.org/who-we-are/what-is-a-case-manager/.

Centers for Medicare and Medicaid Services (CMS). (2019). *Hospital CAHPS (HCAHPS). https://www.cms.gov/Research-Statistics-Data-and-Systems/Research/CAHPS/HCAHPS1.*

Centers for Medicare & Medicaid Services. (CMS). (2020). *CAHPS® Hospital Survey.* https://hcahpsonline.org/.

Churchill, S., Leo, M., Brennan, E., Sellmaier, C., Kendall, J., & Houck, G. (2018). Longitudinal impact of a randomized clinical trial to improve family function, reduce maternal stress and improve child outcomes in families of children with ADHD. *Maternal & Child Health Journal, 22*(8), 1172–1182.

Cicolini, G., Comparcini, D., & Simonetti, V. (2014). Workplace empowerment and nurses' job satisfaction: A systematic literature review. *Journal of Nursing Management, 22*(7), 855–871.

Clavelle, J., O'Grady, Porter, T. Weston, M., & Verran, J. (2016). Evolution of structural empowerment: Moving from shared to professional governance. *Journal of Nursing Administration, 46*(6), 308–312.

Clipper, B., Batcheller, J., Thomaz, A., & Rozga, A. (2018). Artificial intelligence and robotics: A nurse leader's primer. *Nurse Leader, 16*(6), 379–384.

Cloyd, B., & Thompson, J. (2020). Virtual care nursing: The wave of the future. *Nurse Leader, 18*(1), 1–4.

Cole, L., & Houston, S. (1999). Linking outcomes management and practice improvement. Structured care methodologies: Evolution and use in patient care delivery. Outcomes Management for Nursing Practice, *3*(2), 53–60.

Cordo, J., & Hill-Rodriguez, D. (2017). The evolution of a nursing professional practice model through leadership support of clinical nurse engagement, empowerment, and shared decision making. *Nurse Leader, 15*(5), 325–330.

Curtis, K., Fry, M., Shaban, R., & Considine, J. (2017). Translating research findings to clinical nursing practice. *Journal of Clinical Nursing, 26*(5–6), 862–872.

Dal Molin, A., Gatta, C., Boggio Gilot, C., Ferrua, R., Cena, T., Manthey, M., & Croso, A. (2018). The impact of primary nursing care pattern: Results from a before–after study. *Journal of Clinical Nursing, 27*(5-6), 1094–1102.

Davenport, T., & Kalakota, R. (2019). The potential for artificial intelligence in healthcare. *Future Healthcare Journal, 6*(2), 94–98.

Dempsey, C., Wojciechowski, S., McConville, E., & Drain, M. (2014). Reducing patient suffering through compassionate connected care. *Journal of Nursing Administration, 44*(10), 517–524.

Denney, S., & Evans, E. (2017). Virtually integrated care: A new paradigm in patient care delivery. *Nursing Administration Quarterly, 41*(4), 288–296.

Dickerson, J., & Latina, A. (2017). Team nursing: A collaborative approach improves patient care. *Nursing, 2019*47(10), 16–17 .

Donabedian, A. (1988). The quality of care. How it can be assessed. *Journal of the American Medical Association, 260*(12), 1743.

Duffy, J. (2016). *Professional Practice Models in Nursing: Successful Health System Implementation.* Springer Publishing Company.

Eva, N., Prajogo, D., & Cooper, B. (2017). The relationship between personal values, organizational formalization and employee work outcomes of compliance and innovation. *International Journal of Manpower, 38*(2), 274–287.

Fairbrother, G., Chiarella, M., & Braithwaite, J. (2015). Models of care choices in today's nursing workplace: Where does team nursing sit?. *Australian Health Review, 39*(5), 489–493.

Fernandez, R., Johnson, M., Tran, D. T., & Miranda, C. (2012). Models of care in nursing: A systematic review. *International Journal of Evidence-Based Healthcare, 10*(4), 324–337.

Fowler, M. (2017). *Guide to Nursing's Social Policy Statement: Understanding the profession from social contract to social covenant.* American Nurses Association.

Gerteis, M., Edgman-Levitan, S., Daley, J., & Delbanco, T. (1993). *Through the patient's eyes: Understanding and promoting patient-centered care.* John Wiley & Sons, Inc.

Glassman, K. (2016). Developing and implementing a professional practice model. *Nursing Science Quarterly, 29*(4), 336–339.

Griffiths P, Maruotti, A., Recio Saucedo, A., Redfern, O., Ball, J., Briggs, J., et al., Missed Care Study Group. (2019). Nurse staffing, nursing assistants and hospital mortality: Retrospective longitudinal cohort study. *BMJ Quality & Safety*, 28, 609–617.

Gulati, R., Mikhail, O., Morgan, R., & Sittig, D. (2016). Vision statement quality and organizational performance in U.S. hospitals. *Journal of Healthcare Management, 61*(5), 335–350.

Halm, M. (2019). The influence of appropriate staffing and healthy work environments on patient and nurse outcomes. *American Journal of Critical Care, 28*(2), 152–156.

Havaei, F., MacPhee, M., & Dahinten, V. (2016). The effect of nursing care delivery models on quality and safety outcomes of care: A cross-sectional survey study of medical-surgical nurses. *Journal of Advanced Nursing, 75*(10), 2144–2155.

Heslop, L., & Lu, S. (2014). Nursing-sensitive indicators: A concept analysis. *Journal of Advanced Nursing, 70*(11), 2469–2482.

Institute of Medicine (IOM). (2001). *Crossing the quality chasm: A new health system for the 21st century.* Washington, DC: National Academies Press.

Institute of Medicine (IOM). (2010). *The future of nursing: Leading change advancing health.* Washington, DC: National Academies Press.

Institute for Patient-and-Family-Centered Care (IPFCC). (n.d.). Patient-and-family-centered care. https://www.ipfcc.org/about/pfcc.html.

Joo, J., & Huber, D. (2018). Barriers in case managers' roles: A qualitative systematic review. *Western Journal of Nursing Research, 40*(10), 1522–1542.

Kaya, N., Turan, N., & Aydın, G.Ö (2016). Innovation in nursing: A concept analysis. *Journal of Community and Public Health Nursing, 2*(1), 108–112.

King, A., Long, L., & Lisy, K. (2015). Effectiveness of team nursing compared with total patient care on staff wellbeing when organizing nursing work in acute care wards: A systematic review. *JBI Database*

of Systematic Reviews and Implementation Reports,
13(11), 128–168.

Kolcaba, K., Tilton, C., & Drouin, C. (2006). Comfort
Theory: A unifying framework to enhance the practice
environment. *Journal of Nursing Administration, 36*(11),
538–544.

Koloroutis, M. (2004). *Relationship-based care: A model for
transforming practice.* Minneapolis: Creative Healthcare
Management.

Lake, E. (2002). Development of the practice environment
scale of the Nursing Work Index. *Research in Nursing &
Health, 25*(3), 176–188.

Lasater, K., Germack, H., Small, D., & McHugh, M. (2016).
Hospitals known for nursing excellence perform better
on value-based purchasing measures. *Policy, Politics, &
Nursing Practice, 17*(4), 177–186.

Ma, C., Shang, J., & Bott, M. (2015). Linking unit
collaboration and nursing leadership to nurse outcomes
and quality of Care. *Journal of Nursing Administration,
45*(9), 435–442.

Manthey, M. (2002). *The practice of primary nursing* (2nd ed.).
Minneapolis, MN: Creative Health Care Management, Inc.

Martin, D., & Weeres, A. (2016). Building nursing role clarity
on a foundation of knowledge and knowledge application.
Healthcare Management Forum, 29(3), 107–110.

Mattei da Silva, Â. T., de Fátima Mantovani, M., Castanho
Moreira, R., Perez Arthur, J., & Molina de Souza, R. (2020).
Nursing case management for people with hypertension
in primary health care: A randomized controlled trial.
Research in Nursing & Health, 43(1), 68–78.

Mattila, E., Pitkänen, A., Alanen, S., Leino, K., Luojus, K.,
Rantanen, A., & Aalto, P. (2014). The effects of the
primary nursing care model: A systematic review. *Journal
of Nursing and Care, 3*(6), 1–12.

Maughan, E., Cowell, J., Engelke, M., McCarthy, A., Bergren,
M., Murphy, M., & Vessey, J. (2018). The vital role of
school nurses in ensuring the health of our nation's
youth. *Nursing Outlook, 66*(1), 94–96.

Muir, K. (2019). Historical perspectives informing modern
day nursing innovation and economics. *Nursing
Economic, 37*(6), 284–293.

Naylor, M., Hirschman, K., Toles, M., Jarrín, O., Shaid, E.,
& Pauly, M. (2018). Adaptations of the evidence-based
Transitional Care Model in the U.S. *Social Science &
Medicine, 213*, 28–36.

Nightingale, F. (1860). *Notes on nursing: What it is, and what
it is not.* New York. Appleton-Century.

Olds, D., Aiken, L., Cimiotti, J., & Lake, E. (2017). Association
of nurse work environment and safety climate on patient
mortality: A cross-sectional study. *International Journal
of Nursing Studies, 74*, 155–161.

Olaronke, I., Oluwaseun, O., & Rhoda, I. (2017). State of the
art: A study of human-robot interaction in healthcare.
*International Journal of Information Engineering and
Electronic Business, 9*(3), 43–55.

Ortiz, M. (2018). Patient-Centered Care: Nursing knowledge
and policy. *Nursing Science Quarterly, 31*(3), 291–295.

Park, S., Gass, S., & Boyle, D. (2016). Comparison of
reasons for nurse turnover in Magnet® and non-
Magnet hospitals. *Journal of Nursing Administration,
46*(5), 284–290.

Polit, D., & Beck, C. (2017). *Nursing research: Generating
and assessing evidence for nursing practice* (11th ed.).
Philadelphia: Wolters Kluwer | Lippincott Williams &
Wilkins.

Porter-O'Grady, T. (2019). Turning the page: Nursing in the
digital age and beyond. *Nursing Management, 50*(9),
40–47.

Pound C., Gelt V., Akiki S., Eady K., Moreau K., Momoli
F., et al. (2017). Nurse-driven clinical pathway for
inpatient asthma: A randomized controlled trial. *Hospital
Pediatrics, 7*(4), 204–213.

Press Ganey. (2014). *Reducing suffering: The path to patient-
centered care.* https://www.pressganey.com/resources/
white-papers/reducing-suffering-the-path-to-patient-
centered-care.

Press Ganey. (2020). *Capture Nursing Specific Measures.*
https://www.pressganey.com/solutions/clinical-
excellence/capture-nursing-specific-measures.

Prokop, J., LaPres, M., Barron, B., & Villasurda, J. (2017).
Implementing a health home: Michigan's experience.
Policy, Politics & Nursing Practice, 18(3), 149–157.

Reverby, S. (1987). *Ordered to care: The dilemma of American
nursing 1850–1945.* Cambridge, MA: Cambridge
University Press.

Robert, N. (2019). How artificial intelligence is changing
nursing. *Nursing Management, 50*(9), 30–39.

Schuelke, S., Aurit, S., Connot, N., & Denney, S. (2019).
Virtual nursing: The new reality in quality care. *Nursing
Administration Quarterly, 43*(4), 322–328.

Schwab, K. (2019). A hospital introduced a robot to help
nurses. They didn't expect it to be so popular. https://www.
fastcompany.com/90372204/a-hospital-introduced-a-robot-
to-help-nurses-they-didnt-expect-it-to-be-so-popular.

Slayter, S., Coventry, L., Twigg, D, & Davis, S. (2016).
Professional practice model for nursing: A review of the
literature and synthesis of key components. *Journal of
Nursing Management, 24*(2), 139–150.

Stallings-Welden, L., & Shirey, M. (2015). Predictability of a
professional practice model to affect nurse and patient
outcomes. *Nursing Administration Quarterly, 39*(3),
199–210.

Stalpers, D., de Brouwer, B., Kaljouw, M., & Schuurmans, M. (2015). Associations between characteristics of the nurse work environment and five nurse-sensitive patient outcomes in hospitals: A systematic review of literature. *International Journal of Nursing Studies, 52*(4), 817–835.

Stimpfel, A., Sloane, D., McHugh, M., & Aiken, L. (2016). Hospitals known for nursing excellence associated with better hospital experience for patients. *Health Services Research, 51*(3), 1120–1134.

Stuart, S. (2019). When nurses are busy, it's Moxi the robot to the rescue. https://www.pcmag.com/news/when-nurses-are-busy-its-moxi-the-robot-to-the-rescue.

Swan, B., Haas, S., & Jessie, A. (2019). Care coordination: Roles of registered nurses across the care continuum. *Nursing Economic, 37*(6), 317–323.

Tang, J., & Hudson, P. (2019). Evidence-based practice guideline: Nurse retention for nurse managers. *Journal of Gerontological Nursing, 45*(11), 11–19.

Tiedeman, M. (2004). Traditional models of care delivery: What have we learned?. *Journal of Nursing Administration, 34*(6), 291–297.

Twigg, D., Kutzer, Y., Jacob, E., & Seaman, K. (2019). A quantitative systematic review of the association between nurse skill mix and nursing-sensitive patient outcomes in the acute care setting. *Journal of Advanced Nursing, 75*(12), 3404–3423.

Ulep, K. (2018). The nurse leader's pivotal role in retaining millennial nurses. *Journal of Nursing Administration, 48*(12), 604–608.

Vogenberg, F., & Santilli, J. (2018). Healthcare trends for 2018. *American Health and Drug Benefits, 11*(1), 48–55.

Weberg, D. (2009). Innovation in healthcare: A concept analysis. *Nursing Administration Quarterly, 33*(3), 227–237.

Wessel, S., & Manthey, M. (2015). *Primary nursing: Person-centered care delivery system design*. Minneapolis, MN: Creative Health Care Management, Inc.

Wharton, G., Berger, J., & Williams, T. (2016). A tale of 2 units: Lessons in changing the care delivery model. *Journal of Nursing Administration, 46*(4), 176–180.

Whelan, J. C. (2012). When the business of nursing was the nursing business: The private duty registry system, 1900–1940. *Online Journal of Issues in Nursing, 17*(2), 1–1.

Winslow, S., Cook, C., Eisner, W., Hahn, D., Maduro, R., & Morgan, K. (2019). Care delivery models: Challenge to change. *Journal of Nursing Management, 27*(7), 1438–1444.

Wolf, A., Vella, R., & Fors, A. (2019). The impact of person-centered care on patients' care experiences in relation to educational level after acute coronary syndrome: Secondary outcome analysis of a randomised controlled trial. *European Journal of Cardiovascular Nursing, 18*(4), 299–308.

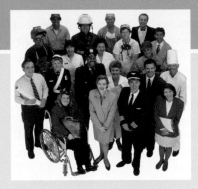

Case and Population Health Management

Ellen Fink-Samnick, Teresa M. Treiger

 http://evolve.elsevier.com/Huber/leadership

Events of recent decades have thrown the health care system into a radical reformation. This revolution continues to unfold in ever-changing ways. Care delivery has shifted from acute institution-based interventional care to a patient-centered primary care model where quality-driven prevention and outpatient management are the preferred method of operating. Case and population health management (PHM) are multidisciplinary by nature. Nurses provide these services and work in these care delivery models, as do many other disciplines (see Chapter 15).

The modern era of case, disease, and PHM began in the early 1990s. The effectiveness of what was called case management (CM) in producing quality and cost containment outcomes began to be noticed anecdotally by providers in the field. More importantly, it was noticed by health insurance companies that came to believe it worked. However, CM services were rarely paid for outside of rehabilitation and some social services areas, which severely limited the widespread implementation of CM and inhibited care integration. Despite funding restrictions, the belief in the effectiveness of CM spurred research and the development of the knowledge base and evidence for practice. Major professional, certification, and trade associations have also grown in this time period.

The field split first into CM and disease management (DM) (Huber, 2005). With the criticism that not all health conditions, such as behavioral health, are "diseases," the term **DM** was dropped in favor of **PHM**. Rigorous research and federal government–funded demonstration grants continued to solidify the evidence base for practice.

When necessary services other than acute care are actually added to/provided for in the mix of health care,

it is difficult to demonstrate cost savings. However, CM, DM, and PHM strategies all have shown positive clinical outcomes. What is clear is that **care coordination** is the core element common to all provider interventions in CM, DM, and PHM.

DEFINITIONS

Case management (CM): "A collaborative process of assessment, planning, facilitation, care coordination, evaluation, and advocacy for options and services to meet an individual's and family's comprehensive health needs through communication and available resources to promote patient safety, quality cost-effective outcomes" (Case Management Society of America, 2017a).

Disease management (DM): Chronic DM is an "integrated care approach to managing illness which includes screenings, check-ups, monitoring and coordinating treatment, and patient education. It can improve your quality of life while reducing your health care costs if you have a chronic disease by preventing or minimizing the effects of a disease" (HealthCare.gov, n.d.).

Population health management (PHM): "A population health management program strives to address health needs at all points along the continuum of health and well-being through participation of, engagement with and targeted interventions for the population. GOAL: Maintain or improve the physical and psychosocial well-being of individuals through cost-effective and tailored health solutions" (Population Health Alliance, n.d.). A more succinct definition is "the process of addressing population health needs and controlling problems at a population level" (Nash et al., 2016).

BACKGROUND

Distinguishing Components of the Health Care Management Continuum

This chapter primarily discusses CM and DM. Before launching into these individual areas, it is essential to frame the health care management continuum and provide perspective on where CM and DM reside within and relate to the whole of PHM.

The health care management continuum (or spectrum as it is sometimes referred) is not synonymous with the continuum of health care practice settings or continuum of care. Although health care management is practiced across the continuum of care, the depth and scope of these services are often driven by the primary purpose of the organization or department (e.g., acute care hospital, emergency department, managed care organization) and the organizational resources available to take on the challenge of these services.

The health care management continuum is better known as PHM. PHM is the overarching umbrella under which CM and DM exist, along with a number of other health management initiatives.

Generally speaking, CM programs serve a smaller percentage of the overall population. Enrollees are complex from a medical–behavioral, health–social vulnerability perspective. Health plans often target the top 5% to 10% high utilizers of their population for CM consideration. The case manager performs an initial screening followed by an in-depth individual assessment involving the client, family caregiver, and other care team members. From the information gathered a CM plan of care is developed. This plan includes highly individualized goals and desired outcomes. DM programs serve a larger percentage of patients whose main problem is one or more chronic condition(s). These individuals generally have similar primary needs regarding health condition education and accommodation strategies. Assessments focus on health condition–specific issues, and programs take a more standardized approach to education and resources. Table 16.1 contains definitions and additional distinguishing characteristics.

CASE MANAGEMENT

CM evolved from a chain of social developments and historical events that made apparent the health, social, and human service needs of disadvantaged, ill, and injured populations through the identification and provision of social services and coordination of care (Treiger and Fink-Samnick, 2013, 2016). Although initially not formally labeled as CM, this history provides a rich context for understanding how CM evolved into what it is today, intertwined with social and legislative events, trends, and changes.

Before government-sponsored interventions, government programs were not addressing the most basic human needs in an organized manner. The federal government had not yet expanded into areas of social support or health care realms, and so efforts to provide social assistance and supportive services for individuals in need were humanitarian and grassroots in nature. Charitable and community-based organizations with wealthy benefactors began to address and fill the local population's needs. The history of caring for the disadvantaged arose from the context of social–political–industrial changes, which piqued more liberal attitudes of social consciousness.

Landmark Legislation

A major influence on CM practice was the continuous stream of socially motivated legislation beginning with the 1935 Social Security Act and extending through to the Patient Protection and Affordable Care Act of (2010) (ACA). These laws put both federal and state governments—as well as newly created regulatory agencies—in a position of responsibility for support and care of the general population. Accompanying these major pieces of legislation was the demand for accountability, service quality, and consumer protection. The role of the case manager (also identified as a service or care coordinator), was first seen in the school setting with the Education for All Handicapped Children Act, (Library of Congress, 1975). Passage of federal and state law mandated CM services for elders (Older Americans Act, 1965), the mentally ill (the Community Mental Health Centers Act, 1963), and the developmentally disabled (the Developmentally Disabled Assistance and Bill of Rights Act, 1975), as noted in the classic resource by Weil and Karls (1985). The ACA further leveraged the concept of case management, envisioning roles within various programs, including the Patient Centered Medical Home (PCMH) and Accountable Care Organizations (ACOs).

CM is not merely the outcome of a single event, piece of legislation, company's risk reduction strategy, or a

TABLE 16.1   Case Management, Disease Management, and Population Health Management Side by Side

Case Management	Disease Management	Population Health Management
"…A collaborative process of assessment, planning, facilitation, care coordination, evaluation, and advocacy for options and services to meet an individual's and family's comprehensive health needs through communication and available resources to promote patient safety, quality cost-effective outcomes."*	Chronic disease management is an "integrated care approach to managing illness which includes screenings, check-ups, monitoring and coordinating treatment, and patient education. It can improve your quality of life while reducing your health care costs if you have a chronic disease by preventing or minimizing the effects of a disease" (HealthCare.gov, n.d.).	Population health management (PHM): "A population health management program strives to address health needs at all points along the continuum of health and well-being through participation of, engagement with and targeted interventions for the population. GOAL: Maintain or improve the physical and psychosocial well-being of individuals through cost-effective and tailored health solutions" (Population Health Alliance, n.d.).
• CMSA definition is used by URAC and NCQA although multiple CM definitions exist • Relies on client-centered assessment, planning, facilitation, care coordination, evaluation, and advocacy • Standards of practice • Individual certifications • Program accreditation and certification available	• Multiple DM definitions • DM program usually focuses on single condition • Relies on a structured system of interventions that focus on a specific condition • No standards of practice • Program content and interventions are evidence and guideline based • Program accreditation and certification available	• Multiple PHM definitions • PHM is a term that overarches the spectrum of health care management • Practice standards exist for components within PHM • Certification and accreditation programs exist for components within PHM

DM, Disease management; *NCQA*, National Committee for Quality Assurance; *PHM*, population health management; *URAC*, Utilization Review Accreditation Commission.
*Data from Case Management Society of America (CMSA). (2016). *Standards of practice for case management.* Little Rock, AR: Author; Disease management. HealthCare.gov. (n.d.). *Chronic disease management.* https://www.healthcare.gov/glossary/chronic-disease-management/; Population health management. Population Health Alliance. (n.d.). *PHM-defined.* https://populationhealthalliance.org/research/understanding-population-health/.

particular professional affiliation. CM is an organically developed practice specialty; it is an insightful response to the interplay of biology, psychology, sociology, health care system factors, and the influences exerted on individuals with complex illnesses and injuries.

Case Management Models

A single and universally accepted CM model does not exist. The diversity of practice models stems from there being multiple definitions of CM. Having infiltrated virtually every practice setting and area of specialization across the health care continuum, it seemed to be an unrealistic expectation that a single model could garner global agreement. However, this assumption hinged on the definition and characteristics of the practice models themselves. Among other influencers is the lack of

title protection for case managers, resulting in the widespread misapplication of the case manager job title.

Contemporary approaches, defined on a foundation of practice competencies, have been introduced. One model sparked the notion that a universal practice paradigm is not only possible but is essential to the continued growth of professional CM practice. This section addresses the background and characteristics of CM models and highlights the current trend of practice models being general to practice settings and competency-based practice models.

Practice Models Background

There are a very large number of identifiable CM practice models. Some are nursing models, others are non-nursing models, and still others are team oriented.

The core elements of CM models center on a case manager who coordinates, and monitors care rendered to clients by multiple health care providers and services in an attempt to decrease service fragmentation and improve the quality of care.

By definition, CM is identified as a cycle. The CM process steps align with components of the nursing process. The CM process identifies needs, risks, and resources, and coordinates care and services while educating the client–caregiver to be better self-advocates for health care. CM is designed to support and foster an individual through the health care system using patient-focused care coordination strategies. "Case management should be considered a bridge, not a crutch" (Treiger, 2012). The CM process may be identified differently because of proprietary branding, and it is affected by legislation, regulation, organizational policy, and care setting. However, at its foundation is an approach that defines the various parts of the CM process. Voluntary practice standards provide a frame for qualifications and expectations in all health care practice settings.

Weil and Karls (1985) identified eight main service components common to all CM models:
1. Client identification and outreach
2. Individual assessment and diagnosis
3. Service planning and resource identification
4. Linking clients to needed services
5. Service implementation and coordination
6. Monitoring service delivery
7. Advocacy
8. Evaluation

These components remain a part of the basic CM process framework to the present day.

CM exists in many contexts, settings, and programs. This includes but is not limited to inpatient care, payer-based, ACOs, employer-based, workers' compensation, social services, independent practice, for-profit companies, non-profit organizations, PCMHs, nursing practice, public health nursing, home health care agencies, maternal–child care, and behavioral health settings.

CM programs incorporate a variety of key activities, some of which vary according to practice setting. These activities include (but are not limited to):
• Identification and screening of participants
• Assessment
• Needs identification
• Planning
• Service and product acquisition and implementation
• Coordination of care
• Ongoing monitoring

These and other activities focus on the achievement of client and organizational outcomes that should be accomplished within effective and appropriate time frames and through efficient utilization of available resources. The time span for CM engagement may be for an episode of care in a single care setting (e.g., acute hospital, rehabilitation) lasting a few days/weeks or may span across care settings (e.g., ACOs) over a number of years or for life. In the setting of patient-centered primary care, a client may engage with a case manager for multiple distinct episodes of care or for years of management due to the client's complexity of needs profile.

A model of CM may be designed for a large, rather generic target group or population (e.g., hospitalized, long-term care, chronic care, rehabilitation) or for a specified segment on the health care continuum (e.g., an episode in one setting, in one organization, or for the whole continuum). Historically, these CM models specify organizational policies and processes for care delivery, resource use, and job responsibilities based on general position descriptions. Depending on the organization's care process, the case manager may or may not be a direct care provider.

Many types of CM models and labels are found in literature. There are discipline-specific models as well as generally accepted overarching models. Two factors are common across all CM models: The core component is coordination of care, and the core principle is advocacy. There are fairly common process elements in CM models in addition to coordination of care, advocacy, brokering of services, and resource management. Models may be tailored to fit unique target groups (e.g., vulnerable populations, care setting) or discipline-specific factors.

Nursing and health care models tend to focus on the management of health/illness or disease, or the rehabilitation needs of an individual or population. These models are sometimes called medical models, medical–social models, acute care nursing CM models, or DM models. There has been some confusion in the nursing literature about whether CM is a care delivery model or an intervention that entails a process. In both nursing and social work, there is a differentiation between CM designed to deliver services and CM designed to coordinate the provision of services. This is a key distinction that impacts staffing and roles.

Several frameworks and other methods of classifying activities have been considered when discussing CM models. Because of the variability in how CM programs are designed and administered, classification into models helps describe—as well as compare and contrast—each type. Using distinctive classifications, CM models may be understood relative to perspective (e.g., organization, setting based), scope (e.g., services delivered within an organization, cross-continuum), and time (e.g., single or multiple episode of care). A methodology for consistent classification of CM practice models has neither been proposed nor accepted. The likelihood of universal acceptance is dim within the current health care context due to the issues associated with the variety of professions practicing CM, competing professional organizations, and the multitude of available individual certifications, among a number of other important influences. Unfortunately, there is no common understanding about what is meant by "doing case management."

Seminal Nursing Case Management Models

There are two historical nursing CM programs cited in nursing literature as forerunners of modern-day nursing CM. These programs are the *New England Medical Center (NEMC) model* and the *Carondelet St. Mary's model*. The NEMC model is considered to be acute care nursing CM, whereas the Carondelet model is a community-based model.

The NEMC model is an extension of primary nursing methodology referred to as nursing CM. It focuses on the acute care episode and is a hospital-based model of CM. It leverages principles of planning and management from engineering and other fields to extend primary nursing into outcomes management.

Carondelet St. Mary's Community Nursing Network, or the Arizona Model (Forbes, 1999), used professional nurse case managers (baccalaureate and master's level) organized as a nursing health maintenance organization (HMO) at the hub of a network to broker services. This model type is known as a beyond-the-walls, medical–social, across-the-continuum of care model. It is best known for its innovative work in moving beyond the inpatient episode of care and into across-the-continuum of care (Cline, 1990).

Social Work Models

CM has been integral to social work since the founding of the profession (Herman, 2013). From their roots in charitable efforts there has been considerable evolution in CM models across the social work profession. Originally known as "social casework," the intervention was used to track the growing needs, progress, and changes for each person. The emphasis has traditionally been on society's most vulnerable populations. These persons are at risk of poor physical, psychological, or social health. Examples include individuals with chronic physical and/or mental illness, intellectual and/or physical disability, and housing insufficiency. By the 1980s, use of the term caseworker was on the wane as use of the term case manager was on the rise (Summers, 2016).

The function of CM remains part of most social work jobs and constitutes a core function of—and specialty within—social work practice. In 2013, standards of practice were developed by the National Association of Social Workers (NASW) to further elaborate on the distinctions for CM from the lens of social work. The six guiding principles are (1) person-centered services, (2) primacy of the client–social worker (SW) relationship, (3) person-in-environment framework, (4) strengths perspective, (5) collaborative teamwork, and (6) intervention at the micro, mezzo, and macro levels of practice (NASW, 2013, pp. 17–18).

More than a dozen different models of contemporary social work CM have been identified in the literature (including medical, social advocacy, managed care, outreach, ecological, intensive, and clinical) (Berger, 2015; Herman, 2013; Summers, 2016). Those most commonly mentioned include: brokerage, primary therapist, interdisciplinary team, comprehensive, and strengths.

The **brokerage model** emphasizes the case manager's traditional linkage function. Clients are linked to a network of providers and service coverage using assessment and referral to ensure the availability of service activities. The case manager plans a comprehensive service package and negotiates through barriers that prevent clients from accessing needed services.

In the **primary therapist model**, the case manager's relationship to the client is primarily therapeutic, and CM functions are undertaken as a part or an extension of therapeutic intervention. The client has one person to relate to about treatment, service access, and case coordination. However, the therapist may feel that CM is a secondary activity to therapeutic work (Weil and Karls, 1985).

The **interdisciplinary team model** uses a specialized team of various professional disciplines in which each member has a specific responsibility for service activities in their area of expertise. Team structures vary considerably. In some, all case managers on the team are interchangeable and serve the total group of clients. Other programs consist of multidisciplinary teams of up to six different professions, often driven by client-specific issues and needs. One team member is identified as the lead, with the other members combining their knowledge to share information about the client.

The **comprehensive service center model** is used in agencies that provide comprehensive services and community-based programming that can include psychosocial support, vocational training, rehabilitation, and care coordination. Examples of settings include community health centers, community-focused programs, continuing care communities (e.g., nursing homes, assisted living facilities), and public housing programs. Case managers in these practice settings may engage in high levels of advocacy, often interacting with members of the client's health care team from other agencies and/or programs.

Interdisciplinary Models

A growing number of interdisciplinary models for CM collaboration exist across practice settings. These models blend the unique competencies and knowledge that underlie nursing and social work education, a full listing of which are shown in Box 16.1. The strength of the social work profession lies in its ability to assess human behavior of patient and families in the context of the social environment. Social work's lens encompasses a multidimensional perspective, which incorporates the biological, psychological, sociological, and spiritual domains (Ashford and LeCroy, 2017). Skilled in psychopathology, and the clinical minutia of behavioral health symptoms, SWs are able to evaluate the premorbid condition of a client's unique situation. In addition, they possess understanding of available community resources and how to access them. Nursing addresses understanding of the pathophysiology of illness with the core of practice to deliver holistic patient-focused care incorporating assessment, diagnosis, outcomes/planning, implementation, and evaluation.

The CM **dyad team model**—composed of a nurse case manager and SW—has been found in hospitals.

BOX 16.1   Professional Competencies of Nursing and Social Work

Nursing
- Clinical judgment
- Advocacy and moral agency
- Caring practices
- Collaboration
- Systems thinking
- Response to diversity
- Facilitation of learning
- Clinical inquiry

Social Work
- Demonstrate ethical and professional behavior
- Engage diversity and difference in practice
- Advance human rights and social, economic, and environmental justice
- Engage in practice-informed research and research-informed practice
- Engage in policy practice
- Engage with individuals, families, groups, organizations, and communities
- Assess individuals, families, groups, organizations, and communities
- Intervene with individuals, families, groups, organizations, and communities
- Evaluate practice with individuals, families, groups, organizations, and communities

Data from American Association of Critical-Care Nurses (AACN). (n.d.). *AACN Synergy Model for patient care.* https://www.aacn.org/nursing-excellence/aacn-standards/synergy-model; Council on Social Work Education. (2015). *Educational policy and accreditation standards for baccalaureate and master's social work programs.* Alexandria, VA: Council on Social Work Education Commission on Accreditation, Commission on Educational Policy.

The dyad structure presents an opportunity for nurses and SWs to integrate their strengths and expertise in a collaborative patient-centered effort (Carr, 2009). These two helping professions align the power of their respective clinical knowledge: social work's proficiency in psychopathology, psychosocial issues, and resource linkage with nursing's emphasis on pathophysiology and the disease process. Both disciplines share the innate value of expertise in empathic listening, advocacy, and critical thinking. This skill set is a forceful combination when used to collaborate with team members in their efforts to evaluate, manage, plan, treat, and coordinate important aspects of the patient's care (Carr, 2009). There is some variation in roles and functions assigned to each discipline, with the distinct scope of job responsibilities defined by each organization.

Through its unique structure, the nurse and social work dyad provides the implementation of collaborative interventions that focus on (1) minimization of inpatient transitions, (2) reduction of cost by decreasing the length of stay, (3) promotion of patient and family satisfaction through efforts of advocacy, and (4) enhanced discharge planning (Carr, 2009).

Hospitals are also increasingly motivated to address readmissions and safe care transitions. Both of these issues are greatly affected by *social determinants*. Social determinants of health (SDoH) are defined by the World Health Organization (2019) as "the conditions in which people are born, grow, live, work and age. These circumstances are shaped by the distribution of money, power, and resources at global, national and local levels. The social determinants of health are mostly responsible for health inequities—the unfair and avoidable differences in health status seen within and between countries." The five domains associated with these non-clinical social service needs, are among the costliest and most complex for health care organizations to care for:

1. Economic stability
2. Education
3. Health care access and quality
4. Neighborhood and built environment
5. Social and community content (HealthyPeople.gov, 2019a)

Current literature has identified that inclusion of these factors, and attention to the SDoH, can lead to a pronounced effect on calculated hospital readmission rates for patients across disease states (Fink-Samnick, 2019b; Gillespie, 2016; Hu et al., 2014; Nagasako et al., 2014; Rice, 2016). When barriers to access to care (e.g., poverty, housing insufficiency, health literacy, medication adherence) are clearly identified by the nurse and SW, specific goals can be established, system processes can be developed or changed, and initiatives can be set into motion to provide patients with safe transitions (Ellsworth, 2015).

Healthy People 2020

The government-sponsored program known as Healthy People "provides science-based, 10-year national objectives for improving the health of all Americans. For 3 decades, Healthy People has established benchmarks and monitored progress over time in order to:

- Encourage collaborations across communities and sectors.
- Empower individuals toward making informed health decisions.
- Measure the impact of prevention activities (HealthyPeople.gov, 2019b).

Healthy People 2020 is a 10-year agenda for improving the nation's health and is the result of local, state, and federal planning processes. A key feature is the engagement of local and state communities to reflect the input from diverse groups (HealthyPeople.gov, 2019b).

The Chronic Care Model

The one general, overarching interdisciplinary model that is becoming widely accepted as the generic CM model is Wagner's **Chronic Care Model** (Improving Chronic Illness Care, 2006–2019). The Chronic Care Model addresses concerns about how to manage chronic illnesses. The six elements of the health care system that encourage quality chronic illness care are the community, the health system, self-management support, delivery system design, decision support, and clinical information systems. The specific concepts related to the six elements are patient safety, cultural competency, care coordination, community policies, and CM. CM is an attractive strategy because it is aimed at care coordination and decreased system-related fragmentation.

A close relative of the Chronic Care Model is the **Collaborative Care Model**. The latter is actively being implemented in primary care practices to address the increased costs for and numbers of patients with co-occurring physical and mental health needs. Patients who have a co-occurring behavioral health condition receive intervention from the health care system significantly more frequently, with bills that are anywhere from 50% to 175% higher than similarly ill patients without a behavioral health condition (Gupta, 2015; Milliman, 2014). Collaborative models for mental and physical health use a team approach to deliver care. The general features of Collaborative Care models are (Bullock et al., 2017):

- Screening for mental health conditions
- Assessing and documenting baseline symptoms using valid instruments for mental health
- Provision of patient and family education to support self-management
- Provision of clinical support and supervision

In the Collaborative Care Model, dedicated team members address the needs of patients though a comprehensive and strategic care delivery process. Included in the team are a primary care provider, a case manager who is trained in behavioral health, and psychiatric consultants and/or behavioral health specialists (Unützer et al., 2013). This comprehensive approach to care serves as a proactive means to screen and track mental health conditions within the primary care setting.

Outcomes indicate that the Collaborative Care Model is clinically sound and cost effective in treating patients with comorbid conditions, including depression and/or anxiety, along with a chronic medical condition (e.g., diabetes, congestive heart failure) (Eghaneyan et al., 2014; Fortney et al., 2015; Robert Wood Johnson Foundation, 2011; Unützer et al., 2013). Hospital readmissions have been reduced by nearly 40%, with a significant decrease in associated costs of care (Epstein Becker Green, 2015).

The new generation of interprofessional teams. The concept of the interprofessional team is rapidly emerging in the literature. The Health and Medicine Division of the National Academies of Sciences, Engineering, and Medicine (formally the Institute of Medicine) discussed the obligation of academic health centers to conduct interdisciplinary education and patient care. This triggered an emphasis on interdisciplinary collaboration toward population health (Interprofessional Education Collaborative [IPEC], 2016).

Concerns have been raised about how the terminology of multidisciplinary, interdisciplinary, and related team approaches were used interchangeably. IPEC discusses Interprofessional Collaboration as the term of art and a unique domain (IPEC, 2016; Treiger and Fink-Samnick, 2016). The goal is to prepare health professions students for deliberately working together, with the common aim of building a safer and better patient-centered and population-oriented US health care system (IPEC, 2016).

Interprofessional teams refer to care delivered by intentionally created, usually relatively small work groups in health care. The teams are recognized by others, as well as by themselves, as having a collective identity and shared responsibility for a patient or group of patients. Examples include distinct teams for rapid response, palliative care, and primary care (IPEC, 2016). These teams are different from many teams found in interdisciplinary models, where members of only two different disciplines (such as nurses and doctors) might partner with or communicate with each other about the care of select patients. The four competencies identified for interprofessional teams are: values/ethics for interprofessional practice, roles/responsibilities, interprofessional communication, and teams and teamwork (IPEC, 2016).

Outcomes demonstrating the success of interprofessional teams are in the early stages, with the verdict still out on long-term acceptance across the industry. The implications for CM are vast, particularly with close alignment of its standards of practice with the IPEC principles. Sustainability will ultimately be driven by how the health care sector and its unique stakeholders interpret and operationalize the new term *interprofessional* as a construct (Treiger and Fink-Samnick, 2016). A number of demonstration projects are in process. Reports and funding opportunities are available on the IPEC website (https://www.ipecollaborative.org/about-ipec.html).

Competency-Based Models

In order for CM practice to progress in step with or ahead of general health care evolution, thought leaders must continuously generate theoretical frameworks and practical solutions to address the challenges of health care delivery, including definition of best practice, terminology (e.g., common language), dedication of resources (e.g., dosage), expected outcomes, and qualifications for professional practice (e.g., education, experience, credentials). In order to provide high quality care continuity, case managers need to speak the same language across the care continuum (Treiger and Fink-Samnick, 2016).

Rather than focus on care setting or organizational priorities as the driver of CM scope and practice, competency-based models approach practice through a lens of qualities and characteristics that contribute to practice excellence. As noted by the Case Management Society of America (CMSA, 2017b), case managers require specific knowledge of the CM process as well as a variety of skills in order to apply their expertise effectively. The most recognizable CM-specific competency framework is COLLABORATE.

The COLLABORATE model. This model builds and supports competent professional practice through the identification and application of essential skills, behaviors, and characteristics. Because it is a model based on characteristics and key elements, the paradigm integrates into existing CM processes and programs across the entire care continuum. COLLABORATE is an acronym identifying the competencies that are important to master for professional CM practice. The acronym stands for *C*ritical thinking, *O*utcomes-driven, *L*ifelong learning, *L*eadership, *A*dvocacy, *B*ig picture orientation, *O*rganized, *R*esource awareness, *A*nticipatory, *T*ransdisciplinary, and *E*thical–Legal (Treiger and Fink-Samnick, 2013; 2016).

Independent of health care's ongoing challenges, case managers must be sufficiently agile to frame (and reframe) professional practice in order to facilitate a client's best outcomes. This is why defining a competency-based CM model, which fits into any setting of care and applies to all populations, is essential. Ultimately, this competency-based model elevates the quality of practice and contributes to optimal CM and health care outcomes (Treiger and Fink-Samnick, 2013). Each competency and the associated key elements of the COLLABORATE model are displayed in Table 16.2.

Other Case Management Models

CM is practiced across the transitions of care, including but not limited to:

- ACOs,
- PCMHs,
- primary care,
- long-term care,
- rehabilitation,
- occupational health,
- workers' compensation, and
- pharmacies.

There are many care settings in which CM is practiced. However, a different setting of care does not necessarily mean another CM model has been created. In some models, the functions of CM, utilization review (UR), and disease management (DM) overlap. The overlap and distinctions between these areas result in organizational challenges. Policies, procedures, and processes are designed to clarify desired work flow in order to eliminate the risk of redundancy.

Insurance models may be divided into **brokerage, gatekeeper**, catastrophic, managed care, and government models. The brokerage model includes an emphasis on linkage to resources but with no provision of direct services. It is similar to the broker in other social work models except for a strong emphasis on conserving benefits utilization.

A **gatekeeper** model is defined as an informal, though widely used, primary care CM model health plan. In this model, all care from providers other than the primary care provider (except for true emergencies) must be authorized by the primary care provider before care is rendered (Kongstvedt, 2013). Cost savings are realized by managing care, including advocating for less costly but more appropriate services by not authorizing the requested higher-cost services. Rather than facilitating access, gatekeepers restrict access as a means to control utilization, which ostensibly controls costs but may just control short-term expenditures. Although there are variations in department configuration, many managed care plans have a medical management department under which a complex—also referred to as catastrophic—CM team exists.

Catastrophic CM is focused on complex and **catastrophic** illness or injury (e.g., spinal cord injury, traumatic brain injury, chronic degenerative neurological disease, medical–behavioral health dual diagnoses) and applies primarily to managed care, workers' compensation, and life-care planning. It is designed to manage and maximize insurance and health care benefits, which may be capped at a lifetime maximum. Screening, data mining, referrals, and other red flag strategies are leveraged to detect the potential for high-cost cases and to interact with clients and service providers proactively to optimize and economize the health services used (CMSA, 2016).

In **managed care** models, prospective or capitated reimbursement systems often place providers in the position of carrying financial risk. This creates pressure on providers to control total costs, provide and promote prevention-oriented services, and substitute lower-cost services, preferably without sacrificing quality. The type of managed care organization dictates the degree to which case managers directly interface with clients and providers.

In the **government model**, federal, state, and local agencies manage and reimburse health care via programs such as Medicare, Medicaid, and workers' compensation. Often management of these programs is handled by established health plans that create separate lines of business for government plans.

Case Management's Established Resources of Accountability

CM practice includes established resources of accountability that set both a context and hierarchy for CM practice. Included in this grouping are state licensure boards, accreditation organizations offering organizational credentialing, plus credentialing bodies, employers, and professional associations. This scope of this listing

TABLE 16.2   COLLABORATE Competencies and Key Elements

Acronym	Competency	Key Elements
C	Critical thinking	Out of the box creativity Analytical Methodical approach
O	Outcome driven	Patient outcomes Strategic goal setting Evidence-based practice
L	Lifelong learning	Valuing • Academia and advanced degrees • Professional development • Evolution of knowledge requirements for new and emerging trends (e.g., technology, innovation, reimbursement) • Practicing at top of licensure and/or certification • Acknowledging no one case manager can and does know all
L	Leadership	Professional identity Self-awareness Professional communication: verbal/non-verbal Team coordinator: a unifier rather than a divider
A	Advocacy	Patient Family Professional
B	Big picture orientation	Bio-psycho-social-spiritual assessment Macro (policy) impact on micro (individual) intervention
O	Organized	Efficient Effective
R	Resource awareness	Utilization management Condition/population specific Management of expectations per setting
A	Anticipatory	Forward thinking Proactive versus reactive practice Self-directed
T	Transdisciplinary	Transcending • Professional disciplines • Across teams • Across the continuum
E	Ethical–legal	Licensure Certification Administrative standards Organizational policies and procedures Ethical codes of conduct

Data from Treiger, T.M., & Fink-Samnick, E. (2016). *COLLABORATE for professional case management: A universal competency-based paradigm.* Philadelphia, PA: Wolters Kluwer.

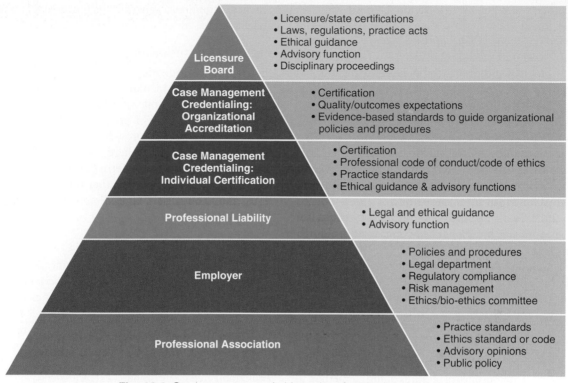

Fig. 16.1 Case management's hierarchy of authority oversight.

encompasses professional regulations and practice acts, codes of ethics, standards of practice, and employer policies and procedures. The actions of each entity inform the foundational pillars of CM practice (Fink-Samnick, 2019a). A graphic presentation of the official hierarchy of oversight for case managers appears in Fig. 16.1.

Case Management Practice Standards, Code of Conduct, and Program Accreditation
Practice Standards

CM practice has expanded at an accelerated rate in order to meet the evolving needs of health care and social services and proliferated across various health care and payer settings and practice models. As it grew and developed, it is essential to recognize that although these programs were frequently referred to as CM, the actual functions and activities of staff were often not reflective of the full scope of CM practice. Department and job titles were often grouped together within overarching care management strategies due, in part, to name recognition. It appears that little attention was given to ensuring CM

departments and jobs were aligned with CM practice standards (Treiger and Fink-Samnick, 2013).

Two CM-specific **standards of practice** are offered by CMSA and the American Case Management Association (ACMA). Additional CM practice standards are offered by the US Department of Veterans Affairs (VA), which apply to CM practice within the VA system, and the NASW, which apply only to SWs. The American Nurses Association (ANA) offers overarching standards and scope of practice for nurses but does not offer CM-specific practice standards.

CMSA's *Standards of Practice for Case Management*, originally released in 1995, has undergone multiple revisions. Each revision was undertaken to address ongoing growth and expansion of CM across the continuum of care and into virtually every care setting. In addition to the standards, the document addresses definition, philosophy and guiding principles, practice settings, roles and responsibilities, and components of the CM process (CMSA, 2016).

ACMA developed professional standards resources for their certificants, holders of the Accredited Case Manager (ACM™) designation. The designation has regulatory oversight by the National Board for Case Management (NBCM). ACMA's *Standards of practice & scope of services for health care delivery system case management and transitions of care (TOC) professionals* (2013) includes professional principles for the areas of education, care coordination, compliance, transition management, utilization management, and standards of practice (including accountability, professionalism, collaboration, care coordination, resource management, and certification). ACMA focused on CM practiced within the health care delivery system, inclusive of transition management. As a result, the standards are applicable to a limited array of care settings.

In 2019, ACMA joined with 15 industry entities to publish *National transitions of care standards and a consensus measures crosswalk.* "The ACMA Transitions of Care Standards were designed with input from 15 collaborating organizations representing 10 practice settings across the industry: acute care, primary care, ambulatory, home care and hospice, managed care pharmacy, healthcare pharmacy, primary care, long-term care, behavioral health and payers." The standards include fundamental and aspirational benchmarks that guide successful care transitions. The consensus measures outline a method to assess a health care organization's performance as transitions are executed (Cobb, 2019).

Although adherence to practice standards is often considered to be voluntary, one exception is the Commission for Case Manager Certification's *Code of professional conduct* (CCMC, 2015). Adherence to this code is mandated for individuals possessing the Certified Case Manager (CCM) credential. It is important to recognize that in a situation where legal action against a case manager occurs, attorneys and the court look at practice standards (in addition to other documents and guidelines) as a means of determining whether the actions of a case manager were aligned with accepted practice. In the case of a nurse case manager, these additional documents include one's own state practice act or remote practice act (when practice involves the Nurse Licensure Compact), applicable nursing standards of practice, CM standards of practice, and organizational policies and procedures.

The most recognizable code of conduct for case managers is the *Code of professional conduct for case managers with standards, rules, procedures, and penalties,* produced by the CCMC (CCMC, 2015). The objective of the code is to protect the public interest. The code is divided into sections, including principles, rules of conduct, scope of practice, definitions, standards for board-CCM conduct, and procedures for processing complaints (CCMC, 2015).

Program Accreditation

In addition to individual certification, organizations, such as the National Committee for Quality Assurance (NCQA) and URAC, offer accreditation and/or distinction recognitions for CM programs. CM accreditation evaluates programs in provider, payer, or community-based organizations. There are also programs for CM rendered in the Long-Term Services and Supports (LTSS) sector. NCQA offers either full accreditation or distinction recognition depending upon the organization's need (NCQA, 2019).

The Case Management Process

The **CM process** focuses on the identification of individuals who would benefit from CM services and the activities of assessment, problem identification, care planning, care delivery, advocacy, monitoring, and evaluation of the care provided, specifically for its relevance to the needs of the patient and caregiver as well as for the health care team's ability to meet the desired outcomes and established goals (Tahan, 2017).

Although the process is presented as having a different number of phases, both CMSA and CCMC have supported following an organized iterative process. A consideration relating to the CM process is that of care setting. Care setting often dictates the type of interaction between case manager and client. For example, the acute care setting generally ensures face-to-face interaction, whereas the managed care setting varies and may be a combination of telephonic, face-to-face and/or Internet chat. The manner in which each case manager interacts with a client not only affects the ability to objectively assess that person but also influences how the relationship will evolve.

Commission for Case Manager Certification (CCMC)

CCMC defines the CM process as it applies to case managers who have achieved the CCM credential as being collaborative in nature. The phases of this process meld seamlessly and aim to support the patient, caregiver, support system, and care team members in addressing health and related issues (CCMC, 2016).

According to CCMC (2016), the process is divided into nine phases: screening, assessing, stratifying risk, planning, implementing (care coordination), following up, transitioning (transitional care), communicating post transition, and evaluating. The CCM navigates CM process being cognizant of the client and caregivers' cultural beliefs, interests, wishes, needs, and values. Because the CM process is an iterative cycle, each phase is revisited as necessary until desired outcomes are achieved and the client's interests are met (CCMC, 2016).

Case Management Society of America (CMSA)

CMSA also stipulates that the CM process is cyclical and recurrent, rather than linear or unidirectional. The CM process incorporates critical thinking and evidence-based knowledge and is carried out within the ethical and legal constructs of a case manager's scope of practice. The steps of the CM process as defined in the CMSA's *Standards of practice for case management* (2016) are client identification and selection, assessment and opportunity identification, development of the CM plan, implementation and coordination of CM plan interventions, monitoring and evaluation of the CM plan, and closing of the CM engagement. Table 16.3 elaborates the CM process phases and notes the similarities between CMSA, CCMC CM, and nursing processes.

Case Management Program Development and Implementation

Case Management Program Development

CM programs are structured around roles and functions of case managers. The case manager's role balances the

TABLE 16.3 Nursing and Case Management Processes

Nursing	CCMC	CMSA	Comments
	Screening	Client identification and selection	Screening and/or selection is specific to case management (CM) where access to a case manager is limited according to the capacity, policy, or practice scope of an organization or department.
Assessment	Assessing	Assessment and opportunity identification	
Diagnosis	Stratifying Risk		The CM process does not include a diagnosis phase, but there are some similarities that align in the opportunity identification and planning phases. • CCMC defines stratifying risk as the classification of a client into one of three risk categories (low, moderate, and high) in order to determine the appropriate level of intervention based on the client's situation and interests.* • In some CM settings, each client's stratification risk is set by the use of predictive modeling software. Subsequent risk score may be edited by the case manager based on client's current status (e.g., health, psychological health, social needs, complexity of care).
Outcomes/planning	Planning	Development of the CM plan	• Despite minute differences, a planning phase is intended to assimilate assessment findings into a workable plan of care for both nurse and case manager. • A CM plan includes overall goals and desired outcomes for identified needs.
Implementation	Implementing (care coordination)	Implementation and coordination of CM plan interventions	The implementation phase puts the plan into action.

CCMC, Commission for Case Manager Certification; *CMSA*, Case Management Society of America.
*Data from American Nurses Association (ANA). (2016). The nursing process. Retrieved May 22, 2016 http://www.nursingworld.org/EspeciallyforYou/StudentNurses/Thenursingprocess.aspx.; Commission for Case Manager Certification (CCMC). (2016). Case Management Body of Knowledge (CMBOK). Mount Laurel, NJ: Author. And Case Management Society of America (CMSA). (2016b). CMSA standards of practice for case management. Little Rock, AR: Author.

aspects of provider, care coordinator, and financial manager. Frequently identified case manager roles are advocate, facilitator, provider, liaison, coordinator, collaborator, broker, educator, negotiator, evaluator, communicator, risk manager, mentor, consultant, and researcher. CM functions are often identified as care coordination, facilitation and linkage, education, advocacy, discharge planning, resource management, and outcomes management.

For provider-based case managers, a CM program may be built based on CMSA's *Standards of practice for case management* (2016). The practice components identified in these standards are authoritative statements that are reflective of the unique roles and responsibilities for which case managers are held accountable. As a result, they can be used as an outline to establish step-by-step processes. In addition, the standards reflect how exclusive values and priorities of practitioners are operationalized and understood by mutual stakeholders (Treiger and Fink-Samnick, 2016).

CM programs are developed using a number of situation-specific elements. Two initial assessments are helpful: assessment of the organization and assessment of client populations. The *organizational assessment* focuses on identification of resources, whereas the client population assessment focuses on how care is experienced by clients and the characteristics of client populations served by the organizations. Box 16.2 lists related assessment questions. If CM is used for specific client populations, priority would go to clients who have a high rate of recidivism or frequent emergency department encounters; have unpredictable needs for care; have significant complications, comorbidities, or variances in usual care patterns; fall into high-risk profiles; and/or are high cost.

The general process for the development of a CM program is to:

1. Assess the organization and the client population served. This assessment provides a baseline for implementation.
2. Identify high-volume or high-risk case types. This assessment will indicate priority areas for care coordination.
3. Determine the usual client care problems, issues, or difficulties related to the high-volume or high-risk case types, with desired goals.
4. Form an interdisciplinary care team of the interrelated care providers who will be involved with the case types.

> ### BOX 16.2   Case Management Assessment Questions
>
> **Organizational Assessment**
> - What clinical and support services are needed?
> - When in the client experience are services most appropriately provided?
> - How should services be provided?
> - Where are services best delivered?
> - Who are the most appropriate providers?
> - Where and by whom are services best managed?
>
> **Client Assessment**
> - What are the major client populations served by the organizations—by volume, diagnosis, cost, payer mix, and high-intensity/resource use outliers?
> - What is the service path followed by client populations—by entry point, internal flow, discharge, and recidivism?
> - What groups of clients fall into high-risk categories—by volume?
> - What clients are at risk for less-than-desired outcomes—by morbidity, mortality, infection rates, falls, and clinical outcomes?

---

5. Develop and design an interdisciplinary critical pathway for each selected case type. The path should outline and specify measurable clinical outcomes, key professional care processes, and exact corresponding timelines as based on practice patterns, professional standards of care, and length-of-stay parameters. The input and involvement of the client and each provider group needs to be clearly specified in relation to actions for achieving client outcomes. The pathway would mark the occurrence of routine treatments, tests, consults, client activities, medications, diet, educational interventions, and discharge planning. Variance from the path triggers analysis and intervention.
6. Develop a pilot program or trial site.
7. Evaluate the pilot program and consider system-wide implementation. Review the pilot program's articulation with the existing mode of nursing care delivery.

CM program development processes emphasize the potential of interprofessional team approaches by involving engaged disciplines in establishing treatment plans and completion of outcomes. They also highlight the importance of preparing patients, professionals, and the organization to facilitate success.

CM has become a popular and effective means to manage patients across populations and practice settings. In hospitals, it has decreased length of stay and secured important outcomes (Daniels, 2015; Watson, 2016). In the newest generation of CM settings, including primary care practices, ACOs, and PCMHs, quality and outcomes are being emphasized more than ever (Watson, 2016). Persuasive arguments exist for implementing CM programming. For example, close follow-up, continuous reinforcement, and systematic treatment adjustments facilitated by case managers contributed to improvement for adult clients with diabetes, heart failure, and comorbid physical and mental health conditions (Advancing Integrated Mental Health Solutions [AIMS] Center, 2019; Stellefson et al., 2013; Takeda et al., 2012; Unützer et al., 2013).

CM has equally been identified as a major strategy for cost containment, which also incorporates quality control. Given the vast financial impact for all practice settings, the case manager shoulders significant responsibilities for tracking both quality and outcomes in addition to targeting improvements. These actions are completed as a means to verify the case manager's own performance, the performance of the team, and to some extent the entire organization (Watson, 2016). Research has emerged over the past decade to substantiate savings from CM interventions, including studies on effectiveness from across the industry (Kolbasovsky et al., 2012; Stellefson et al., 2013).

Case Management Outcomes

Two basic outcomes categories to be captured are clinical outcomes and financial outcomes. For clinical outcomes, Braden (2002) identified these six direct outcomes of CM: (1) patient knowledge, (2) patient involvement, (3) patient participation in care, (4) patient empowerment, (5) patient adherence, and (6) coordination of care.

Improvement in a key indicator (e.g., patient knowledge) can be a direct measure of the clinical effectiveness of a CM intervention. The effectiveness of CM is further strengthened when the outcome of improved patient knowledge is linked to research evidence pertaining to improved patient knowledge reducing chronic relapse or use of health care resources.

Proving financial gain has been somewhat more problematic for CM, although the tide is turning. There has been acknowledged value and acceptance of CM in some areas, such as diabetes, congestive heart failure, and other chronic diseases (Kolbasovsky et al., 2012; Stellefson et al., 2013). In mental health and substance use, the outcomes are becoming more visible (Fortney et al., 2015; Unützer et al., 2013). A robust amount of literature has emerged courtesy of demonstration projects associated with the Collaborative Care Model out of the University of Washington's Advancing Integrated Mental Health Solutions (AIMS) Center (2019). A full listing of these programs is available on the AIMS Center website (http://aims.uw.edu/projects).

DISEASE MANAGEMENT

DM has been acknowledged as a payer strategy to prevent or manage one or more chronic conditions, improve care quality, and reduce costs (Ahmed, 2016; Walters et al., 2012). Since DM's entrance into the health care market, the term has experienced a fair level of transition. DM advanced from identification of persons at risk for one chronic condition to reflect a more comprehensive view of the customer base and is indicative of a global focus on care for entire populations (Ahmed, 2016; Goodman et al., 2014; Rushton, 2015; Walters et al., 2012).

The terms DM and PHM appear throughout this section. However, on the health care management continuum, the overall umbrella concept is better known as PHM. Both CM and DM are segments of the PHM spectrum.

History and Background

DM programs were developed and implemented largely as managed care health plan initiatives. The rise of DM occurred in the late 1980s and into the 1990s in the US health care delivery system. Nested within the general evolution of CM practice, managed care organizations and health plans began to look closely at DM after initial CM programs had been active for decades. Further refinements in program quality and cost savings were desired by employer group purchasers of health coverage. The unique challenges of chronic conditions occurring on a large scale needed to be addressed. Prior experiences with CM became the platform. In pharmaceutical companies, DM emerged as a way to encourage medication adherence.

Growth of Managed Care Systems and a Focus on Quality Care

Two major forces triggered the rise of a DM perspective: (1) a period of growth in managed care systems as a prevailing form of organized health care delivery (the influence of health plans), and (2) the national attention generated by *Crossing the quality chasm*, a health care quality initiative of the Institute of Medicine (IOM, now called the National Academies of Sciences, Engineering, and Medicine, Health and Medicine Division). Health plans led the charge to address the care coordination and service integration needs of clusters of members who had identifiable health conditions that are generally chronic in nature. In 1996, the Health and Medicine Division of the National Academies of Sciences, Engineering, and Medicine launched an ongoing effort focused on the assessment and improvement of the quality of health care in the United States. Their 2001 report *Crossing the quality chasm: A new health system for the 21st century* (IOM, 2001) highlighted the need for profound changes in the environment of care, including revamping practices that fragment the care system. The coordination of care across patient conditions, services, and settings was viewed over time as a major organizational challenge, yet a key dimension of patient-centered care.

DM evolved into proven and effective strategies to make groups of individuals who had a "disease" such as mental health or diabetes healthier while saving scarce health care coverage dollars. In the early 2000s, the federal government's Centers for Medicare & Medicaid Services (CMS, 2003) took notice of DM programs, sponsored DM demonstration projects, and encouraged contracting with DM vendors for outsourced medical management programs because DM was found to be effective in select populations.

Disease Management Transitions to Population Health Management

Moving into the 21st century, DM's identity shifted because of societal transitions. The community had become a more viable focus for health care services, prompting the need to expand DM's perspective. Social and economic pressures demanded that health care organizations focus on ways to provide cost-effective, population-based care. Roughly 40% of deaths were found to be caused by behaviors that could be modified by preventive, population-based intervention. Although these cases only accounted for a small percentage of health spending, the death and disability prevention aspects were important (Shaljian and Nielsen, 2013).

The next generation of health care began to explore the care process across the entire continuum. **Continuum**

of care is a concept involving a system that guides and tracks patients over time through a comprehensive array of health services to span all levels and intensity of care (Young et al., 2014). The services incorporated in each patient's unique continuum vary based on the individualized health and/or behavioral health needs of each person.

Prevention and early detection programs (e.g., parenting, wellness), family and community services, pharmacies, behavioral health, and end-of-life care have also been incorporated as components of the continuum of care. Persons who are homeless and those on domestic and/or international travels are also factored into the equation, as are the services incurred during their experience (Young et al., 2014).

Building an effective continuum of care involves understanding the true health needs of an individual community. Emphasis on the health of a community is anchored in a rich history of innovations in community and public health methods and programs directed at reducing risk factor prevalence, decreasing acute and chronic disease burden and injury occurrence, and promoting health (Goodman et al., 2014). These factors also set a context and rationale for addressing the SDoH. As case managers often possess the prime responsibility in their organizations for care coordination, they face mounting pressures to reconcile client engagement, treatment adherence, and successful short and long-term wellness. As a result, attention to developing strategic partnerships with a responsive continuum of care will promote sound and effective CM intervention and contribute to more positive health outcomes (Fink-Samnick, 2019b).

Community health involves meeting the collective needs of a group or individual community by identifying problems and managing interactions both within the community and between the community and the larger society. Risk factors, health status indicators, functional ability levels, health promotion, health outcomes, and prevention of identified chronic diseases are the focus of data gathering, program planning, and implementation processes and activities. The term *community health* has experienced some evolution in recent years to account for the expansion into public health practice settings and the importance of community engagement as a core element (Goodman et al., 2014). The evolution is further understood by the need for health care professionals to focus more intentionally on both cultural diversity and the SDoH, which are key factors for successful patient engagement and activation (Ashford and LeCroy, 2017; Gillespie, 2016; Goodman et al., 2014; Hu et al., 2014).

As the scope of DM grew, a grander scale of attention beckoned for health care professionals interested in addressing societal trends and implications of chronic illness. In the emerging context of wellness and prevention for society, the term population provided a wider lens and presented as a more logical way to refer to the next wave of health management.

A **population** refers to a group of individuals—in contrast to the individuals themselves—organized in many different units of analysis, depending on the research or policy purpose. The **population health** perspective explores beyond a biomedical model of individual health and allows providers to consider what makes some groups of people healthier than other groups of people. The emphasis by the industry on the impact of socioeconomic factors on hospital readmissions speaks to a population health focus (Hu et al., 2014). Applying population health across the continuum entails the goals of (Nash et al., 2016, p. xvii):

1. Keeping the well, well
2. Reducing health risks
3. Providing quick access to care for acute illness so that health does not deteriorate
4. Managing chronic illness to prevent complications
5. Getting those with complex or catastrophic illness to centers of excellence or compassionate care settings

Accomplishing these goals involves both community participation and partnership, which are key concepts to PHM. Active participation in decision-making processes through a concerted and combined effort induces a vested interest in the success of any effort to improve the health of a community. For nurses, the concept of community as client directs the focus to the collective or common good instead of individual health. Population-based care draws on partnership and community-as-client concepts.

Chronic Health Conditions Align with Population Health Management

Chronic health conditions have long posed a formidable challenge to the health care delivery system. They affect almost half of the adult US population, with 25% having more than one chronic illness (Ward et al., 2013). The management of chronic conditions has been a particular burden for health care payers and employers. Chronic disease creates two particular difficulties for businesses. First, these conditions in the workforce lead to diminished productivity. Second, these conditions result in a greater portion of the business's revenue being diverted to health care expenditures. Further effects have an impact on the health care delivery system, society, and individuals' functioning and activities.

Population and health trends are tracked by governmental agencies such as the US Census Bureau, Centers for Disease Control and Prevention (CDC), Bureau of Labor Statistics (BLS), and Health Resources and Services Administration (HRSA), as well as private foundations and health care organizations. Clearly, health and health care delivery systems data are continually in flux. However, the available statistics are impressive. Costs are a considerable pressure, because on average individuals with chronic conditions cost 3.5 times as much to serve as others, and they account for a large proportion of services. According to the CDC (2019) chronic diseases, inclusive of heart disease, cancer, and diabetes, are the leading causes of death and disability in the United States. These illnesses affect approximately 133 million Americans, representing more than 40% of the total population of this country. These figures are projected to grow to an estimated 157 million, with 81 million having multiple conditions. Six out of 10 adults have at least one chronic disease, with 4 of 10 having two or more chronic diseases (CDC, 2019; National Health Council, 2014).

The chronic conditions that pose a particular economic burden but can be helped by PHM are characterized by high prevalence, high expense, relatively standardized treatment guidelines, and a significant role played by the individual's behavior on the progression of the condition. It is widely recognized that health care delivery can and must be improved. The pressures to provide access to care, maintain a high level of quality, and control expenditures are converging on a traditionally fragmented and acute care–focused system. Projections are that sociodemographic and economic tidal waves are set to converge in a "perfect storm" of crisis over health care in the near future. These tidal waves include the aging of the US population, the effect of the maturing of the baby boom generation, high pharmaceutical costs, advancing medical technology, dramatic increases in chronic health conditions, and US government budget deficits.

The solutions are not easy or obvious. However, PHM is now being viewed as a major health care strategy to improve health outcomes across multiple populations while lowering costs and improving patient satisfaction. It is one of the Institute for Healthcare Improvement's (2017) Triple Aims and is an important aspect of ACOs. PHM has demonstrated effectiveness across disease states, including integrated behavioral health, chronic illness (e.g., diabetes, congestive heart failure), and assorted payers (e.g., Medicare, Medicaid, third party populations) (Fortney et al., 2015; Lyles, 2016; Rushton, 2015; Sidorov & Romney, 2016). Attractive features include effective population management, coordination of care for chronic conditions, consistency of care for at-risk populations, customization of care support, encouragement of adherence to treatment, and proactive interventions. Although chronic diseases are among the most common and costly health problems, they are also among the most preventable. Adopting healthy behaviors such as eating nutritious foods, being physically active, and avoiding tobacco use can prevent or control the devastating effects of these diseases.

Population Health Management Practice Approaches

Early DM programs offered by health plans were developed in-house or purchased either from a vendor or another organization such as a hospital. The newest generation of PHM programs involves proactive outreach. Nursing outreach programs are the core element. Personal communications (usually via telephone) between an expert nurse and the health plan participant build a personal relationship, help identify knowledge deficits and counseling needs, facilitate close monitoring and progress toward goals, enhance treatment adherence, and promote clinical and cost stabilization.

Functioning as a personal health advisor, the health coach, case manager, or care coordinator establishes a single point of contact and coordination of care and service for patients having health problems and promotes a trusting relationship. Whether employed by a health plan or a contracted outside vendor, the PHM provided by nurses functioning as personal health advisors and advocates is central to effective outcomes.

The core of the DM concept was to comprehensively integrate care and reimbursement based on a disease or health condition's natural course. Both clinical and non-clinical interventions are timed to occur where and when they are most likely to have the greatest impact. This sequencing and targeting ideally prevents occurrences or exacerbations, decreases the use of expensive resources, and creates positive health outcomes through the use of prevention and proactive CM strategies. Chronic conditions are the focus, and the methods use systematic ways of delivering health care interventions to patients with similar characteristics. PHM models focus on the identification, standardization, and coordination of services across the continuum of care and for populations with the same or similar health care needs. Several program examples are discussed in the following sections.

The Population Care Coordination Process

Rushton's (2015) *Population care coordination process* provides a scalable framework for providers and/or organizations (e.g., single offices or larger ACOs) to provide multilevel care based on population- and patient-centered principles. It involves care coordination, CM, and PHM to maximize health outcomes and resource utilization for populations and the individuals within them. The process involves six phases to focus on coordinating care for the entire population with individualization of that care: data analysis, selection, assessment, multidisciplinary planning, implementation/intervention, and monitoring/evaluation (Rushton, 2015).

Care of Mental, Physical, and Substance Use Syndromes

Identified as one of the largest Collaborative Care population health implementation initiatives, the Care of Mental, Physical and Substance Use Syndromes (COMPASS) initiative included over 4000 Medicare and Medicaid patients across 187 clinics in seven states: California, Colorado, Massachusetts, Michigan, Minnesota, Pennsylvania, and Washington (Fortney et al., 2015). A core systematic case review (SCR) team intervened with chronically ill patients who were diagnosed with uncontrolled depression and uncontrolled diabetes and/or heart disease. The following program components were included:

- An initial evaluation to measure condition severity and assess the patient's readiness for self-management
- A computerized registry to track and monitor the patient's progress
- A care manager to provide patient education and self-management support, coordinate care with the

primary care physician and consultants, and provide active follow-up.

- A consulting psychiatrist and consulting medical physician to review cases with the care manager and recommend changes in treatment to the primary care physician
- Treatment intensification when there is a lack of improvement
- Relapse and exacerbation prevention

Overall aggregated results from all 18 participating regional groups demonstrated that goals were exceeded for depression, heart disease, and diabetes improvement (Advancing Integrated Mental Health Solutions, 2019; Fortney et al., 2015).

Evolving Practice Standards and Guidelines

Unlike the clear and prevalent industry practice standards for CM, PHM is just achieving its stride with respect to established professional guidelines. The *Population Health Alliance Outcomes Guidelines, Vol. 6* was released in 2015 and serves as a basis for many PHM programs throughout the industry (Population Health Alliance [PHA], 2015). For professional certification, the Chronic Care Professional (CCP) Certification has been offered since 2004 to eligible professionals working in health care or a health-related field. Non-clinical team members (e.g., community health educators, program leaders, or consultants who support health and chronic care improvement) may also apply (Health Sciences Institute, 2016).

Since 2002, The Joint Commission (TJC, 2019) has offered Disease-Specific Care (DSC) Certification to provide a framework for continuously reliable care. TJC accredited health care organizations may seek a 2-year certification for care and services programs that provide for a long list of chronic diseases or conditions. In addition, an advanced level of certification is available to programs that meet the requirements for DSC certification plus additional clinically specific requirements and expectations. The available advanced certification programs are listed by setting on the TJC website (https://www.jointcommission.org/accreditation-and-certification/certification/certifications-by-setting/).

The American Organization of Nurse Executives (now called the American Organization for Nursing Leadership [AONL]) (AONE, 2015) developed *Nurse executive competencies: Population health*. Leadership from the nurse executive is viewed as vital to the

development, execution, and refinement of PHM programming. As an advocate for community health needs and patient populations, the nurse executive in his or her role as an agent of change is viewed as paramount (AONE, 2015).

The National Association of Chronic Disease Directors (NACDD, 2016) is a non-profit public health organization committed to serving chronic disease program directors of each state and US jurisdiction. NACDD works to provide educational and training, develop legislative materials, educate policymakers, provide technical assistance, develop partnerships and collaborations, and advocate for the use of epidemiological approaches in chronic disease services planning and chronic disease data. Moving forward, it is expected that the industry will see the further development and evolution of more standards, organizations, and certifications specific to PHM.

Disease Management Process, Program Development and Implementation

The goal of DM is to maintain or improve the current state of chronic disease(s) through the systematic use of evidence-based interventions. DM uses risk assessment, education, and risk factor reduction strategies to influence behaviors toward the goals of improving outcomes and reducing cost (Ahmed, 2016). DM has been a pivotal health care strategy for decades. However, unlike CM, there does not appear to be a single endorsed DM process that is consistently referenced in texts or journals. The general components associated with a DM program include population risk analysis, identification, stratification, enrollment and engagement, program delivery, outcomes and effectiveness evaluation, and reporting. Each of these components is displayed in Fig. 16.2 and is amplified further in this section.

Before identification of a specific population eligible for a DM program, health plans and DM companies analyze claims data to identify the conditions that are prevalent in a given population. This is completed using coding conventions such as the International Classification of Diagnosis (ICD) and Current Procedural Terminology (CPT). This, combined with claims expenditure data, reveals disease classifications that most affect a covered population. From this perspective an organization is able to determine its strategic and tactical priorities for program development.

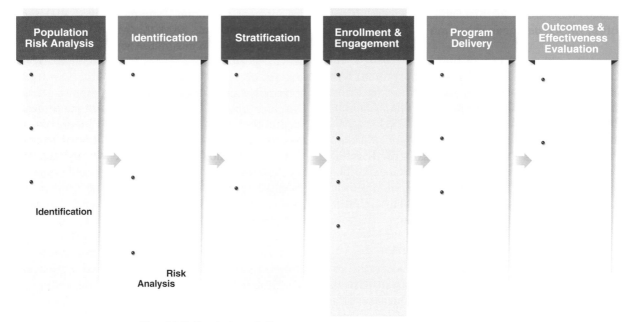

Fig. 16.2 Depiction of disease management program components.

Disease Management Program Components
Population Risk Assessment

The aggregate health care costs of chronic conditions increase yearly as individuals grow older. Older individuals tend to have chronic conditions that require complex care. It is estimated that one-third to one-half of all health care spending is consumed by the elderly. With the shift in demographic trends toward increasing numbers of elderly, there is a shift in the need for preventive care and chronic illness management services. To meet this challenge, managed care organizations have created infrastructures of population-based risk assessment, demand management (self-management and decision support systems such as call centers), DM, and CM.

To be effective at individual and population-based care management, both CM and DM programs need to identify, assess, and define the populations to be served early in the program planning effort. This component represents the effort to assess the health of a specific population (e.g., patient panel, enrollment). This assessment typically "triangulates" by drawing on available types of information (e.g., self-reported health questionnaires, health insurance claims, laboratory and pharmacy data, and clinician documentation). Once the population is defined, individuals within the population must be selected and assessed as to which program and level of intervention will optimally meet the most pressing needs. Factors that are included in an individual profile include age, number of chronic illnesses, and number of medications (Care Continuum Alliance [CCA], 2012a).

Identification

The participant identification process is driven by algorithms or other logic frameworks that are applied to claims data and look for specific diagnosis codes. In addition, predictive modeling tools (e.g., artificial intelligence, neural net logic) are leveraged to harvest information beyond simple diagnosis. *Predictive modeling* is "a commonly used statistical technique to predict future behavior. Predictive modeling solutions are a form of data-mining technology that works by analyzing historical and current data and generating a model to help predict future outcomes" (Gartner, 2016). Predictive models have been used in other industries and businesses, such as credit card companies and retailers, for years. In health care, these methodologies look for experience and other red flags that indicate an individual is at risk and to what extent. The case-finding techniques help to identify individuals who appear to be in most need of additional support in order to stem worsening health conditions and resource expenditures. The identified individuals are then screened by intake specialists to determine the best match between program intensity and client need (Ahmed, 2016).

Additional cycles of predictive modeling help to stratify each person's risk level (e.g., low, medium, high), as well as to look at care patterns and care gaps. These programs also have the ability to identify when an individual is not receiving optimal pharmaceutical therapy, is not having provider visits at the proper interval, or is not receiving the proper immunizations. This information is available to the DM nurse when reaching out to clients, providers, pharmacies, or other providers involved with the individual's care. These results also drive the intensity of intervention (e.g., reminders, risk reduction measures, DM program, or CM interventions) that an individual may be offered (Plocher, 2013).

Stratification

The next step in the population health process is to stratify patients into meaningful categories for patient-centered intervention targeting that uses information collected in health assessments (CCA, 2012a). In population health management, **stratification** has two meanings (PHA, 2015): a method of randomization and a process for sorting a population of eligible members into groups relating to their relative need for total population management interventions. Stratification may be based on the integration of a variety of data, if available, including claims, pharmacy, laboratory, health risks, or consumer-reported data such as health assessments. The stratification process harvests information that can be used to divide the patient population into different levels to ensure a return on investment (ROI) based on resources allowed.

Enrolment and Engagement

Once individuals are identified and stratified, those who appear to qualify for DM intervention receive an outreach notification (e.g., telephone call). The opportunity to enroll in a condition-specific program is offered during this initial contact. The program is explained, and consent to participate is requested. Although the enrollment process sounds straightforward, there are a number of barriers to overcome in getting individuals on-boarded into a program, such as inaccurate data, incorrect contact information, and outright refusal (Plocher, 2013).

One factor that is at the root of some non-enrollment is consumer mistrust of the insurance company's motives for contact. This concept contributes to unwillingness to participate in programs offered by the insurance company. Consumer mistrust is especially important when one considers the cost of delivering a DM program. The cost relating to a DM program is frequently reported at a per-member-per-month (PMPM) level. The expense of creating and maintaining such programs is borne by the insurance company regardless of whether the individual actively participates in the program (Ahmed, 2016).

Historically, program engagement has been a challenge, as typically only about 20% of those eligible participate in these programs (Brown et al., 2012). Despite these programs being established for decades, research on why people opt out or do not participate is limited (Hawkins et al., 2014).

The results of a 2014 study that examined factors driving engagement suggest that individuals most motivated to engage are those who are well informed of the program benefits and have a perceived need that would benefit from said program (e.g., living alone, needing a supportive person to discuss ideas) (Hawkins et al., 2014). Recruitment and engagement strategies continue to evolve, but the challenges facing this component of DM programming include privacy, meaningful engagement, and physician integration (Plocher, 2013).

Program Delivery

Whenever possible, the components of DM should be delivered by leveraging a variety of communications and interventions. This mixed mode approach optimizes the resources and outreach and accommodates the preferences and technological abilities of recipients with the ultimate goal of increased engagement and self-management (CCA, 2012b). This also takes into account that communication preferences vary based on generational differences. Although demographic splitting by age groups may not lead to absolute accuracy, it is generally accepted that communicating with a baby boomer versus a millennial requires consideration of a variety of channels (e.g., social media, hard copy print, telephone calls).

Interaction and management. Communication is a means of interaction and management for program delivery. It mostly involves the program participants, primary care providers, and program staff. There are a number of communication channels used to enhance interaction between the plan and both member and provider. The choice of modes used depends on the organization's ability to maintain compliance with the Health Insurance Portability and Accountability Act of 1996 (HIPAA) across each channel, financial resources to establish and maintain each channel, understanding of a given population's communication preferences, and other factors. Examples of communication options include (Plocher, 2013):

- Mailings
- Information to enrollee: welcome packet, interval updates and results, reminders
- Information to provider: orientation packet, periodic progress updates, periodic guideline recommendations
- Outbound telephone calls and interactive voice response (IVR) (e.g., initial welcome, assessments, progress checks, coaching)
- Inbound calls from participants to address condition and DM care plan questions
- Internet-based text and video chats for progress updates, reminders, condition and DM care plan questions
- Home telemonitoring devices for home device connection to monitor real time results. Frequently transmitted biometrics are weight, vital signs, and pulse oximetry.
- Medication adherence tools with pill box monitoring support for complex medication regimens
- Technology platforms (e.g., web portals) for secure messaging
- Face-to-face conversation for assessment, progress updates, and coaching

As technology continues to develop, so too will communication options. Technology is a core expectation of DM programs. Organizations have invested millions in developing technology to support DM programs from front (e.g., population assessment to identify prevalence, risk stratification) to back (e.g., reporting, effectiveness, outcomes analysis).

Outcomes and Effectiveness Evaluation

Program outcomes and effectiveness reports are an evolving source of information. Before-and-after program enrollment comparison is a common method of demonstrating program impact, but these often require at least a year of continuous participant enrollment to be deemed significant. In addition, the Healthcare Effectiveness Data Information Set (HEDIS®) requires this time span for data collection. These metrics look at testing frequency or certain drugs being prescribed, instead of test result improvement, such as hemoglobin A_1C, low density lipoprotein (LDL) cholesterol, appropriately prescribed angiotensin converting enzyme inhibitor, and appropriately prescribed beta blockers.

In today's lightning-fast, results-driven environment, waiting a full year to see results of an investment is difficult to sell. Metrics of interest include PMPM cost, episode-of-care cost, and utilization (e.g., hospital admissions, inpatient days) (Plocher, 2013). This imperative has spurred on the use of "big data" analytics. For example, at Geisinger Clinic in Pennsylvania, the big data approach was viewed as a way to better manage patients with chronic conditions. Big data is defined as the large volume of structured and unstructured data that swamps businesses on a day-to-day basis (SAS, 2016). Much of the data collected about patients lies dormant and is not used in routine analytic methods. Geisinger undertook a process redesign with its coronary artery disease (CAD) program that eliminated waste, automated processes where possible, and delegated tasks to appropriate staff. Geisinger accelerated the delivery of care through continuous use of data and informatics and addressed nine patient-oriented goals focused on improving the health of nearly 17,000 patients with CAD. The goals were measured in an "all or none" bundle to encourage team-based workflows rather than using measures that focused on a particular team member's performance (e.g., prescribing rate). The measures addressed care issues faced by all patients with CAD. The bundled approach to care measures realized a 300% improvement. The use of big data analytics was anticipated to harvest even more significant improvements in patient care (Graf et al., 2014). The use of big data is poised to flourish in all areas of health care, translating massive amounts of unusable data into useable information.

Reporting

In their 2015 joint report, the Health Enhancement Research Organization (HERO) and Population Health Alliance (PHA) published a core guide to metrics, the *Program measurement & evaluation guide: Core metrics for employee health management.* The categories included financial, health outcomes, participation, satisfaction, organizational support, productivity and performance, and value on investment framework. The report was framed by the following statement, "HERO and PHA are responding to employers who seek a greater level of clarity regarding the value of their wellness efforts. Thus we recommend an initial set of measures to assess the impact of the health management programs offered to employees. The results are better informed business decisions and boardroom discussions" (HERO-PHA, 2015). Although aimed at employer groups, these metrics are solid indicators of PHM program impacts. These metric categories may be applied in whole or in part to measure program impacts and as a means for classifying areas requiring further performance improvement.

When designing and implementing a DM program, use of a detailed project plan is essential to develop and maintain. This is done to track progress toward completion and hold stakeholders accountable for completing assigned tasks. Once implemented, in addition to program metrics, the project plan gives way to more simplified tools such as checklists. Table 16.4 depicts one such checklist. It is strongly recommended that tools such as this be customized to each unique program.

TABLE 16.4 Checklist to Evaluate Disease Management Programs

Component	Present (Yes); Absent (No)	Specific Method or Metric Used

Population identification and selection
  Risk assessment
  Risk stratification		

Use of evidence-based practice guidelines
  Type of practice model
  Collaborative mechanism
  Single discipline predominates (identify)		

Patient self-management
  Education
  Primary prevention
  Behavior modification
  Lifestyle change motivation
  Telephone contact
  Health advocates
  Compliance/adherence
  Surveillance		

Process, outcomes management
  Process identification and measurement
  Process evaluation
  Outcomes identification and measurement
  Outcomes evaluation
  Process and outcomes management		

Feedback loop
  Communication to:
    Patient
    Physician
    Health plan
    Ancillary providers		

Practice profiling		

From D.L. Huber. (2017). *Care for the total population.* Iowa City, IA.

LEADERSHIP AND MANAGEMENT IMPLICATIONS

Nurses who manage client care are clinical managers. The shift to managed care in integrated health systems and ever-expanding care settings (e.g., ACO, PCMH) highlights CM as a key strategy for nursing practice management and empowerment of nurses. It also has made care team collaboration an imperative. Leadership roles for nurses are essential because of the need for care continuity.

Future CM effectiveness is thought to be based on decisions about what types of organizational structures and nursing care delivery systems best enable nurse-managed client care and best support nurses in practice. One related question is, "How much management structure does a nurse require to be effective?" One assessment is the extent to which a nurse provides client care or manages the care of clients. CM is one specific approach to redesigning care delivery for client care improvement. This may mean that some traditional management practices need to be changed or discarded. CM has come to be a part of care delivery management that emphasizes the expertise of nurses.

CM is practiced beyond the walls of the acute care setting. There is no single way to go about identifying how much management structure is necessary because of the variety of care settings and associated bureaucracy. CM leader-managers need to examine the state of health care management in their organizations and develop strategies to implement coordination of care models to best meet client, organizational, societal, and professional priorities, often referred to as patient-and-family-centered models. Given the interdisciplinary nature of CM, model development and success may require a buy-in by other health care disciplines and other organizational stakeholders. Physicians and hospital administrators are crucial stakeholders for the success of CM programs. The CM leader-manager needs to master communication, collaboration, and advocacy skills in order to effect changes within their own department as well as across the organization.

Partnering With Human Resources

Another CM leader-manager challenge is the human resources department itself. Now more than ever the question "Who is qualified to be hired as a case manager?" is one that needs careful consideration. In today's outcomes-driven health care environment, it is important to have the right people in the right positions to maximize their experience, knowledge, and skills. In short, competence should be the driver of personnel changes.

The CM leader-manager works closely with a human resource specialist (HRS) to clarify department structure, mission, and vision. Job descriptions should clearly distinguish position types and grade levels. New position descriptions should provide the required experience, knowledge, and skills that a qualified candidate should possess. CM position descriptions need to reflect education level and credential requirements, being mindful to distinguish requirements from preferences so as to simplify the candidate screening process.

Individual Suitability for Case Management

CM leader-managers need to evaluate employees in existing positions who are considered as case managers. In many situations, job titles and/or responsibilities change over the years regardless of whether the employees are well suited for their new scope of work. In other instances, department reorganizations have allowed people to retain the coveted case manager job title despite the position's purpose having changed significantly. There needs to be an objective process in place in order to fairly evaluate existing employees. Reassignments may be necessary after such an evaluation process. The evaluation process is stressful on staff and management. The CM leader-manager needs to have a clear vision, strategy, and a proactive communication plan in order to move the department through the change management process.

It is important to clarify the requisite experience and credentialing required to fill the CM job. Certification is typically an official credential awarded to an individual by a nationally recognized professional organization based on eligibility and passing a standardized examination. The credential affirms a baseline degree of education, experience, and knowledge. Individual certification is a mark of professional achievement, and although it is difficult to attain, certification is a floor—not a ceiling—of achievement.

CURRENT ISSUES AND TRENDS

There are constant pressures that affect CM practice, including the lack of title protection, which allows misuse of the case manager designation; the inflow of unlicensed and inexperienced individuals performing CM tasks; and challenges with licensure portability affecting individuals' ability to work seamlessly to provide care coordination services across state lines. This section is devoted to select challenges currently challenging the CM workforce.

Branding and Lack of Universal Definition

Health care reform has amplified the number of career options for the CM workforce, especially with the expansion of ACOs, PCMHs, and integrated behavioral health programs. These opportunities span business models, practice settings, professional disciplines, and across the transitions of care. Yet a double-edged sword exists with regard to the vast number of CM-associated titles, roles, functions, and job descriptions that have followed suit. Experts challenge that this expansion has contributed to a paradoxical effect on CM's identity (Treiger & Fink-Samnick, 2013; 2016).

Patients and family caregivers, employers, and other stakeholders with a vested interest are consistently challenged to comprehend the similarities and differences among the many job titles for CM (e.g., case manager, care manager, geriatric care manager, care coordinator, case worker, care advocate, advanced life care planner, patient advocate, patient navigator, health care coach). This role multiplicity is one more obstacle to CM's maturity from advanced practice to established profession (Treiger & Fink-Samnick, 2013; 2016). It also serves to splinter rather than forge a strong foundation for professional CM practice.

Leveraging the Non-Clinical Workforce

Maintaining a workforce consisting primarily of licensed and/or certified clinical professionals is an expensive proposition. In spite of geographical variation, RNs and SWs are justifiably compensated for their clinical and health care system knowledge. Historically, organizations employed RNs and SWs in CM positions. Later, when organizations became more focused on cost-savings and efficiency, they began to use non-clinical staff to perform CM activities or applied the case manager job title indiscriminately in order to attract candidates with a desirable position. The impact of this staffing methodology on care quality or value for service delivered has not been clearly or consistently demonstrated (Treiger, 2011).

Organizations are recognizing the need to hire increasing numbers of non-clinical professionals to leverage the professional CM workforce. The influx of concrete and non-clinical service needs has prompted more primary level CM tasks (e.g., social service referrals, resource coordination, financial services, arranging transportation). To this end, the use of emerging roles, such as community health workers and health service coordinators, is being rapidly integrated into existing CM models across practice settings.

The economics of maintaining a workforce largely made up of clinical professionals continues to force review of hiring practices and raises questions pertaining to required qualifications of individuals working in CM. To reduce program costs, some organizations opt to hire individuals for care coordination positions who lack a professional degree and/or have limited if any clinical experience necessary to handle the complexity of CM functions. In one Midwestern health system, this hiring strategy was brought to an abrupt halt when leaders realized that the staff hired to coordinate care were not qualified to perform an independent assessment, unable to clearly identify patient care challenges and needs as an outcome of the independent assessment, and unqualified to develop a CM care plan to address individual challenges and needs. The failure was corrected by hiring appropriate staff (e.g., RN, SW) for CM positions. However, this was not without some pain and lost time in having to rework an otherwise well-considered corporate revitalization. CM leader-managers need to advocate for a tiered, yet collaborative CM workforce comprised of varying positions within their departments to best address both clinical and non-clinical needs of patient populations. Emphasis must also be on assuring sound partnerships among all members of the workforce to achieve successful patient outcomes.

Legislative and Regulatory Disruptors
Licensure Portability and the Nurse Licensure Compact

Current regulations continue to be grossly out of sync with practice realities for health care professionals, particularly nurses engaged in CM. Many case managers experience huge challenges and potential violations for practicing without a license in a state where the patient is located. The case manager may not be licensed to practice in that particular state and/or their scope of practice fails to allow for telehealth practice (Fink-Samnick & Muller, 2015). This has been a chronic issue, particularly for those nurses employed by national managed care and/or workers' compensation organizations, multihospital systems, or other health and behavioral health providers. For example, tele-management assessment is not permitted consistently across all professional disciplines or states. As a result, nurses are encouraged to check the websites for their respective individual professional state licensure boards and/or certifications on a regular basis to accurately define their individual scope of practice (Fink-Samnick & Muller, 2015).

The **Nurse Licensure Compact** (NLC) and the newer enhanced version, the eNLC, give multistate rights to RNs and licensed practical/vocational nurses (LPN/VN) residing in a member state. The eNLC addressed concerns voiced by several states that declined to join the Compact. The eNCL includes uniform licensure requirements, the authority to submit and obtain background checks, and reporting to participating in alternative to discipline programs in NURSYS® (National Council of State Boards of Nursing, 2016a). Advance practice nurses (APNs) maintain a separate compact. The eNLC allows nurses to have one multistate license with the ability to practice in both their home state and other compact states (National Council of State Boards of Nursing, 2016b). The advancement of the NLC across states has been a vital factor to promote the legal practice of CM across state lines. A current map of NLC member states is available at *https://www.ncsbn.org/nurse-licensure-compact.htm*.

Measuring and Sharing Case Management Outcomes

In 2010, the Agency for Healthcare Research and Quality (AHRQ) issued the comparative effectiveness report *Outpatient case management for adults with medical illness and complex care needs* (Hickam et al., 2013). The report focused on this single segment of practice and specific questions pertaining to CM as an intervention strategy for chronic illness outpatient management. The findings clearly note that there was a wide diversity in the included study populations, interventions, and outcomes. That notwithstanding, the overall conclusion was that CM demonstrated limited impact on patient-centered outcomes, quality of care, and resource utilization among patients with chronic medical illness (Hickam et al., 2013). It is important to sort out the conflicting literature on CM outcomes because direct cause-and-effect may not capture the actual importance of CM to clients and because cost reduction or ROI is hard to demonstrate when a labor-intensive service like CM is added.

These findings need to be leveraged to identify and implement program modifications as well as determine measures that accurately capture CM as value-added irrespective of monetary ROI. Sharing of program metrics across the health care continuum is one way in which research-generated evidence will influence practice moving forward. CM leader-managers undertaking quality and process improvements within a CM department must remain mindful of the importance of the evidence generated from these efforts because it is valuable to the entire CM community.

Treatment Adherence

Treatment adherence continues to be a driver of disease cost and a needed focus of intervention with patients. Medication adherence alone is estimated to have an annual cost of $100 billion in the United States (Lee, 2016). *Adherence* refers to the extent to which the patient continues a negotiated treatment. The topics of treatment adherence and patient engagement are major drivers in ensuring successful outcomes and establishing a PHM program's ROI.

Health risk behaviors (e.g., smoking, inactivity, poor diets, or nonadherence to prescribed therapies) significantly contribute to a population's overall morbidity, disability, mortality, reduced productivity, and escalating health care costs (Lee, 2016; Prochaska & Prochaska, 2016). Intense employer focus on wellness and prevention has escalated the importance of and growth of PHM programs. Studies show as many as 73% of companies are offering workplace or employee wellness to incentivize engagement in healthy lifestyles (Lee, 2016). Identified reasons for low ROI for early DM programs have included late identification of patients, turnover rate, lack of benefit coordination (especially when using an outside DM vendor), and the presence of comorbidities (Ahmed, 2016).

More engaged patients incur lower costs, whereas less engaged patients can generate up to 21% higher health care costs (Calhoun et al., 2016). Successful interventions with nonadherent patient populations include using the transtheoretical model of behavior change, which integrates advising, guiding, and supporting patients through the six stages of health behavior change: precontemplation, contemplation, preparation, action, maintenance, and termination. Key strategies and processes have been identified that work best at each stage to reduce resistance, facilitate progress, and minimize relapse (Prochaska & Prochaska, 2016).

There are planned updates to popular health risk assessments over the next few years toward a more conclusive assessment that takes into account determinants of health and performance (e.g., advances in technology, use of smartphones, and new research) (Edington et al., 2016). All health care professionals, especially nurses, can develop the skills to engage patients in the care process through leveraging meaningful use goals (e.g., health IT) and delivering adherence interventions (Calhoun et al., 2016; Prochaska & Prochaska, 2016).

CONCLUSION

Health care's strong fiscal imperatives have the industry well aligned with the business sector. Organizations strive to align overall goals, financial drivers of care, and department staffing in way that demonstrates ROI as a marker for financial viability. As a result, leaders need to ensure solid processes are in place to guide the development of department programming, provide clear job descriptions for those to be hired, and render a comprehensive means to identify and promote performance quality.

Despite the widespread dissemination of CM and DM as an intervention and system-wide strategy, a number of challenges remain specific to program development and implementation. Organizations struggle with a number of issues including whether and how to internally combine or separate functions. With an emphasis on financial viability or profit margin, CM and DM programs have been analyzed, challenged, redesigned, and reinvented under different labels in order to justify the allocation of scarce resources to them. Where CM is concerned, continued confusion over definitions, evolution and expansion of titles, and ongoing licensure and reimbursement challenges further contribute to constant changes within CM departments and programs.

RESEARCH NOTE

Source
Joo, J.Y., & Liu, M.F. (2019). Effectiveness of nurse-led case management in cancer care: Systematic review. *Clinical Nursing Research, 28*(8), 968–991.

Purpose
The purpose of this research article is to systematically examine the evidence for the effectiveness of nurse-led case management (CM) in adults with cancer. Because cancer is deadly, expensive, requires a high level of care, and care is often uncoordinated and fragmented, CM has been used to increase the efficiency and effectiveness of cancer care. CM has been shown to promote quality of life but is more commonly studied in high-risk or chronic illness populations.

Discussion
Using systematic review principles, the Cochrane processes and PRISMA statements were employed, and nine experimental studies published from 2008–2017 were retrieved from four electronic databases. Across all of the studies, CM interventions were palliative care, supportive services, and regular follow-ups. Three domains of outcomes were psycho-behavioral, hospital access, and health care costs. The results demonstrated that positive case management improved the quality of life for patients and significantly decreased hospital readmission rates. When looking at health care costs and other hospital access measures, the results were mixed. This demonstrates that there is some evidence for the effectiveness of nurse-led CM in cancer care.

Application to Practice
Consistent with other studies, when research is systematically reviewed, there is strong evidence for the fact that for patients with nurse-led CM interventions, there was improved quality of life and significantly decreased hospital readmission rates. Thus, CM is effective for these two outcomes. Other outcomes were mixed, and this may be due to imprecision in standardization of intervention protocols or in measurement of intervention effects on outcomes. Overall, nurse case managers play a pivotal role in cancer treatment, producing some important outcome results. The practice of nurse-led CM needs to be taught to nurses, nurse practitioners, and nurse managers.

CASE STUDY

Ramona St. Rose, RN, was hired to facilitate the Healthy Habits Advisory Group and Ministry at St. Patrick Church in Iowa City for a bilingual community. One third of the population was Latino and two-thirds were White Americans. She worked collaboratively with a team of parishioner volunteers. The team consisted of three physicians, a nurse attorney, two faculty members, prelicensure students in a public health practicum, and the mobile clinic at the local university. Pearl, one volunteer, offered a proactive role called the self-care transition coach. This role would allow discharged parishioners, especially those with chronic diseases, to contact her to manage their discharge instructions at home. The team identified, assessed, and defined the populations to be served early in the planning effort. What methods would Ramona use to define and assess the population? As the demand for services grows, what strategies can be used to avoid overwhelming Pearl and Ramona?

■ CRITICAL THINKING EXERCISE

Nurse Gloria Davis just got her dream job as a case manager for diabetes care in a large integrated delivery system. Nurse Davis is deeply committed to high-quality client care. She has structured an excellent teaching program that is administered through the ambulatory clinics. She has instituted population data collection using the SF-36 and Diabetes Quality of Life tools. Nurse Davis has begun to collect trend data on HbA_{1c} values and frequency of blood glucose instability or complications. The next outcome to measure is client satisfaction. Nurse Davis assumes that client satisfaction is related to adherence with treatment. The first step is a small focus group. In the focus group meeting, Nurse Davis discovers that client interactions with a health care provider are becoming more impersonal. The clients have fewer choices about to whom and where they can go for services, must get complicated authorizations, there is an increasing need to fill out more forms, listen to recorded messages, and are wait longer for appointments. On clinic days they wait a long time to see their provider briefly. The process of coming in for care actually makes many of these clients feel worse. Discuss the following questions based on the content presented:

1. Identify the problem(s).
2. Prioritize what Nurse Davis should do first, and why.
3. How should Nurse Davis analyze this situation?
4. How could Nurse Davis apply the COLLABORATE competencies to this situation?
5. How should Nurse Davis evaluate her final actions?
6. Outline leadership and management strategies that would be useful to Nurse Davis.

REFERENCES

Advancing Integrated Mental Health Solutions (AIMS) Center. (2019). *Our projects.* University of Washington, Psychiatry and Behavioral Sciences Division of Integrated Care and Public Health. http://aims.uw.edu/projects.

Affordable Care Act (ACA). (2010). *ACA the About.* https://www.hhs.gov/healthcare/about-the-aca/index.html.

Ahmed, O. I. (2016). Disease management, case management, care management, and care coordination: A framework and brief manual for care programs and staff. *Professional Case Management, 21*(3), 137–146.

American Association of Critical-Care Nurses (AACN). (2019). *AACN Synergy Model for patient care.* https://www.aacn.org/nursing-excellence/aacn-standards/synergy-model.

American Case Management Association (ACMA). (2013). *Standards of practice & scope of services for health care delivery system case management and transitions of care (TOC) professionals.*

American Organization of Nurse Executives (AONE). (2015). *Nurse executive competencies: Population health.*

Ashford, J. B., & LeCroy, C. W. (2017). *Human behavior in the social environment: A multi-dimensional perspective* (6th ed.): Cengage Learning.

Berger, C. S. (2015). Social work case management in medical settings. In K. Corcoran, & A. R. Roberts (Eds.), *Social workers' desk reference* (3rd ed., pp. 866–878). Oxford University Press.

Braden, C. J. (2002). *State of the science paper #2: Involvement/participation, empowerment and knowledge outcome indicators of case management.* Case Management Society of America.

Brown, R. S., Peikes, D., Peterson, G., Schore, J., & Razafindrakoto, C. M. (2012). Six features of Medicare coordinated care demonstration programs that cut hospital admissions of high-risk patients. *Health Affairs, 31*(6), 1156–1166.

Bullock, H. L., Waddell, K., & Wilson, M. G. (2017). *Knowledge synthesis: Identifying and assessing core components of collaborative-care models for treating mental and physical health conditions.* McMaster Health Forum.

Calhoun, C., Hall, L. K., & Kemper, D. (2016). Patient engagement: Engaging patients in the care process by leveraging meaningful use goals. In D. B. Nash, R. J. Fabius, A. Skoufalos, J. L. Clarke, & M. R. Horowitz (Eds.), *Population health: Creating a culture of wellness* (2nd ed., Chapter 7). Jones and Bartlett Learning.

Care Continuum Alliance (CCA). (2012a). *Implementation and evaluation: A population health guide for primary care models.* https://populationhealthalliance.org/population-health-guide-for-primary-care-models/.

Care Continuum Alliance (CCA). (2012). *Participant engagement and the use of incentives considerations.* https://populationhealthalliance.org/wp-content/uploads/2018/02/cca-incentives-document_1.pdf.

Carr, D. (2009). Building collaborative partnerships in critical care: The RN case manager/social work dyad in critical care. *Professional Case Management, 14*(3), 121–132.

Case Management Society of America (CMSA). (2016). *Standards of practice for case management.*

Case Management Society of America (CMSA). (2017a). What is a case manager? https://www.cmsa.org/who-we-are/what-is-a-case-manager/.

Case Management Society of America (CMSA). (2017b). *CMSA core curriculum for case management.*

Centers for Disease Control and Prevention (CDC). (2019). Chronic Diseases in America. https://www.cdc.gov/chronicdisease/resources/infographic/chronic-diseases.htm.

Centers for Medicare & Medicaid Services (CMS). (2003). Medicare program; Demonstration: Capitated disease management for beneficiaries with chronic illnesses. *Federal Register, 68*(40), 9673–9680.

Cline, B. G. (1990). Case management: Organizational models and administrative methods. *Caring: National Association for Home Care Magazine, 9*(7), 14–18.

Cobb, B. (2019). ACMA and 15 Collaborating Organizations Publish National Transitions of Care Standards and a Consensus Measures Crosswalk, Case Management. *Medical Management Plus, Inc.* http://mmplusinc.com/news-articles/item/acma-and-15-collaborating-organizations-publish-national-transitions-of-care-standards-and-a-consensus-measures-crosswalk.

Commission for Case Manager Certification (CCMC). (2015). *Code of professional conduct for case managers with standards, rules, procedures, and penalties.*

Commission for Case Manager Certification (CCMC). (2016). *Case management body of knowledge (CMBOK).*

Community Mental Health Act. (1963). *S. 1576.* https://www.govtrack.us/congress/votes/88-1963/h78.

Council on Social Work Education. (2015). *Educational policy and accreditation standards for baccalaureate and master's social work programs.* Alexandria: VA: Council on Social Work Education Commission on Accreditation, Commission on Educational Policy.

Daniels, S. (2015). Hospital case management: A new view from the C-Suite. *Professional Case Management, 20*(3), 156–158. https://doi.org/10.1097/NCM.0000000000000095.

Developmentally Disabled Assistance and Bill of Rights Act. (1975). *S. 462 (94th).* https://www.govtrack.us/congress/bills/94/s462.

Edington, D. W., Schultz, A. B., & Pitts, J. S. (2016). The future of population health at the workplace: Trends, technology, and the role of mind-body and behavioral science. In D. B. Nash, R. J. Fabius, A. Skoufalos, J. L. Clarke, & M. R. Horowitz (Eds.), *Population health: Creating a culture of wellness* (2nd ed., Chapter 20). Jones and Bartlett Learning.

Eghaneyan, B. H., Sanchez, K., & Mitschke, D. B. (2014). Implementation of a collaborative care model for the treatment of depression and anxiety in a community health center: Results from a qualitative case study. *Journal of Multidisciplinary Healthcare, 7,* 503–513. https://doi.org/10.2147/JMDH.S69821.

Ellsworth, J. (2015). Case managers: A key to reducing admissions. *Professional Case Management, 20*(3), 147–149.

Epstein Becker Green. (2015). *The challenges and rewards of integrating behavioral health into primary care.* Webinar. https://www.ebglaw.com/events/the-challenges-and-rewards-of-integrating-behavioral-health-into-primary-care-%e2%80%93-thought-leaders-in-population-health-webinar-series/.

Fink-Samnick, E. (2019). *The Essential Guide to Interprofessional Ethics for Healthcare Case Management*: HCPro.

Fink-Samnick, E. (2019). *The Social Determinants of Health: Case Management's Next Frontier* (1st ed): HCPro.

Fink-Samnick, E., & Muller, L. (2015). Case management practice: Is technology helping or hindering practice in legal and regulatory issues. *Professional Case Management, 20*(2), 98–102.

Forbes, M. A. (1999). The practice of professional nurse case management. *Nursing Case Management, 4*(1), 28–33.

Fortney J., Sladek R., Unützer J., Alfred L., Carneal G., Emmet B., et al. (2015). *Fixing behavioral health care in*

America: A national call for integrating and coordinating specialty behavioral health care with the medical system. The Kennedy Forum in Partnership with Advancing Integrated Mental Health Solutions (AIMS) Center, The Kennedy Center for Mental Health Policy and Research, Satcher Health Leadership Institute, Morehouse School of Medicine. Issue Brief. http://www.thekennedyforum.com.

Gartner, Inc. (2016). Predictive modeling. http://www.gartner.com/it-glossary/predictive-modeling/.

Gillespie, L. (2016). *Hospitals push Medicare to soften readmission penalties in light of socioeconomic risks.* Modern Healthcare. http://www.modernhealthcare.com/article/20160521/MAGAZINE/305219914.

Goodman, R. A., Bunnell, R., & Posner, S. F. (2014). What is "community health"? Examining the meaning of an evolving field in public health. *Preventive Medicine, 67*(Supp. 1), S58–S61. https://doi.org/10.1016/j.ypmed.2014.07.028 https://doi.org/.

Graf, T., Erskine, A., & Steele, G. D. (2014). Leveraging data to systematically improve care coronary artery disease management at Geisinger. *Journal of Ambulatory Care Management, 37*(3), 199–205.

Gupta, A. (2015). *Tech is driving collaboration in behavioral health.* TechCrunch. http://techcrunch.com/2015/09/19/tech-is-driving-collaboration-in-behavioral-health/.

Hawkins, K., Wells, T. S., Hommer, C. E., Ozminkowski, R. J., Richards, D. M., & Yeh, C. S. (2014). Factors driving engagement decisions in care coordination programs. *Professional Case Management, 19*(5), 216–223.

Health Enhancement Research Organization (HERO) and Population Health Alliance (PHA). (2015). *Program measurement & evaluation guide: Core metrics for employee health management.* https://populationhealthalliance.org/wp-content/uploads/2018/02/pha-hero-overview-handout_v4.pdf.

HealthCare.gov. (n.d.). *Chronic disease management.* https://www.healthcare.gov/glossary/chronic-disease-management/.

Health Sciences Institute. (2016). *Chronic care professional (CCP) certification.* http://healthsciences.org/Chronic-Care-Professional-Certification.

HealthyPeople.gov (2019a). *Approach to the social determinants.* https://www.healthypeople.gov/2020/topics-objectives/topic-social-determinants-of-health.

HealthyPeople.gov. (2019b). *About healthy people.* https://www.healthypeople.gov/2020/About-Healthy-People.

Herman, C. (2013). *The evolving context of social work case management: NASW releases revised standards of practice, practice perspective.* National Association of Social Workers.

Hickam D. H., Weiss J. W., Guise J-M., Buckley D., Motu'apuaka M., Graham E., et al. (2013). *Outpatient case management for adults with medical illness and complex care needs.* Comparative Effectiveness Review No. 99. (Prepared by the Oregon Evidence based Practice Center under Contract No. 290-2007-10057-I.) AHRQ Publication No.13-EHC031-EF. Rockville, MD: Agency for Healthcare Research and Quality. http://effectivehealthcare.ahrq.gov/index.cfm/search-for-guides-reviews-and-reports/?pageaction=displayproduct&productid=1369.

Hu, J., Gonsahn, M. D., & Nerenz, D. R. (2014). Socioeconomic status and readmissions: Evidence from an urban teaching hospital. *Health Affairs, 33*(5), 778–785. https://doi.org/10.1377/hlthaff.2013.0816 https://doi.org/.

Huber, D. L. (2005). The diversity of service delivery models. In D. Huber (Ed.), *Disease management: A guide for case managers* (pp. 55–67). Saunders.

Huber, D.L. (2017). *Care for the total population.* Iowa City, IA.

Improving Chronic Illness Care. (2006–2019). *The chronic care model.* http://www.improvingchroniccare.org/index.php?p=The_Chronic_CareModel&s=2.

Institute for Healthcare Improvement (IHI). (2017). *Triple aim for populations.* http://www.ihi.org/Topics/TripleAim/Pages/default.aspx.

Institute of Medicine (IOM). (2001). *Crossing the quality chasm: A new health system for the 21st century*: National Academies Press.

Interprofessional Education Collaborative (IPEC). (2016). *Core competencies for interprofessional collaborative practice: 2016 update.*

Kolbasovsky, A., Zeitlin, J., & Gillespie, W. (2012). Impact of point-of-care case management on readmissions and costs. *The American Journal of Managed Care, 18*(8), 300–306.

Kongstvedt, P. R. (2013). *Essentials of managed health care* (6th ed.). Jones and Bartlett.

Lee, J. (2016). Behavioral economics: How BE influences and changes health. In D. B. Nash, R. J. Fabius, A. Skoufalos, J. L. Clarke, & M. R. Horowitz (Eds.), *Population health: Creating a culture of wellness* (2nd ed., Chapter 8). Jones and Bartlett Learning.

Library of Congress (1975). *Education for all handicapped children act.* https://www.govtrack.us/congress/bills/94/s6/summary.

Lyles, C. A. (2016). The political landscape in relation to the health and wealth of nations. In D. B. Nash, R. J. Fabius, A. Skoufalos, J. L. Clarke, & M. R. Horowitz (Eds.), *Population health: Creating a culture of wellness* (2nd ed., Chapter 5). Jones and Bartlett Learning.

Milliman, Inc. (2014). *Economic impact of integrated medical-behavioral healthcare: Implications for psychiatry.* Milliman American Psychiatric Association Report. Denver, CO.

Nagasako, E., Waterman, B., & Dunagan, W. C. (2014). Adding socioeconomic data to hospital readmissions calculations may produce more useful results. *Health Affairs, 33*(5), 786–791. https://doi.org/10.1377/hlthaff.2013.1148.

Nash, D., Fabius, R. J., Skoufalos, A., Clarke, J. L., & Horowitz, M. R. (2016). *Preface. Population health: Creating a culture of wellness* (2nd ed.). Jones and Bartlett Learning.

National Association of Social Workers (NASW). (2013). *Standards for social work case management.*

National Association of Chronic Disease Directors (NACDD). (2016). *About NACDD.* http://www.chronicdisease.org/?page=AboutUs.

National Health Council (2014) About Chronic Diseases.

National Committee for Quality Assurance (NCQA). (2019). *About NCQA.* https://www.ncqa.org/about-ncqa/.

National Council of State Boards of Nursing (NCSBN). (2016a). *The nurse licensure compact: An overview.* https://www.ncsbn.org/9331.htm.

National Council of State Boards of Nursing (NCSBN). (2016b). *Nurse licensure compact.* https://www.ncsbn.org/nurse-licensure-compact.htm.

Older Americans Act. (1965). *42 U.S.C. 3056.* http://www.gpo.gov/fdsys/pkg/STATUTE-79/pdf/STATUTE-79-Pg218.pdf.

Patient Care and Affordable Care Act. (2010). *Public Law 111–148.* http://housedocs.house.gov/energycommerce/ppacacon.pdf.

Plocher, D. W. (2013). Fundamentals and core competencies of disease management. In P. R. Kongstvedt (Ed.), *Essentials of managed health care* (6th ed., Chapter 8). Jones and Bartlett.

Population Health Alliance (PHA). (2015). *2015 Population health alliance outcomes guidelines report.*

Population Health Alliance. (n.d.). *PHM-defined.* https://populationhealthalliance.org/research/understanding-population-health/.

Prochaska, J. O., & Prochaska, J. M. (2016). *Behavior change, population health: Creating a culture of wellness* (2nd ed.). Jones and Bartlett Learning.

Rice, S. (2016). Adjusting for social determinants in value-based payments still fuzzy. *Modern Healthcare.* http://www.modernhealthcare.com/article/20160112/NEWS/160119972.

Robert Wood Johnson Foundation. (2011). *Mental disorders and medical co-morbidity, research synthesis.* Report 21.

Rushton, S. (2015). The population care coordination process. *Professional Case Management, 20*(5), 230–238.

SAS. (2016). *What is Big Data?* http://www.sas.com/en_us/insights/big-data.html.

Shaljian, M., & Nielsen, M. (2013). *Managing populations, maximizing technology: Population health management in the medical neighborhood.* Patient-Centered Primary Care Collaborative.

Sidorov, J., & Romney, M. (2016). The spectrum of care. In D. B. Nash, R. J. Fabius, A. Skoufalos, J. L. Clarke, &
M. R. Horowitz (Eds.), *Population health: Creating a culture of wellness* (2nd ed., Chapter 2). Jones and Bartlett Learning.

Social Security Act of 1935. (2013). *Legislative history.* http://www.ssa.gov/history/35act.html.

Stellefson, M., Dipnarine, K., & Stopka, C. (2013). The chronic care model and diabetes management in US primary care settings: A systematic review. *Preventing Chronic Disease, 10*, 1–21. https://doi.org/10.5888/pcd10.120180 https://doi.org/.

Summers, N. (2016). *Fundamentals of case management practice: Skills for the human services* (5th ed.). Cengage Learning.

Tahan, H. A. (2017). The case management process. In H. A. Tahan, & T. M. Treiger (Eds.), *CMSA core curriculum for case management* (3rd ed.). Wolters Kluwer.

Takeda, A., Taylor, S. J. C., Taylor, R. S., Kahn, F., Krum, H., & Underwood, M. (2012). Clinical service organisation for heart failure. *Cochrane Database of Systematic Reviews,* (9), CD002752. https://doi.org/10.1002/14651858.CD002752.pub3.

The Joint Commission (TJC). (2019). *Certifications by health care setting.* https://www.jointcommission.org/accreditation-and-certification/certification/certifications-by-setting/.

Treiger, T. M. (2011). Case management: Prospects in definition, education, and settings of practice. *The Remington Report, 19*(1), 46–48.

Treiger, T. M. (2012). Helping clients bridge gaps to self-advocacy, self-management. *Healthcare Intelligence Network.* [interview] http://hin.com/blog/2012/09/14/meet-healthcare-case-management-manager-teresa-treiger-helping-clients-bridge-gaps-to-self-advocacy-self-management.

Treiger, T. M., & Fink-Samnick, E. (2013). COLLABORATE: A universal competency based paradigm for professional case management, part I: Introduction, historical validation, and competency presentation. *Professional Case Management, 18*(3), 122–135.

Treiger, T. M., & Fink-Samnick, E. (2016). *COLLABORATE for professional case management: A universal competency-based paradigm*: Wolters Kluwer.

Unützer, J., Harbin, H., Schoenbaum, M., & Druss, B. (2013). *The collaborative care model: An approach to integrating physical and mental health care in Medicaid health homesCenter for Health Care Strategies and Mathematica Policy Research*: Centers for Medicare and Medicaid Services. CMS.

Walters, B. H., Adams, S. A., Nieboer, A. P., & Bal, R. (2012). Disease management projects and the Chronic Care Model in action: Baseline qualitative research. *BMC Health Services Research, 12*(1), 114. https://doi.org/10.1186/1472-6963-12-114.

Ward, B. W., Schiller, J. S., & Goodman, R. A. (2013). Multiple chronic conditions among US adults: A 2012 update. *Preventing Chronic Disease, 11*, E62.

Watson, A. (2016). Evaluating and measuring quality and outcomes: A new "essential activity" of case management practice. *Professional Case Management, 21*(1), 51–52.

Weil, M., & Karls, J. M. (1985). *Case management in human service practice: A systematic approach to mobilizing resources for clients.* Jossey-Bass.

World Health Organization (WHO). (2019). *About social determinants of health.* Retrieved from https://www.who.int/social_determinants/sdh_definition/en/.

Young, B., Clark, C., Kansky, J., & Pupo, E. (2014). *Health information exchange committee ambulatory toolkit.* Chicago, IL: Health Information Management and Systems Society (HIMSS).

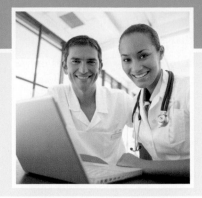

17

Nursing Leadership for Evidence-Based Practice

Laura Cullen, Kirsten Hanrahan, Erin M. Steffen, Michele Farrington, Cindy J. Dawson

 http://evolve.elsevier.com/Huber/leadership

Nurse leaders have responsibility for building and expanding use of evidence-based practice (EBP) in care delivery to improve patient and organizational outcomes (Bunger et al., 2019; Gifford et al., 2018; Melnyk et al., 2016; Stetler et al., 2014). A number of models are available to provide direction for the EBP process. Implementing EBP changes as an organization and unit or clinic requires additional strategies for success. A growing body of research is available to build EBP programs within health care organizations and close the research-to-practice gap (Borsky et al., 2018). Application of EBP is the responsibility of every nursing leader, especially those in the nurse manager role. This chapter outlines the ways nurse leaders can grow the EBP culture in an organization and tactics to create a nurturing climate in the practice setting.

Processes to improve care include quality or performance improvement, EBP, and conduct of research. The best process to use depends on the question at hand, the intent (i.e., knowledge generation or local improvement), and the extent of research and other evidence available on the topic. For questions best addressed through quality improvement (e.g., efficient throughput), improvements may be brought directly to practice. EBP offers the benefit of using existing evidence for designing effective interventions, adapting them for local adoption, planning implementation, and guidance for avoiding unintended consequences. Clinical questions with little or no research that may include patient risk may be appropriate to answer by conducting research.

DEFINITIONS

An understanding of EBP and related concepts requires knowledge of a variety of terms. **Evidence-based practice** (EBP) is a process of shared decision-making in a partnership between patients and clinicians that involves the integration of research and other best evidence with clinical expertise and patient values and preferences in making shared health care decisions (Sackett et al., 2000; Sigma Theta Tau International Research Scholarship Advisory Committee, 2008). EBP is a scholarly process for improving health care quality and safety by building on what is learned from—and also influencing— the conduct of research and quality improvement.

Additional terms are also important to understand. **Knowledge translation** is defined as the process of putting scientific knowledge into practice (Harrison et al., 2013; Straus et al., 2011) and is synonymous with EBP in some regions across the globe. **Best practice** is a popular term, but the definition remains elusive. Use of the term may describe innovative practices that are recognized by peer organizations and that contribute to quality or fiscal goals. Although "best practice," "best evidence," and "evidence-based practice" are sometimes used interchangeably, the extent that "best practices" are based on "best evidence" is often unclear. To promote understanding, it is recommended that when using scientific evidence for guidance, the term evidence-based practice provides the most clarity.

Evidence-based interventions (EBI) are treatments that are supported by empirical evidence from research. EBI are expected to improve outcomes; if not, failure may be related to design of the practice change, related to a poor fit within the local context, not staying true to the treatment procedure (fidelity), or failed implementation.

A **clinical practice guideline** is a report designed to assist clinicians and clients in making decisions about appropriate health care for specific clinical circumstances (Institute of Medicine, 2011). Guidelines are systematically developed, link evidence with health outcomes (benefits and harms), and continue to require subjective judgments and local adaption to apply to patient care. Guidelines are developed with the intent to influence clinician behavior by making clear practice recommendations.

Implementation is the process of putting an idea or process change into practice. The implementation process uses strategies to promote adoption of EBP in a specific setting to improve outcomes (Brownson et al., 2018a). Integration involves the infusion of an innovation until that change is a practice routine. Implementation strategies are tactics used to impact the rate of integration into practice to achieve adoption and sustainability. Strategies that are data driven and evidence based are more likely to result in a sustainable practice change. A Precision Implementation Approach™ uses local data to drive selection of strategies for the most effective and efficient implementation, integration, and sustainability (Cullen et al., 2019b). After initial pilot implementation and evaluation, the boost used to promote integration of EBP is called **reinfusion**.

Implementation science is the "study of methods to promote the adoption and integration of evidence-based practices, interventions and policies, into routine health care and public health settings" (NIH, 2019), and offers great opportunity to learn effective strategies to promote EBP as the standard for health care delivery. Implementation research identifies enablers and barriers to effective health programming and policymaking (NIH, 2019), creating new knowledge that can be leveraged in the application of EBP.

Translation science may be a more confusing term, as it can be defined two ways (Rubio et al., 2010). First, to describe the process of moving knowledge from bench research to patient care (Titler, 2018), translational science is also defined as "the field of investigation focused on understanding the scientific and operational principles underlying each step of the translational process" (Institute of Translational Health Sciences, 2019a). The translation process, as defined by the Institute of

Translational Health Sciences (ITHS), includes five interactive nonlinear phases (T_0–T_4):

"T_0 is characterized by the identification of opportunities and approaches to health problems. T1 seeks to move basic discovery into a candidate health application. T2 assesses the value of application for health practice leading to the development of evidence-based guidelines. T3 attempts to move evidence-based guidelines into health care, through delivery, dissemination, and diffusion research. T4 seeks to evaluate the 'real world' health outcomes of population health practice" (Institute of Translational Health Sciences, 2019b).

The second definition is consistent with implementation science, testing the effect of interventions that promote the rate and extent of adoption of EBP by nurses, physicians, and other health care providers and describing organizational, unit, and individual variables that affect the use of evidence in clinical and operational decision-making (Institute of Translational Health Sciences, 2019a; Titler, 2018). Translational research provides guidance about what strategies are effective, for whom, and in what setting when implementing EBP. In this sense, *the term translational research is often used interchangeably with implementation science.* **Sustainment**, the goal of EBP implementation, is the long-term use of the practice recommendation and indicates the EBI has been hardwired as the new standard (Ament et al., 2015; NHS Institute for Innovation and Improvement, 2010). A comprehensive definition of **sustainability** encompasses five components: (1) the EBI or program, (2) that maintains a change in individual behavior, (3) over a defined time period, (4) in which the EBI may evolve or be adapted, but (5) continues to produce the expected benefits (Moore et al., 2017). Additional rollout or **scaling up** is the systematic process used to expand the reach of effective clinical interventions in one setting to other similar areas or populations; whereas, **scaling out** refers to when EBIs are adapted either to new populations or new delivery systems, or both (Aarons et al., 2017).

In contrast to EBP are **sacred cows**, old practice habits considered routine, above dispute, and particularly resistant to change (Hanrahan et al., 2015). **De-implementation** or de-adoption is needed to reverse, stop, undo, or remove current practices that are not evidence-based, do not improve care, are ineffective, or may be harmful (Helfrich et al., 2018; Patey et al., 2018; Wang et al., 2018). Strategies needed for de-implementation may be different from implementation strategies; theories and research are just emerging.

Organizational context refers to the health system environment in which the proposed EBP is to be implemented. Six contextual features synergistically influence EBP implementation within an organization: (1) organizational culture (e.g., patient centered, innovative), (2) networks and communications (e.g., collaborations and teamwork), (3) leadership (e.g., transformational leadership that gives rise to clear role delineation and teamwork), (4) resources (including financial, staffing, time, and training), (5) evaluation, monitoring, and feedback (e.g., soliciting feedback and ongoing communication with point-of-care clinicians), and (6) champions (i.e., individuals with key attributes including EBP expertise, peer influence, and ability to troubleshoot) (Li et al., 2018).

BACKGROUND MODELS

A variety of knowledge translation theories, models, and frameworks exist to guide both application in practice (EBP) and implementation science (research) (Strifler et al., 2018). Nilsen (2015) described three overarching theoretical approaches in implementation science that aim to (1) describe or guide the EBP process (process models), (2) understand the determinants influencing implementation outcomes (determinant frameworks, classic theories, and implementation theories), and (3) evaluate implementation (evaluation frameworks) (Table 17.1). Process models give step-by-step guidance for planning and executing change. EBP process models may be best suited for guiding the team through organizational change. These models

TABLE 17.1   Select Evidence-Based Practice Models: Implementation Science Theories, Models, and Frameworks

Type	Examples	Citation	Sample of application
EBP Process Models	ACE Star Model of Knowledge Transformation	Stevens (2013)	Farra et al. (2015)
	Advancing Research and Clinical Practice Through Close Collaboration (ARCC) Model	Melnyk et al. (2017)	Little et al. (2017)
	Iowa Model Revised: Evidence-Based Practice to Promote Excellence in Health Care	Iowa Model Collaborative (2017)	Huether et al. (2016)
	Johns Hopkins Nursing Evidence-Based Practice (JHNEBP) Model	Dang & Dearholt (2017)	Pittman et al. (2019)
	Knowledge-to-Action Model (K2A)	Morton et al. (2018)	
	Stetler Model	Stetler (2001)	Stetler et al. (2014)
Determinant Frameworks	EBP Implementation Guide	Cullen & Adams (2012)	Abbott & Hooke (2017)
	Consolidated Framework for Implementation Research (CFIR)	Damschroder & Hagedorn (2011)	Damschroder & Lowery (2013)
	Promoting Action on Research Implementation in Health Services (PARIHS) Framework	Harvey & Kitson (2015)	Lewis et al. (2019)
Classic Theories	Diffusion of Innovation	Rogers (2003)	Zhao et al. (2018)
	Social Learning Theory	Bandura (1977)	Ishikawa et al. (2019)
Implementation Theories	Normalization Process Theory	May et al. (2009)	Mishuris et al. (2019)
	Capabilities, Opportunities, Motivations and Behaviour (COM-B) model	Michie et al. (2014)	Muhwava et al. (2019)

have been used successfully to improve adoption of EBP recommendations and improve patient and health care outcomes (Gawlinski & Rutledge, 2008; Strifler et al., 2018). For example, the *Iowa Model-Revised: Evidence-Based Practice to Promote Excellence in Health Care* (Iowa Model Collaborative, 2017) reflects the current environment in health care and uses implementation science to guide clinician decision-making in a variety of health care settings (Coleman et al., 2018; Huether et al., 2016). Additional details and comparisons of theories, models, and frameworks are summarized elsewhere (Camargo et al., 2017; Cullen et al., 2019a; Dang et al., 2019; Davis et al., 2015; Nilsen, 2015; Schaffer et al., 2013; Strifler et al., 2018).

The challenge for leaders is to identify a model that guides the EBP process and promotes successful adoption of EBP (Dang et al., 2019; Gawlinski & Rutledge, 2008). Adoption of one EBP model across an organization for interprofessional initiatives (Abbott & Hooke, 2017; Cullen et al., 2018a; Hanrahan et al., 2015; Huether et al., 2016) is one strategy for promoting continuous learning and coordination of efforts across a system. EBP models tend to follow a basic problem-solving process with step-by-step guidance, just as do some other quality improvement processes (e.g., Six Sigma). Senior leadership support for EBP can be leveraged by outlining the similarities between EBP and quality improvement processes, structures, and resources for comprehensive improvement in clinical and organizational outcomes (Djulbegovic et al., 2019; Mondoux & Shojania, 2019).

Determinant frameworks identify multi-level facilitators and barriers that influence implementation outcomes and are often linked to classic theories drawn from psychology, sociology, and organizational theory. For example, Cullen and Adams Implementation Strategies for EBP guide (Cullen & Adams, 2012), based on Rogers' Diffusion of Innovations Theory (Rogers, 2003) identifies strategies for clinicians and organizations across four phases of implementation (Fig. 17.1). A multitude of implementation theories and evaluation frameworks have been used to guide research, but most may lack the step-by-step guidance that clinicians need to achieve sustainability (Strifler et al., 2018).

STEPS FOR PERFORMING EVIDENCE-BASED PRACTICE

Nurses across the career continuum can learn and practice the basic steps for EBP. It begins with a question that arises out of practice (QSEN Institute, 2019). Formulate a purpose statement or clinical question by using the PICOT elements: P (patient population, problem, patient perspective, and pilot area), I (intervention), C (comparison), O (outcome desired). Including T is a variation some find helpful (T = time or anticipated completion date). Consider each of these elements in detail. Next, appropriate resources to search for evidence are determined and a search strategy developed. There are many bibliographic databases to use such as PubMed, MEDLINE, CINAHL, OVID, and the Cochrane Database of Systematic Reviews. Use keywords or Medical Subject Heading (MeSH) headings from the purpose statement to help focus the search. A librarian can be very helpful at this stage. If a librarian is not available, database websites often offer user-training modules. Once the search is conducted, there is a need to evaluate the yield from the search for further refinement, such as expanding or narrowing keywords.

Nurses need to have confidence in the evidence used for making decisions about practice. The search methodology that yields the best evidence changes as a clinical issue is analyzed. A focus on randomized controlled trials (RCT) and systematic reviews or meta-analysis for the most desirable study designs is often too limited. Instead, use a systematic process to evaluate the body of evidence in a stepwise manner, and consider appropriate research designs (Cullen et al., 2019a) as follows:
1. Prevalence of the issue—expect descriptive or cohort studies;
2. Risk or risk factors associated with this issue—look for descriptive or cohort studies;
3. Patients and caregiver perspectives, preferences, and values—likely reported in qualitative studies;
4. Assessment for accurate diagnosis—look for psychometric and descriptive studies;
5. Effective interventions—usually experimental and possibly RCT studies. Also consider synthesis reports such as clinical practice guidelines and systematic reviews;
6. Unintended consequences—often missed in RCT studies, look for these in descriptive and qualitative studies.

Implementation Strategies for Evidence-Based Practice

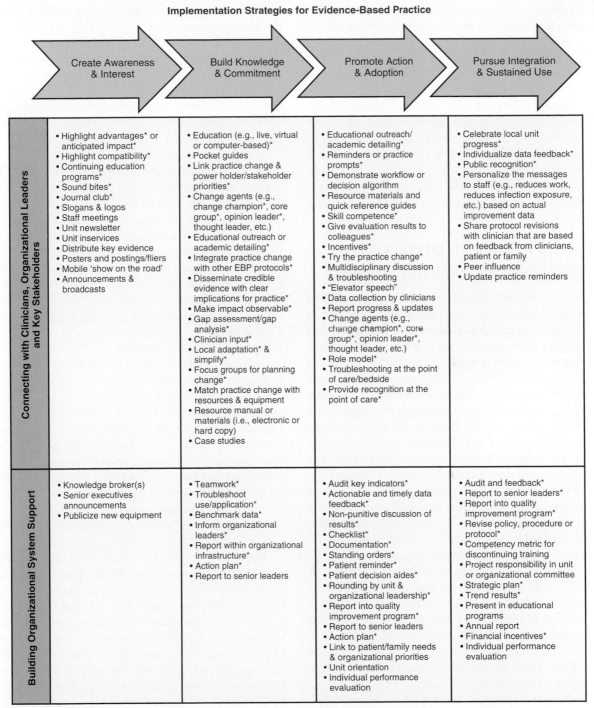

Fig. 17.1 Evidence-based practice implementation guide. (Reproduced with permission from Laura Cullen, DNP, RN, FAAN, and the University of Iowa Hospitals and Clinics. From Cullen, L., & Adams, S. [2012]. Planning for implementation of evidence-based practice. Journal of Nursing Administration, 42[4], 222–230.)

Depending on the desired outcome and the situation, a search for documents from relevant professional organizations may be important.

Use the evidence to design the practice change and evaluation plan (Cullen et al., 2018b). When designing the EBI use the evidence to identify the core elements essential for achieving the desired outcome. Match the practice to patient preferences, values, and needs. Consider interprofessional perspectives, being broadly inclusive, to create a good fit for the local setting. Create a clear procedure, with specific inclusion and exclusion criteria, and decision points. Supporting documents—policies and algorithms—can be useful to promote adoption.

IMPLEMENTING AND SUSTAINING EVIDENCE-BASED PRACTICE CHANGES

Implementation of EBP changes can be challenging in complex health care settings. Baseline evaluation occurs before implementation so that baseline data can incorporate the evidence and locally adapted EBI can be used for implementation planning. Following a *Precision Implementation Approach*™ (Cullen et al., 2019b) leaders used baseline data to select implementation strategies matching local needs. For example, informational and educational strategies can focus specifically on a local clinician's knowledge gap. This avoids using resources on education where knowledge already exists. Likewise, implementation strategies can be selected to target local patient and clinician perceptions and behaviors. Data on outcomes and unintended consequences (balancing measures) can be used during implementation to identify if a midstream correction is warranted or if efforts can move toward integration and sustained use.

Strategies for implementing EBPs occur at the unit or clinic level (Moreno-Poyato et al., 2019), and also at the organizational/systems level (Hanrahan et al., 2015; Li et al., 2018; Sarkies et al., 2017; Stetler et al., 2014), as illustrated in the exemplar in the following section. A large variety of implementation strategies support adoption of EBP and need to target clinicians, patients, and the health care system (Cullen & Adams, 2012; Lewis et al., 2018; Perry et al., 2019; Powell et al., 2015; Rogers, 2003).

The Diffusion of Innovation Theory (Rogers, 2003) provides a well-recognized model with strong research support guiding the hard work of implementation (Davis et al., 2015; Goldstein & Olswang, 2017; Greenhalgh, 2018;

Mohammadi et al., 2018). The *Implementation Strategies for Evidence-Based Practice* guide (see Fig. 17.1) was developed based on Rogers' Innovation-Decision Process Model to assist nurse leaders with planning for use of effective implementation strategies through a process of active diffusion: creating awareness and interest; building knowledge and commitment; promoting action and adoption; and pursuing integration and sustained use (Cullen & Adams, 2012).

Multiple interactive and reinforcing strategies, as outlined, promote adoption of EBP recommendations (Cullen & Adams, 2012; Cullen et al., 2018b; Mohammadi et al., 2018). Strategies to capture a busy clinician's attention are important to include early in the implementation. Nurse leaders can identify additional strategies when working across phases (Bunger et al., 2019). Strategies are added to create a cumulative and comprehensive implementation plan to garner momentum before, during, and after starting an EBP pilot change. The *Implementation Strategies for EBP* guide is a planning tool to be used in combination with an EBP process model (Cullen et al., 2018b).

Early in the EBP process, a fluid action plan is useful to keep the team on task and collectively moving forward (Gude et al., 2019). Implementation and creating sustainability are two of the most difficult steps in the EBP process. Common strategies used for sustaining EBP include adapting the practice recommendation, trending evaluative data, ongoing training, having champions and leaders across all levels, aligning project work with organizational priorities, having sufficient resources allocated, and communicating and partnering with stakeholders (Cullen et al., 2020; Li et al., 2018; Seneski & Stack, 2019; Valim et al., 2019).

Audit and feedback of key indicators remains a necessary component of an integration plan (Li et al., 2018). Key indicators to monitor are drawn from the pilot data and include process (i.e., knowledge, attitudes, and behaviors) and outcomes, including unintended consequences (Cullen et al., 2019b; Norton et al., 2016; Parry et al., 2018). Integration also requires linkages across the governance structure (Cullen et al., 2017, 2020). An important strategy is to link within the quality improvement infrastructure (Fleiszer et al., 2016; Harvey et al., 2019; Norton et al., 2016; Seneski & Stack, 2019) to promote essential influence needed from senior leaders (Li et al., 2018; Taylor et al., 2015).

Change can only be complete and sustained using a combination of implementation strategies (Cullen et al., 2018b; Hanrahan et al., 2015; Seneski & Stack, 2019; Staines et al., 2018; Valim et al., 2019). These principles are highlighted in the following EBP exemplar.

AN EVIDENCE-BASED PRACTICE EXEMPLAR

Title
Strategies for Reducing Reliance on Agency Nursing Staff Equate to $7.7 Million in Savings.

Purpose, Rationale, and Framework
The purpose of this strategic effort was to recruit and hire permanent nursing staff in fiscal year 18 in order to reduce the number of agency nursing staff and trim overall costs (Farrington et al., 2020). Faced with a 12% vacancy rate, a large academic health system opted to hire 224 full-time equivalent (FTE) agency nursing staff to fill the existing gaps while opening a new children's hospital and expanding adult inpatient bed capacity. Although this strategy helped to fill the short-term need, the expense was massive. At the time, the hourly rate the hospital paid for agency nursing staff ranged from $69 to $110, based on specialty. The organization's nursing team rallied to come up with innovative and creative solutions to reduce agency nursing staff to less than 75 FTEs, a two-thirds reduction, in just 6 months. The Iowa Model (Iowa Model Collaborative, 2017) provided the project framework.

Synthesis of Evidence
The ongoing nursing shortage, increasing vacancy rates, and need for expansion are a few challenges facing health care organizations today (Halter et al., 2017). To combat these challenges, hospitals often turn to agency nursing staff to fill the gaps (Warren et al., 2016; Xue et al., 2015). Competition between the public and private sectors to recruit and retain the same nurses forces employers to implement incentives such as higher pay, better benefits, and signing bonuses (Willis et al., 2016). Vacancy rates and replacing nurses place a financial burden on an organization and the health care industry (Huddleston & Gray, 2016b; Warren et al., 2016).

In May 2018 the median annual salary for a nurse in the United States was $71,730 (US Bureau of Labor Statistics,

2019). Using this number, combined with reports of turnover costs being 0.75 to 2 times the annual salary of a nurse, equates to a turnover cost between $53,798 and $143,460 per nurse. At the same time, lower nurse vacancy rates benefit health care consumers through improved patient outcomes and quality of care (Connor et al., 2018; Ducharme et al., 2017; Hairr et al., 2014; Kalisch & Lee, 2014; Martin, 2015). The conditions in which nurses work are critical, as shown by higher nurse retention occurring in "healthy work environments" (American Association of Critical-Care Nurses, 2005). Establishing and maintaining a healthy work environment requires organizations to make strategic investments aimed at improving care delivery, patient satisfaction, clinician satisfaction, patient safety/outcomes, and the culture of nursing practice (Ducharme et al., 2017; Huddleston & Gray, 2016a, 2016b; Huddleston et al., 2017).

There is currently no consistent strategy regarding how best to drive recruitment and retention (Gorman, 2019). A creative and comprehensive approach to recruitment and retention must be deployed at the organizational level and tailored to the unit or clinic.

Practice Change
A four-pronged recruitment approach was used. Focus was first placed on partnering with marketing and communications to improve the social media presence, next was website optimization, third hosting recruitment fairs with onsite interviews, and fourth considered the transition for nurses new to the organization. Since 2009 the organization has provided a nurse residency program (NRP), first accredited in 2012, to smooth the transition from school to hospital-based nursing practice (Hosking et al., 2016). Yet even the most experienced nurses may encounter stress and undergo a difficult professional transition to a new role. The Experienced Nurse Fellowship (ENF) program started in 2015 to support the transition of experienced nurses into new practice environments, increase job satisfaction, and reduce nursing turnover, all designed to positively impact patient outcomes. Advertising the availability of these programs for transitioning nurses, along with spotlighting the organization's Magnet® status as part of the recruitment efforts was critical.

New retention strategies focused on enhanced benefits for current and incoming permanent nursing staff including increased annual inpatient differential from $1000 to $2500; initiating reimbursement for moving expenses; creating a referral incentive for current nurses who recruited experienced nurses into the organization; and introduction of preceptor pay to recognize the time experienced nurses invested in training the incoming nurses.

Implementation Strategies

A comprehensive, phased approach to implementation (Cullen & Adams, 2012) was used as part of this initiative. Creating awareness and interest to get the attention of busy clinicians was accomplished by highlighting the advantages and compatibility; sharing the new initiatives at staff meetings, unit in-services, and in-unit newsletters; displaying posters and postings/fliers; and utilizing announcements and broadcasts by senior executives. Preparing clinicians for the change was critical to build knowledge and commitment. Implementation strategies in this phase included education, change agents, making the impact observable, gap assessment/gap analysis, clinician input, focus groups for planning change, teamwork, and reporting within the organizational infrastructure. Actual behavior change occurred during phase three as part of promoting action and adoption during the "go live" timeframes. Action and adoption strategies included reminders or practice prompts, resource materials and quick reference guides, reporting progress and updates, change agents, actionable and timely data feedback, reporting to senior leaders, and linking to patient/family needs and organizational priorities. In order to hardwire the process, the final stage of pursuing integration and sustained use involved celebrating local unit progress, individualizing data feedback, public recognition, personalizing the messages to staff based on actual improvement data, continuing to audit and provide feedback, reporting to senior leaders, trending results, and presenting in educational programs. The multifaceted content and messaging were widely disseminated via the well-established shared governance structure (Cullen et al., 2017).

Evaluation

Collective efforts resulted in the hiring of more than 800 registered nurses (RNs) in 1 year and reducing agency FTEs by 203 in a little over 5 months (Fig. 17.2), leading to a $7.7 million-dollar savings. Increasing the inpatient differential affected over 2100 RNs with a financial impact of almost $5 million dollars. Reimbursement for moving expenses impacted 21 newly hired nurses, who received almost $54,000. Twenty-four nurses benefited from the referral incentive, equating to $46,000, and 727 RNs financially benefited from disbursement of preceptor pay. The overall vacancy rate simultaneously fell to less than 5% by the end of the fiscal year and has been sustained since that time. Finally, the organization's annual turnover rate remains well below the NSI Nursing Solutions, Inc. benchmark (NSI Nursing Solutions Inc., 2019).

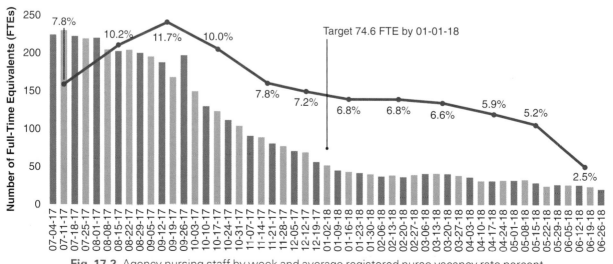

Fig. 17.2 Agency nursing staff by week and average registered nurse vacancy rate percent by month.

Conclusion

Collaborative efforts focused on innovative and aggressive recruitment and retention strategies leading to the reduction of agency nursing staff, recruitment of permanent nurses, and a cost savings of $7.7 million dollars in one fiscal year. These cost savings have allowed for ongoing strategic development in order to continue to positively impact recruitment and retention efforts throughout this large academic **health system**.

ORGANIZATIONAL INFRASTRUCTURE AND CONTEXT

Nurse leaders are in key positions responsible for developing and sustaining an organizational infrastructure and creating an environment that promotes adoption of EBPs and improves patient outcomes (McKay et al., 2018; Melnyk et al., 2016; Shuman et al., 2018; Stetler et al., 2014; Storey et al., 2019). In fact, organizational culture and climate are critical predictors of clinicians' knowledge of and attitudes towards EBP (Powell et al., 2017; Shuman et al., 2018; Yoo et al., 2019). A supportive organizational culture promotes use of evidence, values nurses questioning their practice, provides training about EBP, adopts an EBP model, and recognizes and rewards the work. Evidence-based decision-making is facilitated by roles that promote EBP within the organization, collaborative ties to researchers and networking with other opinion leaders outside the organization, a technical infrastructure to meet informational and data needs, and training programs for building capacity (Brownson et al., 2018b).

It is important to periodically evaluate the infrastructure and context for EBP in the organization. Assessment of EBP leadership, the work environment, and individual and organizational readiness for change may be helpful (Allen et al., 2017; Li et al., 2018; Pittman et al., 2019; Powell et al., 2017; Yoo et al., 2019). Standards for a professional practice environment, such as those outlined through the Magnet Recognition Program®, provide guidance when evaluating an EBP program (https://www.nursingworld.org/organizational-programs/magnet/). A strategic, systematic approach is needed for building EBP capacity (Everett & Sitterding, 2011; Fitzgerald & Harvey, 2015; Shuman et al., 2018; Stetler et al., 2014) at the organization or health system level, building the infrastructure, and creating a culture for change.

Mission, Vision, and Strategic Plan

A mission, vision, and strategic plan inclusive of EBP language provides a sturdy foundation for EBP work at all levels of the organization and begins the process of building a culture in which evidence-based care is the expected norm (Birken et al., 2018; Stetler et al., 2014). A **mission** statement defines the purpose and reflects the values of the organization. When a mission statement is developed, it should be clear that EBP and patient care outcomes are fundamental to why the organization exists (Gifford et al., 2018; Lahey & Nelson, 2020). The mission statement can create a foundation for a culture of inquiry and set the expectation that clinicians will make decisions based on evidence. The **vision** statement can further stretch the current boundaries by promoting EBP work that leads staff to reach for a higher standard. An example of a vision statement might be to develop a center of excellence for EBP within the organization or to be a leader in evidence-based care delivery. The **strategic plan** uses a continuous and systematic planning process to make the mission actionable and outcomes achievable. The strategic plan includes clearly articulated and measurable goals, objectives for meeting outcomes, metrics for measuring progress, a list of resources needed, and a timeline for completion. Attainment of strategic goals should be aimed at positioning the organization for success in a competitive, complex, rapidly changing health care environment (Robertson-Malt & Norton-Westwood, 2017). Goals and objectives should be consistent with the vision and values of the organization. Specific goals for EBP in the strategic plan provide structure for nurse leaders (Lahey & Nelson, 2020; Robertson-Malt & Norton-Westwood, 2017). Action steps are included for creating a culture that values inquiry and innovation and provides leaders with a foundation of support for EBP.

Shared Governance is designed to support the mission, vision, and strategic plan, and provides the infrastructure that integrates the work of EBP. A shared governance system is based on the belief that nurses own their practice and are best informed for making decisions about their practice (Clavelle et al., 2016; Goedhart et al., 2017; Stetler et al., 2014). The right committee or council structure will vary in each organization, but should include point-of-care clinicians and reflect the expertise, functions, and responsibility needed to promote EBP (Cullen et al., 2017; Stetler et al., 2014). Practice change is facilitated when documentation, policies and procedures, and education are based on EBP recommendations. Clinical experts can provide an excellent critique of a new policy or procedure and make recommendations so that policies link practices with evidence and support adaptation of evidence-based policies to fit the organization. Operationalizing communication within the governance structure creates internal peer networking to promote uptake of EBP (Gifford et al., 2018; Li et al., 2018). A clear path for communicating EBP work and necessary approvals between committees within the governance structure needs to be outlined (Cullen et al., 2017). Discussion during committee meetings can stimulate interest in—and use of—EBP, so include an EBP item on each agenda. Another key strategy is having a nurse leader on the Institutional Review Board and a clear process for determining research on human subjects, differentiated from EBP, with a clear process for organizational approvals (Cullen et al., 2018b; Lee et al., 2016; Office of Human Research Protections, U.S. Department of Health & Human Services, n.d.).

Performance Expectations and Appraisal

The value of EBP must be evident through the expected behaviors of nurses at every level in the organization (Taylor et al., 2015). Critical skills for shared governance committee members, include clinical experts, skill with appraisal and synthesis of the evidence, development of an implementation and evaluation plan, basic statistical analysis, and reporting of results (Cullen et al., 2017). Additional expertise can be developed through consultation and collaborations within a practice network, partnerships with academic institutions, or hiring nurse scientists (Sadeghnezhad et al., 2018). Performance appraisals based on job descriptions with EBP components are important for setting behavioral expectations. Inclusion of EBP components in performance appraisals across all job classifications—from top executives to the frontline—promotes positive reinforcement and priority setting in the busy work environment. Providing personal or group performance feedback helps clinicians have ownership of EBP and improves outcomes (Brown et al., 2019; Fleiszer et al., 2016; Hageman et al., 2015; Hysong et al., 2017).

Resources

EBP resources, including time, must be allocated by nurse executives, distributed fairly by managers, and be accessible to clinicians (Birken et al., 2018; Li et al., 2018). The organization can begin to build an EBP culture during orientation for new hires, competency review for current employees, and ongoing training for senior leaders and clinicians. Recruiting and hiring nurses with interest in EBP will help build the capacity. Orientation can contain basic EBP concepts and protocols, with new staff learning from colleagues who share experiences from EBP teamwork on their unit. This provides recognition for completed work, sets the expectation that EBP is important, and demonstrates that nurses have authority over their practice. New graduates have developed skills that support EBP (QSEN Institute, 2019). Nurses in new graduate residency programs can stimulate new—or support existing—EBP work using their creativity, technical skills, and dedicated work time (Hosking et al., 2016). Training opportunities for nurses and interprofessional teams across their career fosters improved outcomes (Cullen et al., 2020; Storey et al., 2019). EBP mentors can be developed from successful projects and used to nurture the next generation of clinical leaders (Abdullah et al., 2014; Gagliardi et al., 2014; Saunders & Vehvilainen-Julkunen, 2017; Spiva et al., 2017; Storey et al., 2019).

Organizational information systems need to be designed to incorporate EBP into clinical workflow if adoption for better outcomes is to be achieved (Renolen et al., 2018). Electronic documentation systems, designed to support clinical practice, need to capture essential elements of clinical practice guidelines that clinicians are expected to perform. The documentation system can serve as a reminder for new practices (Van de Velde et al., 2018). When done right, clinical decision support, such as order sets and interactive documentation prompts, facilitates integrating EBP into daily workflow, making EBP easy for clinicians (Fischer, 2016; Heekin et al., 2018; NAM, 2017; Patel et al., 2017).

Reporting

Internal and external dissemination of EBP results is essential to promote adoption, share learning, garner continued support, and recognize success from the institution's EBP program (Dembe et al., 2014; Esposito et al., 2015; Iowa Model Collaborative, 2017). Internal sharing of anticipated outcomes found in research reports can be helpful early in the EBP process by creating awareness and interest (Cullen & Adams, 2012). Outcomes that target patients and families, staff, and finances are valued by the team and organization, and need to be considered in evaluation planning (Cullen et al., 2018b; Dembe et al., 2014; Esposito et al., 2015; Institute for Healthcare Improvement, 2015; Parry et al., 2018). Cost savings or cost avoidance may not be achieved with every project but should be calculated and reported whenever possible (Sadler et al., 2009; Scott 2nd et al., 2019). Cost data may be available in the literature for estimating cost savings (AHRQ, 2017a; Hollenbeak & Schilling, 2018) and generating interest in EBP changes (Cullen et al., 2020).

Nursing leaders have a responsibility to clearly articulate EBP work in a way that will be heard by decision makers. Structural empowerment through shared governance has been associated with better patient outcomes (Goedhart et al., 2017). Shared governance provides a mechanism for sharing results with bidirectional communication among point-of-care nurses and senior leaders, so leaders can recognize great work while reporting the business case for EBP within governing boards (Abel & Hand, 2018; Murt et al., 2019). Communication with boards about EBP goals and initiatives is an important strategy (Cullen et al., 2017; Institute for Healthcare Improvement, 2016; Mason et al., 2013). Specific actions include sharing three to five brief talking points or takeaway messages and including reporting of the links between EBP and the organization's mission, vision, values, and strategic plan.

Capturing EBP within the quality improvement program (Djulbegovic et al., 2019; Mondoux & Shojania, 2019) is another way to build a strong organizational context. EBP can use the existing quality improvement program's standardized forms, reporting system, and established goals for improving care processes (Allen et al., 2017; Cullen et al., 2017; Harvey et al., 2019). Using the quality improvement system for reporting EBP provides efficient communication within the existing organizational infrastructure. The quality improvement process also supports ongoing planning, monitoring, and reinfusion of expected care delivery, supporting successful integration of EBPs.

Rewards

EBP successes need to be recognized and rewarded along the way (Birken et al., 2018; Sveinsdottir et al., 2016). Celebrations help build a culture that supports and expects use of evidence in practice. Rewards need to include formal recognition from senior leaders, visibility for interprofessional teams and EBP change champions, and clear demonstration of the benefits of EBP. Celebrations provide an opportunity to put clinicians in the spotlight for doing great work and articulate the standard for excellence based on EBP. Recognition can highlight the benefits to, and commitment of, the organization and strengthens the foundation for future efforts.

LEADERSHIP ROLES IN PROMOTING EVIDENCE-BASED PRACTICE

Leaders play a critical role establishing operational support so nurses can learn about and implement EBP (Allen et al., 2017; Gifford et al., 2018; Kowalski et al., 2019; Warren et al., 2016). Leadership is essential to initiate EBP and facilitate sustained change (Li et al., 2018). Clinical nursing and leadership roles complement each other (e.g., chief nurse executives, nurse managers, advanced practice nurses, and point-of-care nurses) to promote EBP and achieve desired outcomes (Harvey et al., 2019). Core groups that include nurses in roles with local leadership can match needed skills with opinion leaders from relevant disciplines, creating an effective EBP team (Chauhan et al., 2017; Cullen et al., 2018a,b; Huether et al., 2016).

Point-of-Care Nurse

Patient care outcomes are directly impacted by point-of-care nurse engagement in EBP (Goedhart et al., 2017; Saunders & Vehvilainen-Julkunen, 2017). Point-of-care nurses are in the ideal position to question practice and identify patient and family needs. Having the confidence to challenge the status quo and ask the question "Why do we practice this way?" is foundational to the success of EBP changes in a continually changing environment (Porter-O'Grady & Malloch, 2008). Staying current in both EBP and a clinical specialty throughout the career continuum occurs through conference attendance, reading scholarly journal articles, continued academic coursework, and professional networking.

The success of many EBP initiatives is contingent on the knowledge, clinical expertise, and passion of the point-of-care nurses. Many organizations provide training opportunities so that point-of-care nurses can get guidance and mentoring through the EBP process (Gifford et al., 2018; Spiva et al., 2017; Storey et al., 2019). EBP training provides nurses with the knowledge and confidence to inquire about best evidence and pursue change, building upon clinical expertise, collaboration and problem-solving. Point-of-care nurses often identify creative solutions to improve adoption of EBP, and can function as EBP change champions and core group members (Chauhan et al., 2017; Cullen et al., 2018b, 2020). They can also engage the team in designing and integrating change into their practice (Chauhan et al., 2017). A positive working environment elevates point-of-care nurses to be able to provide evidence-based care and improve patient outcomes (Goedhart et al., 2017).

Clinical Nurse Leader

Ensuring EBP initiatives are in place to improve quality is a national standard (American Nurses Credentialing Center, n.d.; Royer et al., 2018; The Joint Commission, n.d.). To increase the adoption of EBI, it is important to have technical support and training from a designated leader (Leeman et al., 2017). A key role in bridging the gap between the point-of-care nurse and the leadership team is the clinical nurse leader (CNL) (Bender, 2016; Clavo-Hall et al., 2018). The CNL helps foster learning and supports implementation of an EBP change by using clinical expertise in conjunction with personal connections with the interprofessional team. CNL responsibilities include project management, leading the EBP process, evaluating the impact, and reporting to unit or clinic leaders. Doing so involves understanding opportunities for improvement, constructing interdisciplinary collaboration to create a team approach to improving care processes, role modeling, mentoring, and successfully sustaining the practice change (Bender, 2016).

Advanced Practice Registered Nurse

The Advance Practice Registered Nurse (APRN) (e.g., advanced registered nurse practitioners, clinical nurse specialists, unit practice leaders) plays a strong supportive role in promoting EBP among clinical teams (Patterson et al., 2017). Essential EBP steps offered by this role are helping the team to identify opportunities, successfully implement a practice change and provide ongoing mentorship to sustain the change (Patterson et al., 2017; Royer et al., 2018; Saunders & Vehvilainen-Julkunen, 2017). Having the evidence to support a change in practice is important; however, having the knowledge to implement the change successfully is also essential (Spiva et al., 2017). As a clinical expert and a respected resource, the APRN enhances the knowledge of team members and calls the team to continuously question practice and improve quality through the EBP process. The APRN can lead the EBP process, design the EBI, and provide project management (Stewart et al., 2017). Pivotal roles of APRNs are in the development of policies based on the best evidence and adapted to the local setting. They also serve as change agents with strong leadership skills and organizational knowledge to help motivate and support others delivering EBP (Hole et al., 2016). Active participation in mentoring and modeling the EBP change are important for facilitating change. Role modeling the change, being actively engaged, in addition to being in a leadership role on an interprofessional team, provides resources for point-of-care nurses and enhances the team's willingness to implement the change (Warren et al., 2016).

Nurse Manager

Point-of-care managers have a key role in making EBP the norm for their area (Gifford et al., 2018; Renolen et al., 2020; Shuman et al., 2018; Warren et al., 2016). In order for a team to successfully provide excellent care, managers need to support point-of-care nurses as drivers of change, while also giving and seeking input (Gifford et al., 2018). This promotes superior clinical performance, accountability, and ownership by the team (Porter-O'Grady & Malloch, 2008). Unit or clinic leaders have a responsibility to clear the path so clinicians can have ownership of their work in a way that makes EBP possible (Birken et al., 2018; Kouzes & Posner, 2012). The nurse manager juggles several roles including leading, coaching, addressing concerns, empowering, and overcoming obstacles (Birken et al., 2018; Gifford et al., 2018). Support from the nurse manager enables point-of-care nurses to use EBP by cultivating a shared vision for EBP, being transparent about the value of EBP, and providing resources for EBP (Caramanica & Spiva, 2018). The attitude of the nurse manager sets the tone for how EBP is perceived. It is important to help staff understand the reason for change associated with the EBP recommendations (Birken et al., 2018). In addition, staying mission driven with EBP means "keep the patient and family at the center of all your decisions and you'll always make the right decision" (C. Mentz, personal communication, April 14, 2017).

Managers leading EBP among point-of-care nurses promote a continuous culture of improvement that requires resources (i.e., people, training, supplies, and time) dedicated to EBP (Birken et al., 2018; Gifford et al., 2018). Learning to promote EBP is fostered by answering questions; guiding and resourcing before, during, and after piloting; describing the benefits; setting norms; and providing feedback to internal and external stakeholders (Birken et al., 2018; Gifford et al., 2018). Attention needs to be paid to building EBP into the daily workflow (Renolen et al., 2018). Actions include addressing EBP during daily huddles, staff meetings, and with the EBP team in conjunction with communicating regularly with stakeholders to promote both adoption and sustainability (Harvey et al., 2019), and addressing concerns and acknowledging efforts to change (Gifford et al., 2018). In addition, effectively communicating face-to-face with those hesitant about the change is most productive for addressing concerns and obtaining buy-in (Gifford et al., 2018; C. Mentz, personal communication, November 4, 2019).

By having a strong interest in EBP and being supportive of the time commitment, managers help by maintaining a positive perception of the process and impact (Jansson & Forsberg, 2016). Creating a culture of open dialogue and constructive, professional feedback is imperative. When unit leaders reinforce expectations and maintain priorities, the sustainability of EBP improves (Fleiszer et al., 2016).

Nurse Executive

Nurse executives are key to managers understanding and having ownership of EBP, while also allocating resources (Birken et al., 2018). The nurse executive has a unique opportunity to promote change, set expectations, provide resources and training, and open doors for successful EBP (Gifford et al., 2018). Aligning the infrastructure and strategic plan of the organization with EBP lays the groundwork for successful EBP implementation (Goedhart et al., 2017; Luckson et al., 2018; Stetler et al., 2014). To navigate the ever-changing paradigms of health care, the nurse executive needs to make EBP their priority and an expectation for clinicians, interprofessional teams, and the organization as a whole. By providing opportunities for EBP training, professional development, and growth along the career continuum, the institution can see sustained improvements while building the capacity for the future (Crawford et al., 2017).

Committed leadership and daily resources for EBP require support from senior executives (Balakas et al., 2013; Gifford et al., 2018; Luckson et al., 2018; Melnyk et al., 2016). Walking rounds encourage others and track progress through discussions with clinicians and patients (Harvey et al., 2019). When the nurse executive is passionate about EBP and has a consistent mission and philosophical goals to achieve excellence through EBP and incentivizes EBP, it is reflected in the nursing care provided (Leeman et al., 2017; Yoo et al., 2019). Additionally, it is important to support internal and external dissemination of the EBP work done through local, regional, national, and international oral and poster presentations, along with peer-reviewed publications.

LEADERSHIP AND MANAGEMENT IMPLICATIONS

Change is often difficult, yet challenges can be anticipated. Therefore use of a multifaceted approach by nurse leaders across roles is imperative to integrate and sustain EBP at the unit and organizational level. Empowering all nurses is pivotal to adoption. Transformational leadership can be used to focus nurses on being "leaders" to initiate and sustain EBP by fostering a culture and climate through leadership to provide EBP (Shuman et al., 2018).

Culture

The primary mechanism to drive culture is leadership, more specifically in how the leader "walks the talk." Culture is reinforced by the actions and behavior of the leader, what gets rewarded and punished, and where resources are allocated (Schein & Schein, 2016). Culture then translates to the expectations and behavioral norms that differentiate a work environment and shape the way in which employees' approach and prioritize their work (Glisson, 2015). The secondary drivers of culture are norms and expectations articulated in the organizational mission, vision, values, and documents such as policies and job descriptions (Schein & Schein, 2016; Shuman, 2017). A culture that expects the integration of EBP into practice to provide high-quality patient care is essential for nursing to thrive (Storey et al., 2019). Proficiency is based on having institutions with expectations to maintain the most current knowledge and skills to respond to the unique needs of their patients (Galdikiene et al., 2016; Glisson, 2015).

Climate

Climate refers to the shared perceptions created by employees of the psychological influence of their environment on their personal performance and well-being. Team perceptions represent personal assessments of the significance and value of their work, engagement, and functions (Galdikiene et al., 2016; Glisson, 2015). The EBP climate refers to the clinician's perceptions at the local unit or clinic level, which are influenced by expectations, rewards, and organizational support (Shuman, 2017). Having humble leadership creates a positive organizational climate with increased involvement, constructive feedback, and optimal outcomes (Aarons et al., 2017).

Transformational Leadership

Transformational leadership has been defined as leadership that empowers others, facilitates growth and learning of team members, translates EBP into practice with local application, critically reflects and communicates, and uses problem-solving (Fischer, 2016). Practices of transformational leaders have been described by Kouzes and Posner (2012) as modeling the way, inspiring a shared vision, challenging the process, enabling others to act, and encouraging the heart. Empowering nurses to provide EBP in their daily care through transformational nursing leadership includes a vision that drives organizational change (Hauck et al., 2013). Leaders use transformational leadership to motivate others and inspire their team to provide EBP (Gifford et al., 2018). Partnering with clinical staff to provide opportunities to learn about EBP in conjunction with time to execute new practices highlights the importance of and value placed on EBP. Using transformational leadership to commit to the culture and climate of a unit that supports EBP will achieve a return on investment for patients, families, nurses, and the organization.

Leaders influence an organization's capacity for EBP. Leadership that demonstrates and expects EBP will promote its use in clinical and operational decision-making at the unit or clinic and organizational level. Prioritizing and facilitating leaders' and clinicians' ownership of EBP work is essential. Helping clinicians provide EBP requires leaders to be change-oriented, communicate to build relationships, involve positive and influential team members, address concerns, and acknowledge efforts; management is required to distribute work, arrange for dedicated time, provide needed equipment, and monitor progress (Gifford et al., 2018).

CURRENT ISSUES AND TRENDS

There is a growing demand for evidence-based and patient-centered care, with increasing public accountability and transparency for quality and safety (Centers for Medicare & Medicaid Services, 2019). Reimbursement structures reflect the importance of system redesign to improve coordination, efficiency, and provision of EBP for improved population health. Pay for performance through the Centers for Medicare & Medicaid Services' value-based purchasing and accountable care organization alignment has mixed indications of improving quality and cost of care (Ouayogode et al., 2019; Rutledge et al., 2019; Zhang et al., 2019). Total waste in the US health care system is estimated to be $760–$935 billion, and an estimated 25% could be saved through providing evidence-based care (Shrank et al., 2019). National patient safety goals established by The Joint Commission include a growing number of evidence-based standards. For example, standards for catheter-associated urinary tract infections reflect a growing intolerance for hospital-acquired infections (The Joint Commission, 2016). Likewise, national benchmarks (https://data.medicare.gov/) promote transparency for quality. The financial pressure for provision of EBP will continue to grow with demand from payers and patients.

Patient engagement and provision of patient-centered care is central to the national and international health care agenda (AHRQ, 2017b, 2018; American Academy of Nursing, 2019; American Board of Internal Medicine, 2019). Research is still needed to understand how best to facilitate shared decision-making (Durand et al., 2014; Prochaska & Sanders-Jackson, 2016).

Doctoral preparation continues to grow, as nurse leaders want skills that improve application of scholarship and leadership (American Association of Colleges of Nursing, 2018a). The Doctor of Nursing practice final project is designed as EBP impacting quality in a local setting (American Association of Colleges of Nursing, 2018b). Student work is best done in coordination and with approval of the clinical setting. Integrating student work within the organizational system creates student learning about how organizations work and may facilitate sustainment of their practice changes. Unfortunately, these student projects often conclude with numerous key steps not completed (Minnick et al., 2019). In fact, as many as 82% of final student projects have been found to have insufficient rigor and even fatal flaws (Minnick et al., 2019; Roush & Tesoro, 2018). Basic standards have been published and work is needed to establish and apply standards for these EBP initiatives (Lee et al., 2013; SQUIRE, 2017). The result creates a win–win for students and organizations, which ultimately create a win for patients and families.

A continuing priority for implementation science is to better understand how nurse leaders can promote adoption of evidence-based health care to improve quality and reduce costs (Hollenbeak & Schilling, 2018; Sadler et al., 2009). Understanding how to scale up and sustain EBP improvements is a critical priority (Seneski & Stack, 2019; Valim et al., 2019).

Nurses want to work in an organization that promotes innovation and EBP. An exhaustive body of research consistently finds that leadership support is essential to an organization's ability to consistently use evidence in practice (Gifford et al., 2018; Kowalski et al., 2019). The organizational context within which clinicians work is a complex and dynamic culture unique to each practice setting. Leaders are responsible for providing resources, structures, and processes that move teams beyond barriers to facilitate EBP (Li et al., 2018). Research is still needed to better understand infrastructure design and effective strategies to affect organizational context and capacity, encouraging adoption and delivery of evidence-based care (Clavelle et al., 2016; Goedhart et al., 2017; Stetler et al., 2014).

CONCLUSION

Nursing has a long history of valuing and using the best evidence to improve care quality. However, there continue to be challenges in using evidence-based care within the current health care environment. Nurses in leadership positions have responsibility for supporting evidence-based clinical care and evidence-based operational decision-making. Models outline the process for updating practices when addressing clinical and operational issues. Implementation is one of the most challenging steps in the EBP process. A phased approach using multiple reinforcing and interactive strategies is needed for implementation and sustained improvement. An effective, data-driven implementation approach can be used to create a targeted and highly influential implementation plan.

Nursing leaders can systematically build a strong program supporting evidence-based care delivery. Implementing EBPs is best accomplished by understanding the interplay between organizational and unit factors supported through the organizational infrastructure. Nurse leaders need to connect their evidence-based initiatives to the organization's vision, mission, values, and infrastructure to garner support and resources for EBP care delivery. The leadership and infrastructure to support EBP is essential for creating the desired organizational culture, capacity, and unit climate. Communicating the business case for EBP will help nurses articulate their impact in a way that will be heard by senior leaders. Complementary skills are needed within all nursing roles to create effective EBP teams. Every nurse has a responsibility to lead evidence-based care delivery to improve outcomes for patients and their families, staff, and the organization.

RESEARCH NOTE

Source

Harvey, G., Gifford, W., Cummings, G., Kelly, J., Kislov, R., Kitson, A., et al. (2019). Mobilising evidence to improve nursing practice: A qualitative study of leadership roles and processes in four countries. International Journal of Nursing Studies, 90, 21–30. https://doi.org/10-1016/j.ijnurstu.2018.09.017.

Purpose

The purpose of this qualitative study was to describe senior and frontline leader roles in promoting evidence-based practice (EBP) and identify factors in the practice setting that influence leadership and the implementation process. Participants were nurse executives, nurse managers, and facilitators (i.e., educators or practice development specialists) within acute and community care settings in Australia, Canada, England, and Sweden.

Discussion

Varying roles and structures were used to support evidence-based health care in practice settings. Senior executives were strategic and visionary. Important elements of their role were to establish the infrastructure and create collaborations and processes that support

◢ RESEARCH NOTE—cont'd

EBP. Executives had a local focus while also maintaining links at the regional and national level. Managers had a "gate keeper" role that is pivotal for operationalizing EBP, providing information and directions, role modeling, monitoring progress, and creating policies. The role of facilitation was to increase capacity for EBP and focus on support, including providing education, coaching, linking evidence to practice, providing skill development, and addressing barriers. Facilitators were important for communication and coordination while building practice networks.

The influence of national policy and regulatory monitoring varied across countries, reflecting the environment of the practice settings. Organizations supported EBP through a culture of continuous learning. Core to continuous learning was integration of quality improvement, benchmarks, and local data, as part of the evidence used to guide nursing practice, nursing standards, and accreditation. Inherent differences were reported when working in a health care organization compared with a person's home. Community care clinicians were challenged to audit use of EBP due to their responsiveness to the living situation of individual patients and a lack of electronic health records. Linking EBP to quality improvement processes facilitated adoption. Although participants could describe their role, educational preparation in implementation and the EBP process were limited. Other concerns were time and workload pressures, a deference to a dominant medical model, and focused adherence to policies that contributed to a lack of critical thinking by nurses.

Application to Practice

Leadership roles are complementary and cumulative, supporting evidence-based health care. Senior executives create a vision for the future, a culture of continuous improvement, and build an infrastructure and capacity to achieve EBP. Senior leaders provide support, resources, and training opportunities (Gifford et al., 2018). Managers' focus is operational and pivotal to enabling or obstructing EBP. Managers must commit to providing EBP with consistent messaging that links practice changes to organizational expectations. Managers are information conduits providing information and seeking input, while monitoring, encouraging, and recognizing clinicians (Gifford et al., 2018). Facilitator roles may fall under a variety of headings but were central to EBP capacity building, developing clinicians' knowledge and skills, and supporting ongoing learning, coaching, coordinating, and collaborating. Managers and facilitators should work consistently and collaboratively to garner commitment, navigate changing conditions, and encourage progress to provide evidence-based care (van der Zijpp et al., 2016).

From the perspective of the practice setting, there are several essential elements for EBP. The organization must provide training, resources, technology, expert facilitation, and a supportive infrastructure. Organizations must focus on continuous learning and integration of EBP within quality methods while using local data. Monitoring progress through audit and feedback are a foundational part of a comprehensive implementation plan (Brown et al., 2019; Phelan et al., 2018). The availability of guidelines, policies, practice registries, benchmarks, an electronic health record, and resources for training and development of local clinician leaders may be determined by government regulations.

CASE STUDY

Updated recommendations were published for cleaning endoscopes and preventing pathogen transmission, creating an opportunity to evaluate the organization's infection prevention policy related to cleaning, transporting, and storage. An ambulatory nursing leader recognized this as a chance to infuse evidence-based practice (EBP) into the Ambulatory Nursing division (Association for the Advancement of Medical Instrumentation—Endoscope Reprocessing Work Group, 2015; Office of Public Health Preparedness and Response, 2015). The following benefits were anticipated:

- Decreased risk of pathogen transmission
- Decreased endoscope cleaning time

- Decreased costs
- Empowered point-of-care nursing staff to use evidence-based recommendations
- Expanded culture in the Ambulatory Nursing division regarding use of evidence in daily practice

Next Steps

Essential steps are to recognize the need to form an interprofessional team; review and synthesize available evidence; revise the current policy and procedure; and create comprehensive implementation and evaluation plans. Collaborating with key stakeholders (e.g., nursing, infection prevention, central sterilizing services) throughout the

CASE STUDY—cont'd

organization was needed to match the skills and expertise required. The Nurse Manager (NM) of the Otolaryngology-Head and Neck Surgery Clinic had an identified need with over 700 patients getting scoped each month. The NM was already an opinion leader and ideally suited to lead the team. The team developed an action plan and divided responsibility for project work. Team members completed each of the following:

- Reviewed and synthesized the literature
- Developed a comprehensive implementation plan comprised of strategies to promote adoption of the practice change
- Developed an initial orientation and annual competency checklist where clinicians verbalize key components of the revised policy and procedure and completed a hands-on demonstration of the process for cleaning, transporting, and storing endoscopes
- Developed a standard workflow document for each type of endoscope
- Developed an educational presentation, visual learning tools, content for a just-in-time nursing education, and a poster based on the literature review
- Developed a process to monitor ongoing compliance with the practice change to ensure sustainability

The practice change involved precleaning endoscopes immediately following removal from patient care at the bedside or in the procedure or exam room. Clinicians performed hand hygiene and wore appropriate personal protective equipment, then used a lint-free sponge or towel to preclean the endoscope, which was placed in biohazard containers. In addition, endoscopes were not precleaned in handwashing sinks and only approved precleaning products were used. The date, time, and initials of the clinician performing the precleaning were written on the lid of the biohazard-labeled container. Finally, every endoscope was linked by a unique identification number to the patient's medical record number in the electronic health record.

Endoscopes were transported to the flexible endoscope reprocessing center to be reprocessed within 60 minutes of the completed precleaning procedure. After reprocessing, endoscopes were stored in unit- or clinic-based cabinets with continuous high-efficiency particulate air (HEPA) filtration, hung completely extended (no looping of insertion tubes), and not touching one another. Clean,

ready-to-use endoscopes were used within 30 days or reprocessed.

This ambulatory nursing-led, and subsequent house-wide practice change required multiple strategies for implementation (Cullen & Adams, 2012). The team used the following implementation strategies: highlight anticipated impact; highlight compatibility; discuss at staff meetings/unit in-services/huddles; distribute key evidence; use posters and postings/fliers; publicize new equipment; use education, change agents, and gap assessment/gap analysis; match practice change with resources and equipment; troubleshoot use/application; have an action plan; create resource materials and quick reference guides; verify skill competence; audit key indicators; use actionable and timely data feedback, checklists, and documentation changes in the electronic health record; have unit orientation; and revise the current policy and procedure.

Process and outcome indicators were included in the evaluation (Cullen et al., 2019b; Institute for Healthcare Improvement, 2019; Parry et al., 2018). Data captured those performing the precleaning, the number of scopes processed per month for each clinical area, the number of scopes that required an extended reprocessing time each month, when no precleaning time was noted, when extra equipment was sent with the endoscope to the reprocessing center, and incidents of pathogen transmission, all of which were measured and trended.

This EBP filled a critical gap in patient safety related to properly maintaining, cleaning, and disinfecting endoscopes according to established industry guidelines and manufacturer's instructions. Identification of key stakeholders, who could continue to dedicate time to this practice change, was warranted to ensure sustainability and compliance with ever-evolving regulatory standards. To meet this need, the organization chose to form an Endoscope Life Cycle Committee. A revised process was introduced, and patient care improvements occurred through the EBP changes. The ambulatory NM facilitated project work and integration of the practice change by serving as the project director to establish the priority, find resources, and guide the team to maneuver through the system for adoption and dissemination (Dawson, 2012; 2013; 2016; 2018) of the practice change.

CRITICAL THINKING EXERCISE

As the nurse manager on a general surgery unit, questions about practice frequently come your way. At a staff meeting, a newer nurse, Emily, asks, "Why don't we perform end-tidal CO_2 (EtCO$_2$) monitoring for patients receiving opioid medications to help prevent opioid-induced respiratory depression? I have read about the benefits of EtCO$_2$ monitoring in the literature (Jungquist et al., 2019), and I think this would be a good fit for the patients on our unit. Plus, the current bedside monitors could easily be adapted to include the capnography component." Mary, an experienced nurse on the unit, states, "We already monitor our patients receiving opioid medications for unintended sedation and respiratory depression using a modified POSS (Pasero Opioid-Induced Sedation Scale) scale (Pasero, 2009). And, we do not want to hear more monitors alarming each shift just to say we are using more technology, especially when it is not needed." Others attending the staff meeting nod their heads in agreement with Mary. You ask those present if they know about the emerging evidence about the benefits of EtCO$_2$ monitoring that Emily referenced and if they are interested in learning more to ensure provision of safe, high-quality patient care while at the same time preventing adverse events. You realize this topic could result in an EBP initiative. How will you engage the team in this EBP project?

1. What issues do you anticipate with regards to an EBP project related to EtCO2 monitoring for postsurgical patients receiving opioid medications?
2. Who is an emerging leader, to assume the project director role and manage the project? Why was this person your top candidate to be the project director?

3. How can you help the project team determine whether EtCO$_2$ monitoring for postsurgical patients is a priority for the organization?
4. Who will be key stakeholders and potential team members?
5. How will you, as the nurse manager, be involved in the project?
6. What is the benefit of a current literature review specific to EtCO$_2$ monitoring for post-surgical patients receiving opioid medications?
7. Why is it important to adapt the practice change to fit into the unit workflow?
8. How might the core project team learn more about and incorporate patient and family preferences when designing the practice change and implementation?
9. After designing an EBP change to incorporate the use of EtCO$_2$ monitoring for post-surgical patients receiving opioid medications:
   a. How can you create awareness and interest about the need for a practice change?
   b. What education is needed and what other strategies would help you build knowledge and commitment among the health care team?
   c. How can the change agent role enhance adoption of the practice change?
   d. What key process and outcome indicators should be measured?
   e. How should the key indicators be measured?
   f. Who is going to provide actionable and timely data feedback to the frontline clinicians?
   g. Who can assist with ongoing monitoring of compliance with the practice change to ensure sustainability is achieved?

REFERENCES

Aarons, G. A., Ehrhart, M. G., Torres, E. M., Finn, N. K., & Beidas, R. S. (2017). The humble leader: Association of discrepancies in leader and follower ratings of implementation leadership with organizational climate in mental health. *Psychiatric Services, 68*(2), 115–122. https://doi.org/10.1176/appi.ps.201600062.

Aarons, G. A., Sklar, M., Mustanski, B., Benbow, N., & Brown, C. H. (2017). "Scaling-out" evidence-based interventions to new populations or new health care delivery systems. *Implementation Science, 12*(1), 111. https://doi.org/10.1186/s13012-017-0640-6.

Abbott, L., & Hooke, M. C. (2017). Energy through motion: An activity intervention for cancer-related fatigue in an ambulatory infusion center. *Clinical Journal of Oncology Nursing, 21*(5), 618–626. https://doi.org/10.1188/17.CJON.618-626.

Abdullah, G., Rossy, D., Ploeg, J., Davies, B., Higuchi, K., Sikora, L., et al. (2014). Measuring the effectiveness of mentoring as a knowledge translation intervention for implementing empirical evidence: A systematic review. *Worldviews on Evidence-Based Nursing, 11*(5), 284–300. https://doi.org/10.1111/wvn.12060.

Abel, S. E., & Hand, M. W. (2018). Exploring, defining, and illustrating a concept: Structural and psychological empowerment in the workplace. *Nursing Forum, 53*(4), 579–584. https://doi.org/10.1111/nuf.12289.

AHRQ. (2017a). *Estimating the additional hospital inpatient cost and mortality associated with selected hospital-acquired conditions.* https://www.ahrq.gov/hai/pfp/haccost2017-results.html.

AHRQ. (2017b). *Strategy 6I: Shared decisionmaking.* https://www.ahrq.gov/cahps/quality-improvement/improvement-guide/6-strategies-for-improving/communication/strategy6i-shared-decisionmaking.html.

AHRQ. (2018). *The guide to improving patient safety in primary care settings by engaging patients and families.* https://www.ahrq.gov/sites/default/files/wysiwyg/professionals/quality-patient-safety/patient-family-engagement/pfeprimarycare/pfepc-fullguide-final508.pdf.

Allen, J. D., Towne, S. D., Jr., Maxwell, A. E., DiMartino, L., Leyva, B., Bowen, D. J., et al. (2017). Measures of organizational characteristics associated with adoption and/or implementation of innovations: A systematic review. *BMC Health Services Research, 17*(1), 591. https://doi.org/10.1186/s12913-017-2459-x.

Ament, S. M., de Groot, J. J., Maessen, J. M., Dirksen, C. D., van der Weijden, T., & Kleijnen, J. (2015). Sustainability of professionals' adherence to clinical practice guidelines in medical care: A systematic review. *BMJ Open, 5*(12), Article e008073. https://doi.org/10.1136/bmjopen-2015-008073.

American Academy of Nursing. (2019). *Twenty-five things nurses and patients should question.* https://www.choosingwisely.org/societies/american-academy-of-nursing/.

American Association of Colleges of Nursing. (2018a). *2017–2018 enrollment and graduations in baccalaureate and graduate programs in nursing.* Author. Washington: DC.

American Association of Colleges of Nursing. (2018b). *Defining scholarship for academic nursing. Report from the task force for consensus position statement.* Author. Washington: DC.

American Association of Critical-Care Nurses (AACN). (2005). AACN standards for establishing and sustaining healthy work environments: A journey to excellence. *American Journal of Critical Care, 14*(3), 187–197.

American Board of Internal Medicine. (2019). *Choosing wisely.* https://abimfoundation.org/what-we-do/choosing-wisely.

American Nurses Credentialing Center. (n.d.). *Magnet recognition program.* https://www.nursingworld.org/organizational-programs/magnet/.

Association for the Advancement of Medical Instrumentation—Endoscope Reprocessing Work Group. (2015). *Flexible and semi-rigid endoscope reprocessing in health care facilities.* Arlington, VA: Association for the Advancement of Medical Instrumentation.

Balakas, K., Sparks, L., Steurer, L., & Bryant, T. (2013). An outcome of evidence-based practice education: sustained clinical decision making among bedside nurses. *Journal of Pediatric Nursing, 28*(5), 479–485. https://doi.org/10.1016/j.pedn.2012.08.007.

Bandura, A. (1977). *Social learning theory.* Englewood Cliffs, NJ: Prentice-Hall.

Bender, M. (2016). Clinical nurse leader integration into practice: Developing theory to guide best practice. *Journal of Professional Nursing, 32*(1), 32–40. https://doi.org/10.1016/j.profnurs.2015.06.007.

Birken, S., Clary, A., Tabriz, A. A., Turner, K., Meza, R., Zizzi, A., et al. (2018). Middle managers' role in implementing evidence-based practices in healthcare: A systematic review. *Implementation Science, 13*(1), 149. https://doi.org/10.1186/s13012-018-0843-5.

Borsky, A., Zhan, C., Miller, T., Ngo-Metzger, Q., Bierman, A. S., & Meyers, D. (2018). Few Americans receive all high-priority, appropriate clinical preventive services. *Health Affairs, 37*(6), 925–928. https://doi.org/10.1377/hlthaff.2017.1248.

Brown, B., Gude, W. T., Blakeman, T., van der Veer, S. N., Ivers, N., Francis, J. J., et al. (2019a). Clinical performance feedback intervention theory (CP-FIT): A new theory for designing, implementing, and evaluating feedback in health care based on a systematic review and meta-synthesis of qualitative research. *Implementation Science, 14*(1), 40. https://doi.org/10.1186/s13012-019-0883-5.

Brownson, R. C., Colditz, G. A., & Proctor, E. K. (2018a). *Dissemination and implementation research in health: Translating science to practice* (2nd ed.). Oxford: Oxford University Press.

Brownson, R. C., Fielding, J. E., & Green, L. W. (2018b). Building capacity for evidence-based public health: Reconciling the pulls of practice and the push of research. *Annual Review of Public Health, 39*, 27–53. https://doi.org/10.1146/annurev-publhealth-040617-014746.

Bunger, A. C., Birken, S. A., Hoffman, J. A., MacDowell, H., Choy-Brown, M., & Magier, E. (2019). Elucidating the influence of supervisors' roles on implementation climate. *Implementation Science, 14*(1), 93. https://doi.org/10.1186/s13012-019-0939-6.

Camargo, F. C., Iwamoto, H. H., Galvão, C. M., Monteiro, D. A. T., Goulart, M. B., & Garcia, L. A. A. (2017). Models for the implementation of evidence-based practice in hospital based nursing: A narrative review. *Texto & Contexto - Enfermagem, 26*(4), Article e2070017. https://doi.org/10.1590/0104-07072017002070017.

Caramanica, L., & Spiva, L. (2018). Exploring nurse manager support of evidence-based practice: Clinical nurse perceptions. *Journal of Nursing*

Administration, 48(5), 272–278. https://doi.org/10.1097/NNA.0000000000000612.

Centers for Medicare & Medicaid Services. (2019). *Sharing savings program.* https://www.cms.gov/Medicare/Medicare-Fee-for-Service-Payment/sharedsavingsprogram/index.

Chauhan, B. F., Jeyaraman, M. M., Mann, A. S., Lys, J., Skidmore, B., Sibley, K. M., et al. (2017). Behavior change interventions and policies influencing primary healthcare professionals' practice-an overview of reviews. *Implementation Science, 12*(1), 3. https://doi.org/10.1186/s13012-016-0538-8.

Clavelle, J. T., Porter O'Grady, T., Weston, M. J., & Verran, J. A. (2016). Evolution of structural empowerment: Moving from shared to professional governance. *Journal of Nursing Administration, 46*(6), 308–312. https://doi.org/10.1097/NNA.0000000000000350.

Clavo-Hall, J. A., Bender, M., & Harvath, T. A. (2018). Roles enacted by clinical nurse leaders across the healthcare spectrum: A systematic literature review. *Journal of Professional Nursing, 34*(4), 259–268. https://doi.org/10.1016/j.profnurs.2017.11.007.

Coleman, D. E., Kamai, S., & Davis, K. F. (2018). Impact of a collaborative evidence-based practice nursing education program on clinical operations. *Journal of Hospital Librarianship, 18*(4), 323–330. https://doi.org/10.1080/15323269.2018.1509194.

Connor, J. A., Ziniel, S. I., Porter, C., Doherty, D., Moonan, M., Dwyer, P., et al. (2018). Interprofessional use and validation of the AACN healthy work environment assessment tool. *American Journal of Critical Care, 27*(5), 363–371. https://doi.org/10.4037/ajcc2018179.

Crawford, C. L., Omery, A., & Spicer, J. (2017). An integrative review of 21st-century roles, responsibilities, characteristics, and competencies of chief nurse executives: A blueprint for the next generation. *Nursing Administration Quarterly, 41*(4), 297–309. https://doi.org/10.1097/NAQ.0000000000000245.

Cullen, L., & Adams, S. L. (2012). Planning for implementation of evidence-based practice. *Journal of Nursing Administration, 42*(4), 222–230. https://doi.org/10.1097/NNA.0b013e31824ccd0a.

Cullen, L., Baumler, S., Farrington, M., Dawson, C., Folkmann, P., & Brenner, L. (2018). CE: Oral care for head and neck cancer symptom management. *American Journal of Nursing, 118*(1), 24–34. https://doi.org/10.1097/01.NAJ.0000529694.30568.41.

Cullen, L., DeBerg, J., & Hanrahan, K. (2019a). *Turning the evidence pyramid upside down.* Poster session presented at the 2019 Fuld Institute for EBP National Summit. The Ohio State University.

Cullen, L., Hanrahan, K., Farrington, M., Anderson, R., Dimmer, E., Miner, R., et al. (2020). Evidence-based practice change champions program improves quality care. *Journal of Nursing Administration, 50*(3), 128–134.

Cullen, L., Hanrahan, K., Farrington, M., Deberg, J., Tucker, S., & Kleiber, C. (2018). *Evidence-based practice in action: Comprehensive strategies, tools and tips from the University of Iowa Hospitals and Clinics.* Iowa City: Sigma: Theta Tau International.

Cullen, L., Hanrahan, K., Tucker, S. J., & Gallagher-Ford, L. (2019b). Data-driven precision implementation approach. *American Journal of Nursing, 119*(8), 60–63. https://doi.org/10.1097/01.NAJ.0000577460.00222.32.

Cullen, L., Wagner, M., Matthews, G., & Farrington, M. (2017). Evidence into practice: Integration within an organizational infrastructure. *Journal of PeriAnesthesia Nursing, 32*(3), 247–256. https://doi.org/10.1016/j.jopan.2017.02.003.

Damschroder, L. J., & Hagedorn, H. J. (2011). A guiding framework and approach for implementation research in substance use disorders treatment. *Psychology of Addictive Behaviors, 25*(2), 194–205. https://doi.org/10.1037/a0022284.

Damschroder, L. J., & Lowery, J. C. (2013). Evaluation of a large-scale weight management program using the consolidated framework for implementation research (CFIR). *Implementation Science, 8*(51). https://doi.org/10.1186/1748-5908-8-51.

Dang, D., & Dearholt, S. L. (2017). *Johns Hopkins nursing evidence-based practice: model and guidelines* (3rd ed). Indianapolis, IN: Sigma: Theta Tau International.

Dang, D., Melnyk, B., Fineout-Overholt, E., Yost, J., Cullen, L., Cvach, M., et al. (2019). Models to guide implementation and sustainability of evidence-based practice. In B. Melnyk, & E. Fineout-Overholt (Eds.), *Evidence-based practice in nursing & healthcare: A guide to best practice* (4th ed.) (pp. 378–427). Philadelphia, PA: Lippincott, Williams & Wilkins.

Davis, R., Campbell, R., Hildon, Z., Hobbs, L., & Michie, S. (2015). Theories of behaviour and behaviour change across the social and behavioural sciences: A scoping review. *Health Psychology Review, 9*(3), 323–344. https://doi.org/10.1080/17437199.2014.941722.09.

Dawson, C. (2012, September). *An EBP project: High level disinfection of scopes,* Poster session presented at the 36th Annual Society of Otorhinolaryngology and Head-Neck Nurses Congress and Nursing Symposium, Washington, DC.

Dawson, C. (2013). *Cleaning and high-level disinfection (HLD) of flexible and rigid semi-critical medical scopes (without internal channels) using ortho-phthalaldehyde (Cidex OPA).* Poster session presented at the 20th National Evidence-Based Practice Conference, University of Iowa Hospitals and Clinics, Iowa City, IA.

Dawson, C. (2016, September). *High level disinfection of scopes update*. Paper presented at the 40th Annual Society of Otorhinolaryngology and Head-Neck Nurses Congress and Nursing Symposium, San Diego, CA.

Dawson, C. (2018, October). *Disinfection and cleaning of scopes/instruments*. Paper presented at the 42nd Annual Society of Otorhinolaryngology and Head-Neck Nurses Congress and Nursing Symposium, Atlanta, GA.

Dembe, A. E., Lynch, M. S., Gugiu, P. C., & Jackson, R. D. (2014). The translational research impact scale: development, construct validity, and reliability testing. *Evaluation & the Health Professions, 37*(1), 50–70. https://doi.org/10.1177/0163278713506112.

Djulbegovic, B., Bennett, C. L., & Guyatt, G. (2019). Failure to place evidence at the centre of quality improvement remains a major barrier for advances in quality improvement. *Journal of Evaluation in Clinical Practice, 25*(3), 369–372. https://doi.org/10.1111/jep.13146.

Ducharme, M. P., Bernhardt, J. M., Padula, C. A., & Adams, J. M. (2017). Leader influence, the professional practice environment, and nurse engagement in essential nursing practice. *Journal of Nursing Administration, 47*(7/8), 367–375. https://doi.org/10.1097/NNA.0000000000000497.

Durand, M. A., Carpenter, L., Dolan, H., Bravo, P., Mann, M., Bunn, F., & Elwyn, G. (2014). Do interventions designed to support shared decision making reduce health inequalities? A systematic review and meta-analysis. *PLoS One, 9*(4), e94670. https://doi.org/10.1371/journal.pone.0094670.

Esposito, D., Heeringa, J., Bradley, K., Croake, S., & Kimmey, L. (2015). *PCORI dissemination and implementation framework*. Washington, DC: Patient-Centered Outcomes Research Institute. https://www.pcori.org/sites/default/files/PCORI-Dissemination-Implementation-Framework.pdf.

Everett, L. Q., & Sitterding, M. C. (2011). Transformational leadership required to design and sustain evidence-based practice: A system exemplar. *Western Journal of Nursing Research, 33*(3), 398–426. https://doi.org/10.1177/0193945910383056.

Farra, S. L., Miller, E. T., & Hodgson, E. (2015). Virtual reality disaster training: Translation to practice. *Nurse Education in Practice, 15*(1), 53–57. https://doi.org/10.1016/j.nepr.2013.08.017.

Farrington, M., Ward, E., & Dawson, C. (2020). Reducing Reliance on Agency Staff = $7.7 Million in Savings and Improved Nurse Engagement. *Journal of perianesthesia nursing : official journal of the American Society of PeriAnesthesia Nurses, 35*(3), 333–336. https://doi.org/10.1016/j.jopan.2020.02.006.

Fischer, S. A. (2016). Transformational leadership in nursing: A concept analysis. *Journal of Advanced Nursing, 72*(11), 2644–2653. https://doi.org/10.1111/jan.13049.

Fitzgerald, L., & Harvey, G. (2015). Translational networks in healthcare? Evidence on the design and initiation of organizational networks for knowledge mobilization. *Social Science & Medicine, 138*, 192–200. https://doi.org/10.1016/j.socscimed.2015.06.015.

Fleiszer, A. R., Semenic, S. E., Ritchie, J. A., Richer, M. C., & Denis, J. L. (2016). Nursing unit leaders' influence on the long-term sustainability of evidence-based practice improvements. *Journal of Nursing Management, 24*(3), 309–318. https://doi.org/10.1111/jonm.12320.

Gagliardi, A. R., Webster, F., Perrier, L., Bell, M., & Straus, S. (2014). Exploring mentorship as a strategy to build capacity for knowledge translation research and practice: A scoping systematic review. *Implementation Science, 9*, 122. https://doi.org/10.1186/s13012-014-0122-z.

Galdikiene, N., Asikainen, P., Rostila, I., Green, P., Balciunas, S., & Suominen, T. (2016). Organizational social context in primary health care. *Nordic Journal of Nursing Research, 36*(2), 103–111. https://doi.org/10.1177/2057158516628728.

Gawlinski, A., & Rutledge, D. (2008). Selecting a model for evidence-based practice changes: A practical approach. *AACN Advanced Critical Care, 19*(3), 291 300. https://doi.org/10.1097/01.AACN.0000330380.41766.63.

Gifford, W. A., Squires, J. E., Angus, D. E., Ashley, L. A., Brosseau, L., Craik, J. M., et al. (2018). Managerial leadership for research use in nursing and allied health care professions: A systematic review. *Implementation Science, 13*(1), 127. https://doi.org/10.1186/s13012-018-0817-7.

Glisson, C. (2015). The role of organizational culture and climate in innovation and effectiveness. *Human Service Organizations, Management, Leadership & Governance, 39*(4), 245–250. https://doi.org/10.1080/23303131.2015.1087770.

Goedhart, N. S., van Oostveen, C. J., & Vermeulen, H. (2017). The effect of structural empowerment of nurses on quality outcomes in hospitals: A scoping review. *Journal of Nursing Management, 25*(3), 194–206. https://doi.org/10.1111/jonm.12455.

Goldstein, H., & Olswang, L. (2017). Is there a science to facilitate implementation of evidence-based practices and programs? *Evidence-Based Communication Assessment and Intervention, 11*(3-4), 55–60. https://doi.org/10.1080/17489539.2017.1416768.

Gorman, V. L. (2019). Future emergency nursing workforce: What the evidence is telling us. *Journal of Emergency Nursing, 45*(2), 132–136. https://doi.org/10.1016/j.jen.2018.09.009.

Greenhalgh, T. (2018). *How to implement evidence-based healthcare*. Hoboken, NJ: Wiley & Sons.

Gude, W. T., Roos-Blom, M. J., van der Veer, S. N., Dongelmans, D. A., de Jonge, E., Peek, N., & de Keizer,

N. F. (2019). Facilitating action planning within audit and feedback interventions: A mixed-methods process evaluation of an action implementation toolbox in intensive care. *Implementation Science, 14*(1), 90. https://doi.org/10.1186/s13012-019-0937-8.

Hageman, M. G., Ring, D. C., Gregory, P. J., Rubash, H. E., & Harmon, L. (2015). Do 360-degree feedback survey results relate to patient satisfaction measures? *Clinical Orthopaedics and Related Research, 473*(5), 1590–1597. https://doi.org/10.1007/s11999-014-3981-3.

Hairr, D. C., Salisbury, H., Johannsson, M., & Redfern-Vance, N. (2014). Nurse staffing and the relationship to job satisfaction and retention. *Nursing Economic, 32*(3), 142–147.

Halter, M., Boiko, O., Pelone, F., Beighton, C., Harris, R., Gale, J., et al. (2017). The determinants and consequences of adult nursing staff turnover: A systematic review of systematic reviews. *BMC Health Services Research, 17*(1), 824. https://doi.org/10.1186/s12913-017-2707-0.

Hanrahan, K., Wagner, M., Matthews, G., Stewart, S., Dawson, C., Greiner, J., et al. (2015). Sacred cow gone to pasture: A systematic evaluation and integration of evidence-based practice. *Worldviews on Evidence-Based Nursing, 12*(1), 3–11. https://doi.org/10.1111/wvn.12072.

Harrison, M. B., Graham, I. D., van den Hoek, J., Dogherty, E. J., Carley, M. E., & Angus, V. (2013). Guideline adaptation and implementation planning: A prospective observational study. *Implementation Science, 8*(49). https://doi.org/10.1186/1748-5908-8-49.

Harvey, G., Gifford, W., Cummings, G., Kelly, J., Kislov, R., Kitson, A., et al. (2019). Mobilising evidence to improve nursing practice: A qualitative study of leadership roles and processes in four countries. *International Journal of Nursing Studies, 90*, 21–30. https://doi.org/10.1016/j.ijnurstu.2018.09.017.

Harvey, G., & Kitson, A. (2015). *Implementing evidence-based practice in healthcare: A facilitation guide*. London: Routledge.

Hauck, S., Winsett, R. P., & Kuric, J. (2013). Leadership facilitation strategies to establish evidence-based practice in an acute care hospital. *Journal of Advanced Nursing, 69*(3), 664–674. https://doi.org/10.1111/j.1365-2648.2012.06053.x.

Heekin, A. M., Kontor, J., Sax, H. C., Keller, M. S., Wellington, A., & Weingarten, S. (2018). Choosing wisely clinical decision support adherence and associated inpatient outcomes. *American Journal of Managed Care, 24*(8), 361–366.

Helfrich, C. D., Rose, A. J., Hartmann, C. W., van Bodegom-Vos, L., Graham, I. D., Wood, S. J., et al. (2018). How the dual process model of human cognition can inform efforts to de-implement ineffective and harmful clinical practices: A preliminary model of unlearning and

substitution. *Journal of Evaluation in Clinical Practice, 24*(1), 198–205. https://doi.org/10.1111/jep.12855.

Hole, G. O., Brenna, S. J., Graverholt, B., Ciliska, D., & Nortvedt, M. W. (2016). Educating change agents: A qualitative descriptive study of graduates of a Master's program in evidence-based practice. *BMC Medical Education, 16*(71). https://doi.org/10.1186/s12909-016-0597-1.

Hollenbeak, C. S., & Schilling, A. L. (2018). The attributable cost of catheter-associated urinary tract infections in the United States: A systematic review. *American Journal of Infection Control, 46*(7), 751–757. https://doi.org/10.1016/j.ajic.2018.01.015.

Hosking, J., Knox, K., Forman, J., Montgomery, L. A., Valde, J. G., & Cullen, L. (2016). Evidence into practice: Leading new graduate nurses to evidence-based practice through a nurse residency program. *Journal of PeriAnesthesia Nursing, 31*(3), 260–265. https://doi.org/10.1016/j.jopan.2016.02.006.

Huddleston, P., & Gray, J. (2016a). Measuring nurse leaders' and direct care nurses' perceptions of a healthy work environment in an acute care setting, part 1: A pilot study. *Journal of Nursing Administration, 46*(7-8), 373–378. https://doi.org/10.1097/NNA.0000000000000361.

Huddleston, P., & Gray, J. (2016b). Describing nurse leaders' and direct care nurses' perceptions of a healthy work environment in acute care settings, part 2. *Journal of Nursing Administration, 46*(9), 462–467. https://doi.org/10.1097/NNA.0000000000000376.

Huddleston, P., Mancini, M. E., & Gray, J. (2017). Measuring nurse leaders' and direct care nurses' perceptions of a healthy work environment in acute care settings, part 3: Healthy work environment scales for nurse leaders and direct care nurses. *Journal of Nursing Administration, 47*(3), 140–146. https://doi.org/10.1097/NNA.0000000000000456.

Huether, K., Abbott, L., Cullen, L., Cullen, L., & Gaarde, A. (2016). Energy through motion: An evidence-based exercise program to reduce cancer-related fatigue and improve quality of life. *Clinical Journal of Oncology Nursing, 20*(3), E60–E70. https://doi.org/10.1188/16.CJON.E60-E70.

Hysong, S. J., Kell, H. J., Petersen, L. A., Campbell, B. A., & Trautner, B. W. (2017). Theory-based and evidence-based design of audit and feedback programmes: Examples from two clinical intervention studies. *BMJ Quality & Safety, 26*(4), 323–334. https://doi.org/10.1136/bmjqs-2015-004796.

Institute for Healthcare Improvement. (2015). *The Science of Improvement on a Whiteboard!*. http://www.ihi.org/education/IHIOpenSchool/resources/Pages/BobLloydWhiteboard.aspx.

Institute for Healthcare Improvement. (2016). *Governance Leadership of Safety and Improvement.* http://www.ihi. org/Topics/GovernanceLeadership/Pages/default.aspx.

Institute for Healthcare Improvement. (2019). *Family of Measures.* http://www.ihi.org/education/IHIOpenSchool/ resources/Pages/AudioandVideo/Whiteboard15.aspx.

Institute of Medicine. (2011). *Clinical Practice Guidelines we can Trust.* Washington, DC: The National Acadmies Press.

Institute of Translational Health Sciences. (2019a). *Definitions of Clinical and Translational Research.* https://www.iths. org/investigators/definitions/definitions-of-clinical-and- translational-research/.

Institute of Translational Health Sciences. (2019b). *T-phases of Translational Health Record.* https://www.iths.org/ investigators/definitions/translational-research/.

Iowa Model Collaborative. (2017). Iowa model of evidence- based practice: Revisions and validation. *Worldviews on Evidence-Based Nursing, 14*(3), 175–182. https://doi. org/10.1111/wvn.12223.

Ishikawa, S. I., Kishida, K., Oka, T., Saito, A., Shimotsu, S., Watanabe, N., et al. (2019). Developing the universal unified prevention program for diverse disorders for school-aged children. *Child and Adolescent Psychiatry and Mental Health, 13*(44). https://doi.org/10.1186/ s13034-019-0303-2.

Jansson, I., & Forsberg, A. (2016). How do nurses and ward managers perceive that evidence-based sources are obtained to inform relevant nursing interventions?–An exploratory study. *Journal of Clinical Nursing, 25*(5-6), 769–776. https://doi.org/10.1111/jocn.13095.

Jungquist, C. R., Chandola, V., Spulecki, C., Nguyen, K. V., Crescenzi, P., Tekeste, D., et al. (2019). Identifying patients experiencing opioid-induced respiratory depression during recovery from anesthesia: The application of electronic monitoring devices. *Worldviews on Evidence-Based Nursing, 16*(3), 186–194. https://doi. org/10.1111/wvn.12362.

Kalisch, B., & Lee, K. H. (2014). Staffing and job satisfaction: Nurses and nursing assistants. *Journal of Nursing Management, 22*(4), 465–471. https://doi.org/10.1111/ jonm.12012.

Kouzes, J. M., & Posner, B. Z. (2012). *The Leadership Challenge: How to Make Extraordinary Things Happen in Organizations.* San Fransisco, CA: Jossey-Bass.

Kowalski, M. O., Basile, C., Bersick, E., Cole, D. A., McClure, D. E., & Weaver, S. H. (2019). What do nurses need to practice effectively in the hospital environment? An integrative review with implications for nurse leaders. *Worldviews on Evidence-Based Nursing.* https://doi. org/10.1111/wvn.12401.

Lahey, T., & Nelson, W. (2020). A dashboard to improve the alignment of healthcare organization decisionmaking to core values and mission statement. *Cambridge Quarterly of Healthcare Ethics, 29*(1), 156–162. https://doi. org/10.1017/S0963180119000884.

Lee, M. C., Johnson, K. L., Newhouse, R. P., & Warren, J. I. (2013). Evidence-based practice process quality assessment: EPQA guidelines. *Worldviews on Evidence- Based Nursing, 10*(3), 140–149. https://doi.org/10.1111/ j.1741-6787.2012.00264.x.

Lee, S. S., Kelley, M., Cho, M. K., Kraft, S. A., James, C., Constantine M., et al. (2016). Adrift in the gray zone: IRB perspectives on research in the learning health system. *AJOB Empirical Bioethics, 7*(2), 125–134. https://doi.org/1 0.1080/23294515.2016.1155674.

Leeman, J., Calancie, L., Kegler, M. C., Escoffery, C. T., Herrmann, A. K., Thatcher E., et al. (2017). Developing theory to guide building practitioners' capacity to implement evidence-based interventions. *Health Education & Behavior, 44*(1), 59–69. https://doi. org/10.1177/1090198115610572.

Lewis, A., Harvey, G., Hogan, M., & Kitson, A. (2019). Can oral healthcare for older people be embedded into routine community aged care practice? A realist evaluation using normalisation process theory. *International Journal of Nursing Studies, 94*, 32–41. https://doi.org/10.1016/j. ijnurstu.2018.12.016.

Lewis, C. C., Klasnja, P., Powell, B. J., Lyon, A. R., Tuzzio, L., Jones, S., et al. (2018). From classification to causality: Advancing understanding of mechanisms of change in implementation science. *Frontiers in Public Health, 6*(136). https://doi.org/10.3389/ fpubh.2018.00136.

Li, S. A., Jeffs, L., Barwick, M., & Stevens, B. (2018). Organizational contextual features that influence the implementation of evidence-based practices across healthcare settings: A systematic integrative review. *Systematic Reviews, 7*(1), 72. https://doi.org/10.1186/ s13643-018-0734-5.

Little, S. H., Dickerson, P. S., Randolph, G., Rocco, P., & Short, N. (2017). Using the ARCC model to implement the 2015 ANCC COA criteria: A North Carolina public health nursing project. *Journal of Continuing Education in Nursing, 48*(11), 501–507. https://doi. org/10.3928/00220124-20171017-07.

Luckson, M., Duncan, F., Rajai, A., & Haigh, C. (2018). Exploring the research culture of nurses and allied health professionals (AHPs) in a research-focused and a non-research-focused healthcare organisation in the UK. *Journal of Clinical Nursing, 27*(7-8), e1462–e1476. https:// doi.org/10.1111/jocn.14264.

Martin, C. J. (2015). The effects of nurse staffing on quality of care. *Medsurg Nursing, 24*(2), 4–6 Suppl.

Mason, D. J., Keepnews, D., Holmberg, J., & Murray, E. (2013). The representation of health professionals on governing boards of health care organizations in New York City. *Journal of Urban Health: Bulletin of the New York Academy of Medicine, 90*(5), 888–901. https://doi.org/10.1007/s11524-012-9772-9.

May, C. R., Mair, F., Finch, T., MacFarlane, A., Dowrick, C., Treweek, S., et al. (2009). Development of a theory of implementation and integration: Normalization process theory. *Implementation Science, 4*(29). https://doi.org/10.1186/1748-5908-4-29.

McKay, V. R., Hoffer, L. D., Combs, T. B., & Margaret Dolcini, M. (2018). The dynamic influence of human resources on evidence-based intervention sustainability and population outcomes: An agent-based modeling approach. *Implementation Science, 13*(1), 77. https://doi.org/10.1186/s13012-018-0767-0.

Melnyk, B. M., Fineout-Overholt, E., Giggleman, M., & Choy, K. (2017). A test of the ARCC© model improves implementation of evidence-based practice, healthcare culture, and patient outcomes. *Worldviews on Evidence-Based Nursing, 14*(1), 5–9. https://doi.org/10.1111/wvn.12188.

Melnyk, B. M., Gallagher-Ford, L., Thomas, B. K., Troseth, M., Wyngarden, K., & Szalacha, L. (2016). A study of chief nurse executives indicates low prioritization of evidence-based practice and shortcomings in hospital performance metrics across the United States. *Worldviews on Evidence-Based Nursing, 13*(1), 6–14. https://doi.org/10.1111/wvn.12133.

Michie, S., Atkins, L., & West, R. (2014). *The behaviour change wheel: A guide to designing interventions.* London: Silverback Publishing.

Minnick, A. F., Kleinpell, R., & Allison, T. L. (2019). Reports of three organizations' members about doctor of nursing practice project experiences and outcomes. *Nursing Outlook, 67*(6), 671–679. https://doi.org/10.1016/j.outlook.2019.05.012.

Mishuris, R. G., Palmisano, J., McCullagh, L., Hess, R., Feldstein, D. A., Smith, P. D., et al. (2019). Using normalisation process theory to understand workflow implications of decision support implementation across diverse primary care settings. *BMJ Health & Care Informatics, 26*(1), Article e100088. https://doi.org/10.1136/bmjhci-2019-100088.

Mohammadi, M. M., Poursaberi, R., & Salahshoor, M. R. (2018). Evaluating the adoption of evidence-based practice using Rogers's diffusion of innovation theory: A model testing study. *Health Promotion Perspectives, 8*(1), 25–32. https://doi.org/10.15171/hpp.2018.03.

Mondoux, S., & Shojania, K. G. (2019). Evidence-based medicine: A cornerstone for clinical care but not for quality improvement. *Journal of Evaluation in Clinical Practice, 25*(3), 363–368. https://doi.org/10.1111/jep.13135.

Moore, J. E., Mascarenhas, A., Bain, J., & Straus, S. E. (2017). Developing a comprehensive definition of sustainability. *Implementation Science, 12*(1), 110. https://doi.org/10.1186/s13012-017-0637-1.

Moreno-Poyato, A. R., Delgado-Hito, P., Leyva-Moral, J. M., Casanova-Garrigos, G., & Monteso-Curto, P. (2019). Implementing evidence-based practices on the therapeutic relationship in inpatient psychiatric care: A participatory action research. *Journal of Clinical Nursing, 28*(9-10), 1614–1622. https://doi.org/10.1111/jocn.14759.

Morton, S., Wilson, S., Inglis, S., Ritchie, K., & Wales, A. (2018). Developing a framework to evaluate knowledge into action interventions. *BMC Health Services Research, 18*(1), 133. https://doi.org/10.1186/s12913-018-2930-3.

Muhwava, L. S., Murphy, K., Zarowsky, C., & Levitt, N. (2019). Experiences of lifestyle change among women with gestational diabetes mellitus (GDM): A behavioural diagnosis using the COM-B model in a low-income setting. *PLoS One, 14*(11), Article e0225431. https://doi.org/10.1371/journal.pone.0225431.

Murt, M. F., Krouse, A. M., Baumberger-Henry, M. L., & Drayton-Brooks, S. M. (2019). Nurses at the table: A naturalistic inquiry of nurses on governing boards. *Nursing Forum, 54*(4), 575–581. https://doi.org/10.1111/nuf.12372.

NAM. (2017). *Optimizing Strategies for Clinical Decision Support: Summary of a Meeting Series.* https://nam.edu/optimizing-strategies-clinical-decision-support/.

NHS Institute for Innovation and Improvemen. (2010). *Sustainability Model.* https://improvement.nhs.uk/documents/2174/sustainability-model.pdf.

NIH. (2019). *Implementation Science News, Resources and Funding for Global Health Researchers.* https://www.fic.nih.gov/ResearchTopics/Pages/ImplementationScience.aspx.

Nilsen, P. (2015). Making sense of implementation theories, models and frameworks. *Implementation Science, 10*(1), 53. https://doi.org/10.1186/s13012-015-0242-0.

Norton, S., Milat, A., Edwards, B., & Giffin, M. (2016). Narrative review of strategies by organizations for building evaluation capacity. *Evaluation and Program Planning, 58*, 1–19. https://doi.org/10.1016/j.evalprogplan.2016.04.004.

NSI Nursing Solutions Inc. (2019). *2019 National Health Care Retention & RN Staffing Report.* http://www.nsinursingsolutions.com/Files/assets/library/retentioninstitute/2019%20National%20Health%20Care%20Retention%20Report.pdf.

Office of Human Research Protections, U.S. Department of Health & Human Services. (n.d.). *Quality improvement activities FAQs.* https://www.hhs.gov/ohrp/regulations-and-policy/guidance/faq/quality-improvement-activities/index.html.

Office of Public Health Preparedness and Response. (2015). *Immediate need for healthcare facilities to review procedures for cleaning, disinfecting, and sterilizing reusable medical devices.* Atlanta, GA: U.S: Department of Health & Human Services.

Ouayogode, M. H., Mainor, A. J., Meara, E., Bynum, J. P. W., & Colla, C. H. (2019). Association between care management and outcomes among patients with complex needs in Medicare accountable care organizations. *JAMA Network Open, 2*(7), Article e196939. https://doi.org/10.1001/jamanetworkopen.2019.6939.

Parry, G., Coly, A., Goldmann, D., Rowe, A. K., Chattu, V., Logiudice, D., et al. (2018). Practical recommendations for the evaluation of improvement initiatives. *International Journal for Quality in Health Care, 30*(suppl 1), 29–36. https://doi.org/10.1093/intqhc/mzy021.

Pasero, C. (2009). Assessment of sedation during opioid administration for pain management. *Journal of PeriAnesthesia Nursing, 24*(3), 186–190. https://doi.org/10.1016/j.jopan.2009.03.005.

Patel, M. S., Volpp, K. G., Small, D. S., Wynne, C., Zhu, J., Yang, L., et al. (2017). Using active choice within the electronic health record to increase influenza vaccination rates. *Journal of General Internal Medicine, 32*(7), 790–795. https://doi.org/10.1007/s11606-017-4046-6.

Patey, A. M., Hurt, C. S., Grimshaw, J. M., & Francis, J. J. (2018). Changing behaviour 'more or less'-do theories of behaviour inform strategies for implementation and de-implementation? A critical interpretive synthesis. *Implementation Science, 13*(1), 134. https://doi.org/10.1186/s13012-018-0826-6.

Patterson, A. E., Mason, T. M., & Duncan, P. (2017). Enhancing a culture of inquiry: The role of a clinical nurse specialist in supporting the adoption of evidence. *Journal of Nursing Administration, 47*(3), 154–158. https://doi.org/10.1097/NNA.0000000000000458.

Perry, C. K., Damschroder, L. J., Hemler, J. R., Woodson, T. T., Ono, S. S., & Cohen, D. J. (2019). Specifying and comparing implementation strategies across seven large implementation interventions: A practical application of theory. *Implementation Science, 14*(1), 32. https://doi.org/10.1186/s13012-019-0876-4.

Phelan, S., Lin, F., Mitchell, M., & Chaboyer, W. (2018). Implementing early mobilisation in the intensive care unit: An integrative review. *International Journal of Nursing Studies, 77*, 91–105. https://doi.org/10.1016/j.ijnurstu.2017.09.019.

Pittman, J., Cohee, A., Storey, S., LaMothe, J., Gilbert, J., Bakoyannis, G., et al. (2019). A multisite health system survey to assess organizational context to support evidence-based practice. *Worldviews on Evidence-Based Nursing, 16*(4), 271–280. https://doi.org/10.1111/wvn.12375.

Porter-O'Grady, T., & Malloch, K. (2008). Beyond myth and magic: The future of evidence-based leadership. *Nursing Administration Quarterly, 32*(3), 176–187. https://doi.org/10.1097/01.NAQ.0000325174.30923.b6.

Powell, B. J., Mandell, D. S., Hadley, T. R., Rubin, R. M., Evans, A. C., Hurford, M. O., et al. (2017). Are general and strategic measures of organizational context and leadership associated with knowledge and attitudes toward evidence-based practices in public behavioral health settings? A cross-sectional observational study. *Implementation Science, 12*(1), 64. https://doi.org/10.1186/s13012-017-0593-9.

Powell, B. J., Waltz, T. J., Chinman, M. J., Damschroder, L. J., Smith, J. L., Matthieu, M. M., et al. (2015). A refined compilation of implementation strategies: Results from the expert recommendations for implementing change (ERIC) project. *Implementation Science, 10*(21). https://doi.org/10.1186/s13012-015-0209-1.

Prochaska, J. J., & Sanders-Jackson, A. (2016). Patient decision aids for discouraging low-value health care procedures: Null findings and lessons learned. *JAMA Internal Medicine, 176*(1), 41–42. https://doi.org/10.1001/jamainternmed.2015.7347.

QSEN Institute. (2019). *Quality and Safety Education for Nurses.* http://qsen.org/competencies/.

Renolen, A., Hjalmhult, E., Hoye, S., Danbolt, L. J., & Kirkevold, M. (2020). Creating room for evidence-based practice: Leader behavior in hospital wards. *Research in Nursing & Health.* https://doi.org/10.1002/nur.21981.

Renolen, A., Hoye, S., Hjalmhult, E., Danbolt, L. J., & Kirkevold, M. (2018). "Keeping on track"-Hospital nurses' struggles with maintaining workflow while seeking to integrate evidence-based practice into their daily work: A grounded theory study. *International Journal of Nursing Studies, 77*, 179–188. https://doi.org/10.1016/j.ijnurstu.2017.09.006.

Robertson-Malt, S., & Norton-Westwood, D. (2017). Framework of care: Communicating the structure and processes of care. *International Journal of Evidence-Based Healthcare, 15*(3), 82–89. https://doi.org/10.1097/XEB.0000000000000114.

Rogers, E. (2003). *Diffusion of innovations* (5th ed.). New York: The Free Press.

Roush, K., & Tesoro, M. (2018). An examination of the rigor and value of final scholarly projects completed by DNP nursing students. *Journal of Professional Nursing, 34*(6), 437–443. https://doi.org/10.1016/j.profnurs.2018.03.003.

Royer, H. R., Crary, P., Fayram, E., & Heidrich, S. M. (2018). Five-year program evaluation of an evidence-based practice scholars program. *Journal of Continuation Education in Nursing, 49*(12), 547–554. https://doi.org/10.3928/00220124-20181116-05.

Rubio, D. M., Schoenbaum, E. E., Lee, L. S., Schteingart, D. E., Marantz, P. R., Anderson, K. E., et al. (2010). Defining translational research: implications for training. *Academic Medicine, 85*(3), 470–475. https://doi.org/10.1097/ACM.0b013e3181ccd618.

Rutledge, R. I., Romaire, M. A., Hersey, C. L., Parish, W. J., Kissam, S. M., & Lloyd, J. T. (2019). Medicaid accountable care organizations in four states: Implementation and early impacts. *Milbank Quarterly, 97*(2), 583–619. https://doi.org/10.1111/1468-0009.12386.

Sackett, D. L., Strauss, S. E., Richardson, W. S., Rosenberg, W., & Haynes, R. B. (2000). *Evidence-based medicine: How to practice and team EBM* (2nd ed.). Edinburgh: Churchill Livingstone.

Sadeghnezhad, M., Heshmati Nabavi, F., Najafi, F., Kareshki, H., & Esmaily, H. (2018). Mutual benefits in academic-service partnership: An integrative review. *Nurse Education Today, 68*, 78–85. https://doi.org/10.1016/j.nedt.2018.05.019.

Sadler, B. L., Joseph, A., Keller, A., & Rostenberg, B. (2009). *Using evidence-based environmental design to enhance safety and quality*. IHI Innovation Series white Paper. Institute for Healthcare Improvement. www.IHI.org.

Sarkies, M. N., Bowles, K. A., Skinner, E. H., Haas, R., Lane, H., & Haines, T. P. (2017). The effectiveness of research implementation strategies for promoting evidence-informed policy and management decisions in healthcare: A systematic review. *Implementation Science, 12*(1), 132. https://doi.org/10.1186/s13012-017-0662-0.

Saunders, H., & Vehvilainen-Julkunen, K. (2017). Nurses' evidence-based practice beliefs and the role of evidence-based practice mentors at University Hospitals in Finland. *Worldviews on Evidence-Based Nursing, 14*(1), 35–45. https://doi.org/10.1111/wvn.12189.

Schaffer, M. A., Sandau, K. E., & Diedrick, L. (2013). Evidence-based practice models for organizational change: Overview and practical applications. *Journal of Advanced Nursing, 69*(5), 1197–1209. https://doi.org/10.1111/j.1365-2648.2012.06122.x.

Schein, E. H., & Schein, P. (2016). *Organizational culture and leadership* (5th ed.): Hoboken, NJ: John Wiley & Sons Inc.

Scott 2nd, R.D., Culler, S. D., & Rask, K. J. (2019). Understanding the economic impact of health care-associated infections: A cost perspective analysis. *Journal of Infusion Nursing, 42*(2), 61–69. https://doi.org/10.1097/NAN.0000000000000313.

Seneski, A., & Stack, A. M. (2019). A framework for maintenance and scaling of an evidence-based guideline program. *Pediatric Quality & Safety, 4*(2), e153. https://doi.org/10.1097/pq9.0000000000000153.

Shrank, W. H., Rogstad, T. L., & Parekh, N. (2019). Waste in the US health care system: Estimated costs and potential for savings. *JAMA, 322*(15), 1501–1509. https://doi.org/10.1001/jama.2019.13978.

Shuman, C. J. (2017). *Addressing the practice context in evidence-based practice implementation: Leadership and climate* (PhD thesis). Ann Arbor, MI: University of Michigan.

Shuman, C. J., Liu, X., Aebersold, M. L., Tschannen, D., Banaszak-Holl, J., & Titler, M. G. (2018). Associations among unit leadership and unit climates for implementation in acute care: A cross-sectional study. *Implementation Science, 13*(1), 62. https://doi.org/10.1186/s13012-018-0753-6.

Sigma Theta Tau International Research Scholarship Advisory Committee. (2008). Sigma Theta Tau International position statement on evidence-based practice February 2007 summary. *Worldviews on Evidence-Based Nursing, 5*(2), 57–59. https://doi.org/10.1111/j.1741-6787.2008.00118.x.

Spiva, L., Hart, P. L., Patrick, S., Waggoner, J., Jackson, C., & Threatt, J. L. (2017). Effectiveness of an evidence-based practice nurse mentor training program. *Worldviews on Evidence-Based Nursing, 14*(3), 183–191. https://doi.org/10.1111/wvn.12219.

SQUIRE. (2017). *SQUIRE 2.0 guidelines*. http://squire-statement.org/index.cfm?fuseaction=Page.ViewPage&PageID=471.

Staines, A., Vanderavero, P., Duvillard, B., Deriaz, P., Erard, P., Kundig, F., et al. (2018). Sustained improvement in hand hygiene compliance using a multi-modal improvement programme at a Swiss multi-site regional hospital. *Journal of Hospital Infection, 100*(2), 176–182. https://doi.org/10.1016/j.jhin.2018.04.010.

Stetler, C. B. (2001). Updating the Stetler Model of research utilization to facilitate evidence-based practice. *Nursing Outlook, 49*(6), 272–279. https://doi.org/10.1067/mno.2001.120517.

Stetler, C. B., Ritchie, J. A., Rycroft-Malone, J., & Charns, M. P. (2014). Leadership for evidence-based practice: strategic and functional behaviors for institutionalizing EBP. *Worldviews on Evidence-Based Nursing, 11*(4), 219–226. https://doi.org/10.1111/wvn.12044.

Stevens, K. R. (2013). The impact of evidence-based practice in nursing and the next big ideas. *OJIN: Online Journal of Issues in Nursing, 18*(2), 4.

Stewart, R. E., Adams, D. R., Mandell, D. S., Nangia G., Shaffer, L., Evans A. C., et al. (2017). Non-participant,s in policy efforts to promote evidence-based practices in a large behavioral health system. *Implementation Science, 12*(1), 70. https://doi.org/10.1186/s13012-017-0598-4.

Storey, S., Wagnes, L., LaMothe, J., Pittman, J., Cohee, A., & Newhouse, R. (2019). Building evidence-based nursing practice capacity in a large statewide health system: A multimodal approach. *Journal of Nursing*

Administration, 49(4), 208–214. https://doi.org/10.1097/NNA.0000000000000739.

Straus, S. E., Tetroe, J. M., & Graham, I. D. (2011). Knowledge translation is the use of knowledge in health care decision making. *Journal of Clinical Epidemiology, 64*(1), 6–10. https://doi.org/10.1016/j.jclinepi.2009.08.016.

Strifler, L., Cardoso, R., McGowan, J., Cogo, E., Nincic, V., Khan, P. A., et al. (2018). Scoping review identifies significant number of knowledge translation theories, models, and frameworks with limited use. *Journal of Clinical Epidemiology, 100*, 92–102. https://doi.org/10.1016/j.jclinepi.2018.04.008.

Sveinsdottir, H., Ragnarsdottir, E. D., & Blondal, K. (2016). Praise matters: The influence of nurse unit managers' praise on nurses' practice, work environment and job satisfaction: a questionnaire study. *Journal of Advanced Nursing, 72*(3), 558–568. https://doi.org/10.1111/jan.12849.

Taylor, N., Clay-Williams, R., Hogden, E., Braithwaite, J., & Groene, O. (2015). High performing hospitals: A qualitative systematic review of associated factors and practical strategies for improvement. *BMC Health Services Research, 15*(244). https://doi.org/10.1186/s12913-015-0879-z.

The Joint Commission. (2016). *R3 report issue 2: CAUTI.* https://www.jointcommission.org/standards/r3-report/r3-report-issue-2-cauti/.

The Joint Commission. (n.d.). ORYX performance measures. https://www.jointcommission.org/the_joint_commission_measures_effective_january_1_2019/.

Titler, M. G. (2018). Translation research in practice: An introduction. *OJIN: The Online Journal of Issues in Nursing, 23*(2). Manuscript 1. https://doi.org/10.3912/OJIN.Vol23No02Man01.

U.S. Bureau of Labor Statistics. (2019). *Occupational outlook handbook.* https://www.bls.gov/ooh/.

Valim, M. D., Rocha, I. L. S., Souza, T. P. M., Cruz, Y. A. D., Bezerra, T. B., Baggio, E., et al. (2019). Efficacy of the multimodal strategy for Hand Hygiene compliance: An integrative review. *Revista Brasileira de Enfermagem, 72*(2), 552–565. https://doi.org/10.1590/0034-7167-2018-0584.

Van de Velde, S., Heselmans A., Delvaux N., Brandt L., Marco-Ruiz L., Spitaels D., et al. (2018). A systematic review of trials evaluating success factors of interventions with computerised clinical decision support. *Implementation Science, 13*(1), 114. https://doi.org/10.1186/s13012-018-0790-1.

van der Zijpp, T. J., Niessen, T., Eldh, A. C., Hawkes, C., McMullan, C., Mockford, C., et al. (2016). A bridge over turbulent waters: Illustrating the interaction between managerial leaders and facilitators when implementing research evidence. *Worldviews on Evidence-Based Nursing, 13*(1), 25–31. https://doi.org/10.1111/wvn.12138.

Wang, V., Maciejewski, M. L., Helfrich, C. D., & Weiner, B. J. (2018). Working smarter not harder: Coupling implementation to de-implementation. *Healthcare (Amsterdam, Netherlands), 6*(2), 104–107. https://doi.org/10.1016/j.hjdsi.2017.12.004.

Warren, J. I., Montgomery, K. L., & Friedmann, E. (2016). Three-year pre-post analysis of EBP integration in a Magnet-designated community hospital. *Worldviews on Evidence-Based Nursing, 13*(1), 50–58. https://doi.org/10.1111/wvn.12148.

Willis, W. K., Muslin, I., & Timko, K. N. (2016). A house divided: Cooperative and competitive recruitment in vital industries. *Journal of Nursing Management, 24*(2), 253–260. https://doi.org/10.1111/jonm.12308.

Xue, Y., Chappel, A. R., Freund, D. A., Aiken, L. H., & Noyes, K. (2015). Cost outcomes of supplemental nurse staffing in a large medical center. *Journal of Nursing Care Quality, 30*(2), 130–137. https://doi.org/10.1097/NCQ.0000000000000100.

Yoo, J. Y., Kim, J. H., Kim, J. S., Kim, H. L., & Ki, J. S. (2019). Clinical nurses' beliefs, knowledge, organizational readiness and level of implementation of evidence-based practice: The first step to creating an evidence-based practice culture. *PLoS One, 14*(12), Article e0226742. https://doi.org/10.1371/journal.pone.0226742.

Zhang, H., Cowling, D. W., Graham, J. M., & Taylor, E. (2019). Five-year impact of a commercial accountable care Organization on health care spending, utilization, and quality of care. *Medical Care, 57*(11), 845–854. https://doi.org/10.1097/MLR.0000000000001179.

Zhao, Q., Yang, M. M., Huang, Y. Y., & Chen, W. (2018). How to make hand hygiene interventions more attractive to nurses: A discrete choice experiment. *PLoS One, 13*(8), Article e0202014. https://doi.org/10.1371/journal.pone.0202014.

18

Quality and Safety

Luc R. Pelletier

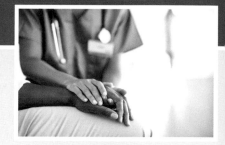

 http://evolve.elsevier.com/Huber/leadership

Quality and safety share center stage in value-driven health care. Quality and safety principles and practices form the foundation of an accessible, reliable health care enterprise. Health care quality is an art and science that continues to evolve. Its relevance was heightened with ongoing reports from the American Academy of Nursing, National Academy of Medicine, and other national organizations related to health care and health care quality. Well before these reports were published, however, professional nurses assumed key roles in the business of measuring, monitoring, and improving health care quality and safety. Nurses have typically taken a leadership role in performance and quality improvement and continue to do so in their roles as board members, chief executives, experience officers, chief quality officers, health care quality professionals, enterprise risk managers, and safety officers. It is important to note that identifying opportunities for improvement and continuously improving services is every health care professional's responsibility. Patients and their families also have rights and responsibilities related to quality and safety. Where once there were dedicated quality departments in health care organizations, now best-in-class health care organizations train everyone in performance improvement models and techniques (e.g., *Plan-Do-Study-Act [PDSA]*, Lean, Six Sigma). It would be difficult to describe the entire field of health care quality and patient safety in one chapter. In this chapter a large amount of information and emerging trends have been distilled, and specific content has been targeted toward nurse leaders. This system overview includes definitions of commonly used terms; health care quality in a new millennium; interprofessional collaboration, patient engagement, and self-care as professional nursing imperatives; industrial models and standards of quality; quality and safety performance improvement models; costs associated with waste in health care; and issues and trends in leadership and management. Resources are provided throughout for nurse leaders to use in their everyday practice.

DEFINITIONS

There are many concepts and terms related to health care quality and safety. Definitions are as follows:

Benchmarking "includes routinely comparing indicators (structure, process, and outcomes) against best performance and seeking out ways to make improvements with the greatest impact on outcomes. Ideally, the reference point is a demonstrated best practice" (Rosati, 2018, p. 234).

Continuous quality improvement (CQI) is defined by the American Society for Quality (ASQ) as "a philosophy and attitude for analyzing capabilities and processes and improving them repeatedly to achieve customer satisfaction" (ASQ, 2019a, p. 71). **Evidence-based practice** was originally defined by Sackett et al. (1996) as "the conscientious, explicit, and judicious use of current best evidence in making decisions about the care of individual patients" (p. 71). A **fair and just culture** is defined as "organizational accountability for the systems they've designed and employee accountability for the choices they make" (Paradiso & Sweeney, 2019, p. 40).

Lean originated in manufacturing before being applied to health care. It is "a set of management practices to improve efficiency and effectiveness by eliminating waste. The core principle of lean is to reduce and eliminate non value-adding activities and waste" (ASQ, 2019b, p. 1). **Six Sigma** is achieved when the organization reaches an error or defect rate of 3.4 or less per one million. Six Sigma in health care "reduces the number of errors made by physicians, nurses and technicians; improving lab turnaround times; reducing appointment times; decreasing steps in the supply chain; accelerating reimbursement for insurance claims; and improving patient outcomes" (Villanova University, 2019, p. 5).

Patient engagement is defined as "the desire and capability to actively choose to participate in care in a way uniquely appropriate to the individual in cooperation with a healthcare provider or institution for the purposes of maximizing outcomes or experiences of care" (Higgins et al., 2017, p. 33). **Patient activation** describes the four degrees of engagement, including "Level 1—Disengaged and overwhelmed; Level 2—Becoming aware, but still struggling; Level 3—Taking action; and Level 4—Maintaining behaviors and pushing further" (Insignia Health, 2018, p. 1). Patient activation "is a proxy for terms such as self-care, self-management or readiness for discharge" (Stichler & Pelletier, 2020, p. 3).

Patient safety practices are "a type of process or structure whose application reduces the probability of adverse events resulting from exposure to the healthcare system across a range of diseases and procedures" (Shojania et al., 2001, p. 13).

A **performance measure** is "a quantitative tool (for example, rate, ratio, index, percentage) that provides an indication of an organization's performance in relation to a specified process or outcome" (The Joint Commission [TJC], 2019a, p. 110). A **performance measurement system** is a systems-based approach to quality and safety where "the organization uses evidence-based medicine and clinical decision support tools, engages in performance measurement and improvement, measures and responds to patient experiences and satisfaction, practices population health management, and publicly shares robust quality and safety data and improvement activities" (The Joint Commission, 2019b, p. 6).

A **performance/quality improvement program** is an overarching organizational strategy to ensure accountability of all employees, incorporating evidence-based health care quality indicators to continuously improve care delivered to various populations. It is the

organization's blueprint for achieving and maintaining performance excellence. **PDSA** is an acronym for an improvement model for testing change, which includes "developing a plan to test the change (Plan), carrying out the test (Do), observing and learning from the consequences (Study), and determining what modifications should be made to the test (Act)" (Institute for Healthcare Improvement [IHI], 2020a, p.1).

Quality refers to characteristics of and the pursuit of excellence. **Health care quality** is classically defined as "the degree to which health services for individuals and populations increase the likelihood of desired health outcomes and are consistent with current professional knowledge" (Institute of Medicine, 2000, pp. 128–129). Inpatient **quality indicators** are "standardized, evidence-based measures of health care quality that can be used with readily available hospital inpatient administrative data to measure and track clinical performance and outcomes" (AHRQ, n.d.a., p. 3). The Agency for Healthcare Research and Quality (AHRQ) also has quality indicators for prevention, inpatient quality, patient safety, and pediatric care. A high **reliability organization** is "an organization operating in an industry that is complex and has high risk for harm that consistently performs at high levels of safety over long periods of time" (Pelletier & Beaudin, 2018, p. 252).

Risk adjustment is a process in which differences among clients or variables such as age or disease severity are weighted or adjusted for outcomes analyses or benchmarking efforts. **Enterprise risk management (ERM)** "in healthcare promotes a comprehensive framework for making risk management decisions which maximize value protection and creation by managing risk and uncertainty and their connection to total value" (Carroll, 2014, p. 5). An **ERM program** includes components of culture, strategy, objectives, appetite/tolerance, ERM structure and plans, communication and reporting plans, and oversight (Carroll, 2014, pp. 6–8).

A **sentinel event** "is a patient safety event that reaches a patient and results in any of the following: death, permanent harm, or severe temporary harm and intervention required. Such events are called 'sentinel' because they signal the need for immediate investigation and response" (TJC, 2019c, pp. 5–7).

Standards are defined as written value statements. These statements form the rules that apply to key processes and the results that can be expected when the processes are performed according to specifications.

The three basic types of standards for health care quality are (1) structure, (2) process, and (3) outcome, following Donabedian's (1980) quality framework. **Structure standards and measures** focus on the internal characteristics of the organization and its personnel. **Process standards and measures** focus on whether the activities within an organization are being conducted appropriately, effectively, and efficiently. **Outcome standards and measures** refer to a change in the patient's current or future health status that is attributed to antecedent health care and client attributes of health care.

BACKGROUND

HEALTH CARE QUALITY IN A NEW MILLENNIUM

Professional nurses have an obligation to reasonably ensure that the care they provide is evidence based (Sackett et al., 1996) and that work processes are consumer and family centric. Their interventions should be conscious and intentional (Waddill-Goad & Langster, 2016). Providing "quality" health care is "the degree to which health services for individuals and populations increase the likelihood of desired health outcomes and are consistent with current professional knowledge" (Institute of Medicine, 2000, pp. 128–129). As clinical leaders and managers, nurses have served as health care quality professionals and have promoted standardization, measurement, and continuous quality improvement in a variety of care delivery settings. Professional nurses have consistently held the practice of quality and safety management in high regard and have the effective care of clients and families as their primary focus. Nurses are bound by their professional association's *Code of Ethics* (American Nurses Association [ANA], 2015) and scope of professional standards to participate in the continuous improvement of the services they provide. Specifically, in Provision 3, the "nurse promotes, advocates for, and protects the rights, health, and *safety* of the patient" (Hegge, 2015, Set 2: slide 45). Recent health reform legislation serves as a call to action for professional nurses—from frontline clinicians to executives—to be actively involved in health care transformation. This includes nursing taking a leadership role in ensuring patients and families receive safe

and effective person-centered health care (Institute of Medicine [IOM], 2011, p. 228).

Although the manufacturing industry has dutifully explored ways to enhance its business practices, health care has lagged behind, and only within the past half century has it embraced improvement concepts. Health care has borrowed and applied models of continuous quality improvement that contained principles and practices originally developed for the manufacturing industry. *Continuous quality improvement (CQI)* is defined by the American Society for Quality (ASQ) as "a philosophy and attitude for analyzing capabilities and processes and improving them repeatedly to achieve customer satisfaction" (ASQ, 2019a, p. 69). As industry has had its quality gurus, so too has the health care quality and safety movement been fostered by health care professionals who have focused on continuous improvement.

Donald M. Berwick, MD, coauthor of the book *Curing Health Care: New Strategies for Quality Improvement* (Berwick et al., 1990), was an early pioneer in identifying how the concepts of CQI programs could apply to health care. In 1991 the National Demonstration Project on Quality Improvement in Health Care was conducted as a collaboration between members of the John A. Hartford Foundation, the Harvard Community Health Plan, the Juran Institute, the Hospital Corporation of America, and other health care organizations (IHI, 2004). The goal was to apply the methods and tools of industrial quality improvement in a variety of organizations to determine whether they could apply to a service industry. Berwick was a principal investigator for this project. As a result of this endeavor, the IHI was founded and became an early advocate for the concepts of process improvement and team problem-solving in health care organizations. In 2010 Berwick was appointed by President Obama as administrator of the Centers for Medicare & Medicaid Services (CMS). He served for 18 months and was responsible for introducing the "Triple Aim": improving the patient care experience, improving population health, and reducing health costs (Berwick et al., 2008). In 2015, a fourth aim was introduced to rename it the "quadruple aim." This additional aim was proposed to address improving the experience of workforce environments, safety, and engagement (Sikka et al., 2015). Berwick's administration was also responsible for initiating major transformative changes under health reform legislation *(Affordable Care Act)*.

In the mid-1990s The Joint Commission (TJC), a health care accreditation organization, began incorporating the principles of CQI in its revised standards. Starting in 1996 the IOM, through its Committee on Quality of Health Care in America (CQHCA), convened the nation's quality leaders and other public and private stakeholders to assess and improve health care for all. These leaders have promoted CQI in health care through education, research, and evaluation. Tenets promoted by these health care leaders and organizations—and embraced by health care professionals—include:

- Processes and systems are the problems, not people.
- Standardization of core processes is key to managing work and people.
- Quality can be enhanced only in safe, nonpunitive, fair, and just work cultures.

- Quality and safety measurement, monitoring, and improvement are everyone's job.
- The impetus for quality monitoring is not primarily for accreditation or regulatory compliance, but as a planned part of an organization's learning culture to continuously enhance and improve its services based on continuous feedback from employees and customers.
- Consumers and stakeholders must be included in all phases of quality improvement planning.
- Consensus among all stakeholders must be gained to have an impact on quality and safety.
- Health policy should include a focus on continuous enhancement of quality and safety.

A framework for understanding health care improvement was proposed by the IOM Committee on Quality of Health Care in America (2001) (Box 18.1). These six aims for health care quality improvement propose that health care systems ensure that care is safe, effective, patient centered, timely, efficient, and equitable.

BOX 18.1 Institute of Medicine's Specific Aims for Health Care Quality Improvement

- *Safe:* "Patients should not be harmed by the care that is intended to help them, nor should harm come to those who work in health care" (IOM, Committee on the National Quality Report on Health Care Delivery, 2001, p. 47).
- *Effective:* "Refers to care that is based on the use of systematically acquired evidence to determine whether an intervention, such as a preventive service, diagnostic test, or therapy, produces better outcomes than do alternatives—including the alternative to do nothing" (IOM, Committee on the National Quality Report on Health Care Delivery, 2001, p. 49). Evidence-based practice requires that those who give care consistently avoid both underuse of effective care and overuse of ineffective care that is more likely to harm than help the patient (Chassin, 1997).
- *Patient-centered:* "Refers to health care that establishes a partnership among practitioners, patients, and their families (when appropriate) to ensure that decisions respect patients' wants, needs, and preferences; and that patients have the education and support they need to make decisions and participate in their own care" (IOM, Committee on the National Quality Report on Health Care Delivery, 2001, p. 50).
- *Timeliness:* "Refers to obtaining needed care and minimizing unnecessary delays in getting that care" (IOM, Committee on the National Quality Report on Health Care Delivery, 2001, p. 53).
- *Efficient:* "Refers to a health care system where resources are used to get the best value for the money spent" (Palmer & Torgerson, 1999, p. 1136). "The opposite of efficiency is waste; the use of resources without benefit to the patients a system is intended to help. There are at least two ways to improve efficiency: (a) reduce quality waste and (b) reduce administrative or production costs" (IOM, CQHCA, 2001, p. 54).
- *Equitable:* "Providing care that does not vary in quality because of personal characteristics such as gender, ethnicity, geographical location, and socioeconomic status" (IOM, CQHCA, 2001, p. 6).

From Pelletier, L.R., & Hoffman, J.A. (2002). A framework for selecting performance measures for opioid treatment programs. *Journal for Healthcare Quality, 24*(3), 25. Reprinted with permission from the National Association for Healthcare Quality.

LEADERSHIP AND MANAGEMENT IMPLICATIONS

Interprofessional Collaboration

Collaboration should be a goal of any interaction, regardless of the workplace or situation. Collaboration is an imperative set by the American Nurses Association (ANA). The ANA, in its current *Guide to the Code of Ethics for Nurses with Interpretive Statements*, proposed that "the nurse collaborates with other health professionals and the public to protect human rights, promote health diplomacy, and reduce health disparities" (Hegge, 2015, Set 3: slide 12). Collaborative partnerships are part of this imperative and shape the way professional nurses act clinically and how they participate in performance and quality improvement efforts. As the complexity of care increases, multidisciplinary and interprofessional teamwork is used to solve complex problems in practice. For example, nursing, medicine, pharmacy, and information technology (IT) personnel may form a team or committee to develop a risk screen and smart alert for patients at risk for delirium in hospital settings.

Collaboration is about relationships. Conflict may be the result of an undeveloped or poor interpersonal relationship with a colleague. To overcome conflicts, it is necessary to strengthen, not shy away from, the relationship of the two opposing parties. As early as the late 1990s, the Pew Health Professions Commission (PHPC) talked about practicing relationship-centered care as one of 21 health profession competencies for the twenty-first century (O'Neil & PHPC, 1998). Relationship-centered care in this context surely involves nurse and client/family interactions, but it also stresses the importance of collaborative interprofessional relationships. These 21 competencies are necessary ingredients for effective professional relationships and can become guideposts for successful professional working relationships within a continuous improvement framework.

The 21 competencies also include a professional nurse's responsibility and accountability for health care quality. The specific statements related to health care quality include "take responsibility for quality of care and health outcomes at all levels" and "contribute to continuous improvement of the health care system" (O'Neill & PHPC, 1998, p. vii) (Box 18.2). Four core competencies specific to interprofessional collaborative practice have also been developed (Interprofessional Education Collaborative, 2016, p. 10). They include:

1. *Values/ethics for interprofessional practice:* work with individuals of other professions to maintain a climate of mutual respect and shared values.

BOX 18.2   Twenty-One Competencies for the Twenty-First Century

1. Embrace a personal ethic of social responsibility and service.
2. Exhibit ethical behavior in all professional activities.
3. Provide evidence-based, clinically competent care.
4. Incorporate the multiple determinants of health in clinical care.
5. Apply knowledge of the new sciences.
6. Demonstrate critical thinking, reflection, and problem-solving skills.
7. Understand the role of primary care.
8. Rigorously practice preventive health care.
9. Integrate population-based care and services into practice.
10. Improve access to health care for those with unmet health needs.
11. Practice relationship-centered care with individuals and families.
12. Provide culturally sensitive care to a diverse society.
13. Partner with communities in health care decisions.
14. Use communication and information technology effectively and appropriately.
15. Work in interdisciplinary teams.
16. Ensure care that balances individual, professional, system, and societal needs.
17. Practice leadership.
18. Take responsibility for quality of care and health outcomes at all levels.
19. Contribute to continuous improvement of the health care system.
20. Advocate for public policy that promotes and protects the health of the public.
21. Continue to learn and help others learn.

From O'Neil, E.H., & the Pew Health Professions Commission (PHPC). (1998). *Recreating health professional practice for a new century: The fourth report of the Pew Health Professions Commission.* San Francisco, CA: PHPC.

2. *Roles/responsibilities:* use the knowledge of one's own role and those of other professions to appropriately assess and address the health care needs of patients and to promote and advance the health of populations.

3. *Interprofessional communication:* communicate with patients, families, communities, and professionals in health and other fields in a responsive and responsible manner that supports a team approach to the promotion and maintenance of health, and the prevention and treatment of disease.

4. *Teams and teamwork:* apply relationship-building values and the principles of team dynamics to perform effectively in different team roles to plan, deliver, and evaluate patient/population-centered care and population health programs and policies that are safe, timely, efficient, effective, and equitable.

Patient Engagement

Health care reform brings a heightened focus on accountability for health care professionals. A critical component of reform includes an emphasis on patient-centered care and patient engagement. The American Academy of Nursing has declared patient engagement and activation a health reform imperative for nursing (Pelletier & Stichler, 2013). *Patient engagement* is defined as "the desire and capability to actively choose to participate in care in a way uniquely appropriate to the individual in cooperation with a healthcare provider or institution for the purposes of maximizing outcomes or experiences of care" (Higgins, et al., 2017, p. 33). Emphasis is on the actions of patients and families and their self-care behaviors. Engaging patients in their own care can affect inpatient safety in psychiatric inpatient settings (Pelletier, 2015; Polacek et al., 2015). Patient engagement in this context involves an active process of synthesizing health information, recommendations of health care professionals, and personal beliefs and preferences to manage one's illness.

Nurse leaders continue to play an important role in designing care delivery systems that promote patient and family engagement (Pelletier & Stichler, 2014a). Various toolkits have been developed to assist staff nurses and managers who desire to engage patients and their families in hospitals (AHRQ, 2017a; AHRQ, 2017b; Pelletier & Stichler, 2014b), and ambulatory and primary care (Caplan et al., 2014; Robert Wood Johnson Foundation, 2014). *Patient activation* describes the four degrees of engagement, including "Level 1—Disengaged and overwhelmed; Level 2—Becoming aware, but still struggling; Level 3—Taking action and gaining control; and Level 4—Maintaining behaviors and pushing further" (Insignia Health, 2020, p. 1). Patient activation "is a proxy for terms such as self-care, self-management or readiness for discharge" (Stichler & Pelletier, 2019, p. 3). Patient/consumer satisfaction is but one common outcome measure of patient engagement, along with desired clinical outcomes.

Self-Care and Resilience

Aligned with the quadruple aim of healthy workplaces (Sikka et al., 2015), burnout is seen as an "unrecognized threat to safe, quality care" (Dyrbye et al., 2017, p. 791). Burnout, compassion fatigue, and secondary trauma are all personal consequences of caregiving (Kelly, 2020; McCann et al., 2013). Clinician burnout can negatively influence levels of patient satisfaction, clinical outcomes, and patient safety (Brigham et al., 2018). The National Academy of Medicine Action Collaborative on Clinician Well-being and Resilience has developed resources, including a conceptual model and evidence-based solutions, to promote clinician well-being and reduce burnout (National Academy of Medicine, 2019). The Joint Commission also published a brief on developing resilience to combat nurse burnout. They identified five leadership empowering behaviors to promote workplace empowerment. These include:

1. Enhancing the meaningfulness of work;
2. Fostering opportunity to participate in decision-making;
3. Expressing confidence in high performance;
4. Facilitating the attainment of organizational goals;
5. Providing autonomy and freedom from bureaucratic restrictions (The Joint Commission, 2019c, p. 2).

The Advisory Board (2018) proposed that unmet needs form "cracks in the foundation" of health care. They targeted four "cracks" and recommended specific nurse manager/executive strategies to foster nurse resilience to prevent burnout as follows:

1. Since violence and point-of-care safety threats are now commonplace, reduce response time to routine point-of-care threats.
2. Since nurses feel they have to make compromises in care delivery, surface and address frontline perceptions of "unsafe" staffing.

3. Since staff bounce from traumatic experiences to other care activities with no time to recover, make emotional support "opt-out" only.
4. Since new technology, responsibilities, and care protocols cause nurses to feel "isolated in a crowd," reconnect nurses through storytelling (pp. 1–4).

Nurse leaders can use these resources, concepts, assessment tools, and methods in ensuring an engaged, well, and effective workforce.

INDUSTRIAL MODELS OF QUALITY

Industrial models have heavily influenced the way quality is currently understood and measured in health care settings across the continuum. Industry leaders who have influenced nursing's understanding of health care quality include Walter Shewhart, Joseph Juran, Philip Crosby, and W. Edwards Deming. These leaders provided blueprints from which nursing performance and quality improvement programs have been derived. Understanding quality in health care is enhanced by understanding the development of industrial models of quality.

Shewhart explored causes of variation in core work processes. He quantified these variations, categorizing variables as common or special cause. His *Plan, Do, Check, Act (PDCA)* model was updated to the PDSA cycle and is probably the most frequently used improvement tool in health care quality settings today, as follows (Fig. 18.1): developing a plan to test the change (Plan), carrying out the test (Do), observing and learning from the consequences (Study), and determining what modifications should be made to the test (Act) (IHI, 2020a, p. 1). Shewhart also provided the industrial community

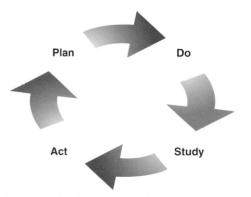

Fig. 18.1 PDSA (Plan, Do, Study, Act) cycle.

with statistical process control techniques that are used widely today. Deming (2000a, b) adopted his work and refined it.

Juran (1989) defined quality as "fitness for use." In his work, quality was defined as freedom from defects plus value and continuously meeting customer expectations. His approach to quality centered on the use of interdisciplinary teams that used diagnostic tools to understand why industrial processes produce a product not fit for use. His framework included a three-pronged approach: quality planning, quality control, and quality improvement. Quality planning "establishes the design of a product, service, or process that will meet customer, business, and operational needs to produce the product before it is produced. Quality planning follows a universal sequence of steps, as follows:

- Identify customers and target markets
- Discover hidden and unmet customer needs
- Translate these needs into product or service requirements: a means to meet their needs (new standards, specifications, etc.)
- Develop a service or product that exceeds customers' needs
- Develop the processes that will provide the service, or create the product, in the most efficient way
- Transfer these designs to the organization and the operating forces to be carried out." (Juran Institute, 2009, pp. 1–2).

Crosby viewed quality in production terms of zero defects and measured quality in relation to conformance to requirements. He believed that the results or products of a company are made by people. He focused on systems and the consequences of poor quality. He emphasized doing the right thing the first time to prevent waste. Waste and rework were seen as costly, and good managers were those who prevented costly mistakes. The cost of waste in health care is discussed later in this chapter.

In addition to PDSA, Deming focused on statistical process control techniques and on continuous quality improvement through a culture of quality. He is credited as being influential in the success of Japanese industries post–World War II. He proposed 14 points to help management understand and commit to quality. These points are listed in Box 18.3 (Deming, 2000a, b) and have heavily influenced health care's adoption of quality and safety improvement principles.

BOX 18.3   Deming's 14 Points for Quality

1. Create constancy of purpose toward improving products and services.
2. Adopt the new philosophy.
3. Cease dependence on inspection to achieve quality.
4. End the practice of awarding business on the basis of cost alone.
5. Improve constantly and forever every process for planning, production, and service.
6. Institute training on the job.
7. Adopt and institute leadership aimed at helping people do their jobs better.
8. Drive out fear by promoting two-way communication.
9. Break down barriers between departments.
10. Eliminate exhortations for the workforce in such forms as posters and slogans; these methods tend to create adversarial relationships.
11. Eliminate numerical quotas for productivity; instead have leaders promote continuous quality improvement (CQI).
12. Permit pride of workmanship by removing the barriers that prevent this.
13. Encourage education and self-improvement for all workers.
14. Define management's commitment to CQI and their obligation to implement these points.

From Deming, W.E. (2000a). *The new economics for industry, government, education.* Cambridge, MA: MIT Center for Advanced Engineering Studies; and Deming, W.E. (2000b). *Out of the crisis.* Cambridge, MA: MIT Center for Advanced Engineering Studies.

STANDARDS OF QUALITY

Donabedian (1980) developed the initial theoretical model of health care quality standards: structure, process, and outcomes, which identified that quality can be measured using these three aspects. Donabedian's framework is the most widely referenced model of quality; professional nurses have used this model to develop performance and quality improvement programs and conduct evidence-based improvement studies and nursing research. *Standards*, or written value statements, essentially define quality, against which performance and outcomes are measured. Standards and measures are typically developed from *benchmarking* activities and reviews of best practices in best-in-class organizations. Therefore the selection of standards and measures is a critical activity in the performance and quality improvement process. Actually, standards establish the baseline against which measurement and evaluation are conducted. It is also critical to decide who determines the standards and which standards are selected to define quality. Over the past 70 years, national groups have been formed to gain consensus on health care performance standards and measures. One such entity is the National Quality Forum (NQF), a not-for-profit, public–private membership organization created in 1999 to develop and implement a national strategy for health care quality measurement and reporting.

Structure Standards and Measures

Structure standards and measures focus on the internal characteristics of the organization and its personnel. They answer the following questions. Is an infrastructure in place and tools accessible to allow quality to exist? Is the structure of the organization set up to allow for the effective, efficient delivery of services? For example, a structural standard for a long-term care facility might be to have an adequate mix of registered nurses (RNs), licensed vocational/practical nurses (LVNs, LPNs), and nursing assistants on site to ensure that comprehensive care is delivered. For specialized areas, structure standards may address whether there are enough specialists, hospitalists, or intensivists to ensure quality care. Certain committees, policy statements, rules and regulations, or manuals, forms, or contracts may be needed. Structure standards regulate the environment to ensure quality. Human, organizational, and physical resources, and environmental characteristics, are examples of structure elements.

Process Standards and Measures

Process standards and measures focus on whether the activities within an organization are being conducted appropriately, effectively, and efficiently. Process measures focus on the behaviors of the professional nurse as a provider of care. The interventions recommended in a clinical practice guideline or best practice are examples of process standards. They relate to what the nurse will be doing and the process the nurse should follow to ensure effective, *evidence-based care*. Process standards look at activities, interventions, and the sequence of caregiving events, sometimes referred to as workflow. Typically, processes are assessed by audits, observational studies, or workflow analyses. Examples of process standards include the following: a nursing assessment is completed within 24 hours of admission, client calls are returned within 1 hour of the initial call, or a face-to-face assessment is completed within 1 hour by appropriate personnel for seclusion and restraints in a behavioral health setting.

Outcome Standards and Measures

Outcome standards and measures refer to whether the services provided by the organization make any difference. Were they effective? They answer important questions about the services that nurses provide. Did those services make a difference to the clients or to the health status of the population? Outcome standards address physical health status, mental health status, social and physical function, health attitudes/knowledge/behavior, utilization of services, and the client's perception and satisfaction with the care received. *Outcome process and measures* refer to a change in the current or future health status attributed to antecedent health care and client attributes of health care. Outcome standards present the possibility of measuring the effectiveness, quality, time, and resources allocated for care. Outcomes are reported as a rate per unit of measurement. Examples of outcome measures include the following: percentage of patients whose activities of daily living have improved by 80%, percentage of clients who have stopped smoking after 12 weeks of intensive psychoeducational therapy, and falls with injury per 1000 patient days.

In measuring quality, both structure and process parameters are important, but they are not sufficient in determining whether the care led to an effective outcome or whether the client learned, recovered, or improved his or her health status. Over the years, the emphasis on structure, process, and outcome aspects of health care has varied. Ultimately, various stakeholders are interested in knowing whether care resulted in a positive, expected clinical outcome, based on objective, measurable criteria.

When developing a quality and safety improvement program, nurse leaders are cautioned not to start by creating new standards and measures. Rather, locating the evidence through a literature search or finding a systematic review will most likely yield measures from which to choose. These measures have typically been tested for reliability and validity and have been piloted in the field. National repositories of quality and safety performance measures can be found at:

- Centers for Medicare & Medicaid Services Quality Measures
- The Joint Commission
- National Database for Nursing Quality Indicators (NDNQI) and the CALNOC Registry (Press Ganey, 2020)
- National Quality Forum Quality Positioning System
- National Committee for Quality Assurance Health Effectiveness Data and Information Set (Health plans)
- Leapfrog Group
- The Cochrane Library
- Specialty professional associations and societies (American Psychiatric Association, American Nurses Association).

Selection criteria can then be adopted and measures chosen for a specific intervention or program. A number of selection criteria guideline statements have been developed, including the performance measurement evaluation criteria from the NQF (2012a). The performance measurement attributes common to these entities' guideline statements have been reported in the set of criteria proposed to be used for a national health care quality report (Institute of Medicine [IOM], Committee on the National Quality Report on Health Care Delivery, 2001). Common performance measurement selection criteria are listed in Box 18.4 (Pelletier & Hoffman, 2002). The adoption of these performance measurement selection criteria is the first step in developing a comprehensive *performance measurement system*, which is a systems-based approach to quality and safety where "the organization uses evidence-based medicine and clinical decision support tools, engages in performance measurement and improvement, measures and responds to patient experiences and satisfaction, practices population health management, and publicly shares robust quality and safety data and improvement activities" (The Joint Commission, 2019b, p. 6).

BOX 18.4 Common Performance Measurement Selection Criteria*

- *Relevance:* The measure should address features of the health care system applicable to health professionals, policy makers, and consumers.
- *Meaningfulness and interpretability:* The measure should be understandable to at least one of the audiences. It should help inform them about the important issues or concerns.
- *Scientific or clinical evidence:* The measure should be based on evidence documenting the links between the interventions, clinical processes, and/or outcomes it addresses.
- *Reliability or reproducibility:* The measure should produce the same results when repeated in the same population and setting.

- *Feasibility:* The measure should be specified precisely. Collection of data for the measure should be inexpensive and logistically feasible.
- *Validity:* The measure should make sense (face validity), correlate well with other measures of the same aspects of care (construct validity), and capture meaningful aspects of care (content validity).
- *Health importance:* The measure should include the prevalence of the health condition to which it applies, and the seriousness of the health outcomes affected.

*Criteria are listed in order of their frequency, with the one mentioned most often listed first. The same label for a criterion can have different meanings depending on the framework, because the criteria are not standardized. The definitions, rather than the labels, were used to construct the figure. Feasibility was used as a category covering several criteria in some of the frameworks and as a single criterion in others. Parts of this figure were adapted from NCQA's list of desirable attributes for HEDIS measures (IOM, Committee on the National Quality Report on Health Care Delivery, 2001, p. 81).

From Pelletier, L.R., & Hoffman, J.A. (2002). A framework for selecting performance measures for opioid treatment programs. *Journal for Healthcare Quality, 24*(3), 26. Reprinted with permission from the National Association for Healthcare Quality.

QUALITY AND SAFETY PERFORMANCE IMPROVEMENT MODELS

A number of industry-based models for quality and safety performance management have been adopted by the health care industry. These include Six Sigma, Lean, the Baldrige National Quality Award, high-reliability organizations, American Nurses Credentialing Center's Magnet Recognition Program®, and Planetree. These models are briefly described in the following sections.

Six Sigma

A strategy developed by Motorola and implemented successfully at General Electric (GE) and AlliedSignal Companies provided an innovative approach to reduce variation and error rates. Not surprisingly, the Six Sigma approach that these companies use is similar to tried-and-true approaches historically deployed by health care quality professionals. In the Six Sigma breakthrough strategy, errors are measured in defects per million opportunities (dpmo). *Six Sigma* is achieved when the organization reaches an error or defect rate of 3.4 or less per one million. Application of Six Sigma in health care "reduces the number of errors made by physicians, nurses and technicians; improving lab turnaround

times; reducing appointment wait times; decreasing steps in the supply chain; accelerating reimbursement for insurance claims; and improving patient outcomes" (Villanova University, 2019, p. 5). The Six Sigma strategy of **d**efine, **m**easure, **a**nalyze, **i**mprove, and **c**ontrol (DMAIC) (Harry & Schroeder, 2000) is remarkably similar to Juran's problem-solving strategy (Plsek & Omnias, 1989) that has been applied to health care. Table 18.1 illustrates these similarities (Pelletier, 2000).

Lean

Lean is a model of quality measurement that was originally associated with Deming, but was reintroduced to the United States by Womack in the mid-1990s (Jones & Womack, 2003). The premise of this model is that operational waste in an organization needs to be eliminated. *Lean* originated in manufacturing before being applied to health care. It is "a set of management practices to improve efficiency and effectiveness by eliminating waste. The core principle of lean is to reduce and eliminate non value-adding activities and waste" (ASQ, 2019b, 1). With a focus on core processes, "a perfect process creates precisely the right value for the customer. In a perfect process, every step is valuable (creates value for the customer), capable (produces a good result every

TABLE 18.1   Comparison of Six Sigma Breakthrough Strategy and Juran's Problem-Solving Strategy

SIX SIGMA BREAKTHROUGH STRATEGY		JURAN'S PROBLEM-SOLVING STRATEGY	
Stage	**Step (Objective)**	**Phase**	**Step**
Identification	1. Recognize 2. Define (Identify key business issues)	Project definition and organization	1. List and prioritize problems 2. Define project and team
Characterization	1. Measure 2. Analyze (Understand current performance levels)	Diagnostic journey	1. Analyze symptom 2. Formulate theory of causes 3. Test theories 4. Identify root causes
Optimization	1. Improve 2. Control (Achieve breakthrough improvement)	Remedial journey	1. Consider alternative solutions 2. Design solutions and controls 3. Address resistance to change 4. Implement solutions and controls
Institutionalization	1. Standardize 2. Integrate (Transform how day-to-day business is conducted)	Holding the gains	1. Check performance 2. Monitor control system

From Pelletier, L.R. (2000). On error-free health care: Mission possible! (Editorial). *Journal for Healthcare Quality, 22*(3), 9. Reprinted with permission from the National Association for Healthcare Quality.

time), available (produces the desired output, not just the desired quality, every time), adequate (does not cause delay), flexible, and linked by continuous flow" (IHI, 2005, p. 6). When any of these components are missing, the result is waste, which must be eliminated because it is costly. Lean has wide applicability in health care where there are many opportunities to improve processes such as supply chain management or medication administration. By challenging and analyzing any work process, obvious wasteful rework is flushed out and then the process is redone to be both more efficient and effective. Nurses find it rewarding to reduce or eliminate unnecessary effort; it gives them more time to spend at the bedside.

Baldrige National Quality Award Program

The Baldrige National Quality Award (BNQA) established a set of performance standards that define a total quality organization. Named after the Secretary of Commerce, the BNQA "was established by Congress in 1987 to enhance the competitiveness and performance of US businesses" (Baldrige Foundation, 2020, p. 3). The standards in seven areas of excellence are (1) leadership, (2) strategic planning, (3) customer and market focus,

(4) information and analysis, (5) human resource focus, (6) process management, and (7) business results. A study completed in 2011 found that a return on investment of money spent to implement the Baldrige criteria vis-à-vis economic benefit was 820:1 (Link & Scott, 2011). Organizations committed to quality improvement choose to adopt the BNQA approach as another means of defining and improving their organizational processes to achieve quality outcomes. Manufacturing, service, and small business were the original award categories, but education and health care were added in 1999. With the trend in health care of adopting industry applications and measure sets for quality improvement, it was fitting that the health care industry was recognized as one that could benefit from participating in this program. It is appropriate for health care entities to strive to achieve internationally recognized standards for performance excellence that enable them to benchmark their "best practices" with others in the field. The first health care organization to apply and be awarded the BNQA in health care was the SSM system in St. Louis, MO, in 2002. The most recent health care awardees include Adventist Health White Memorial in Los Angeles, CA and Mary Greeley Medical Center in Ames, IA (National Institute

of Standards and Technology, 2019, p. 3). The Alliance for Performance Excellence is a network of national, state, and local Baldrige-based organizations helping institutions achieve performance excellence using the Baldrige criteria (https://www.baldrigealliance.org/). Various states have also developed quality awards based on the BNQA criteria.

High-Reliability Organizations

In their book *Managing the Unexpected* (2007), Weick and Sutcliffe described high reliability as involving anticipation and containment. They believed that an organization's "collective mindfulness" (Chassin & Loeb, 2013) ensured that potential problems are anticipated and that strategies are in place should an unexpected event occur, and responses are early enough to prevent catastrophic consequences (AHRQ, 2019a, p. 2).

- Anticipation has three elements: (1) preoccupation with failure—being mindful of how complex their operations are and the fact that errors do occur, (2) reluctance to simplify—requiring staff to dig deep in understanding the cause of error versus overly simplified explanations (e.g., staff education), and (3) sensitivity to operations—be aware of structure and processes that are in place to effect desired patient outcomes.
- Containment has two elements: (1) commitment to resilience—having systems in place to return to normal operations quickly, and (2) deference to expertise—relying on and listening to frontline staff for their intimate knowledge about daily operations (Chassin & Loeb, 2013; Weick & Sutcliffe, 2007).

A high reliability organization is "an organization operating in an industry that is complex and has high risk for harm that consistently performs at high levels of safety over long periods of time" (Pelletier & Beaudin, 2018, p. 252). The Institute for Healthcare Improvement (IHI; 2020b), The Joint Commission (Joint Commission Center for Transforming Healthcare, 2020) and AHRQ's Patient Safety Network have a multitude of resources for helping healthcare entities implement HRO concepts and principles (AHRQ, 2019a).

American Nurses Credentialing Center Magnet Designation

The American Nurses Credentialing Center's (ANCC) Magnet Recognition Program® recognizes health care organizations for aligning "their strategic goals to improve the organization's outcomes" (ANCC, n.d., p. 2). Magnet-designated hospitals "attract" staff and retain them due to their characteristics or "forces of magnetism," such as the quality of nursing leadership, professional models of care and quality of care, nursing research, and evidence-based practice (ANCC, n.d.). The Magnet model includes the following components: transformational leadership, structural empowerment, exemplary professional practice, new knowledge, innovations and improvements, and empirical quality outcomes. Hospitals that embark on the Magnet journey first must assess where they are related to preestablished Magnet standards. Typically, nursing leadership staff complete a gap analysis to identify opportunities for improvement before submitting their application for designation. Organizations have used the journey to effect higher patient ratings of their hospital experience (Stimpfel et al., 2016), lower mortality (Bekelis et al., 2017; Missios & Bekelis, 2018), lower central line-associated bloodstream infection rates (Barnes et al., 2016), lower RN turnover (Park et al., 2016), and lower length of stay (Bekelis et al., 2017; Missios & Bekelis, 2017).

Planetree

Since 1978 Planetree has designated health care organizations for person-centered excellence. The Planetree model proposes that "Person-centered care yields internal, external, financial and cultural benefits to healthcare organizations. It engages patients, aligns with today's mandates for better population health management and improves organizational performance in quality, safety and experience" (Planetree, 2018, p. 1). Its standards help organizations increase patient activation, staff engagement, and foster staff and leadership development. Recently a Planetree Higher Education Advisory Council convened to develop person-centered care standards of excellence for universities and colleges preparing the next generation of health care providers. National University in California was one of the first universities to receive Planetree recognition in 2017 (National University, 2020).

COSTS ASSOCIATED WITH WASTE IN HEALTH CARE

According to Shrank et al. (2019), the cost associated with waste in health care ranges from $760 to $935 billion annually and plagues every sector in the health care industry. Berwick and Hackbarth (2012) listed categories of waste as: failures of care delivery, failures of care coordination, overtreatment, administrative complexity, pricing failures, and fraud and abuse. Shrank and colleagues further stated that policy experts have proposed that this waste represents 25% of total health care spending, estimated to be $3.82 trillion in 2019. They believe that aligning payers and providers through current value-based care initiatives can help cut waste.

The number of medical errors was described as unacceptable in *To Err Is Human: Building a Safer Health Care System* (Kohn et al., 2000), an IOM report that has been referenced widely in the professional and consumer press since its release. The IOM report reached the highest levels in the federal government, but response to its findings and recommendations have been lackluster. Health care organizations were slow to adopt its recommendations fully even 20 years later. Several reports on health care quality and safety have followed this landmark report.

The IOM (now called the National Academies of Sciences, Engineering, and Medicine, Health and Medicine Division) reports defined specific strategies that could inform the development and refinement of health care safety systems nationwide. An important component of these reports is the mention of the error-reduction techniques of other industries. The federal reports provided another opportunity to advocate for patients, families, and populations. They gave health care quality professionals the evidence and research with which to defend a quality management budget, enhance information systems and technologies to monitor and track errors, and further develop quality activities and studies using proven tools and techniques. The reports are also models in defining and describing cost/benefit analyses and return-on-investment scenarios for quality and performance improvement programs. In essence, they provided a business case for quality and safety.

The IOM *report Crossing the Quality Chasm: A New Health System for the 21st Century* (IOM, Committee on Quality of Health Care in America [CQHCA], 2001, p. 11) recommended that Congress establish a Health Care Quality Innovation Fund "to support projects targeted at (1) achieving the six aims of safety, effectiveness, patient-centeredness, timeliness, efficiency, and equity; and/or (2) producing substantial improvements in quality for the [15] priority conditions." The overall goal of the funding would be to produce a "public-domain portfolio of programs, tools, and technologies of widespread applicability" (p. 11). The report recommended an initial investment of $1 billion over three to five years to support this goal (p. 11). Health care organizations could take the lead either by enhancing the current resources dedicated to quality and performance improvement in their organizations, or by using the funds to finance regional collaborative health care quality projects. These successes could then be described in the literature for wider application.

Leadership by Example: Coordinating Government Roles in Improving Health Care Quality, the third in a series of IOM quality chasm reports, was released in 2002 (Corrigan et al., 2002). The original charge of the IOM Committee on Enhancing Federal Healthcare Quality Programs (CEFHQP) was to acknowledge that "The current federal quality oversight programs represent a patchwork of requirements and processes that have evolved over the last 30 to 35 years" (IOM, CEFHQP, 2002, p. 1). The committee was convened "to re-examine the various federal quality improvement and oversight programs to assess whether changes are needed to (1) provide adequate protection to beneficiaries, (2) provide strong incentives to providers to improve quality, and (3) improve the efficiency of the oversight processes by reducing redundancy" (IOM, CEFHQP, 2002, p. 1). In doing their work, the committee held workshops to obtain perspectives and information from various stakeholders with expertise in the fields of quality measurement, improvement, oversight, and research on ways to improve current federal programs (e.g., Medicare, Children's Health Insurance Program, Tricare, and Veterans Affairs).

These findings were not a surprise to many nurses and health care quality professionals who have been burdened with duplicative reporting such as licensing and accreditation for years. The positive message was that strong recommendations from this committee were sent to the federal government's leadership, asking them to attack these problems with a good deal of muscle to shape performance measurement for the whole health care sector. Standardization of protocols and measures is not a new idea (Pelletier, 1998). Reducing administrative burden and duplicative reporting would provide more time for clinical responsibilities and direct health care services to individuals, families, and populations/communities.

Clinical standardization has become the focus of efforts to reduce variability in practice and health care costs. However, a lack of centralization and absence of enforced universal standards have led to the development of guidelines not based on evidence (Benavidez & Frakt, 2019, p. 6). These authors proposed two steps to strengthen clinical practice guidelines: (1) restore funding for the Agency for Healthcare Research and Quality's National Guideline Clearinghouse, or establish a similar central guidelines repository, and (2) enforce a rigorous, universal methodology for creating guidelines (pp. 22–28).

CURRENT ISSUES AND TRENDS

Mission, Vision, and Core Values

An organization that adopts and nurtures a continuous quality and safety improvement culture (and rewards those who identify opportunities for improvement and their solutions) recognizes that change is an everyday event. One of the ways that change can be managed is to acknowledge it and make it a part of the organization's strategic planning process. Just as an organization defines its mission, vision, and core values, so too must change agents and teams define the purpose of the change (expected outcomes), the mission and vision of the change process, and the core values of the group that will be responsible for managing the change.

An organization's mission is a concise statement that answers the question: What business are we in today? For example, Sharp HealthCare, a San Diego-based not-for-profit integrated regional health care delivery system that was the recipient of the BNQA in 2007, stated that its mission is "to improve the health of those we serve with a commitment to excellence in all that we do. Our goal is to offer quality care and programs that set community standards, exceed patients' expectations and are provided in a caring, convenient, cost-effective and accessible manner" (Sharp HealthCare, 2020, p. 1). The Visiting Nursing Service of New York's (VNSNY) mission is "to improve the health and well-being of people through high-quality, cost-effective healthcare in the home and community" (VNSNY, 2020, p. 1).

An organization's vision should accurately depict what the company is striving to become. For example, Sharp HealthCare's vision is "to be the best health system in the universe" (Sharp HealthCare, 2020, p. 2).

VNSNY's vision "...continues to draw strength from this mission to care for vulnerable individuals and families. We strive to be the most significant, best-in-class, not-for-profit community-based health care organization, providing superior care coordination and health care services to vulnerable New Yorkers across a broad regional footprint" (VNSNY, 2020, p. 2).

It is critical for mission and vision statements to be communicated effectively and widely to internal stakeholders (employees and management personnel) and to external stakeholders (investors, clients, patients, vendors, and accreditation agencies). In this way the statements keep employees on a path to an attainable goal such as quality outcomes. Mission, vision, and value statements form the foundation for quality and safety and their management and improvement. Departmental mission and vision statements need to be aligned with the organization's core value statements.

Core value statements frame the organization's culture in the same way mission and vision statements do; they remain constant in an ever-changing landscape. "Values are operational qualities used by organizations to maintain or enhance performance" (Harmon, 1997, p. 246). Values consciously and unconsciously guide a professional nurse's personal and professional behavior. His Holiness the Dalai Lama and Cutler (1998) said the following about values: "Higher stages of growth and development depend on an underlying set of values that can guide us. A value system that can provide continuity and coherence to our lives, by which we can measure our experiences. A value system that can help us decide which goals are truly worthwhile and which pursuits are meaningless. Values help us with the challenges of everyday life" (pp. 192–193).

Nurses' personal and professional values come from the experiences they have shared with others in interpersonal exchanges at work and at home. To identify a group's core values, investigate these questions: Which three people have had the greatest influence in your personal and professional life? What are the three most important values these influential people taught you? The answers to these questions can help inform the development of mission, vision, and core value statements. An example is a set of core values or "core principles" from the Mayo Clinic, as outlined in Table 18.2.

TABLE 18.2 Mayo Clinic Value Statements

These values, which guide Mayo Clinic's mission to this day, are an expression of the vision and intent of our founders, the original Mayo physicians, and the Sisters of Saint Francis.

Respect	Treat everyone in our diverse community, including patients, their families, and colleagues with dignity.
Integrity	Adhere to the highest standards of professionalism, ethics, and personal responsibility, worthy of the trust our patients place in us.
Compassion	Provide the best care, treating patients and family members with sensitivity and empathy.
Healing	Inspire hope and nurture the well-being of the whole person, respecting physical, emotional, and spiritual needs.
Teamwork	Value the contributions of all, blending the skills of individual staff members in unsurpassed collaboration.
Innovation	Infuse and energize the organization, enhancing the lives of those we serve, through the creative ideas and unique talents of each employee.
Excellence	Deliver the best outcomes and highest quality service through the dedicated effort of every team member.
Stewardship	Sustain and reinvest in our mission and extended communities by wisely managing our human, natural, and material resources.

From Mayo Foundation for Medical Research and Education. (2020). *About Mayo Clinic: Mayo Clinic mission and values.* Rochester, MN: Author. http://www.mayoclinic.org/about-mayo-clinic/mission-values.

A Nurse Leader's Health Care Quality Toolbox

Along with the paradigm shift from quality assurance to organizational performance improvement came the expectation that accredited organizations become skilled at the art and science of CQI. This included the concepts of leadership involvement, a commitment to customers' needs (i.e., patients and families), an understanding of the principle of process versus people, a devotion to data collection and analysis as the foundation for problem-solving, and the recognition that interprofessional study teams are the experts and are best equipped to drive change and improvement.

Nurses are frequently tapped to participate in organization-wide improvement teams designed to address overarching problem resolution or process redesign projects. Many of the early quality leaders received training in facilitation and group meeting techniques in addition to the performance and quality improvement (PQI) tools. This enabled them to promote the team-based model of cross-functional and interprofessional problem-solving that became the standard for most organizations. Nurses in the new millennium continue to need skills and expertise in the concepts of team building, conflict resolution, statistical process control, customer service, and process improvement.

Nurse leaders in accredited organizations are expected to learn principles and tools for quality improvement, educate all staff on these techniques, collaboratively identify improvement opportunities on nursing units, and use data analyses to demonstrate the impact of change initiatives.

Nurses at all levels are affected by organizational quality efforts. Knowledge through continuous learning forms the backdrop for quality and safety. New nurses in nurse residency programs may undertake a small-scale, unit-based quality initiative, or change projects. Often the impetus arises from seeing a problem in practice and then pursuing an evidence-based quality improvement approach (Melnyk et al., 2015), and using PQI tools to analyze, plan, and take action through interprofessional teams and shared governance structures.

Health care quality professionals and nurses involved in quality and safety improvement activities have an enormous set of resources available to them as they plan for an enterprise-wide quality and safety program. Tools and techniques that nurses can readily use are shown in Table 18.3 and Figs. 18.2 through 18.7, which illustrate examples of templates and forms to be included in a nurse leader's quality "toolbox."

Two excellent resources for hospital-based and ambulatory quality programs are the National Database of Nursing Quality Indicators (NDNQI) and the CALNOC Registry, owned by Press Ganey (Press Ganey, 2020). NDNQI was originally developed by the ANA. This database is composed of nurse-sensitive indicators collected at the nursing unit level and provides the ability for participants to benchmark performance with national

TABLE 18.3	A Nurse Manager's Health Care Quality Toolbox	
Tool	**Description of the Tool**	**Example**
Data-collection tools	Check sheets and checklists facilitate the gathering of data for eventual analysis and reporting. Good data collection tools can help to count and categorize data.	Sample data collection sheet for a nurse manager's quality toolbox (see Fig. 18.2).
Control chart	This tool includes data points and their placement on a graph to depict variation. Its purpose is to illustrate whether the process variation is expected ("common cause") or an unexpected or unusual variation ("special cause"). Included are three lines—the mean, an upper control limit (UCL), and a lower control limit (LCL). Generally, a process is considered "out of control" when the data points stray outside of the control limits or a series of data points follow a defined pattern that illustrates a lack of control in the process.	Sample control chart for a nurse manager's quality toolbox (see Fig. 18.3).
Cause-and-effect (or fishbone) diagram	This tool resembles diagramming sentences. The "effect" is illustrated in a box at the end of a midline (or "head" of the fish). The "causes" are generally four or five categories of elements that might contribute to the effect (e.g., machines, methods, people, materials, and measurements) and the specific activities. Under each of these category headings, individual items that might lead to the effect are listed. By diagramming all of the possible contributors, the predominant or root causes may be found more readily.	Sample cause-and-effect diagram for a nurse manager's quality toolbox (see Fig. 18.4).
Detailed flowchart	Using various shapes, this tool is used to depict a work process, from start to finish, illustrating all of the processes' action steps, decision points, handoffs, or waiting stages. Flowcharts form the cornerstone of process improvement planning and analysis. The entire process must first be accurately defined to identify problems or process improvement opportunities.	Sample detailed flowchart for a nurse manager's quality toolbox (see Fig. 18.5).
Pareto chart	This bar graph can help depict the "80/20" rule. In the nineteenth century, it was used to show that 80% of the wealth was held by 20% of the people. In health care, typically 20% of the issues cause 80% of the problems. The use of this tool allows a performance improvement team to focus on the "vital few" causes of the problems in a process under study.	Example of a Pareto chart for a nurse manager's quality toolbox (see Fig. 18.6).
Scatter diagram	This graph describes the relationship between two variables that are continuous. It is used when the potential causes of effects under study cannot be easily categorized, such as in a Pareto chart or cause-and-effect diagram. Data points are plotted along the vertical and horizontal axes of the graph, and a correlation between the two variables can either be weak or strong, based on the pattern of the data points.	Example of a scatter diagram for a nurse manager's quality toolbox. (see Fig. 18.7).

Data Collection Sheet

Organization/Unit: _____   Date: _____

Process: _____

MEASURE	DATE	TIME	WHERE	WHEN

Fig. 18.2 Sample data collection sheet for a nurse manager's quality toolbox.

averages. The CALNOC Registry is the first database registry of inpatient and ambulatory nurse-sensitive quality indicators, now managed by Press Ganey, a company that partners with more than 26,000 organizations to better the patient experience. The NQF, in collaboration with the Robert Wood Johnson Foundation, has developed nurse-sensitive performance measures under its Core Measures for Nursing Care Performance Project (NQF, 2012a). Some of these measures have since been endorsed by the NQF. They include falls and falls with injury, hospital-acquired pressure ulcers, health care–associated infections, nursing care hours per patient day, nursing care hours, nursing turnover, physical restraints, RN engagement survey, and skill mix (Press Ganey, 2020). These "nurse-sensitive" indicators refer to the structure, process, and outcomes of professional

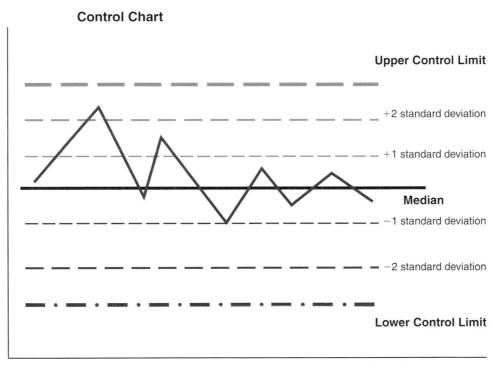

Control Chart

Upper Control Limit

+2 standard deviation

+1 standard deviation

Median

−1 standard deviation

−2 standard deviation

Lower Control Limit

Fig. 18.3 Sample control chart for a nurse manager's quality toolbox.

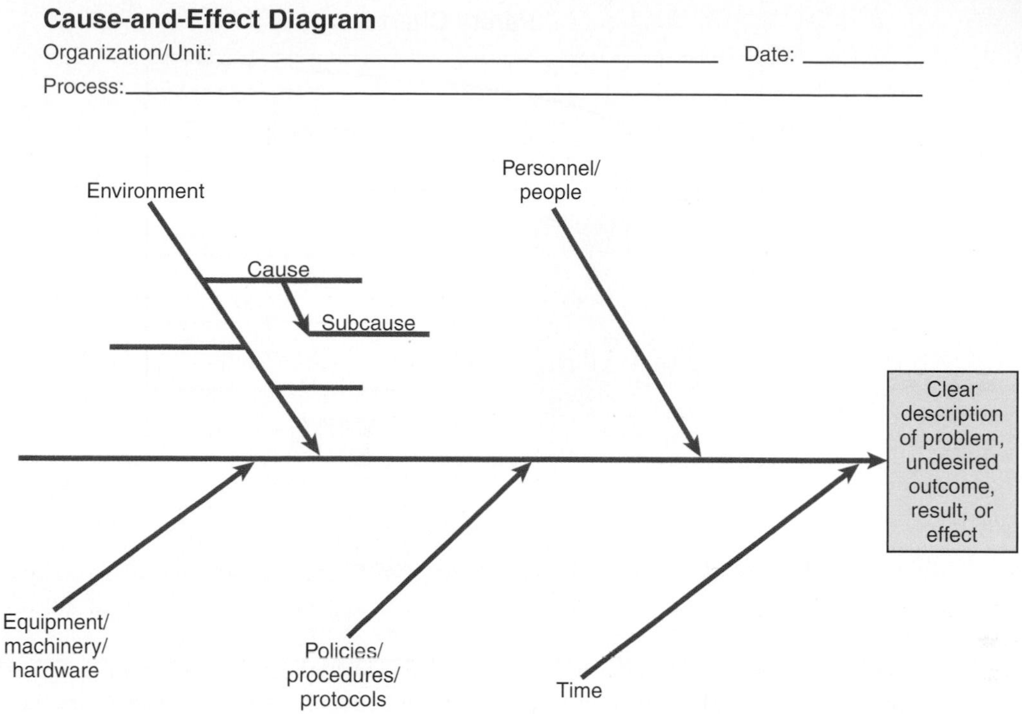

Cause-and-Effect Diagram

Organization/Unit: _____ Date: _____

Process:_____

Fig. 18.4 Sample cause-and-effect diagram for a nurse manager's quality toolbox.

nursing care. Because nursing care influences these outcomes (positively or negatively), they are called nurse sensitive.

The most frequently cited factor in medical errors is poor or inadequate communication. TeamSTEPPS 2.0, an evidence-based teamwork system, was designed for health care professionals by the US Department of Defense and the Agency for Healthcare Research and Quality (AHRQ) to improve communication and teamwork skills among health care professionals

Detailed Flowchart

Organization/Unit: _____ Date: _____ Process owner: _____

Process:_____

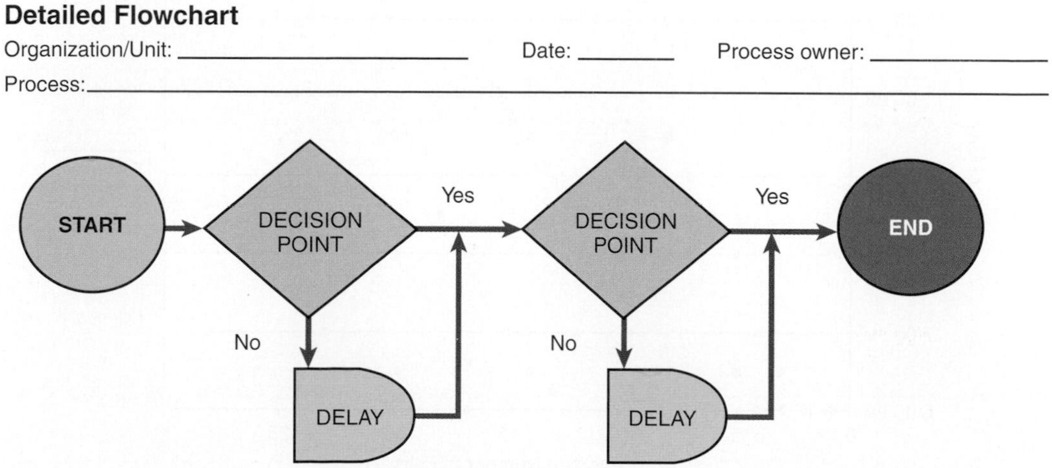

Fig. 18.5 Sample detailed flowchart for a nurse manager's quality toolbox.

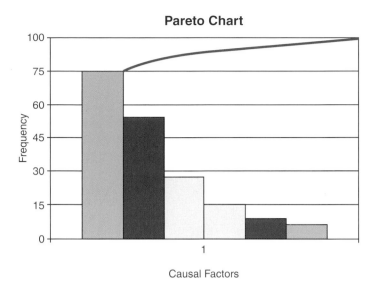

Fig. 18.6 Example of a Pareto chart for a nurse manager's quality toolbox.

(AHRQ, n.d.b.). The program provides a comprehensive suite of ready-to-use materials and a training curriculum to successfully integrate teamwork principles in all areas of a health care system. In addition, the Internet can provide professional nurses with administrative and clinical tools to support a quality and performance improvement program regardless of the delivery setting. A health care quality glossary can also assist professional nurse managers in navigating the health care quality field. A glossary of frequently used terms in this chapter is discussed in the Definitions section.

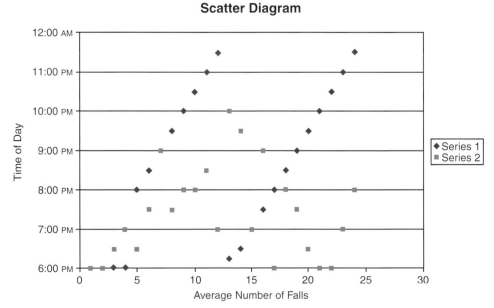

Fig. 18.7 Example of a scatter diagram for a nurse manager's quality toolbox.

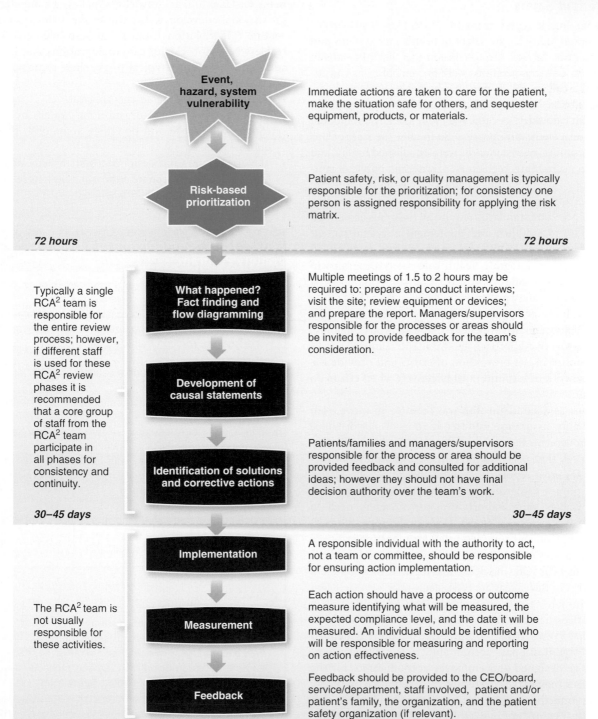

Fig. 18.8 NPSF Root Cause Analysis and Action (RCA²) Process. Reprinted from www.IHI.org with permission of the Institute for Healthcare Improvement, ©2019.

Patient Safety

A landmark report from the IOM launched a major national focus on the safety of health care systems and processes. In fact, the conclusion that 98,000 deaths in health care organizations were preventable was considered a call to action not only by health care providers but also by business and government. Not surprisingly, health care safety became the focus as a key component of the accreditation process. Soon after the start of this millennium, new standards were established by TJC and other accrediting, regulatory, private, and public organizations to address the issue of safety within health care organizations.

Since 2001 standards require all hospitals accredited by TJC to establish and implement a formal patient safety program. Additional standards have been added over time to integrate health care safety programs in organization-wide processes. The components of a health care safety program are listed in Box 18.5. Those individuals and organizations committed to health care safety initiatives believe that a rigorous, ongoing, and proactive approach to the identification of risks will result in the prevention of errors and provide the framework to respond most effectively when errors do occur.

Just as a paradigm shift was required to move from a quality assurance mindset to one of performance improvement, the new paradigm for health care safety requires that organizations create a nonpunitive culture for error reporting. Systems that single out, blame, and punish caregivers who commit errors are no longer viable. More importantly, nurse leaders need to learn the principles of the nonpunitive approach (i.e., they applaud and commend staff for reporting errors or "near misses"). In fact, in some industrial models, those managers or staff who detect and report errors or system failures in their areas are rewarded.

Human resources management regarding safety practices has generated the concept of a *fair and just culture* (Wise, 2014). A fair and just culture is defined as "organizational accountability for the systems they've designed and employee accountability for the choices they make" (Paradiso & Sweeney, 2019, p. 40). Everyone throughout the organization is aware that medical errors are inevitable, but all errors and unintended events are reported—even when the events may not cause patient injury. This culture can make the system safer as it recognizes that competent professionals make mistakes and acknowledges that even competent professionals develop unhealthy norms (shortcuts or routine rule violations), but it has zero tolerance for reckless behavior. Health care organizations that have adopted a just culture typically have these characteristics (Wise, 2014):

- Mission and value statements are clear.
- Employees protect the organization's values by the choices they make and how they accomplish their duties.
- The organization has designed a system that catches errors before they become critical and designs recoveries to stop or reduce bad outcomes.

BOX 18.5 Components of a Health Care Safety Program

- Leadership commitment as evidenced through the allocation of resources for health care safety
- Assignment of individual(s) to manage the program
- Interdisciplinary (cross-organizational) participation, coordination, and communication about safety activities
- Education and involvement of patients and families in health care safety issues
- Disclosure of unanticipated outcomes of care to patients and families
- Education of staff on safety-related topics and training in team communication techniques
- Data collection and analysis in safety-related areas, including the following:
  - Incident/variance reporting
  - Medication errors, near misses
  - Infection surveillance and prevention; outbreak management
  - Facility/environmental surveillance
  - Staff willingness to report errors
  - Staff perceptions of and suggestions for improving safety
  - Patient and family perceptions and/or suggestions for improvement regarding safety
- Definition of terms related to safety, including sentinel events, "near misses," and what is reportable, and the development of policies and procedures to address each category of patient safety event
- Management of sentinel events
- Adherence to The Joint Commission National Patient Safety Goals
- Establishment of a risk reduction process to include Healthcare Failure Modes Effects Analysis (HFMEA)

• The organization continuously refines its core processes from employee feedback and is always learning; employees feel safe in reporting errors or potential errors.

Health care organizations that embrace a fair and just culture identify and correct the systems or processes of care that contributed to the medical error or near miss. Nurse leaders believe that more health care professionals will report more errors and near misses when they are protected by a nonpunitive culture of medical error reporting, and this will further improve patient safety through opportunities for improvement and lessons learned (Paradiso & Sweeney, 2019). The American Nurses Association has endorsed just culture as a means of ensuring safe care (ANA, 2010).

The Veterans Affairs (VA) National Center for Patient Safety (NCPS) is an example of a large organization that has created health care safety programs. The NCPS is committed to the reduction of error and improvement of quality through proactive approaches to risk reduction (US Department of Veterans Affairs, 2018a). This is accomplished through focusing on prevention, creating nonpunitive environments, and conducting safety research through such concepts as human factors analysis, and studying HROs in other industries such as aviation and nuclear energy.

In 1998 the VA created a VA Quality Scholars Program to train leaders and scholars in health care improvement for the VA who are prepared to lead change nationally and internationally. The program consists of 11 sites across the United States and has affiliate sites in Toronto and Canada. Each site in the US consists of a partnership between a VA hospital and an academic institution. It has an interprofessional emphasis with physicians, nurses educated nurses to doctoral level, clinical psychologists, and pharmacists as fellows and faculty (US Department of Veterans Affairs, 2018b). The VA has created numerous educational programs through the NCPS and freely shares them with all health care providers who want to learn about health care safety tools and techniques. They have taken the lead in adopting the methodology and tools of Healthcare Failure Modes and Effects Analysis (HFMEA).

The National Quality Forum is a consortium of public–private organizations that work collaboratively to address health care quality and safety. In 2003 the NQF published a list of 30 consensus standards to address safe practices that, if implemented, would yield improvements in the safety of health care. Examples of this initial list included establishment of a culture for safety, adoption of protocols to prevent wrong-side surgery, and implementation of effective admission assessments to identify and treat underlying conditions early in the care process. The NQF Safety Practices were updated in 2006, and a total of 34 practices were included in 2009 Safe Practices. New Safe Practices in the 2009 set were added in areas such as pediatric imaging, glycemic control, organ donation, catheter-associated urinary tract infection, and multidrug-resistant organisms. A number of previously endorsed practices were updated based on new evidence, including the pharmacist's role in medication management, pressure ulcers, and an entire chapter on health care associated infections (NQF, 2012b). Current safety topics that the NQF has endorsed and recommend include implementation of effective handoff communication, initiation of rapid response teams, and management of methicillin-resistant *Staphylococcus* aureus (MRSA) infection.

Nurses and nurse leaders can personally create an environment that is devoted to health care safety by doing the following:

• Learning the concepts and tools related to risk identification, analysis, and error reduction;
• Adopting and embracing the concept of nonpunitive error reporting;
• Advocating for the establishment of a nonpunitive culture if it is not currently a strong ideal within the organization;
• Encouraging staff to be constantly vigilant in identifying potential risks in the care environment;
• Creating a sense of partnership with patients and families to promote communication about safety concerns and soliciting their suggestions to correct and prevent potential risks;
• Being a role model and coach for staff and peers in practicing health care safety concepts.

National Patient Safety Goals

Since the late 1990s, TJC has collected data on sentinel events and the outcomes of their root cause analyses (RCAs) for the purpose of sharing those data with health care organizations to prevent similar sentinel events from occurring. The results of the aggregation of these data are published by TJC in a series of newsletters titled *Sentinel Event Alerts*. These *Sentinel Event Alerts* address events such as preventing unintended retained foreign objects, preventing infection from the misuse of vials, safe use of health information technology, preventing falls and fall-related injuries in health care facilities, and detecting and treating suicide ideation in all settings (TJC, 2020c). The original intent of these alerts was for health care organizations to review the "lessons learned" from facilities that had experienced these sentinel events. With the emphasis on health care patient safety (including the adoption of their own set of patient safety standards), the impact of the IOM reports, and the industry-wide emphasis on error prevention as a backdrop, TJC formalized the information contained in their sentinel event database into a new accreditation requirement called the *National Patient Safety Goals* (TJC, 2020d).

In 2002 TJC's Board of Commissioners approved an initial list of six National Patient Safety Goals (NPSGs) that represented the most commonly occurring and/or serious events from its sentinel event database, combined with the recommendations of an interdisciplinary task force. Each goal has evidence-based or expert-based recommendations to define how to implement the goal successfully. The Joint Commission board reevaluates the goals annually. New goals are added to the list if necessary, and/or existing goals may be replaced with new goals that reflect processes in which there are safety concerns (e.g., hand hygiene, goals for medication reconciliation and handoff communications, and a goal for anticoagulation therapy). Each organization must demonstrate compliance with all applicable NPSG recommendations during the time of their accreditation survey (there are specific goals for ambulatory health, behavioral health, critical access hospitals, home care, hospitals, laboratories, nursing care centers, and office-based surgery centers). These goals have become the underpinning of the survey process. Those organizations that effectively implement the NPSGs find that they are more apt to have a successful survey outcome in this era of unannounced surveys.

Nurse leaders can serve as role models by fully committing to the NPSGs on their units/departments and communicating their belief that implementation of these standards leads to safer patient care. They are key to successful design and implementation of processes to address NPSGs.

Accreditation and Regulatory Influences on Quality and Safety

Quality and safety are crucial aspects of health care delivery. Yet how do consumers know if an organization is safe and of high quality? Health care organizations have always been required to meet standards for federal and state reimbursement regulations (Medicare and Medicaid) and state licensure rules and regulations in order to operate. These regulations have traditionally defined requirements for quality. However, the private accreditation process has probably had the most significant impact on the development of quality improvement systems in health care. It has been through organizations such as The Joint Commission (TJC), Accreditation Association for Ambulatory Health Care (AAAHC), Community Health Accreditation Partner (CHAP), The American Osteopathic Association's Healthcare Facilities Accreditation Program (HFAP), CARF International, URAC, and the National Committee for Quality Assurance (NCQA) that performance standards have been promulgated and universally adopted. In each of these accreditation processes, the concept of system-wide quality improvement provides the framework for the standards. Although accreditation is not mandatory, eligibility to participate in and receive reimbursement from managed care organizations or federal and state program funding sources such as Medicare is often tied to the achievement of accreditation by one or more of the voluntary accreditation organizations.

Of all of these voluntary accreditation programs, TJC has had the greatest degree of impact on the health care industry. Founded in 1951, it led the way in establishing a set of performance standards for hospitals to follow to become accredited. Over the years its accreditation standards and programs have evolved to reflect the many types of providers that now constitute the health care system, thus expanding its role beyond hospital accreditation. Currently TJC sponsors accreditation programs for organizations that provide services in the areas of ambulatory care, assisted living, behavioral health, critical access hospitals, health care networks, hospitals, home care, laboratory, long-term care, and office-based surgery.

TJC has continually adjusted its performance standards for quality throughout its evolution. During the 1980s and the early 1990s, TJC promoted a "10-Step Process for Quality Assurance" that provided the framework for quality in hospitals. In 1994 TJC identified the need to enhance overall quality of care via an improvement in its own accreditation processes, and it completely revised the accreditation standards for all programs. Instead of chapters organized by department, the new approach revised and reorganized the requirements into cross-functional processes of care and services (e.g., Patients' Rights, Patient Assessment, Patient Family Education) to more appropriately reflect the manner in which care is delivered. A new chapter titled "Improving Organizational Performance" was introduced that created specific standards focused on quality that were based on the principle of continuous improvement rather than on preestablished thresholds for performance of individual health care quality indicators. This change reflected the influence of the industrial quality movement on health care in the early 1990s.

With this major restructuring of TJC standards, the new era of thinking in terms of *process improvement* rather than quality assurance began not only for TJC-accredited organizations, but also for other accrediting bodies. The description for this organization-wide programmatic approach, or *performance improvement* (PI), established the expectation that quality initiatives in the organization were no longer the responsibility of a single quality assurance nurse or department but instead the responsibility of the enterprise's leaders. Standards in the newly developed "Leadership" chapter established the expectation that the outcomes of performance improvement measures be elevated to review by the administrative and clinical leaders of the organization. This review of performance measurement at senior levels of the organization supplies the information that leaders require to provide oversight to the quality of care being delivered to all patients and families (customers).

The Joint Commission's PI standards delineate specific requirements for data collection in high-risk areas such as medication management, restraints, and blood transfusions. Beyond these mandatory quality indicators, the leaders of each organization are expected to set their own priorities for measurement that reflect the types of services provided to the various populations served by the organization. The PI and Leadership standards also expect that the outcomes of data analysis and the actions taken to address improvement opportunities should be communicated to staff. It is in this arena that a nurse leader can make the PI process come alive for

nursing staff. Staff can relate to and understand data outcomes that are based on measurement of the everyday processes in which they work. The nurse leader needs to involve staff in identifying relevant and significant data collection measures for their unit/department that will have a direct impact on changing and continuously improving care processes. A sample data collection sheet is displayed in Fig. 18.2.

Nurse leaders need to stay abreast of changes in the standards of their organization's primary accrediting and state and federal regulatory agencies to ensure that quality outcome measures for their units/departments remain current and viable. In addition to keeping up with these requirements, as previously described, many hospitals are pursuing or have plans to pursue Magnet designation of their hospital's nursing practice as awarded by the American Nurses Credentialing Center through its Magnet Recognition Program® (ANCC, n.d.). To be positioned to score well on an application for the Magnet Recognition Program, nurse leaders need to take an active role in the management (monitoring and improving) of robust and effective quality measures (nurse-sensitive patient outcomes, patient and staff satisfaction and engagement, etc.). A step further might be to participate in local, regional, and national committees that set performance standards. This can be done through professional associations such as the American Nurses Association, the National Association for Healthcare Quality and the American Society for Professionals in Patient Safety. Certification programs are available through these professional associations.

Policies and procedures and guidelines of care at the unit/department level must be updated and/or revised as new standards are introduced, either through participation in voluntary accreditation programs or because of regulatory requirements. Staff need to be educated about the impact and meaning of the standards that are applicable to the care they provide. Documentation requirements may change, and this may affect the outcome of clinical data measures and/or reimbursement. Nurse managers need to provide leadership in adopting and adapting to ongoing changes in these arenas. Many organizations do not have the luxury of devoting one individual or department solely to managing accreditation or regulatory compliance processes. At best, in those organizations that have dedicated individuals or departments for this purpose, they serve as facilitators and coaches for the accreditation and licensing processes. TJC conducts accreditation surveys on an unannounced basis. This requires that leaders and managers throughout the organization be in a continual state of readiness (i.e., to have their departments and staff in compliance with all applicable standards at all times). Thus the onus of responsibility and accountability for continuous readiness has moved from a single regulatory or quality department to all leaders and managers in the organization.

Data Collection and Public Reporting of Quality Outcomes

TJC requires accredited organizations to participate in its core measure initiative. This program requires accredited health care organizations to select outcome measures that reflect the operations of their organizations and to choose a performance measurement vendor to aggregate and analyze the data and submit them on a quarterly basis to TJC. Similarly, the National Committee for Quality Assurance's (NCQA) Healthcare Effectiveness Data and Information Set (HEDIS) outcomes have been an integral part of the NCQA accreditation process for health plans. Of note, CARF International has required both program evaluation and quality outcomes measurement as components of its accreditation process since the 1980s, about a decade before the other accreditors.

An initial drawback to TJC's initial performance measurement process—and that of the quality reporting required by other accreditors—was an inability to compare performance outcomes across and among health care organizations. This was due primarily to the variability allowed in selection of measures and reporting systems. To remedy this critical flaw, TJC devised its Core Measures program. The initial measures in 2001 were acute myocardial infarction (AMI), community-acquired pneumonia (PN), and heart failure (HF) and comprised 10 process measures, often referred to as the "starter set." The current Core Measure sets include: cardiac care, emergency department, health care staffing services, hospital outpatient department, hospital-based inpatient psychiatric services, immunization, palliative care, perinatal care, stroke, substance use, tobacco treatment, total hip and knee replacement, and venous thromboembolism (TJC, 2020a); see Box 18.6 for sample Core Measures from the Hospital Compare database (CMS, n.d.). Consumers are able to access these data and compare hospital performance.

CMS has historically mandated data submission programs for health care organizations to qualify for participation in their Medicare programs. *The Specification Manual for National Hospital Inpatient Quality Measures* is a guide that combines both the CMS measures and the TJC Core Measure sets "to minimize data collection efforts for these common measures and focus efforts on the use of data to improve the health care delivery process" (TJC, 2020a, p. 3). For long-term care hospitals (LTCH), CMS requires the submission

---

BOX 18.6   Selected Measures Reported on the Hospital Compare Website

Survey of Patients' Experiences
- *Hospital Outpatient Department Consumer Assessment of Healthcare Providers and Systems (CAHPS)*
- Patients who reported that staff definitely gave care in a professional way
- Patients who reported that staff definitely communicated about what to expect during and after the procedure
- Patients who reported YES they would definitely recommend the facility to family or friends

Timely and Effective Care
Sepsis Care
- Percentage of patients who received appropriate care for severe sepsis and septic shock
- *Heart Attack Care*

- Average (median) number of minutes before outpatients with chest pain or possible heart attack who needed specialized care were transferred to another hospital

Complications & Deaths
Infections
- Catheter-associated urinary tract infections (CAUTI) in ICUs and select wards
- Surgical site infections (SSI) from colon surgery

Payment and Value of Care
- *Value of care for heart attack patients*
- Death rate for heart attack patients
- Payment for heart attack patients

From Centers for Medicare & Medicaid Services. (CMS, n.d.). *Hospital Compare: Compare hospitals.* https://www.medicare.gov/hospitalcompare/search.html.

of data through its LTCH Quality Reporting Program. For home health care, CMS requires submission of data to the Home Health Quality Reporting Program, which includes data from the Outcome and Assessment Information Set (OASIS; patient outcome measures) and the Home Health Consumer Assessment for Healthcare Providers and Systems (HHCAHPS; patient survey results) (CMS, 2019a). In both these initiatives, the results for individual health care organizations also were not originally made public. In fall 2001 the US Secretary of Health and Human Services announced the George W. Bush administration's commitment to quality health care through the publication of consumer information. Various Centers for Medicare & Medicaid Services quality programs allow consumers to make informed choices about their health care providers and encourage providers to improve their care.

In 2011 CMS developed the Hospital Value-Based Purchasing Program. Under the program, CMS makes value-based incentive payments to 2700 acute care hospitals based either on how well the hospitals perform on certain quality measures or how much the hospitals' performance improves on certain quality measures from their performance during a baseline period. Reimbursement is based on quality of care, not quantity. The higher a hospital's performance or improvement during the performance period for a fiscal year, the higher the hospital's value-based incentive payment for the fiscal year (FY) would be (CMS, 2019b). The measurement domains for FY2020 are clinical outcomes, safety, person and community engagement, and efficiency and cost reduction. It is estimated that $1.9 billion is available for value-based incentive payments in FY2019 (CMS, 2019c, p. 3).

Initially health care providers were resistant and concerned about issues such as data integrity and the lack of risk adjustments that would ensure that the results were comparable. They were convinced that without safeguards built into state reporting systems, their organizations might look bad to the public. Data analysis systems have evolved and improved over the years to address these concerns. A majority of states have now enacted legislation requiring public reporting. With federal reporting requirements increasingly linked to reimbursement, providers must participate in data submission for public reporting or risk losing accreditation, income, and community status. As an example, organizations must be diligent in

documentation of initial patient assessments, because care for patients with poor outcomes (e.g., skin breakdown) that are not recorded as being present on admission (POA), are no longer reimbursed. Terms like "never events" represent a category of adverse outcomes that, in the view of insurers, should never happen and for which they are no longer willing to pay.

Nurses need to be cognizant of the variety of measures being collected for state, federal, and accreditation purposes that apply to their units and patients. Nurse leaders and their staff often have to participate in the data collection effort and discuss outcomes at unit practice council and/or quality improvement committees. Nurse managers, leaders, and executives are held accountable to implement corrective action plans focused on their unit/department to address issues of noncompliance with quality indicators such as Core Measures (e.g., not documenting education about smoking cessation or offering tobacco replacement therapy for patients with AMI). In the future, patients and families may inquire about the organization's publicly reported outcomes (for example, from Hospital Compare or the Leapfrog Group), so it is imperative that all nurses are engaged in quality initiatives and that managers are conversant with this topic.

Health Care Enterprise Risk Management

The Joint Commission has traditionally required a risk management program for the entire organization as a part of its quality improvement efforts. Risk management is an integral component of an organization's quality and safety programs and a risk manager is one of the "first responders" in a serious or sentinel event situation. A new concept and process called *Enterprise Risk Management* (ERM) addresses the evaluation of all risks confronting an organization in order to maximize safety and risk reduction. The idea is to prevent undesirable events from happening and to minimize the impact of unpreventable risks. The concept of enterprise risk management dovetails with the overall requirements of a comprehensive organization-wide approach to patient safety. ERM "promotes a comprehensive framework for making risk management decisions which maximize value protection and creation by managing risk and uncertainty and their connection to total value" (Carroll, 2014, p. 5). *An ERM program* includes components of culture, strategy, objectives, appetite/tolerance,

ERM structure and plans, communication and reporting plans, and oversight.

- **Culture:** A culture supporting ERM, including programs such as High Reliability Organizations (HROs), Crew Resource Management (CRM), Team-STEPPS, Just Culture, and Mindfulness.
- **Strategy:** Management's game plan for strengthening enterprise performance, with an organizational strategy that is linked to vision, mission, goals, and objectives.
- **Objectives:** Ensuring that ERM objectives are SMART—specific, measureable, achievable, realistic, and timely.
- **Appetite/tolerance:** Determining the desired level of risk the organization will take vis-à-vis its mission and threshold or qualitative range of risks taken in pursuit of the organization's strategy (tolerance).
- **ERM structure and plans:** Organization-wide communication and education plans that describe key roles and committee structures, employee engagement strategies, techniques to update employees on the progress of ERM initiatives, key performance and key risk indicators, and scenarios that highlight the value of ERM to the organization.
- **Oversight:** Acknowledging that the governing body is responsible for ERM oversight, leadership ensures that the governing body is regularly apprised of progress on risk strategies, status of key performance indicators (KPIs) and key risk indicators (KRIs), emerging risks, and recommendations for new projects (Carroll, 2014, pp. 6–8).

Patient Safety Event Reporting

Tools for ongoing risk identification and reporting, incident or variance reports, form the core of organizational reporting from a risk management perspective. An important tool is an incident/variance report. This report provides factual accounting of a patient safety incident or adverse event to ensure that all facts surrounding the incident are recorded. Key attributes of an effective incident reporting system include the following: (1) institution must foster a supportive environment for event reporting that protects the privacy of staff who report occurrences, (2) reports should be received from a broad range of personnel, (3) summaries of reported events must be disseminated in a timely fashion, and (4) a structured mechanism must be in place for reviewing reports and developing action plans (AHRQ, 2019b, p. 3). A successful incident reporting process is one in which the majority of all appropriate incidents/adverse outcomes are reported by various health care professionals.

Fear of disciplinary action continues to be a reason for not reporting, and organizations put an emphasis on data collection versus participative learning (Macrae, 2016, p. 74). Aguilar stated that "healthcare still has a prevalent culture of silence. Frontline workers worried about litigation or job loss cover up mistakes and leaders fail to address medical errors even in a pre-emptive fashion…" (Aguilar, 2019, p. 34). Frequent reporting is more apt to be achieved in those organizations that have adopted a learning, nonpunitive, fair and just culture for reporting errors. Further, "a culture of empowerment enables an organization's frontline staff—the people with the most timely exposure to potential medical errors—to signal the presence of an error or defect and work together with their teams to resolve it" (Virginia Mason Institute, 2016, p. 1).

The data contained in an incident/variance report also alert the nurse leaders and risk managers about facts and circumstances that may contribute to a potential malpractice or lawsuit claim. Similar to quality improvement activities, the analysis of incident reports is the responsibility of the nurse leaders in many organizations. The incident/variance reporting system provides the nurse manager with the opportunity to investigate all serious situations immediately. Data from incident reports are collated, analyzed, and used by unit nurse managers and risk managers to identify risk areas that have ongoing trends or to point to areas that have emerging risk potential. These data can inform the choices that the organization's leaders make in the selection of processes to target for HFMEA projects or to "drill down" further via an RCA to study an adverse outcome or "near miss" more fully. Aggregated data from the organization's health care ERM program are reported through the performance improvement and safety reporting systems to coordinate information about overall organizational risks. New performance measures defined in the action plan resulting from an RCA or HFMEA can be incorporated in a unit's/department's set of quality measures. Nurse managers can set the expectation for reporting of all risk events and "near misses" or "close calls" on their units/departments. Through diligent follow-up and the adoption of a nonpunitive culture, managers can set the tone for a truly proactive and responsive ERM program.

In addition to internal reporting, many states (most via their health care licensure agencies, such as a department of health) have implemented mandatory adverse event reporting requirements, resulting in a new role for many health care risk managers. In organizations in these states, the risk manager is often accountable for the reporting of incidents that are on the mandated list. Most of these mandatory reporting programs also require the submission of formal RCAs as a follow-up to the initial report, including actions taken and assessment of the effectiveness of those actions. If the regulatory agency determines that the organization has not appropriately responded to the identified risks, it may result in further requirements for reporting and follow-up. This expanded role of the health care risk manager in external reporting creates a need for collaboration with the quality professionals in the organization. Working together as a team, the risk manager and quality manager will often share responsibilities for facilitation of RCA and HFMEA teams to meet all of the internal and external accreditation and regulatory reporting requirements.

Sentinel Events

Organizational response to sentinel events is one element included in TJC standards in both the Leadership and Performance Improvement chapters. A *sentinel event* is defined by TJC as "a patient safety event that reaches a patient and results in any of the following: death, permanent harm, or severe temporary harm and intervention required. Such events are called 'sentinel' because they signal the need for immediate investigation and response" (TJC, 2019d, pp. 5–7).

Since 1999 TJC has required health care organizations to respond to sentinel events in a systematic and formal way such as conducting a RCA. The purpose of the RCA is to "drill down" to the most common cause(s), using flowcharting and cause-and-effect diagramming, for the event and determine what process improvements can be made to prevent the sentinel event from occurring in the future.

The detailed requirements for reporting and submitting RCAs are contained in the Sentinel Event policy and can be found on the TJC website (https://www.jointcommission.org/resources/patient-safety-topics/sentinel-event/sentinel-event-policy-and-procedures/). Specific sentinel event outcomes are considered "reviewable" by TJC. Reviewable sentinel events are events that have resulted in an unanticipated death, permanent harm, or severe temporary harm. Examples of events that are considered sentinel:

- Suicide of any patient receiving care, treatment, and services in a staffed-around-the-clock care setting or within 72 hours of discharge, including from the hospital's emergency department (ED)
- Unanticipated death of a full-term infant
- Discharge of an infant to the wrong family
- Abduction of any patient receiving care, treatment, and services
- An elopement (unauthorized departure) of a patient from a staffed-around-the-clock care setting (including the ED), leading to death, permanent harm, or severe temporary harm to the patient
- Administration of blood or blood products having unintended ABO or non-ABO incompatibilities, hemolytic transfusion reactions, or transfusions resulting in severe temporary harm, permanent harm or death
- Rape, assault, or homicide of any patient receiving care, treatment, and services while on site at the hospital
- Rape, assault, or homicide of a staff member, licensed independent practitioner, visitor, or vendor while on site at the hospital
- Surgery or other invasive procedure performed on the wrong site, on the wrong patient, or that is the wrong (unintended) procedure for a patient
- Unintended retention of a foreign object in a patient after an invasive procedure, including surgery
- Severe neonatal hyperbilirubinemia (bilirubin >30 mg/dl)
- Prolonged fluoroscopy with cumulative dose >1500 rads to a single field or any delivery of radiotherapy to the wrong body region or >25% above the planned radiotherapy dose
- Fire, flame, or unanticipated smoke, heat, or flashes occurring during direct patient care caused by equipment operated and used by the hospital
- Any intrapartum (related to the birth process) maternal death
- Severe maternal morbidity (not primarily related to the natural course of the patient's illness or underlying condition) when it reaches a patient and results in any of the following: permanent harm or

severe temporary harm (TJC, 2019d, Hospital, pp. SE1–SE3).

Time frames for concluding this analysis and guidelines for conducting a *thorough* and *credible* process are outlined in the current accreditation standards.

The action plan that results from the RCA must be robust and must be strong enough to sustain the prevention of such events from occurring in the future. The VA NCPS has developed an action hierarchy that outlines strong, intermediate, and weak actions (Box 18.7; US Department of Veterans Affairs, 2015, p. 28).

The National Patient Safety Foundation has also developed a definitive guide on conducting RCAs (NPSF, 2016), which has been endorsed by TJC and other public and private patient safety organizations. The document provides teams with effective techniques to conduct comprehensive systematic reviews (RCAs) and develop sustainable actions to prevent their future occurrence (see Fig. 18.8 for the *NPSF Root Cause Analysis and Action [RCA²] Process*).

Organizations that have initiated comprehensive and robust safety programs are committed to the process of ongoing risk identification and prevention. These organizations encourage the staff to identify potential errors and report any "near misses" or "close calls" that occur. Even if an adverse event is not considered reviewable, such organizations conduct RCAs on these identified risks to prevent similar errors from occurring in the future.

The Joint Commission accreditation standards also require that organizations go a step beyond the RCA process in their health care risk reduction and management programs. A set of standards in the Patient Safety Systems chapter of the accreditation manual (TJC, 2016) encourages leaders to maintain a safety system by promoting learning and motivating staff to uphold a fair and just safety culture, providing a transparent environment in which quality measures and patient harms are freely shared with staff, modeling professional behavior, removing intimidating behavior that might prevent safe behaviors, and providing the resources and training necessary to take on improvement initiatives (TJC, 2020b).

One of the methods for proactive risk assessment that accredited hospitals are expected to implement is the process of HFMEA. The expectation is that an HFMEA will be performed on at least one identified high-risk process annually. The HFMEA is conducted by an interdisciplinary team of professionals who own the process being studied and is facilitated by someone with knowledge and skills in quality improvement tools. The HFMEA begins with flowcharting the steps of the process being studied. The team assesses risk points within the process steps, and these key risk points are ranked in terms of their impact on the potential failure of the system. Scores for severity and probability are calculated to give a "hazard" score to the identified breakdown, and detectability of the failure mode is factored into the analysis of its impact on the overall process. The team then "designs out" the most critical of the potential failures and recommends process improvements for prevention of the failures. Once these prevention strategies are identified, action plans for implementing them are reported to the

---

BOX 18.7   VA National Center for Patient Safety Action Hierarchy

Stronger Actions
- Architectural/physical plant changes
- New devices with usability testing before purchasing
- Engineering control, interlock, forcing functions
- Simplify the process and remove unnecessary steps
- Standardize on equipment or process or care maps
- Tangible involvement and action by leadership in support of patient safety

Intermediate Actions
- Redundancy/back-up systems
- Increase in staffing/decrease in workload

- Software enhancements/modifications
- Eliminate/reduce distractions
- Checklist/cognitive aid
- Eliminate look- and sound-alikes
- Enhanced documentation/communication

Weaker Actions
- Double checks
- Warnings and labels
- New procedure/memorandum/policy

From US Department of Veterans Affairs, VA National Center for Patient Safety, 2015b. http://www.patientsafety.va.gov/docs/joe/rca_tools_2_15.pdf.

enterprise leaders and endorsed for implementation (US Department of Veterans Affairs, 2019).

Educating Nurses about Quality and Safety

Academia has confronted the challenge of educating nurses about quality and safety by developing formal curricula. Quality and Safety Education for Nurses (QSEN), originally funded by the Robert Wood Johnson Foundation, and now managed by the Frances Payne Bolton School of Nursing at Case Western Reserve University, is a comprehensive resource for faculty to help new health care professionals learn the knowledge and skills necessary to lead and support quality and safety initiatives in health care organizations (QSEN Institute, 2020). QSEN has identified six core knowledge, skills, and attitude competencies related to quality and safety:

> "1) Patient-centered care: Recognize the patient or designee as the source of control and full partner in providing compassionate and coordinated care based on respect for patient's preferences, values and needs; 2) Teamwork and collaboration: function effectively within nursing and interprofessional teams, fostering open communication, mutual respect, and shared decision-making to achieve quality patient care; 3) Evidence-based practice (EBP): Integrate best current evidence with clinical expertise and patient/family preferences and values for delivery of optimal health care; 4) Quality improvement (QI): Use data to monitor the outcomes of care processes and use improvement methods to design and test changes to continuously improve the quality and safety of health care systems; 5) Safety: Minimizes risk of harm to patients and providers through both system effectiveness and individual performance; and 6) Informatics: Use information and technology to communicate, manage knowledge, mitigate error, and support decision making" (QSEN Institute, 2020, pp. 5–11).

Regional education sessions have provided the opportunity for the content to spread throughout nursing academia.

Acknowledging the critical role that nurses play in improving the quality and safety of patient care, the AHRQ published *Patient Safety and Quality: An Evidence-Based Handbook for Nurses*, a comprehensive compendium of health care quality resources. Readers are provided with proven techniques and interventions they can use to enhance patient care outcomes (Hughes, 2008).

The Institute for Healthcare Improvement provides an "Open School" for health professionals to learn about quality and safety. The IHI Open School for Health Professions is an interprofessional educational community that gives students the skills to become change agents in health care improvement (IHI, 2020c).

Advancing Quality and Safety Policy

The Nursing Alliance for Quality Care (NAQC) was established in 2010 at the George Washington University School of Nursing and managed by the American Nurses Association since 2013. "It has become the 'go-to' organization in the field for advancing high quality, patient-centered healthcare" (ANA/NAQC, n.d., p. 1). NAQC members include nursing professional associations and consumer groups such as ANA, American Association of Colleges of Nursing, National Council of State Boards of Nursing, American Academy of Nursing, and Mothers Against Medical Error. The group proposes to set policy related to nursing's pivotal role in health care transformation.

CONCLUSION

Clearly, nurses have been accountable for health care quality and safety since the profession's inception. Over the years, nurses have assumed roles in various health care settings for oversight of quality and safety improvement, as well as health care ERM. The IOM reports, the CMS requirements for public data reporting, and recent health care reform legislation initiatives have raised public awareness about quality and safety outcomes in health care organizations. These quality and safety issues have challenged health care quality professionals and nurse leaders for decades. A heightened public awareness, combined with increasingly stringent standards for reporting quality and safety outcomes, are driving the need for health care organizations to address these issues. Professional nurses in direct care and leaders in managerial and executive roles need to continue to be at the forefront, leading the charge in adoption of quality and safety initiatives that continuously enhance the quality of care and services provided to patients/clients, families, and populations/communities.

RESEARCH NOTE

Source
Stichler, J.F., & Pelletier, L.R. (2019). Psychometric testing of a patient empowerment, engagement, and activation survey. *Journal of Nursing Care Quality, 35*(4), E49–E57.

Purpose
Patient or person-centered care has become a widely used philosophical framework and yet has varying definitions and characteristics. Person-centered care has recently been conceptualized as patient empowerment, engagement, and activation with studies citing positive outcomes. This study reports the psychometric properties of the Patient Empowerment, Engagement, and Activation Survey.

Discussion
An instrument development and testing approach was used. A 21-item survey was developed demonstrating respectable Cronbach α coefficients for the total scale ($\alpha = 0.88$) and for each subscale: Empowerment ($\alpha = 0.71$), Engagement ($\alpha = 0.81$), and Activation ($\alpha = 0.76$). A regression analysis with 1 item, "I am ready to be discharged" as the dependent variable and all other items as independent variables explained 65% of the variance in readiness for discharge ($P < .001$). Limitations of the study included: small sample size, not testing the survey in combination with other valid and reliable instruments. This study validates the predictive strength of empowerment and engagement on activation similar to other studies.

Application to Practice
Professional nurses need to be aware of the patient's level of empowerment, engagement, and activation and how these influence outcomes of care. It is also important to be aware of any barriers that may impede the patient's level of empowerment, engagement, and activation (limited health literacy, severe medical illness, altered psychological states, language, and cultural), and determine ways to alleviate these barriers. The Patient Empowerment, Engagement, and Activation Survey (PEEAS) can be used to evaluate patients' perspectives of care quality (empowerment and engagement) and readiness for discharge (activation). Used within 24 hours of discharge, the survey can be used to measure the patient's readiness to leave the hospital and assume responsibility for their own care. Future research could combine this new survey with other similar instruments to gauge convergent and divergent validity of the instrument. Additionally, if this type of scale was programmed within the electronic health record, it could trigger various learning strategies in the individualized plan of care based on the patient's level of empowerment, engagement, and activation.

CASE STUDY

Nurse Manager Jaxson has been asked by his Chief Nursing Officer to spearhead a group to evaluate self-injurious behavior (SIB) on a child and adolescent psychiatric unit. Prevention of injury is aligned with the organization's patient safety goals. Based on incident/variance reports, he determines that there is indeed an improvement opportunity, and he selects nurses and a mental health associate (MHA) for the project team. He asks a pharmacist and physician to join the project team to represent the interprofessional aspects of the issue. Jaxson recruits a family member of one of the patients on the child and adolescent unit to provide their perspective. Jaxson then applies the Define, Measure, Analyze, Improve, and Control (DMAIC) improvement model to conduct a quality and safety improvement project.

- **Define phase:** Jaxson and the project team research the scientific and nursing literature to determine the prevalence of SIB. They also determine that patient safety is a national imperative and review The Joint Commission statements related to self-injurious behavior. They propose an aim of "zero harm" from self-injurious injuries, which has been described in the patient safety literature.
- **Measure phase:** Jaxson and the project team request incident/variance data from the Clinical Effectiveness Department for the past year. They request that the data be stratified by time of day, age of patient, location of incident, type of injury, and whether or not the injury required medical intervention.
- **Analyze phase:** The project team analyzes the data they received from the Clinical Effectiveness

CASE STUDY—cont'd

Department. They use flowcharting to visually illustrate a typical SIB episode. Next the team brainstorms a list of all of the problems that are associated with these incidents. From this list, Jaxson directs the team to categorize these factors in five or six groups using an affinity diagram. Once the categories are defined, the team uses a cause-and-effect (fishbone) diagram to identify all of the potential causes that lead to the eventual effect of a self-injurious injury. From this fishbone diagram, specific factors are considered as potential root causes (e.g., lack of safety check on admission, incomplete admission assessment, poor observation in some areas of the unit, lack of consistent evening programming, staffing and staffing mix, lack of consistent staffing during visiting hours, patient's lack of safety awareness, and poor impulse control). The project team used a Pareto chart to visually illustrate the most frequently occurring problems in descending order. By using this technique, they find that lack of safety check on admission, inadequate admission assessment, poor observation in some areas of the unit, and lack of consistent evening programming are the most common factors in SIB incidents. They also use Pareto charts to further define the stratification categories. When using this tool, they find that female teenagers with a presenting problem of suicidal ideation on admission are the most likely to self-injure. Most of the occurrences are on the evening shift.

- **Improve phase:** Jaxson and the project team design a checklist for nursing assessments, highlighting the admission safety check and admission assessment and reassessments. They collect data for 2 months; they meet to analyze the data to find that compliance with admission assessment processes have improved. They meet with Plant Operations to discuss "blind spots" on the unit; those areas that

are hard to observe because of physical barriers. They discuss a plan for unit renovations; renovations are completed in 6 months. The project team discuss barriers to meeting expectations for evening programming. They identify a lack of knowledge in leading groups. Jaxson meets with the Unit Psychologist, who will provide education on leading and managing groups; the plan is to complete education in 2 months. After education has been completed, the project team develop an evening programming audit to determine which groups were completed weekly; data are collected for a month. Barriers to offering evening programming are also identified. Jaxson hires a 0.5 FTE MHA to ensure evening programming occurs as scheduled. The audit results show that evening programming has improved 90% over the last 6 months.

- **Control phase:** The team reconvenes to evaluate the data collected in the Improve phase. Since they found a 75% improvement in assessments, they plan to implement the assessment checklist once per quarter for 6 months to "hold the gains." They also plan to implement the evening programming audit 1 week per quarter for 6 months. The project team plans to look at incident/variance data for the year to determine if their rates have decreased due to their patient safety interventions.

Jaxson shares the data with the hospital's nursing leadership group using control charts to demonstrate the outcomes. They also present their DMAIC project at the hospital's Quality Council. Jaxson applies for an annual Quality Award based on their successful project. He and his Director have also submitted their project as a poster presentation at the next American Psychiatric Nurses Association annual meeting. They also plan on disseminating their work in a peer-reviewed publication in the near future.

CRITICAL THINKING EXERCISE

Nurse Manager Adeline has been in her current position for 6 months. Her hospital is preparing for their first Magnet designation, and her Director would like Adeline to work on improving nursing engagement on her unit. The Director gives Adeline last year's results of the National Database of Nursing Quality Indicators (NDNQI) RN Engagement Survey (see following table). Since Adeline is not familiar with the Magnet standards, she asks her Director for the standard requirements and information about the survey.

Results of RN Engagement Survey							
	Autonomy	Professional Development	Leadership Access & Responsiveness	Interprofessional Relationships	Fundamentals of Quality Nursing Care	Adequacy of Resources & Staffing	RN–RN Teamwork & Collaboration
Adeline's Unit	3.85	3.17	3.63	4.19	4.15	3.85	4.27
National Benchmark	3.44	3.83	3.82	3.30	3.74	3.73	3.50

1. What should Adeline do first to address this issue (what additional information does she need before she can plan a course of action)?
2. What domains of RN engagement should she target (which domains received scores below the national benchmark)?
3. Should she do a literature search on RN engagement?
4. Who should she include on a team to address RN engagement on her unit?

5. Describe the interventions she will employ to enhance RN engagement on her unit based on a literature review, addressing the domains that have scored below the benchmark.
6. Describe the reports she will write about the project and to whom she would send the reports.

REFERENCES

Advisory Board. (2018). *Cracks in the foundation undermine nurse resilience.* https://www.advisory.com/research/nursing-executive-center/resources/posters/nurse-resilience.

Agency for Healthcare Research and Quality (AHRQ). (2017a). *Guide to patient and family engagement in hospital quality and safety.* http://www.ahrq.gov/professionals/systems/hospital/engagingfamilies/index.html.

Agency for Healthcare Research and Quality. (2017b). *Strategy 3: Nurse bedside shift report implementation handbook.* Rockville, MD: AHRQ. http://www.ahrq.gov/professionals/systems/hospital/engagingfamilies/strategy3/index.html.

Agency for Healthcare Research and Quality (AHRQ). (2019a). *High reliability.* https://psnet.ahrq.gov/primer/high-reliability.

Agency for Healthcare Research and Quality (AHRQ). (2019b). *Patient safety primer: Reporting patient safety events.* https://psnet.ahrq.gov/primer/reporting-patient-safety-events.

Agency for Healthcare Research and Quality (AHRQ). (n.d.a.). *AHRQuality indicators.* https://www.qualityindicators.ahrq.gov/.

Agency for Healthcare Research and Quality (AHRQ). (n.d.b.). *TeamSTEPPS: National implementation.* http://teamstepps.ahrq.gov/.

Aguilar, A. (2019). Culture of silence contributes to lack of progress on patient safety. *Modern Healthcare, 49*(44), 34.

American Nurses Association (ANA). (2010). *Position statement: Just culture.* http://nursingworld.org/psjustculture.

American Nurses Association (ANA). (2015). *Code of ethics for nurses with interpretive statements.* Silver Spring, MD: ANA.

American Nurses Association/Nursing Alliance for Quality Care (NAQC). (n.d.). *About NAQC.* https://www.nursingworld.org/practice-policy/naqc/.

American Nurses Credentialing Center (ANCC). (n.d.). ANCC Magnet Recognition Program®. https://www.nursingworld.org/magnet.

American Society for Quality (ASQ). (2019a). *Quality glossary – C.* https://asq.org/quality-resources/quality-glossary/c.

American Society for Quality (ASQ). (2019b). *What is lean?* https://asq.org/quality-resources/lean.

Baldrige Foundation. (2020). *Baldrige – America's best investment.* https://baldrigefoundation.org/who-we-are/history.html.

Barnes, H., Rearden, J., & McHugh, M. D. (2016). Magnet hospital recognition linked to lower central line-associated bloodstream infection rates. *Research in Nursing & Health, 39*(2), 96–104. https://doi.org/10.1002/nur.21709.

Bekelis, K., Missios, S., & MacKenzie, T. A. (2017). Association of Magnet status with hospitalization outcomes for ischemic stroke patients. *Journal of the American Heart Association, 6*(4), Article e3005880. https://doi.org/ 10.1161/JAHA.117.005880.

Benavidez, G., & Frakt, A. B. (2019). Fixing clinical practice guidelines. *Health Affairs Blog.* https://www.healthaffairs.org/do/10.1377/hblog20190730.874541/full/. https://doi.org/10.1377/hblog20190730.874541.

Berwick, D. M., Godfrey, A. B., & Roessner, J. (1990). *Curing health care: New strategies for quality improvement.* San Francisco, CA: Jossey-Bass.

Berwick, D. M., & Hackbarth, A. D. (2012). Eliminating waste in US health care. *Journal of the American Medical Association, 307*(14), 1513–1516. https://doi.org/10.1001/jama.2012.362.

Berwick, D. M., Nolan, T. W., & Whittington, J. (2008). The triple aim: Care, health and cost. *Health Affairs, 27*(3), 759–769. https://doi.org/10.1377/hlthaff.27.3.759.

Brigham, T., Barden, C., Dopp, A. L., Hengerer, A., Kaplan, J., Malone, B., et al. (2018). *A journey to construct an all-encompassing conceptual model of factors affecting clinical well-being and resilience.* Washington, DC: National Academy of Medicine.

Caplan, W., Davis, S., Kraft, S., Berkson, S., Gaines, M. E., Schwab, W., & Pandhi, N. (2014). Engaging patients at the front lines of primary care redesign: Operational lessons for an effective program. *The Joint Commission Journal on Quality and Patient Safety, 40*(12), 533–540. https://doi.org/10.1016/s1553-7250(14)40069-2.

Carroll, R. (2014). *Enterprise risk management: A framework for success.* Chicago, IL: American Society for Health Risk Management.

Centers for Medicare & Medicaid Services (CMS). (2019a). *Home health quality measures.* https://www.cms.gov/Medicare/Quality-Initiatives-Patient-Assessment-Instruments/HomeHealthQualityInits/Home-Health-Quality-Measures.

Centers for Medicare & Medicaid Services (CMS). (2019b). *The hospital value-based purchasing program.* https://www.cms.gov/Medicare/Quality-Initiatives-Patient-Assessment-Instruments/Value-Based-Programs/HVBP/Hospital-Value-Based-Purchasing.

Centers for Medicare & Medicaid Services (CMS). (2019c). *CMS hospital value-based purchasing program for fiscal year 2020.* https://www.cms.gov/newsroom/fact-sheets/cms-hospital-value-based-purchasing-program-results-fiscal-year-2020.

Centers for Medicare & Medicaid Services (CMS). (n.d.). *Hospital Compare: Compare hospitals.* https://www.medicare.gov/hospitalcompare/search.html.

Chassin, M. R. (1997). Assessing strategies for quality improvement. *Health Affairs, 16*(3), 151–161. https://doi.org/10.1377/hlthaff.16.3.151.

Chassin, M. R., & Loeb, J. M. (2013). High-reliability health care: Getting there from here. *The Milbank Quarterly, 91*(3), 459–490. https://doi.org/10.1111/1468-0009.12023.

Corrigan, J. M., Eden, J., & Smith, B. M. (Eds.). (2002). *Leadership by example: Coordinating government roles in improving health care quality.* Washington, DC: National Academies Press.

Deming, W. E. (2000a). *The new economics for industry, government, education.* Cambridge, MA: MIT Center for Advanced Engineering Studies.

Deming, W. E. (2000b). *Out of the crisis.* Cambridge, MA: MIT Center for Advanced Engineering Studies.

Donabedian, A. (1980). *Explorations in quality assessment and monitoring: The definition of quality and approaches to its assessment* (Vol.1). Ann Arbor, MI: Health Administration Press.

Dyrbye, L. N., Shanafelt, T. D., Sinsky, C. A., Cipriano, P. F., Bhatt, J., Ommaya, A., et al. (2017). Burnout among health care professionals: A call to explore and address this unrecognized threat to safe, quality care. Discussion Paper, *NAM Perspectives.* Washington, DC: National Academy of Medicine.

Harmon, F. G. (1997). Future present. In F. Hesselbein, M. Goldsmith, & R. Beckhard (Eds.), *The organization of the future* (pp. 239–247). San Francisco, CA: Jossey-Bass.

Harry, M., & Schroeder, R. (2000). *Six Sigma: The breakthrough strategy revolutionizing the world's top corporations.* New York: Currency/Doubleday.

Hegge, M. (2015). *Faculty pak: Guide to the code of ethics for nurses with interpretive statements: Development, interpretation and application.* American Nurses Association. http://www.nursingworld.org/MainMenuCategories/EthicsStandards/CodeofEthicsforNurses/Faculty-Pak.

Higgins, T., Larson, E., & Schnall, R. (2017). Unravelling the meaning of patient engagement: A concept analysis. *Patient Education and Counseling, 100*(1), 30–36. https://doi.org/10.1016/j.pec.2016.09.002.

His Holiness the Dalai Lama, & Cutler, H. C. (1998). *The art of happiness.* New York: Penguin Random House, Riverhead Books.

Hughes, R. G. (2008). *Patient safety and quality: An evidence-based handbook for nurses.* Rockville, MD: (AHRQ Publication No. 08-0043). http://archive.ahrq.gov/professionals/clinicians-providers/resources/nursing/resources/nurseshdbk/nurseshdbk.pdf.

Insignia Health. (2020). *Patient activation measure.* https://www.insigniahealth.com/products/pam-survey.

Institute for Healthcare Improvement (IHI). (2004). *About IHI.* http://www.ihi.org/about/Pages/default.aspx.

Institute for Healthcare Improvement (IHI). (2005). *Going lean in health care.* Cambridge, MA: IHI.

Institute for Healthcare Improvement (IHI). (2020a). *Plan-Do-Study-Act (PDSA) worksheet.* http://www.ihi.org/resources/pages/tools/plandostudyactworksheet.aspx.

Institute for Healthcare Improvement (IHI). (2020b). *High reliability* (search). http://www.ihi.org/sites/search/pages/results.aspx?k=high+reliability.

Institute for Healthcare Improvement (IHI). (2020c). IHI Open School: *Overview.* http://www.ihi.org/education/ihiopenschool/overview/Pages/default.aspx.

Institute of Medicine. (2000). *Medicare: A strategy for quality assurance* (Vol.2). Washington, DC: National Academies Press.

Institute of Medicine (IOM), Committee on Enhancing Federal Health Care Quality Programs (CEFHQP). (2002). *Enhancing federal health care quality programs.* https://www8.nationalacademies.org/onpinews/newsitem.aspx?RecordID=0309086163.

Institute of Medicine (IOM), *Committee on Quality of Health Care in America (CQHCA).* (2001). *Crossing the quality chasm: A new health system for the 21st century.* Washington, DC: National Academies Press.

Institute of Medicine (IOM), Committee on the National Quality Report on Health Care Delivery. (2001). *Envisioning the national health care quality report.* Washington, DC: National Academies Press.

Institute of Medicine (IOM), Committee on the Robert Wood Johnson Foundation Initiative on the Future of Nursing. (2011). *The future of nursing: Leading change, advancing health.* Washington, DC: National Academies Press.

Interprofessional Education Collaborative. (2016). *Core competencies for interprofessional collaborative practice: 2016 update.* https://hsc.unm.edu/ipe/resources/ipec-2016-core-competencies.pdf.

Joint Commission Center for Transforming Healthcare. (2020). *High reliability in health care is possible.* https://www.centerfortransforminghealthcare.org/en/high-reliability-in-health-care/.

Jones, D., & Womack, J. (2003). *Lean thinking: Banish waste and create wealth in your corporation, revised and updated.* New York: Free Press.

Juran, J. M. (1989). *Juran on leadership for quality: An executive handbook.* New York: Free Press.

Juran Institute. (2009). *Product store.* https://www.juran.com/resources/.

Kelly, L. (2020). Burnout, compassion fatigue, and secondary trauma in nurses: Recognizing the occupational phenomenon and personal consequences of caregiving. *Critical Care Nursing Quarterly, 43*(1), 73–80. https://doi.org/10.1097/CNQ.0000000000000293.

Kohn, L. T., Corrigan, J. M., & Donaldson, M. S. (Eds.). (2000). *To err is human: Building a safer health care system.* Washington, DC: National Academies Press.

Link, A. N., & Scott, J. T. (2011). *Planning report 11-2: Economic evaluation of the Baldrige Performance Excellence Program.* National Institute of Standards and Technology, US Department of Commerce. https://www.nist.gov/system/files/documents/2017/05/09/report11-2.pdf.

Macrae, C. (2016). The problem with incident reporting. *BMJ Quality & Safety, 25,* 71–75. https://doi.org/10.1136/bmjqs-2015-004732.

McCann, C. M., Beddoe, E., McCormick, K., Huggard, P., Kedge, S., Adamson, C., et al. (2013). Resilience in the health professions: A review of the recent literature. *International Journal of Wellbeing, 3*(1), 60–81. https://doi.org/10.5502/ijw.v3i1.4.

Missios, S., & Bekelis, K. (2018). Association of hospitalization for neurosurgical operations in Magnet hospitals with mortality and length of stay. *Neurosurgery, 82*(3), 372–377. https://doi.org/10.1093/neuros/nyx203.

Melnyk, B., Buck, J., & Gallagher-Ford, L. (2015). Transforming quality improvement into evidence-based quality improvement: A key solution to improve healthcare outcomes. *World Views of Evidence Based Practice, 12*(5), 251–252. https://doi.org/10.1111/wvn.12112.

National Academy of Medicine. (2019). *Action collaborative on clinician well-being and resilience.* https://nam.edu/initiatives/clinician-resilience-and-well-being/.

National Institute of Standards and Technology. (2019). *Six health care, nonprofit and education organizations win Baldrige awards for performance excellence.* https://www.nist.gov/news-events/news/2019/11/six-health-care-nonprofit-and-education-organizations-win-baldrige-awards.

National Patient Safety Foundation. (2016). RCA^2 *Improving root cause analyses and actions to prevent harm.* https://www.ashp.org/-/media/assets/policy-guidelines/docs/endorsed-documents/endorsed-documents-improving-root-cause-analyses-actions-prevent-harm.ashx.

National Quality Forum (NQF). (2012a). *Nursing-sensitive care: Initial measures.* http://www.qualityforum.org/Projects/n-r/Nursing-Sensitive_Care_Initial_Measures/Nursing_Sensitive_Care__Initial_Measures.aspx.

National Quality Forum (NQF). (2012b). *Measure evaluation criteria.* http://www.qualityforum.org/Measuring_Performance/Submitting_Standards/Measure_Evaluation_Criteria.aspx.

National University. (2020). *Planetree.* https://www.nu.edu/planetree/.

O'Neil, E. H., & The Pew Health Professions Commission (PHPC). (1998). *Recreating health professional practice for a new century: The fourth report of the Pew Health Professions Commission.* University of California, San Francisco, CA: PHPC.

Palmer, S., & Torgerson, D. J. (1999). Definition of efficiency. *British Medical Journal, 318,* 1136.

Paradiso, L., & Sweeney, N. (2019). Just culture: It's more than policy. *Nursing Management, 50*(6), 38–45. https://doi.org/10.1097/01.NUMA.0000558482.07815.ae.

Park, S. H., Gass, S., & Boyle, D. K. (2016). Comparison of reasons for nurse turnover in Magnet and non-Magnet hospitals. *Journal of Nursing Administration, 46*(5), 284–290. https://doi.org/10.1097/NNA.0000000000000344.

Pelletier, L. R. (1998). Guest editorial: Standardization. *Journal of Nursing Care Quality, 13*(1), vii.

Pelletier, L. R. (2000). On error-free health care: Mission possible! [Editorial]. *Journal for Healthcare Quality, 22*(3), 2, 9.

Pelletier, L. R. (2015). Commentary on "Engagement as an element of safe inpatient psychiatric environments". *Journal of the American Psychiatric Nurses Association, 21*(3), 191–194. https://doi.org/10.1177/1078390315593061.

Pelletier, L. R., & Beaudin, C. L. (2018). *HQ solutions: Resource for the healthcare quality professional (4th ed.).* Philadelphia: Wolters-Kluwer Health.

Pelletier, L. R., & Hoffman, J. A. (2002). A framework for selecting performance measures for opioid treatment programs. *Journal for Healthcare Quality, 24*(3), 24–35. https://doi.org/10.1111/j.1945-1474.2002.tb00430.x.

Pelletier, L. R., & Stichler, J. F. (2014a). Ensuring patient and family engagement: A professional nurse's toolkit. *Journal of Nursing Care Quality, 29*(2), 110–114. https://doi.org/10.1097/NCQ.0000000000000046.

Pelletier, L. R., & Stichler, J. F. (2014b). Patient-centered care and engagement: Nurse leaders' imperative for health reform. *The Journal of Nursing Administration, 44*(9), 473–480. https://doi.org/10.1097/NNA.0000000000000102.

Pelletier, L. R., & Stichler, J. F. (2013). Action brief: Patient engagement and activation: A health reform imperative and improvement opportunity for nursing. *Nursing Outlook, 61*(1), 51–54. https://doi.org/10.1016/j.outlook.2012.11.003.

Planetree. (2018). *Creating a standard of person-centered care.* https://www.planetree.org/how-we-help.

Plsek, P., & Omnias, A. (1989). *Juran Institute quality improvement tools: Problem solving/glossary.* Wilton, CT: Juran Institute.

Polacek, M. J., Allen, D. E., Damin-Moss, R. S., Schwartz, A. J., & Sharp, D., et al. (2015). Engagement as an element of safe inpatient psychiatric environments-. *Journal of the American Psychiatric Nurses Association, 21*(3), 181–190. https://doi.org/10.1177/1078390315593107.

Press Ganey. (2020). *Capture nursing-specific measures.* https://www.pressganey.com/solutions/clinical-excellence/capture-nursing-specific-measures.

QSEN Institute. (2020). *QSEN competencies.* http://qsen.org/competencies/pre-licensure-ksas/.

Robert Wood Johnson Foundation. (2014). *Aligning forces for quality: Patient engagement toolkit.* http://forces4quality.org/node/6319.html.

Rosati, R. (2018). Health data analytics. In L. R. Pelletier, & C. L. Beaudin (Eds.), *HQ Solutions: Resources for the Healthcare Quality Professional.* Philadelphia, PA: Wolters Kluwer.

Sackett, D. L., Rosenberg, W. M. C., Gray, J. A. M., Haynes, R. B., & Richardson, W. S. (1996). Evidence-based medicine: What it is and what it isn't. *British Medical Journal, 312*(7023), 71. https://doi.org/10.1136/bmj.312.7023.71.

Sharp HealthCare. (2020). *Mission, vision and values.* http://www.sharp.com/about/our-story/mission-vision-values.cfm.

Shojania, K. G., Duncan, B. W., McDonald, K. M., & Wachter, R. M. (2001). *Making health care safer: A clinical analysis of patient safety practices.* Evidence Report/Technology Assessment No. 43. https://archive.ahrq.gov/clinic/ptsafety/pdf/ptsafety.pdf.

Shrank, W. H., Rogstad, T. L., & Parekh, N. (2019). Waste in the US health care system: Estimated costs and potential for savings. *New England Journal of Medicine, 322*(15), 1501–1509. https://doi.org/10.1001/jama.2019.13978.

Sikka, R., Morath, J. M., & Leape, L. (2015). The quadruple aim: Care, health, cost and meaning in work. *BMJ Quality and Safety Online.* http://qualitysafety.bmj.com/content/qhc/24/10/608.full.pdf.

Stichler, J. F., & Pelletier, L. R. (2019). Psychometric testing of a patient empowerment, engagement, and activation survey. *Journal of Nursing Care Quality, 35*(4), E49–E57. https://doi.org/10.1097/NCQ.0000000000000452.

Stimpfel, A. W., Sloane, D. M., McHugh, M. D., & Aiken, L. H. (2016). Hospitals known for nursing excellence associated with better hospital experience for patients. *Health Services Research, 51*(3), 1120–1134. https://doi.org/10.1111/1475-6773.12357.

The Joint Commission (TJC). (2016). *Comprehensive accreditation manual for hospitals: Patient safety systems (Update 2).* http://www.jointcommission.org/assets/1/18/PSC_for_Web.pdf.

The Joint Commission (TJC). (2019a). *Specifications Manual for Joint Commission National Quality Measures.* https://manual.jointcommission.org/releases/TJC2019A1/.

The Joint Commission (TJC). (2019b). *Primary Care Medical Home Certification Program.* https://www.jointcommission.org/accreditation-and-certification/certification/certifications-by-setting/hospital-certifications/primary-care-medical-home-certification/#6013d8e234884e60a1326022ca98c9e4_ae0c115936bd43f98842cd6001c8145f.

The Joint Commission (TJC). (2019c). *Quick Safety: Developing resilience to combat nurse burnout. Issue 50.* Oakbrook Terrace, IL: TJC. https://www.

jointcommission.org/resources/news-and-multimedia/news/2019/07/the-joint-commission-issues-quick-safety-advisory-on-combating-nurse-burnout-through-resilience/.

The Joint Commission (TJC). (2019d). *Sentinel event policy and procedures*. https://www.jointcommission.org/resources/patient-safety-topics/sentinel-event/sentinel-event-policy-and-procedures/.

The Joint Commission (TJC). (2020a). *Measures*. https://www.jointcommission.org/en/measurement/measure/, https://www.jointcommission.org/en/measurement/specification-manuals/chart-abstracted-measures/.

The Joint Commission (TJC). (2020b). *Joint Commission urges healthcare leaders to develop cultures of safety*. https://www.fiercehealthcare.com/healthcare/healthcare-leaders-must-develop-a-culture-safety-joint-commission-says.

The Joint Commission (TJC). (2020c). *Sentinel event alert newsletters*. https://www.jointcommission.org/resources/patient-safety-topics/sentinel-event/sentinel-event-alert-newsletters/.

The Joint Commission (TJC). (2020d). *National patient safety goals*. http://www.jointcommission.org/standards_information/npsgs.aspx.

US Department of Veterans Affairs. (2015). *Root cause analysis tools*. http://www.patientsafety.va.gov/docs/joe/rca_tools_2_15.pdf.

US Department of Veterans Affairs. (2018a). *VA National Center for Patient Safety*. http://www.patientsafety.va.gov/index.asp.

US Department of Veterans Affairs. (2018b). *VA Quality Scholars*. https://www.vaqs.org.

US Department of Veterans Affairs. (2019). *Healthcare failure mode and effect analysis (HFMEA)*. http://www.patientsafety.va.gov/professionals/onthejob/hfmea.asp.

Villanova University. (2019). *A look at Six Sigma's increasing role in improving healthcare*. https://www.villanovau.com/resources/six-sigma/six-sigma-improving-healthcare/. Virginia Mason Institute. (2016). *Leader tools to prevent medical errors*. https://www.virginiamasoninstitute.org/2016/03/health-care-leaders-can-stop-medical-errors/.

Visiting Nursing Service of New York (VNSNY). (2020). *Vision and mission*. https://www.vnsny.org/who-we-are/about-us/mission-vision/.

Waddill-Goad, S. M., & Langster, H. J. (2016). *Nurse burnout: Planning intentional quality and safety*. https://www.reflectionsonnursingleadership.org/features/more-features/Vol42-1-nurse-burnout-planning-intentional-quality-and-safety.

Weick, K. E., & Sutcliffe, K. M. (2007). *Managing the unexpected (2nd ed.)*. San Francisco, CA: Jossey-Bass.

Wise, D. (2014). *Getting to know just culture*. https://www.outcome-eng.com/getting-to-know-just-culture/.

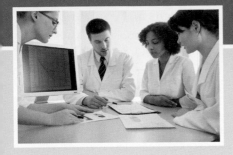

19

Measuring and Managing Outcomes

Christina Dempsey, Mary Jo Assi

http://evolve.elsevier.com/Huber/leadership

Achieving and sustaining quality outcomes is a goal in every health care organization. This effort requires the companion efforts of measuring and managing outcomes as a guide. Measuring important outcomes helps decision makers draw conclusions about new programs, tests, or procedures, and whether to promote the adoption of these new innovations. For example, Wu and colleagues' (2018) literature synthesis indicated that the effectiveness of telehealth interventions in diabetes management was supported by evidence. This bolsters support for advocating for telehealth interventions to policy and decision makers.

Rising costs and demands for accountability in the health care system have led to an increased focus on measuring quality (National Quality Forum [NQF], 2015). Porter (2010) framed outcomes as a key part of value in health care. He defined value as the patient outcomes obtained in a health care setting divided by the costs incurred in providing the services, which places outcomes measurement and management at the heart of health care leadership. In 2001 The Institute of Medicine (IOM) established six aims for care: safe, effective, timely, equitable, patient-centered, and efficient (Agency for Healthcare Research and Quality [AHRQ], 2018). Outcomes research examines variations in the delivery and results of health care services that have particular relevance for clinicians and leaders alike. Health care leaders and researchers understand that quality outcomes related to safety, clinical excellence, and experience of care for both patients and caregivers require a continued effort to quantify the contribution of nurses and nursing interventions in databases that enable benchmarked nursing-related outcomes across units, institutions, systems, regions, and even countries (Jeffs et al., 2015a; Loan et al., 2011; Zrelak et al., 2012). Moreover, Jones (2016) demonstrated that measuring outcomes is part of the social contract nurses have with the community as stewards of health care resources and done to meet the six aims articulated by the IOM. Furthermore, this social obligation to move the profession beyond a task-based, checklist-oriented practice to one that is outcomes-based demonstrates that the value of nursing care depends upon data and evidence (Jones, 2016). This chapter provides an overview of definitions, key concepts in outcomes and outcomes management, defines outcomes research and the challenges it involves, elements of outcome research, leadership and management implications, and current issues and trends.

DEFINITIONS

Key terms related to outcomes and their measurement and management include outcomes, indicators, common data elements (CDEs), measures, nurse-sensitive care, nursing outcomes research, and high reliability.

An **outcome** is the result or results obtained from the efforts to accomplish a goal. In proposing a three-part model of health care quality, Donabedian (1985) described outcomes as changes in the actual or potential health status of individuals, groups, or communities, and contrasted outcomes with processes (what occurs in the delivery of health care) and structures (the organizational context and "raw materials" of health care delivery). Donabedian's classic framework is useful for understanding the relationship between outcomes and the structures and processes that have produced them. This suggests that nurses and nurse managers need to attend to structure and process factors as precursors to patient outcomes (Donabedian, 2005). A patient-focused definition of outcomes considers them "the results people care about most when seeking treatment, including functional improvement and the ability to live normal, productive lives" (International Consortium for Health Outcomes Measurement [ICHOM], 2016; Porter, 2010).

Indicators: Indicators can be used to measure all three of Donabedian's (1985) domains of quality: structure, process, and outcomes. Specifically, structure indicators include the supply, skill level, education, and certification levels of nursing staff; process indicators measure methods of patient assessment and nursing interventions; and outcome indicators reflect both patient clinical and experience outcomes, such as pressure ulcers and falls, and nurse outcomes such as job satisfaction or turnover. Although patient outcomes are the focus of this chapter, other indicators are key to understanding and managing variations in outcomes. AHRQ (2016) has listed a set of three broad desirable attributes of a quality indicator: (1) importance to stakeholders in the health care system, (2) meets rigorous survey science requirements, and (3) feasibility of collection. A variety of accreditation and regulatory bodies and a number of trade and professional associations—as well as health care quality assessment organizations (sometimes alliances of stakeholders)—have developed sets of standardized health care performance indicators for measuring outcomes (see Chapter 18). For example, in 2003 the AHRQ developed a series of measures that help hospitals to identify potential adverse events and provide the opportunity to assess both adverse events and complications through data analysis of the patient record. "Following the seminal 'To Err is Human' report from the Institute of Medicine, the Agency for Healthcare Research and Quality (AHRQ) developed measures that health providers can use to identify potential in-hospital patient safety problems for targeted institution-level quality improvement efforts" (Centers for Medicare & Medicaid Services [CMS], 2019).

Measures: "These Patient Safety Indicators (PSIs) are comprised of 26 measures (including 18 provider-level indicators) that highlight safety-related adverse events occurring in hospitals following operations, procedures, and childbirth. CMS developed the PSIs after a comprehensive literature review, analysis of available

International Classification of Diseases (ICD) codes, review by clinical panels, implementation of risk adjustment, and empirical analyses" (CMS, 2019). Table 19.1 describes examples of provider, populational, and organizational level domain and indicators/measures that specify preventable adverse events and complications that patients may experience in their contacts across the healthcare continuum (CMS, 2019). Although the primary focus and interest of stakeholders is actual outcomes related to care, it is important to note that quality measurement sets in health care have been critiqued for an excessive focus on processes rather than patient outcomes (Porter, 2010).

Nursing-sensitive care measures: Measures to assist in quantifying nursing's contribution to quality and safety; there have been long-standing efforts to develop indicator sets addressing outcomes of care that are believed to be especially nursing specific or nursing sensitive (Doran et al., 2011; Jeffs et al., 2015b; Loan et al., 2011). Among these nursing-sensitive measures are institutionally acquired pressure injuries (formerly pressure ulcers) and falls with injuries. These indicators are called nursing sensitive because there is evidence that they reflect nursing availability, attention, and nurses' clinical judgment. The National Quality Forum (NQF) endorsed (and subsequently re-endorsed) a set of voluntary consensus standards for nursing-sensitive care that quantify the contribution of nursing to patient safety, health care outcomes, and the professional work environment (Frith et al., 2010; Naylor, 2007; NQF, 2004). Expanding measure sets that are potentially linked with nursing may help clinicians and administrators focus on areas of performance possibly tied to the organization of nursing services and processes of care. Outcomes depend largely on the structure that underlies a nursing organization and the scope and standards of its practice. Nursing structure comprises many distinct elements, including staffing ratios, education and certification, availability of resources, nurse engagement, team culture, and skill mix. These elements combine to shape nurses' work environment, which is the foundation for their success. Defects or dysfunction in the nursing work environment can lead to minor local disruptions or major systemic consequences, both of which influence the quality, safety, cost, and patient experience of care.

Common data elements (CDEs): CDEs are defined as variables that are operationalized and measured in identical ways in similar settings and contexts to enable

TABLE 19.1	CMS provider, populational, and organizational level quality domains
Quality Domain	Examples of Structures/Processes/Outcomes in the Domain
Clinical care	"Clinical care measures reflect clinical care processes closely linked to outcomes, based on evidence and practice guidelines from professional clinical societies, or can be measures of person-centered outcomes of disease conditions, including PROMs and measures of functional status."
Safety	"Safety measures reflect the safe delivery of clinical services in all health care settings. These measures address a structure or process that is designed to reduce risk of harm or the occurrence of an untoward outcome in the delivery of health care, such as an adverse event. Safety measures also address complications of procedures, treatments, or similar interventions during health care delivery. Measures of inappropriate use that could harm a patient."
Patient and caregiver experience	"The domain of patient and caregiver experience includes measures that focus on the potential to improve person-centered care and family and caregiver experiences. For example, this domain includes measures of organizational structures or processes that foster the inclusion of persons and family members as active members of the health care team and collaborative partners with clinicians and provider organizations. This domain also includes PROMs that assess patient-reported experiences and outcomes that reflect involvement of persons and families in the care process and demonstrate knowledge, skill, and confidence to self-manage health care."
Care coordination	"Measures assigned to the care coordination domain focus on appropriate and timely sharing of information with patients, caregivers, and families and coordination of services among health professionals. The measures in this domain may also reflect outcomes of successful coordination of care [e.g.] admissions and readmissions to the hospital."
Population health and prevention	"Population health is defined as the health outcomes of a group of individuals, including the distribution of such outcomes within the group. Measures in this domain reflect the use of clinical and preventive services and the achievement of improvements in the health of the population served. Included in this domain are outcome measures that reflect the health of a population or community and process measures that focus on the primary prevention of disease or screening for early detection of disease that is unrelated to a current or prior condition."

PROMs, Patient-reported outcome measures.
Data from Centers for Medicare & Medicaid Services (CMS). (2016). *CMS quality measure development plan: supporting the transition to the merit-based incentive payment system (MIPS) and alternative payment models (APMs).* https://www.cms.gov/Medicare/Quality-Initiatives-Patient-Assessment-Instruments/Value-Based-Programs/MACRA-MIPS-and-APMs/Final-MDP.pdf, pp. 36-40.

comparison of data across datasets or studies in ways that would otherwise be impossible (National Institutes of Health [NIH], 2016; Redeker et al., 2015). CDEs are both a research tool and elements that inform standardized formats for electronic health records to provide comparison data for quality improvement initiatives.

Outcomes management: Outcomes management is a process used to assist managers and others in making rational patient care-oriented decisions based on what is known about the effect of those choices on patient outcomes (Ellwood, 1988). It is defined as "a multidisciplinary process designed to provide quality health care,

decrease fragmentation, enhance outcomes, and constrain costs. The core idea of outcomes management is the use of care process activities to improve outcomes" (Huber & Oermann, 1998, p. 4). In outcomes management, information about client experiences or other endpoints of care is assembled, trends are identified, departures from expectations are examined, and needed modifications are identified. To understand outcomes the process of care across the entire continuum of care needs to be carefully examined, and variations must be analyzed. Outcomes management is a five-step process: (1) data are collected about outcomes, (2) trends are identified from data analysis, (3) variances are investigated, (4) potential service delivery changes are explored and selected, and (5) changes are implemented and their impacts evaluated.

Management of care: Potential changes in care delivery or the management of care are intended to optimize care or reduce undesirable variances in care for a group of patients or a larger population. This is the analytical management of care delivery. Goals of optimization include robust quality improvement within a framework of high reliability and risk reduction (Fig. 19.1). For nurses, variations of interest may mean departures from anticipated clinical trajectories for some or all patients. Variances may be positive or negative, but identifying them is critical.

Outcomes research: a subfield of health services research that "seeks to understand the end results of particular health care practices and interventions" (AHRQ, 2000) or the extent to which services achieve the goals of health care. What makes outcomes research distinct from other bodies of research that examine end points in patients (i.e., much clinically oriented research) is that outcomes researchers seek to tease out the effects of patient-level care and systems-level environments from the background demographic, psychosocial, and clinical characteristics of patients as influences on end points. The goal is to understand which patients or clients fare well and which do not in relation to treatments selected and/or the organizational context of care delivery (Kane, 2006). Examples of variables that might be investigated as a predictor of patient outcomes might be the provider's professional or educational background (e.g., physicians versus advanced practice nurses, registered nurses [RNs] versus licensed practical or vocational nurses [LPNs/LVNs]), or the characteristics of care settings).

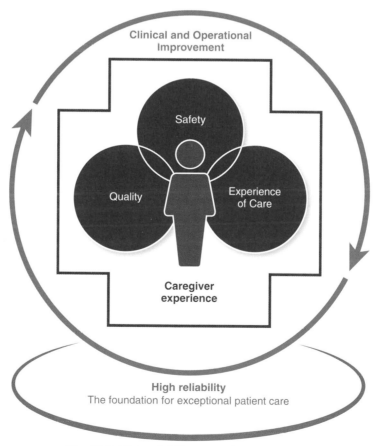

Fig. 19.1 High reliability operating model.

Comparative effectiveness research: A broadening of outcomes research has been the use of comparative effectiveness research (CER) and patient-centered outcomes studies, which include the effects of treatment on health outcomes in different patient populations. The goal is to produce new knowledge and reduce uncertainty about the effects on patient health outcomes of treatments, prevention, or other interventions by investigating on a large scale.

Nursing outcomes research: This is a subspecialty within the larger field of health outcomes research that focuses on determining the effect of different contexts and conditions that are related specifically to nurses and nursing care on the health status of patients. Nursing outcomes researchers are often interested in the structures or management strategies for nursing care delivery and the mix of health care workers best equipped to care for them or the types of patients who benefit most from certain nursing interventions.

Outcomes research: This strategy can help identify interventions that may be the most useful in improving patients' health status, sometimes leading to changes not only in care in the clinic or hospital but also in preparation and coaching of patients for self-management. Ideally clinical care or the management of health services is at least partially guided by research evidence. Although outcomes research has a great deal in common with other forms of research, it involves some special elements. For example, outcomes researchers are especially concerned about understanding "real" (clinically or practically important) differences between expected and observed outcomes and between outcomes on different units, in different institutions, or at different points in time. Outcomes research can provide key data for managerial decision-making to improve quality of care. Data derived from outcomes research can be used to answer the following types of questions:

- What mix of staff types (including education levels among RNs) is most likely to achieve optimal outcomes for a clinical population with a particular level of services?
- Which technologies and blends of technology and staff achieve the best outcomes for high-risk patients?
- What are the optimal organizational structures to maintain efficiency, safety, and patient satisfaction at institutions that provide high volumes of services?

Although the answers to each of these questions depend on individual and institutional contexts and economic considerations, data from outcomes research can be used to inform decision-making. For example, nurse practitioners may be interested in accomplishing outcomes for patients that improve their health yet also reduce costs. Thus they may investigate interventions such as pharmacogenetics testing and profiling to identify the best metabolized pain medication versus those that provide an individual little benefit at a given dose.

BACKGROUND

To measure and manage outcomes, approaches are needed that use appropriate measures and include the experience of care to lead to optimal outcomes for patients and nurses, and in turn, provide a return on investment that aligns with value-based purchasing initiatives driving reimbursement in today's health care environment. Influences on outcomes, measurement of outcomes, and elements of outcomes research will be discussed.

INFLUENCES ON OUTCOMES

It is critical that consumers of outcomes data, including clinical nurses and nurse leaders, understand how to interpret outcomes measures. Nurses and nurse leaders are obviously most interested in the impact of clinical care on patient and population health outcomes. For nurses, the focus is usually on outcomes related to the care delivered by clinical teams and often encompasses the actions of the entire multidisciplinary health team.

MEASUREMENT OF OUTCOMES

Other outcomes indicators incorporate a broader impact of disease and its management on patients' lives. These outcomes, often measured through surveys of patient perceptions and experiences, include quality of life, functional status, health status, and patient experience of care. There are also provider and organizational outcomes. Provider-focused outcomes can include measures of processes and outcomes of care for individual professionals as well as health care work as experienced by workers reflected in such phenomena as nurse burnout, turnover, job satisfaction, work environment, and occupational injuries. Organization-focused outcomes may include patient or provider outcomes that are aggregated to the organizational level, such as rates of hospital-wide inpatient or 30-day mortality, errors, hospital acquired conditions, and other adverse events; or they may examine aspects of the performance of a system that are more of concern to managers than to clinicians or patients. For instance, cost of care indicators are commonly measured at the organizational (hospital-wide) or unit level. A number of health system-level outcomes are also receiving increased attention and include measures of successful movements of patients across settings (i.e., care transitions) (Dusek et al., 2014) and readmission rates (Berkowitz et al., 2013). There is a growing body of evidence linking outcomes to practice environment characteristics such as workplace culture, staffing levels, skill mix, interprofessional collaboration, job satisfaction, burn-out to care quality, productivity, and experience (Aiken et al., 2011; Hinno et al., 2012; McHugh et al., 2011; Nantsupawat 2011; Roche et al., 2012; Trinkoff et al., 2011; Twigg et al., 2013; Van Bogaert et al., 2014; You et al., 2013). Given the breadth of the evidence linking nursing care to patient and organizational outcomes, and the financial stakes associated with value-based incentives and penalties tied to patient outcomes and engagement, the business case for scrutinizing and optimizing nurse work environments is strong (Press Ganey, 2015).

ELEMENTS OF OUTCOMES RESEARCH

Indicators can highlight areas for improvement in structures and processes of nursing care and justify various investments in human and material resources needed to improve outcomes. Nurses can turn to research that has formally examined specific indicators for guidance to understand indicators, how they vary across settings, and the factors that most strongly influence them. Areas to pay particular attention to in outcomes research include the choice of specific measures or variables to address quality and the role of risk adjustment. In addition, the advent of value-based purchasing and values-based reimbursement have added quality and outcomes measures that also drive reimbursement across the continuum of care.

Variable Selection

When interpreting outcomes research, nurses need to be aware that researchers face considerable challenges when selecting outcome measures. For instance, outcomes can either be generic or broadly applicable to many patient groups, or be condition-specific, but they must be clearly defined. An outcome that is not clearly associated with a precise method for gathering and processing of data to measure it is difficult to interpret. Conclusions or decisions based on research results from those data may be flawed. Nurses also need to consider the sources of data used. For example, when evaluating a study examining the association of workload with nurse injuries, it would be important to know whether the injury data were gathered from nurse self-reports, an injury database, manager reports, insurance records, or some other source—and to be aware of the potential limitations or biases of each of these sources.

Risk Adjustment

Risk adjustment analyses of outcomes across groups are meaningful only if relevant individual differences in the patients examined are taken into consideration. Risk adjustment accounts for patient factors, such as the intrinsic risks that a patient brings to the health care encounter in the form of clinical and/or demographic factors, before drawing conclusions about the meaning of different values for indicators. Comparisons of outcomes across settings or time periods are meaningful only when potential differences in the characteristics of patients cared for are taken into account. Risk adjustment can be complicated but is important, because if key patient factors are not considered then differences across units, hospitals, or time periods may or may not be reflective of variations in quality of care. It is important to note that certain types of outcomes are so dramatic and so closely tied to systems failures (e.g., transfusion errors, severe pressure injuries) that risk adjustment is unlikely to alter the interpretation of the relevant indicators. The literature contains some excellent references that discuss the state of the science in risk adjustment techniques (Iezzoni, 2013; Kane, 2006).

LEADERSHIP AND MANAGEMENT IMPLICATIONS

Evidenced-Based Informed Decisions

Health care leaders are accountable for ensuring high quality services that achieve a variety of desired outcomes, including the Institute for Healthcare Improvement's Triple Aim of improving the patient experience of care, improving the health of populations, and reducing the per capita cost of health care. Many organizations have added a fourth aim: attaining joy in work of health care providers (Bodenheimer, 2014; Institute for Healthcare Improvement [IHI], 2016). Outcomes research can provide nurse leaders with evidence to guide decisions around resource allocation and ongoing monitoring of patient safety, quality care outcomes, and a positive work environment for nurses and interprofessional teams (NQF, 2015; Rosen et al., 2018; Westra et al., 2015,). Correctly analyzed and interpreted, local outcomes data help leaders make evidence-based informed decisions around creating healthier work environments and conditions for nurses to provide effective and efficient care, for positive outcomes and experiences for all stakeholders. Managers and executives today have a wealth of information available to them, and they are charged with determining which data indicate a need for action. A significant body of literature from nursing outcomes research continues to grow and is a valuable resource and reference point. For example, a large body of literature suggests that lower staffing levels and skill mix in acute care hospitals are associated with increased risk of negative outcomes. For example, the RN4CAST study involving nine European countries extended earlier findings, and reported that an increase in a nurse's workload by one patient increased the likelihood of an inpatient dying within 30 days of admission by 7% (Aiken et al., 2014). This study also reported that every 10% increase in the proportion of RNs holding bachelor's degrees was associated with a decrease in the likelihood of an inpatient dying within 30 days of admission by 7%. However, the specific context of the care environment and the patient population of interest call for continual monitoring of outcomes against internal and external benchmarks. Several data systems support the monitoring of nursing-sensitive outcomes. For example, the American Nurses Association (ANA) developed a proprietary national database of quality indicators and measures called the National Database for Nursing Quality Indicators (NDNQI). This database, along with the Collaborative Alliance for Nursing Outcomes (CALNOC), both acquired by Press Ganey Associates, LLC in 2013 and 2019 respectively, provide a deep benchmark for unit-specific data on nursing-sensitive indicators. Agencies as diverse as the Centers for Medicare & Medicaid Services (CMS), The Joint Commission, and the Magnet Recognition Program® of the American Nurses Credentialing Center (ANCC) now have outcomes-based reporting requirements that focus on a variety of indicators and outcomes. Many believe that mandated quality reporting has greater potential to improve quality than voluntary reporting (Mukamel et al., 2015). Nurses need to ensure that data-driven patient care improvement strategies are foundational to transformational efforts within organizations (Jeffs et al., 2015b; Murphy et al., 2013; Reichert & Furlong, 2014). Nurse leaders need to guide how nursing data is captured and used. Evidence may be used for (1) improving nursing operations and advancing nursing practice, (2) improving patient, and population health outcomes, and (3) ensuring that data regarding structures, processes, and outcomes of nursing care be integrated into Big Data architecture to facilitate the translation of Big Data into actionable information (Garcia et al., 2015). Nurse leaders also have a critical role in ensuring that nursing perspectives and priorities are represented in collecting, understanding, interpreting, and using performance measures (Murphy et al., 2013), and they are well positioned to develop infrastructure to ensure data are being used to inform decisions about care delivery in health care organizations (Murphy et al., 2013).

High-Reliability Organizations

Press Ganey's research demonstrated the impact of nurse managers on safety, quality, and experience of care. This quantitative and qualitative study found that high performing nurse managers have an unwavering focus on safety and quality, build a culture of respect and interprofessional teamwork, utilize huddles for communication and team building, leverage data for practice, and utilize safe and appropriate staffing (Press Ganey, 2015). High-reliability organizations are those that exhibit these elements of culture. The Agency for Healthcare Research and Quality (AHRQ) defined a highly reliable organization as one that operates in a complex, hazardous environment for extended periods of time without serious accidents or catastrophic failures (AHRQ, 2018). Highly reliable organizations have a proactive approach in which problems are anticipated. There is a preoccupation with failure so that problems are identified early and addressed early enough to prevent catastrophic consequences. These organizations are identified by five characteristics: preoccupation with failure; reluctance to simplify explanations for operations, successes, and failures; situational awareness; deference to frontline expertise; and a commitment to resilience (AHRQ, 2018).

When operating on a foundation of high reliability, health care organizations utilize a skill-based approach to standardizing leader and employee work that enhances communication and ensures consistency in the application of best practices known to improve quality, safety, and the experience of care. Practices that support consistency and standardization include the use of daily management boards, standard leader work, and daily safety huddles. A primary goal of high-reliability organizations, and critical to success, is an enterprise-wide adoption and enculturation of new habits and behaviors that are laser focused on improving quality and safety across all domains of the system.

Big Data Applications

Big Data is a term that is being used to encompass artificial intelligence (AI) and machine learning (the application of AI) as well as predictive analytics. It functions on the principle that collecting and analyzing large amounts of data will allow for relationships that may have been unknown to be identified and studied, thus allowing nurses to make better and more informed decisions (Marr, 2017). With the advent of electronic health records, discrete data points about patient demographics, clinical processes, and outcomes are available. Data from wearables like fitness bands and monitors provide real-time information. Drug and other specialty kinds of databases like that of American College of Cardiology also contribute to the amount of data. In addition, CMS has the Consumer Assessment of Healthcare Providers and Services (CAHPS) programs that offer data relative to the patient's perception of the care they received. Patient reported outcomes measures (PROMS) promises to provide data and insights into the patient's own perceptions of their functional status. With Natural Language Processing (NLP), it is also possible to use patient's comments or sentiment analysis to add to this body of data (Bresnick, 2018). Harnessing all of this data and turning it into insights and improvement is the key. Data without measurement is simply numbers. Measurement without insight is a fool's errand and leads to nothing. Insight without action is stagnation.

Performance Scorecards and Dashboards

Managers and executives often struggle to find a manageable number of data elements and indicators to collect and track to satisfy payers and regulators as well as meet the needs for managing quality related to safety, clinical quality, and the experience of care for both patients and caregivers. Balanced scorecards and dashboards are often used in health care as a part of continuous quality improvement. Balanced scorecards were first introduced in 1992 in the business sector by Kaplan and Norton as a way to review performance more broadly. A balanced scorecard links financial measures with operational measures such as patient experience and outcomes that drive future financial performance. Balanced scorecards help leaders to understand performance by answering four key questions. (1) Financial: What is our financial situation? (2) Internal business: What must we excel at? (3) Innovation and learning: How will we continue to improve and create value? (4) Customer perspective: How do customers see us? (Kaplan & Norton, 1992).

By reviewing measures in this way, leaders are more able to see the interrelationships necessary for success. Dashboards allow clinicians and leaders to view and synthesize multiple sources of data and information simultaneously for improvement efforts. When thoughtfully designed, scorecards and dashboards provide a visual display of critical information so that leaders can quickly grasp performance across multiple domains (Fig. 19.2). Coupled with internal and external best-practice structures and process benchmarks, dashboards provide a robust framework for targeting, implementing, and evaluating improvement activities (Baker, 2015).

CURRENT ISSUES AND TRENDS

Mitigating Cost-Containment Requests

More than ever, decisions involving nursing services need to be justified in terms of their impact on organizational outcomes. Cost-containment strategies sometimes involve targeting human resources expenditures by dropping staff coverage or reducing the proportion of RNs in staff mixes without forethought to the potential consequences for patient outcomes. Outcomes research will be vital for understanding the consequences of deploying various care-delivery models and configurations of staff in different circumstances, especially if circumstances arise where traditional models of care are no longer viable because sufficient numbers of the certain types of nursing staff are no longer available or affordable. Outcomes research can shape the policy environment and can ultimately influence constraints under which managers operate. Since 1999 when California Governor Gray Davis signed Assembly Bill 394 (AB 394)

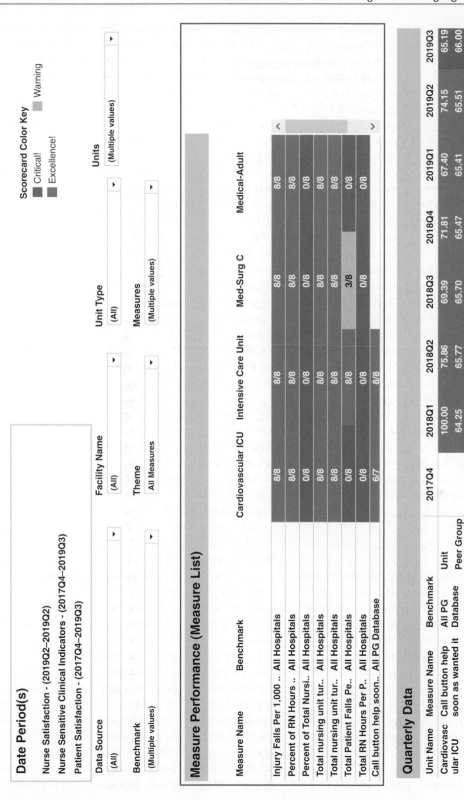

Fig. 19.2 Integrated dashboard.

into law requiring the California Department of Health Care Services to adopt regulations establishing minimum nurse-to-patient ratios, there has been widespread discussion of similar legislation at both the state and federal levels across the United States and elsewhere. The legislative intent behind the California initiative was to improve quality of care, patient safety, and nurse retention. Then and now, proposals to regulate nurse staffing in some way, for example, requiring the reporting of staffing levels, submission of staffing plans, or mandating specific ratios, cite the body of evidence from outcomes research demonstrating links between low nurse staffing and poor outcomes. Evaluation of the impacts of the California experiment continues, and results in terms of net benefits to patients and the state's health care system have been decidedly mixed (Serratt, 2013a, b). Although the continued dialogue does reflect ongoing interest in tracking and perhaps regulating structural elements in health care settings such as staffing, it is important to note that research supports the importance of staffing in the context of the broader work environment. A Press Ganey study (2015) examined the influence of staffing and factors of the work environment on nurse and patient outcomes. And although significant correlations were seen between staffing and nurse and patient outcomes, correlations to the same outcomes were influenced more strongly by factors of the work environment. There is a significant opportunity to evolve and expand research activity to more deeply explore the elements of nursing care, care-delivery models, and factors of the practice and work environment that most strongly impact nurse and patient outcomes.

Population Health

Another trend is heightened interest in measuring and managing outcomes in populations. Population health management is *proactive* care, delivered on an individualized basis. By emphasizing prevention and customization, it optimizes quality while lowering cost and improving value. Population health management is a key feature of the *Affordable Care Act* (ACA). Under this legislation, providers across the health care continuum may form Accountable Care Organizations (ACOs), taking responsibility for a patient population, including the costs and quality of its care. According to Abrams and colleagues, at the Commonwealth Fund (2015), the ACA established the Medicare Shared Savings Program that encouraged the development of ACOs so that if they

met quality benchmarks and kept spending below budget, they would receive half the savings achieved, with the remainder going back to CMS. Policymakers hoped that this kind of bundled payment program would encourage continuity and coordination of care, prompting organizations to focus more on health promotion and disease prevention, which would in turn drive costs down. According to a *Harvard Business Review* profile (Porter & Kaplan, 2016), the bundled payment holds everyone on the health care team accountable for achieving outcomes that matter to patients. This entails the forward-looking management of care. The risk adjustment of bundled payments incentivizes providers to care for even difficult cases. If organizations do not provide care efficiently, or if they provide it inappropriately, the government penalizes them financially. Policymakers hoped that if they held providers accountable for outcomes that encompassed the entire continuum of care, organizations would add new services, interventions, or diagnostic tests that improved outcomes or lowered the cost of care. Porter and Kaplan (2016) suggested that costs could potentially decrease by up to 20% or 30% without compromises in quality.

Management of Nursing Outcomes

As consumers, regulators, and payers increase their focus on outcomes, nurses need to proactively manage outcomes and participate in the ongoing development and implementation of indicators related to nursing care and services. Awareness of advances in outcomes measurement and familiarity with outcomes research findings are essential and will continue to be critical for effective nursing leadership. As health care systems become increasingly outcomes driven, nurse managers and leaders must be involved and spearhead the development of outcomes tracking and management systems appropriate to the setting. The integration of Big Data from electronic health records and other information systems provides opportunities to predict patient outcomes and resource utilization that can be used to guide improvements in patient safety and other outcomes (Westra et al., 2015). Further, Big Data offers a more comprehensive and synthesized understanding of health data across populations that can lead to discovering new knowledge that positively affects nurses and the people they serve with improved health care (Healthcare Information and Management Systems Society [HIMSS], 2015; Westra et al., 2015). Specifically, the profession and its leadership need to contribute to Big Data initiatives by (1) offering definitions and context for data elements, (2) providing expertise in the use of theories to organize variables and interpret analysis results, and (3) creating interventions that assist patients in interpreting and acting on the information afforded through data science investigations (Brennan & Bakken, 2015).

This is crucial to the measurement and management of outcomes. Widespread use of common data elements and measures provides opportunities to compare results across studies and supports the goal of disseminating and translating information into practice (Cohen et al., 2015).

CONCLUSION

Meaningful measurement is key to helping organizations understand what is working well and where opportunities for improvement still exist. For many reasons, outcomes measurement has emphasized health care processes and outcomes that reflect the values and priorities of health professionals, researchers, and administrators. More recently, there has been an important movement by health care thought leaders toward measuring outcomes from the patient's standpoint, especially experiences in receiving health care and quality of life issues (Porter et al., 2016). Researchers and health care leaders are now being pushed to collect meaningful data that can enhance decision-making by health care leaders and policymakers as well as provide patients, families, and the clinicians who work with

them with data that can inform treatment choices. The 2015 CMS Quality Measure Development Plan identified the patient and caregiver experience as one of the five quality domains along with clinical care, safety, care coordination, and population health and prevention to be targeted in quality-oriented reforms to payment structures (CMS, 2015). Integrating these datasets has been a challenge, but tools are evolving that will allow for more sophisticated analytics across different databases that help to demonstrate the impact that safety, quality, experience, and engagement has collectively and in parallel. This integration helps to target improvement efforts in the most effective and efficient manner that can mitigate organizational initiative fatigue—a common pain point for health care leaders and clinicians. Nurse leaders seeking to involve their organizations in indicator benchmarking will have to participate in data-sharing initiatives to align such participation with meaningful quality improvement efforts and other organizational priorities.

Most organizations identify improvement opportunities through data analysis and synthesis. These improvement efforts are often thwarted when they are not sustainable. The evolution of high-reliability science, a well-known framework in the aviation, nuclear, and manufacturing industries, has also moved into the health care arena. In high-reliability organizations scores are not the goal; they are a tool. Meaningful measurement is key to achieving patient, nurse, and organizational outcomes.

RESEARCH NOTE

Source
Press Ganey (2015). *Nursing special report: The influence of nurse work environment on patient, payment and nurse outcomes in acute care settings.* http://healthcare.pressganey.com/2015-Nursing-SR_Influence_Work_Environment

Purpose
As survey science related to the patient and caregiver experience has evolved, so has data analysis methodology. Cross-domain analytics provide organizations with important insights into key drivers and correlations across multiple domains, including patient experience, engagement, safety, and clinical quality. Nursing leaders and clinical

nurses can easily articulate current barriers to creating and sustaining an engaged workforce, as well as challenges that interfere with the ability to provide safe, quality patient-centered care. Today as in the past, nurse staffing continues to be a significant pain point for nurses in many different roles and settings. Responding to overwhelming consensus from the Press Ganey CNO Advisory Council, a study was undertaken in 2015 to better understand critical factors related to staffing, the practice, and the work environment that impact both patient and nurse outcomes.

Discussion
This study combined data from the National Database of Nursing Quality Indicators (NDNQI) and the Press Ganey

Continued

RESEARCH NOTE—cont'd

Patient Experience database to conduct cross-domain analytics to determine the impact of nurse staffing and factors of the work environment on selected outcomes. Key findings demonstrated that overall, although staffing does significantly impact RN perception of quality and job satisfaction, the patient experience global measure (Likelihood to Recommend), clinical outcome measures (i.e., falls, CLABSI, and CAUTI), and key components of the work environment (i.e., nurse intent to remain in current position and perceived status of nursing) are significantly more impactful on nurse and patient outcomes.

Application in Practice

Achieving and sustaining quality outcomes is a goal in every health care organization. Given the vast amount of data that leaders are expected to process and understand at a granular level, improvement efforts can get mired down by initiative fatigue—an ongoing concern of many health care leaders. Thinking about data more holistically, and understanding how factors across the domains of patient experience, clinical quality, engagement and safety influence one another, provides nurse leaders with insights that can focus improvement efforts across all domains.

CASE STUDY

Margaret, the director of quality in an inpatient rehabilitation facility (IRF), recognized a trend upward in the number of patient falls. Data were reviewed to determine opportunities for improvement. She knew that a review of the data was important in order to determine next steps in improvement. After a review of the incident reports she found the following.

Data were stratified by the IRF to evaluate trends by day of week, time the fall occurred, the day of the stay, the fall risk score, diagnosis, whether the policy was enforced, and what the patient was doing prior to the fall. The lowest fall rate by month occurred in December with four falls, while the highest number was in October with 34 falls. These both appeared to be outliers in the data. Average monthly fall volume was 12.5 falls per month or 11.74 with outliers removed. Fall rates by month demonstrated that the fall rate had been less than 8% for three out of six months: January, May, and June. However, the rates for February at 11.64%, March at 11.07%, and April at 16.98% were significantly higher. The breakdown of falls by day of week demonstrate that 40% of patient falls occurred on Tuesdays and Sundays, Wednesdays had the fewest falls at 6%, Mondays accounted for 17% of falls, Thursdays for 10%, and both Friday and Saturday at 13% each. In terms of hour of day, 22% of patient falls occurred between the hours of 3 pm and 6 pm; only 6% occurred between midnight and 3 am; 17% between 6 am and 9 am; 15% for both 9 am to noon and noon to 3 pm; 16% for 6 pm to 9 pm; 2% from 9 pm to midnight. Falls on

day of stay 0–11 accounted for 63% of falls, with 28% of these falling between day 8 and day 11. Of note, this corresponded with the average length of stay of 11 days. Cerebral vascular accident (CVA) diagnosis accounted for 49% of falls but was also the highest volume diagnosis for the facility. The next highest was traumatic brain injury at 17% of falls. Patient falls from a wheelchair occurred in 38% of falls, and 33% fell during transfer or ambulation. Unwitnessed falls accounted for 56% of falls. Fortunately, only two falls with injury were reported from January to June. Despite the policy to perform a post-fall huddle, only 41% of falls had a huddle documented post-incident.

1. What other data should Margaret obtain?
2. Who should be involved in the data review and improvement strategies?

Leaders and clinical staff agreed to completely reframe their approach and thinking by adopting a philosophy of zero harm, which, in turn, required an absolute goal of zero falls. Leaders clearly articulated that the goal of zero harm is a journey and that incremental reductions in falls from the average of 12.5 per month will be expected. The aim was to reduce patient falls in this inpatient rehabilitation hospital from the average of 12.5 per month to at or below the stated goal of 6 per month or less than 8% within 90 days after improvement implementation for the patient population as a first step, and zero falls by the end of the calendar year.

Is this a reasonable aim? Why or why not?

CRITICAL THINKING EXCERCISE

Utilizing the fundamentals of high-reliability organizations, a staff-driven falls team was convened for the inpatient rehabilitation facility noted in the case study. Data were shared demonstrating trends that illustrated the need to reduce falls, and a comprehensive assessment was completed that identified cultural challenges and a lack of consistent processes. The falls team identified and prioritized a bundled approach to nonnegotiable tactics including safety huddles, room signage, patient contracts, transfer training, and purposeful rounding. A skills fair was conducted to include all staff within the facility that focused on each of the bundle components. Further, stark concerns relative to the nursing transfer abilities were identified during the skills fair allowing for changes to orientation and ongoing training. Particular

components of rounding were also identified as opportunities for all staff to understand how to keep patients and staff safe. Falls were reduced during the project with a low of 8.29% in March, closely approximating the goal of 8% and demonstrating a downward trend in falls over the course of the project. The staff-driven nature of this work provided a model that the organization will continue to use for performance improvement going forward.

1. What data measurement and management strategies should be employed to drive sustainability of this work?
2. Describe how the five characteristics of a high-reliability organization were utilized with the proposed change?

REFERENCES

Abrams, M. K., Nuzum, R., Zezza, M. A., Ryan, J., Kiszla, J., & Guterman, S. (2015). *Delivery system reforms: A progress report at five years*. Commonwealth Fund. http://www.commonwealthfund.org/publications/issue-briefs/2015/may/aca-payment-and-delivery-system-reforms-at-5-years.

Agency for Healthcare Research and Quality (AHRQ). (2000). *Outcomes research fact sheet*. http://archive.ahrq.gov/research/findings/factsheets/outcomes/outfact/outcomes-and-research.html.

Agency for Healthcare Research and Quality (AHRQ). (2016). *Desirable attributes of a quality measure*. https://www.qualitymeasures.ahrq.gov/tutorial/attributes.aspx.

Agency for Healthcare Research and Quality (AHRQ). (2018). *Six domains of health care quality*. https://www.ahrq.gov/talkingquality/measures/six-domains.html.

Aiken, L. H., Sloane, D. M., Bruyneel, L., Van den Heede, K., Griffiths, P., Busse, R., et al. (2014). Nurse staffing and education and hospital mortality in nine European countries: A retrospective observational study. *Lancet, 383*(9931), 1824–1830.

Aiken, L. H., Cimiotti, J. P., Sloane, D. M., Smith, H. L., Flynn, L., & Neff, D. F. (2011). Effects of nurse staffing and nurse education on patient deaths in hospitals with different nurse work environments. *Medical Care, (12)*, 1047–1053.

Baker, J. D. (2015). Language of improvement: Metrics, key performance indicators, benchmarks, analytics,

scorecards, and dashboards. *AORN Journal, 102*(3), 223–227.

Berkowitz, R. E., Fang, Z., Helfand, B. K., Jones, R. N., Schreiber, R., & Paasche-Orlow, M. K. (2013). Project ReEngineered Discharge (RED) lowers hospital readmissions of patients discharged from a skilled nursing facility. *Journal of the American Medical Directors Association, 14*(10), 736–740.

Bodenheimer, T., & Sinsky, C. (2014). From triple to quadruple aim: Care of the patient requires care of the provider. *Annals of Family Medicine, 12*(6), 573–576.

Brennan, P. F., & Bakken, S. (2015). Nursing needs big data and big data needs nursing. *Journal of Nursing Scholarship, 47*(5), 477–484.

Bresnick, J. (2018). *EHR users want their time back, and artificial intelligence can help*. Health IT Analytics. https://healthitanalytics.com/features/ehr-users-want-their-time-back-and-artificial-intelligence-can-help.

Centers for Medicare & Medicaid Services (CMS). (2015). *CMS quality measure development plan: Supporting the transition to the merit-based incentive payment system (MIPS) and alternative payment models (APMs)*. https://www.cms.gov/Medicare/Quality-Initiatives-Patient-Assessment-Instruments/Value-Based-Programs/MACRA-MIPS-and-APMs/Draft-CMS-Quality-Measure-Development-Plan-MDP.pdf.

Centers for Medicare & Medicaid Services (CMS). (2019). *CMS Patient Safety Indicators PSI 90 (NQF #0531) National Quality Strategy Domain: Patient Safety.* https://innovation.cms.gov/Files/fact-sheet/bpciadvanced-fs-psi90.pdf.

Cohen, M. Z., Thompson, C. B., Yates, B., Zimmerman, L., & Pullen, C. H. (2015). Implementing common data elements across studies to advance research. *Nursing Outlook, 63*(2), 181–188.

Donabedian, A. (1985). *The methods and findings of quality assessment and monitoring: An illustrated analysis* (Vol 3). Ann Arbor, MI: Health Administration Press.

Donabedian, A. (2005). Evaluating the quality of medical care. (1966. *Milbank Quarterly, 83*(4), 691–729.

Doran, D., Mildon, B., & Clarke, S. (2011). Towards a national report card in nursing: A knowledge synthesis. *Nursing Leadership, 24*(2), 38–57.

Dusek, B., Pearce, N., Harripaul, A., & Lloyd, M. (2014). Care transitions: A systematic review of best practices. *Journal of Nursing Care Quality, 30*(3), 233–239.

Ellwood, P. M. (1988). Shattuck lecture—Outcomes management: A technology of patient experience. *New England Journal of Medicine, 318*(23), 1549–1556.

Frith, K. H., Anderson, F., & Sewell, J. P. (2010). Assessing and selecting data for a nursing services dashboard. *Journal of Nursing Administration, 40*(1), 10–16.

Garcia, A., Caspers, B., Westra, B., Pruinelli, L., & Delaney, C. (2015). Sharable and comparable data for nursing management. *Nursing Administration Quarterly, 39*(4), 297–303.

Healthcare Information and Management Systems Society (HIMSS). (2015). *HIMSS CNO-CNIO vendor roundtable guiding principles for Big Data in nursing: Using Big Data to improve the quality of care and outcomes.* http://www.himss.org/sites/himssorg/files/FileDownloads/HIMSS_Nursing_Big_Data_Group_Principles.pdf.

Hinno, S., Partanen, P., & Vehviläinen-Julkunen, K. (2012). Nursing activities, nurse staffing and adverse patient outcomes as perceived by hospital nurses. *Journal of Clinical Nursing, 21*(11-12), 1584–1593.

Huber, D., & Oermann, M. (1998). The evolution of outcomes management. In D. L. Flarey & S. S. Blancett (Eds.), *Cardiovascular outcomes: Collaborative, path-based approaches* (pp. 3–12). Gaithersburg, MD: Aspen.

Iezzoni, L. I. (Ed.). (2013). *Risk adjustment for measuring health care outcomes* (4th ed.). Chicago, IL: Health Administration Press.

Institute for Healthcare Improvement (IHI). (2016). *Triple Aim for populations.* http://www.ihi.org/Topics/TripleAim/Pages/default.aspx.

International Consortium for Health Outcomes Measurement (ICHOM). (2016). *ICHOM's mission.* http://www.ichom.org/why-we-do-it/.

Jeffs, L., Doran, D., Hayes, L., Mainville, C., VanDeVelde-Coke, S., Lamont, L., & Boal, A. S. (2015a). Implementation of the National Nursing Quality Report initiative in Canada: Insights from pilot participants. *Journal of Nursing Care Quality, 30*(4), E9–E16.

Jeffs, L., Nincic, V., White, P., Hayes, L., & Lo, J. (2015b). Leveraging data to transform nursing care: Insights from nurse leaders. *Journal of Nursing Care Quality, 30*(3), 269–274.

Jones, T. (2016). Outcome measurement in nursing: Imperatives, ideals, history, and challenges. *OJIN: The Online Journal of Issues in Nursing, 21*(2).

Kane, R. L. (2006). Introduction: An outcomes approach. In R. L. Kane (Ed.), *Understanding health care outcomes research* (2nd ed.), (pp. 3–22). Burlington, MA: Jones & Bartlett.

Kaplan, R. S., & Norton, D. P. (1992). The balanced scorecard–measures that drive performance. *Harvard Business Review, 70*(1), 71–79.

Loan, L. A., Patrician, P. A., & McCarthy, M. (2011). Participation in a national nursing outcomes database: Monitoring outcomes over time. *Nursing Administration Quarterly, 35*(1), 72–81.

Marr, B. (2017). *Data strategy: How to profit from a world of big data, analytics and the internet of things.* London: Kogan Page Publishers.

McHugh, M. D., Kutney-Lee, A., Cimiotti, J. P., Sloane, D. M., & Aiken, L. H. (2011). Nurses' widespread job dissatisfaction, burnout, and frustration with health benefits signal problems for patient care. *Health Affairs, 30*(2), 202–210.

Mukamel, D. B., Ye, Z., Glance, L. G., & Li, Y. (2015). Does mandating nursing home participation in quality reporting make a difference? Evidence from Massachusetts. *Medical Care, 53*(8), 713–719.

Murphy, L. S., Wilson, M. L., & Newhouse, R. P. (2013). Data analytics: Making the most of input with strategic output. *Journal of Nursing Administration, 43*(7–8), 367–370.

Nantsupawat, A., Srisuphan, W., Kunaviktikul, W., Wichaikhum, O. A., Aungsuroch, Y., & Aiken, L. H. (2011). Impact of nurse work environment and staffing on hospital nurse and quality of care in Thailand. *Journal of Nursing Scholarship, 43*(4), 426–432.

National Institutes of Health (NIH). (2016). *Common data element (CDE) resource portal.* https://www.nlm.nih.gov/cde/.

National Quality Forum (NQF). (2004). *National voluntary consensus standards for nursing sensitive care: An initial performance measure set—a consensus report.* Author. http://www.qualityforum.org/Publications/2004/10/National_Voluntary_Consensus_Standards_for_Nursing-Sensitive_Care__An_Initial_Performance_Measure_Set.aspx.

National Quality Forum (NQF). (2015). *Data needed for systematically improving healthcare.* http://www.qualityforum.org/Publications/2015/07/Data_for_Systematic_Improvement_Final_White_Paper.aspx.

Naylor, M. D. (2007). Advancing the science in the measurement of health care quality influenced by nurses. *Medical Care Research & Review, 64*(Suppl. 2), S144–S169.

Porter, M. E. (2010). What is value in health care? *New England Journal of Medicine, 363*(26), 2477–2481.

Porter, M. E., Larsson, S., & Lee, T. H. (2016). Standardizing patient outcomes measurement. *New England Journal of Medicine, 374*(6), 504–506.

Porter, M. E., & Kaplan, R. S. (2016). How to Pay for Health Care. *Harvard Business Review, 94*(7-8), 88–134.

Press Ganey. (2015). Nursing special report: The influence of nurse work environment on patient, payment and nurse outcomes in acute care settings. http://healthcare.pressganey.com/2015-Nursing-SR_Influence_Work_Environment.

Redeker, N. S., Anderson, R., Bakken, S., Corwin, E., Docherty, S., Dorsey, S. G., et al. (2015). Advancing symptom science through use of common data elements. *Journal of Nursing Scholarship, 17*(5), 379–388.

Reichert, J., & Furlong, G. (2014). Five key pillars of an analytics center of excellence, which are required to manage populations and transform organizations into the next era of health care. *Nursing Administration Quarterly, 38*(2), 159–165.

Roche, M., Duffield, C., Aisbett, C., Diers, D., & Stasa, H. (2012). Nursing work directions in Australia: Does evidence drive the policy? *Collegian, 19*(4), 231–238.

Rosen, M. A, Diaz-Granados, D., Dietz, A. S., et al. (2018). Teamwork in healthcare: Key discoveries enabling safer, high-quality care. *The American Psychologist, 73*(4), 433–450.

Serratt, T. (2013a). California's nurse-to-patient ratios, Part 2: 8 years later, what do we know about hospital level outcomes? *Journal of Nursing Administration, 43*(10), 549–553.

Serratt, T. (2013b). California's nurse-to-patient ratios, Part 3: Eight years later, what do we know about patient level outcomes? *Journal of Nursing Administration, 43*(11), 581–585.

Trinkoff, A. M., Johantgen, M., Storr, C. L., Gurses, A. P., Liang, Y., & Han, K. (2011). Nurses' work schedule characteristics, nurse staffing, and patient mortality. *Nursing Research, 60*(1), 1–8.

Twigg, D. E, Geelhoed, E. A., Bremner, A. P., & Duffield, C. M. (2013). The economic benefits of increased levels of nursing care in the hospital setting. *Journal of Advanced Nursing, 69*(10), 2253–2261.

Van Bogaert, P., Van Heusden, D., Timmermans, O., & Franck, E. (2014). Nurse work engagement impacts job outcome and nurse-assessed quality of care: model testing with nurse practice environment and nurse work characteristics as predictors. *Frontiers in Psychology,* (5), 1261.

Westra, B., Clancy, T., Sensmeier, J, Warren, J. J., Weaver, C., & Delaney, C. W. (2015). Nursing knowledge: Big data science—implications for nurse leaders. *Nursing Administration Quarterly, 39*(4), 304–310.

Wu, C., Wu, Z., Yang, L., Zhu, W., Zhang, M., Zhu, Q., et al. (2018). Evaluation of the clinical outcomes of telehealth for managing diabetes: A PRISMA-compliant meta-analysis. *Medicine, 97*(43), e12962. doi:10.1097/MD.0000000000012962.

You, L. M., Aiken, L. H., Sloane, D. M, et al. (2013). Hospital nursing, care quality, and patient satisfaction: Cross-sectional surveys of nurses and patients in hospitals in China and Europe. *International Journal of Nursing Studies, 50*(2), 154–161.

Zrelak, P. A., Utter, G. H., Sadeghi, B., Cuny, J., Baron, R., & Romano, P. S. (2012). Using the agency for healthcare research and quality patient safety indicators for targeting nursing quality improvement. *Journal of Nursing Care Quality, 27*(2), 99–108.

20

Workplace Violence and Incivility

Palma D. Iacovitti

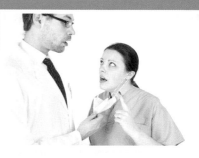

 http://evolve.elsevier.com/Huber/leadership

Nurses expect to be safe at work, especially in health care organizations. Surprisingly, nurses encounter workplace violence and incivility far too commonly. It is important to begin with a general concept of workplace violence and its subsets, workplace bullying and incivility, because they are terms used interchangeably and contain various elements under their definitions. For the purpose of this context, a workplace can be described as a health care organization or setting of any size, location, and type of health care service provided. This also includes care performed outside the health care organization, such as ambulance services or home health care. Any place where such health services are performed will be considered a workplace.

The American Psychological Association (APA, 2020) defined **violence** as an extreme form of aggression, such as assault, rape, or murder. Violence has many causes including, but not limited to, frustration, anger, exposure to violent media, and violence in the home. Certain circumstances can provoke the risk of violent behavior, such as alcohol, drugs, slurs and other irritations, and environmental influences (APA, 2020). This chapter discusses forms of employee violence, health care regulatory bodies to manage violence, leadership roles and responsibilities, de-escalation methods, and current legislation.

DEFINITIONS

The basic terms used in relation to workplace violence and incivility are violence, workplace incivility, workplace violence, and workplace bullying.

Violence is assault, battery, manslaughter, or homicide.

Workplace incivility is violent acts, including physical assaults and threats of assault, directed to persons at work or on duty (Occupational Safety and Health Administration [OSHA], 2015a, p. 1).

Workplace violence is the act or threat of violence, ranging from verbal abuse to physical assaults directed toward persons at work or on duty (National Institute of Occupational Safety and Health [NIOSH], 2019).

Workplace bullying is a situation in which "anyone who uses his perceived strength or power to intimidate another person who he or she think is weaker in order to gain power over that person." (Ciocco, 2018, p. 39).

BACKGROUND

Workplace violence comes in multiple forms. It is defined as the act or threat of violence, ranging from verbal abuse to physical assaults directed toward persons at work or on duty (NIOSH, 2019). There are four types of workplace violence based on the perpetrator's relationship to the workplace. Table 20.1 outlines the types and their description. Health workers all over the world are subject to workplace violence. Between 8% and 38% of health workers are likely to endure physical violence at work. This percentage does not include those who are intimidated or subjected to verbal assault. Most violence is committed by patients and visitors. Groups of health workers who are at high risk, especially in emergency services, include nurses and ancillary staff directly involved in patient care, emergency room staff,

TABLE 20.1	Types of Workplace Violence and Perpetrator Relationship to Workplace	
Type	**Description**	**Example**
I (Criminal intent)	Perpetrator has no legitimate relationship to the business or its employees	A nurse assaulted in the hospital parking garage.
II (Customer/patient) Most common in healthcare environments	Perpetrator is a customer or patient of the workplace or employee	Patient with paranoid schizophrenia kicks nursing personnel.
III (Customer/patient) Commonly referred to as lateral or horizontal violence	Perpetrator is current or former employee	Employee assaults supervisor after receiving performance evaluation.
IV (Personal relationship)	Perpetrator has a relationship to the employee outside of work, no relationship with the organization	Spouse of an employee follows him/her to work, places ultimatums, and makes threats that pose harm.

Source: National Institute of Occupational Safety and Health (NIOSH). 2019. *Occupational violence.* https://www.cdc.gov/niosh/topics/violence/default.html.

and paramedics (World Health Organization, 2020). Workplace violence is a major concern for employers and employees nationwide.

Every year the number of workers who report being a victim of some type of workplace violence increases. In 2017 assaults resulted in 18,400 injuries and 458 fatalities. Seventy-one percent of the assaults occur in health care and social services, amounting to 9% of the US workforce, according to the National Safety Council (NSC, 2019). Further data reveal a median of 5 days of absences for injuries occurring to head, upper extremities, and trunk (NSC, 2019). Fig. 20.1 provides a graph of nonfatal injuries and time away from work trends.

Nurses are at risk for verbal or physical assaults every day. There is a major crisis in our society when nurses are having to confront this type of peril on a regular basis. According to the Bureau of Labor Statistics (BLS, 2019a), the rate of fatal injury overall for hospitals for 2018 was 0.4 per 100,000 full-time equivalent workers. Data are not available by event type. The data further reveal that hospitals in 2018 had a total of 7720 nonfatal reported cases, an incident rate of 19.4 over the year, and employees were off work an average of 6 days (BLS, 2019b).

Risk factors for violence in health care organizations include patient, client, and setting-related risk factors such as (1) working with people who have a history of violence, (2) transporting patients, (3) working alone with patients, (4) unsafe building and parking lot design, (5) lack of means of emergency communication, and (6) availability of items that can be used as weapons. Other risk factors are organizational such as (1) lack of facility policies and training, (2) working when understaffed, (3) high worker turnover, (4) inadequate security personnel, (5) long waits for patients and clients in overcrowded waiting rooms, (6) unrestricted access by the public, and (7) a perception that violence is tolerated (OSHA, 2015b). In addition, an inadequate facility design may contribute to the penetration of violent incidents. Box 20.1 provides a checklist to develop new facilities or mitigate issues with facility designs (OSHA, 2015b).

Regulatory Bodies
Occupational Safety and Health Administration

The Occupational Safety and Health Act of 1970 created the Occupational Safety and Health Administration (OSHA) in the US Department of Labor. This legislation declared that employers have a general duty to provide safe and healthy working conditions. OSHA followed up on the general duty requirement in 1989 with voluntary generic safety and health program management guidelines for all employers to use as a foundation for their safety and health programs. However, the guidelines were not regulations. Nevertheless, under the OSHA Act, employers face fines if an incident of workplace violence occurs. OSHA made it clear that safety and

Assault, nonfatal injuries and illnesses involving days away from work

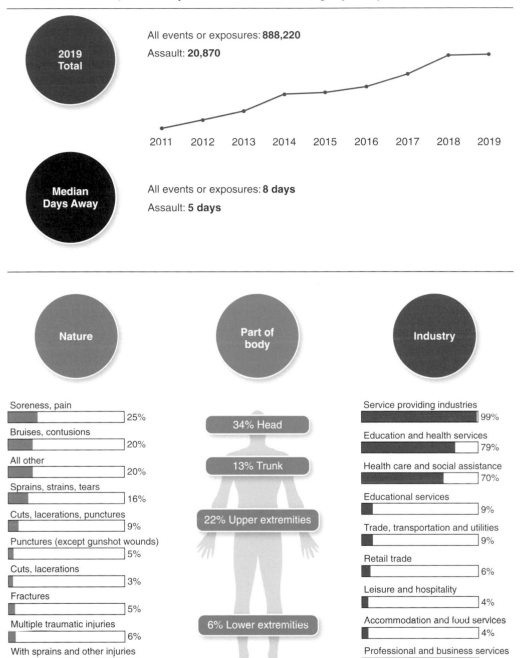

Fig. 20.1 Assault, nonfatal injuries, and illnesses involving days away from work. Permission to reprint/use granted by the National Safety Council © 2020. https://injuryfacts.nsc.org/work/safety-topics/assault/.

BOX 20.1 Facility Design Checklist

- Are there enough exits and adequate routes of escape?
- Can exit doors be opened only from the inside to prevent unauthorized entry?
- Is the lighting adequate to see clearly in indoor areas?
- Are there employee-only work areas that are separate from public areas?
- Is access to work areas only through a reception area?
- Are reception and work areas designed to prevent unauthorized entry?
- Could someone hear a worker call for help?
- Can workers observe patients or clients in waiting areas?
- Do areas used for patient or client interviews allow co-workers to observe any problems?
- Are waiting and work areas free of objects that could be used as weapons?
- Are chairs and furniture secured to prevent their use as weapons?
- Is furniture in waiting and work areas arranged to prevent workers from becoming trapped?
- Are patient or client areas designed to maximize comfort and minimize stress?
- Is a secure place available for workers to store their personal belongings?
- Are private, locked restrooms available for staff?

Modified from Occupational Safety and Health Administration (OSHA) US Department of Labor. (2015b). *Guidelines for preventing workplace violence for healthcare and social service workers.* OSHA publication 3148-04R 2015. https://www.osha.gov/Publications/osha3148.pdf.

health programs could be construed to include workplace violence prevention programs. In 1998 OSHA built on the 1989 generic workplace safety and health guidelines by announcing guidelines designed to identify common risk factors. They also included policy recommendations and practical corrective methods to help prevent and mitigate the effects of workplace violence in the health care industry (OSHA, 2015b). According to OSHA (2015a) an effective workplace violence prevention program includes:

1. **Management commitment and employee participation.** Commitment of all C-suite executives, leaders, and management for a violence prevention initiative including employee feedback in the development process.
2. **Worksite analysis:** Perform needs assessment to gauge an organization's susceptibility to violence.
3. **Hazard prevention and control:** Implement appropriate controls to eliminate or reduce hazards identified through Evaluation of Physical Environment.
4. **Safety and health training:** Strongly recommended for all employees. Content should include but not limited to: definition of workplace violence, prevention policies, risk and warning signs, and de-escalation. NIOSH (2019) offers a video that discusses sensible actions for identifying risk factors for violence at work and tactical actions that can maintain safety.
5. **Record-keeping and program evaluation:** Records maintenance is essential, including data of work-related injuries and illnesses, workers' compensation records, education records, safety committee minutes, and the identification and correction of recognized hazards.

National Institute for Occupation Safety and Health

The Occupational Safety and Health Act of 1970 also created the National Institute for Occupation Safety and Health (NIOSH), located within the Centers for Disease Control & Prevention (CDC) in the Department of Health and Human Services. Through this act, NIOSH was charged with drafting and recommending occupational safety and health standards (NIOSH, 2015).

NIOSH recognized that workplace violence is an issue in the health care industry and recommended the following violence prevention strategies for employers: environmental designs, administrative controls, and behavior modifications. Environmental designs include signaling systems, alarm systems, monitoring systems, security devices, security escorts, lighting, and architectural and furniture modifications to improve worker safety. Administrative controls include (1) adequate staffing patterns to prevent personnel from working alone and to reduce waiting times, (2) controlled access, and (3) development of systems to alert security personnel when violence is threatened. Behavior modifications provide all workers with training in recognizing and managing assaults, resolving conflicts, and maintaining hazard awareness (OSHA, 2015c). NIOSH (2013) has produced a free course on workplace violence prevention that earns three continuing education unit credits for nurses (http://www.cdc.gov/niosh/topics/violence/training_nurses.html). The American Nurses Association also offers education and several resources related to workplace violence (https://www.

nursingworld.org/practice-policy/work-environment/violence-incivility-bullying).

The Joint Commission

The Joint Commission (TJC, 2020a) is an independent, not-for-profit organization that accredits and certifies nearly 21,000 health care organizations and programs in the United States. The mission of TJC is "to continuously improve health care for the public, in collaboration with other stakeholders, by evaluating health care organizations and inspiring them to excel in providing safe and effective care of the highest quality and value." Toward this end, TJC requires the reporting of incidents and causes of workplace violence in the Sentinel Event Database (TJC, 2020b). TJC has recently updated Sentinel Event Alert 45: Preventing violence in the health care setting. It modified causal factors, high-risk areas, prevention strategies, and suggested actions, with emphasis on reporting workplace violence (TJC, 2019a).

Regulatory guidelines for the prevention of workplace violence derive from OSHA, NIOSH, and TJC. OSHA establishes that leaders have a general responsibility to create an awareness, take measures to prevent workplace violence, and promote safety and health in the work environment. NIOSH, OSHA, and TJC all make recommendations for standards to protect workers from violence. All these bodies, including BLS, continuously collect data on injuries, fatalities, and workplace violence. Given the economic strain of workplace violence and the potential legal liability, leaders of health care organizations have a financial responsibility to prevent workplace violence and provide a safe environment in which employees can speak up.

LEADERSHIP AND MANAGEMENT IMPLICATIONS

Leadership Responsibility for Workplace Violence

Organizational leaders have an obligation to protect employees from workplace violence. They must first acknowledge that a risk exists, then be committed to adopting TJC, OSHA, and NIOSH recommendations to increase awareness and implement workplace violence programs, policies and procedures, proper consequences for breaching policies, and encouragement of staff to report any type of workplace violence.

Employees should feel safe going into work without fear of being hurt physically or emotionally. OSHA (2015c) stated, "All employees can bring important knowledge and perspectives to the workplace violence prevention program—especially caregivers who interact directly with patients. A joint management–employee committee can foster a participatory approach where employees and management work together on worksite assessment and solution implementation". This includes (1) acknowledging the value of a safe and healthful, violence-free workplace, (2) distributing appropriate authority and resources to all accountable groups, (3) assigning responsibility and authority for the various aspects of the workplace violence prevention program to ensure that all managers and supervisors understand their duties, (4) maintaining a system of accountability, (5) supporting and implementing appropriate recommendations from safety and health committees, (6) developing medical and psychological therapy and debriefing for employees who have been affected by violent incidents, and (7) creating policies that certify the reporting, recording, and monitoring of incidents and near misses that protect the employee from retribution.

In the 2019 American Nurse Today's third annual Nursing Trends and Salary Survey (Spader, 2019), there were 5262 registered nurse respondents. Over fifty respondents were victims of violence, verbal assault, sexual harassment, or bullying in the workplace. Fifty-nine percent reported verbal assault by a patient in the past 24 months, 43% were verbally assaulted by a patient's family member or visitor, 23% of respondents were physically assaulted by a patient (a 3% increase compared with 2018). Forty-four percent reported being unsatisfied in the management of the events. In the same 2019 survey, 90% of those surveyed reported that policies had been implemented within their organization for workplace violence, 76% have received de-escalation education, with 83% declaring it is beneficial, and 73% were able to apply de-escalation techniques (Spader, 2019).

De-escalation

TJC (2019b) described de-escalation as a combination of strategies, techniques, and methods intended to reduce a patient's agitation and aggression. These can include communication, self-regulation, assessment, actions, and safety maintenance in order to reduce the risk of harm to patients and caregivers, and the use of restraints or seclusion. Annual training should include all employees at all levels within the organization. Additional training is recommended for those staff working in high-risk areas such as hospitals, schools, and food service places. TJC recommended three de-escalation models and four tools for managing workplace violence.

De-escalation models (TJC, 2019b)

- *The Dix and Page* model consists of three interdependent components: assessment, communication, and tactics (ACT).
- *Turnbull et al.* model is similar to Dix and Page's model. However, it describes how the de-escalator evaluates the aggressor's response to their use of de-escalation skills by constantly monitoring and evaluating feedback from the aggressor.
- *Safewards Model* begins with delimiting the situation by moving the patient or other patients to a safe area and maintaining a safe distance, clarifying the reasons for the anger using effective communication, and resolving the problem by finding a mutually agreeable solution.

Tools to Recognize Risk of Workplace Violence

- *STAMP* (Staring, Tone and volume of voice, Anxiety, Mumbling, and Pacing) is a validated tool for use in the emergency department (ED).
- *Overt Aggression Scale* (OAS) is a tool for use in the inpatient setting for children and adults.
- *Broset Violence Checklist* (BVC) is a validated checklist for use in the adult inpatient psychiatric unit.
- *Brief Rating of Aggression by Children and Adolescents* (BRACHA) is a valid tool for the ED to determine the best placement for children and adolescents on an inpatient Psychiatric unit.

A study using questionnaires was conducted by Arnetz and colleagues (2018) to examine the effect of work stress, staff interaction, and safety climate on self-reported workplace violence (see conceptual model, Fig. 20.2). Descriptive and correlational analyses were conducted. Results indicated interpersonal conflict was a risk factor for verbal violence, low work efficiency was a risk factor for physical violence, and poor violence prevention climate was a risk factor for verbal and physical violence. The researchers recommended that interventions should aim at enhancing employee interactions,

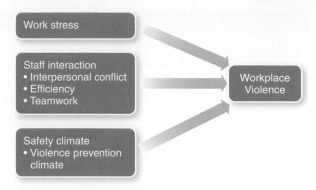

Fig. 20.2 A conceptual model of workplace violence. Source: Arnetz, J., Hamblin, L. E., Sudan, S., & Arnetz, B. (2018). Organizational determinants of workplace violence against hospital workers. *Journal of Occupational and Environmental Medicine*, *60*(8), 693–699. https://doi.org/10.1097/JOM.0000000000001345.

work efficiency, and management endorsement of a violence prevention environment.

Workplace Incivility

Incivility is "one or more rude, discourteous, or disrespectful actions that may or may not have a negative intent behind them" (American Nurses Association [ANA], 2015). The behaviors can be either intentional or unintentional, having the potential to cause long-term effects on the victim. It is a mild form of bullying and unlike incivility, bullying is considered a type of violence. If incivility is not managed in a timely and appropriate manner, it has the potential to escalate into bullying. It is everyone's responsibility to create a culture of safety and well-being. The following behaviors define incivility (Ciocco, 2018):

- Covert
- Direct and blatant aggression
- Overt—more subtle behaviors such as sarcasm, gossiping, or gesturing
- From one person to another or between a group and a targeted person ("mobbing"); this is when a specific person is the victim of rude and discourteous behavior from two or more persons
- Displaying favoritism
- Making verbal insults

Workplace Bullying

Bullying is defined as "anyone who uses his or her perceived strength or power to intimidate another person

TABLE 20.2   Roles in Bullying

Roles	Definitions
Bully/perpetrator	Someone invoking repeated, malicious, intentional arrogant, underhanded behavior
Victim/target	Someone who is the recipient of bully's behavior (unwanted, repeated, malicious, intentional behavior) causing physical and emotional harm
Bystander	Someone who witnesses bullying
Upstander	Someone who witnesses bullying and intervenes

Source: Ciocco, M. 2018. *Fast facts on combating nurse bullying, incivility and workplace violence.* New York: Springer: Pelletier, P. (2015). *Workplace bullying: It's just bad for business.* (p. 54). Diversity Publishing.

who, he or she thinks, is weaker in order to gain power over that person" (Ciocco, 2018, p. 39). Definitions vary among researchers and experts on the topic. However, the underlying themes are similar. The ANA (2015) described bullying as "repeated, unwanted harmful actions intended to humiliate, offend, and cause distress in the recipient, including those that harm, undermine, and degrade." Research on workplace bullying started in the late 1980s in Sweden with Heinz Leymann's seminal works. Subsequently the fields of psychology, occupational health and medicine, epidemiology, violence, and management research have contributed to the knowledge of this area.

Bullying occurs in any type of occupation, not just health care (Namie, 2017); 60.4 million Americans are affected by bullying, and 61% of Americans are aware of abusive conduct in the workplace. Causes of bullying include work culture, workforce mix, and the employer's response to bullying. According to Glambeck and colleagues (2018), bullying can include all members of a team. In addition, intense workplaces promote the greatest occurrences of bullying. In a recent study, these researchers noted that bullying behaviors dismissed by leadership increased the risk of continued abuse by perpetrators (Glambeck et al., 2018). There are various types of bullying including:

- **Verbal bullying:** Slandering, ridiculing, or maligning a person or their family; persistent name-calling that is hurtful, insulting, or humiliating; using a person as the butt of jokes; abusive and offensive remarks.
- **Physical bullying:** Pushing, shoving, kicking, poking, tripping, assault or threat of physical assault, and damage to a person's work area or property.
- **Mobbing:** Mobbing is the bullying or social isolation of a person through collective unjustified accusations, humiliation, general harassment, or emotional abuse.

- **Cyberbullying:** Cyberbullying is bullying that takes place over digital devices like cell phones, computers, and tablets. Cyberbullying includes sending, posting, or sharing negative, harmful, false, or mean content about someone else. It can include sharing personal or private information about someone else causing embarrassment or humiliation.
- **Exclusion:** Socially or physically excluding or disregarding a person in work-related activities.

There are various roles assumed by individuals in the bullying process. These include perpetrator, target, bystander, and upstander. Table 20.2 shows terms and definitions for specific roles in bullying (Cioccio, 2018; Pelletier, 2015).

Pelletier (2015) identified common attributes of victims or targets (Box 20.2). These include independence, technically skilled, go-to workers to whom new staff turn for guidance, successful, better social skills

BOX 20.2   Common Attributes of Victims (Targets)

- Targets are independent
- Targets are more technically skilled than their bullies
- They are the "go-to" workers to whom new staff turn for guidance
- Targets are better liked
- They are successful
- They have more social skills and possess greater emotional awareness and maturity
- Targets are ethical and honest
- Targets are people with personalities founded on a nurturing and social orientation—a desire to help, heal, teach, develop, and nurture others

Pelletier, P. (2015). *Workplace bullying: It's just bad for business.* (p. 54). United States of America: Diversity Publishing.

with a nurturing and social orientation. Ciocco (2018) described bullying in further detail: (1) it can be physical or verbal; (2) it may include threats, exclusion, or violence; (3) it can take place in a single occurrence or over a period of time, by the same person or by a group; (4) it occurs throughout all age ranges and in all places: schools, workplace, and social settings; (5) it can include recurrent efforts to include physical injury, emotional and mental harm; (6) it can occur between strangers, work peers, acquaintances, or friends; (7) it is intentional; (8) it focuses on a specific target or targets; (9) it includes psychological cruelty and well-thought out actions; and (10) it is disruptive and interferes with work.

Organizational Role

Organizational leaders have an instrumental role in managing workplace bullying. Bullying can be perpetrated by nurses on others, or by others on nurses. Although leaders may be aware of toxic behaviors, very little is done to address it. There are multiple reasons for this. Some reasons are due to education, little experience or self-confidence with having difficult conversations with staff, fear of being a victim themselves, or they may have a personal relationship with the bully. All of these factors make it very difficult to promote civility in work environments. In a 2019 survey (Spader, 2019) 35% of respondents had been verbally assaulted by a health care provider in the past 24 months, as compared to 36% in 2018. A total of 64% of respondents reported the event, and only 25% perceived that the issue was well managed. Approximately 46% of nurses spoke up when bullying was witnessed, 77% reported the incident, and less than 50% were content with how the incident was handled (Spader, 2019). Although workplace bullying is widespread, some behaviors do not constitute bullying:

- Reasonable management practices, including performance management and disciplinary procedures;
- A direction to carry out reasonable duties and instructions.

An OSHA report provided through TJC stated that "over 50 percent have been verbally abused (a category that included bullying) in a 12-month period and 59 percent experienced verbal abuse during a seven-day period" (TJC, 2016). Destructive acts cause unhealthy work environments impacting patient care, quality outcomes, and financial loss in organizations. Bullying increases feelings of anxiety and depression, reduces job satisfaction, and increases organizational nursing turnover. Perpetrators thrive on control. They often focus on individuals who are perceived weak, have stronger skills sets, or are well liked by others. Bullying has financial ramifications to organizations, among the array of negative consequences overall for organizations.

The public views nursing as the most trusted, ethical, and honest profession. Behind closed doors, nurses are losing trust and reverence for one another. Bullying is a hidden epidemic. It poses jeopardy to financial stability, job security, and employees' health and well-being. There are health-related risks to bullying such as anxiety, depression, posttraumatic stress disorder, insomnia, panic attacks, and migraine headaches. Because of psychosocial and physical harm to employees, it leads to absenteeism, poor morale, and decreased job satisfaction, which affects hospital outcomes and patient care.

Bullying and incivility in health care are being addressed by many regulatory agencies such as TJC. They published the following Sentinel Alerts:

- Sentinel Event Alert 40 in 2008: Behaviors that undermine a culture of safety,
- Sentinel Event 24 in 2016: Bullying has no place in health care,
- Sentinel Event Alert 57 in 2017: The essential role of leadership in developing a safety culture,
- Sentinel Event Alert 59 in 2018: Physical and verbal violence against health care workers, and the recently updated,
- Sentinel Event Alert 45 in 2019: Preventing violence in the health care setting.

The Magnet® Recognition program within the American Nurses Credentialing Center (ANCC) has taken steps to address these issues. In 2017, within the domain of Exemplary Professional Practice (EP), a culture of safety EP criterion was developed for physical and verbal violence in health care systems. The EP15EO expects organizations pursuing Magnet designation to demonstrate strong data and strategies regarding workplace violence, bullying, and incivility towards nursing (Thompson, 2019, p. 25).

Impact of Workplace Bullying

Hostile work environments can harm patients and the organization's status, decrease employee satisfaction, and greatly affect a company's bottom line due to increased turnover and absenteeism. An unhealthy work culture can lead to increased rates of insomnia, high blood pressure, anxiety, headaches, posttraumatic stress disorder, depression, gastrointestinal disorders, strained personal relationships, mistrust, substance abuse, eating disorders, and suicidal ideations (Ciocco, 2018). Bullying results in companies losing more than $250 million every year from not only employee turnover but lost productivity, workers' compensation claims, recruitment, orientation of new staff, and court costs (American Psychiatric Association Foundation, 2020; Herschcovis et al., 2015).

Employment Assistance Programs

Employee assistance programs (EAPs) provide a range of services to help employees cope with stressors that occur at home and at work. Family counseling might be useful in reducing domestic violence that can spill over into the workplace. Programs that counsel both the victim and the abuser could be instrumental in initiating needed interventions to defuse domestic violence situations that could affect the worksite. Furthermore, individual counseling can help employees cope with personal stressors that might contribute to unpredictable or violent behaviors. EAPs can be useful in preventing or mitigating loss caused by domestic violence that extends to the workplace.

CURRENT ISSUES AND TRENDS

Active Shooter

The deadliest situations involve an active shooter. US Department of Homeland Security (DHS) defined active shooter as someone "actively engaged in killing or attempting to kill people in a confined and populated area" (National Safety Council [NSC], 2019). During a chaotic situation involving an active shooter, DHS suggested avoiding knee-jerk reactions, remaining calm, and doing one of three options (NSC, 2019):

1. If there is an accessible escape route, leave belongings and get out.
2. If evacuation is not possible, find a hiding place where you won't be trapped should the shooter find you, lock and blockade the door, and silence your phone.
3. As a last resort and only when your life is in imminent danger, attempt to incapacitate the shooter by throwing items, improvising weapons, and yelling.

Many organizations have recognized and adopted strategies to navigate active shooters. The following actionable framework is commonly promoted for decision-making during active shootings: (1) run and escape if possible, (2) hide if escape is not possible, or (3) fight as a last resort (see Box 20.3 for more details).

Active shooter training has not only been strongly encouraged by DHS, but it is an expectation by OSHA, TJC, and NIOSH. Active shooter incidents frequently end within 10 to 15 minutes. Therefore prior to law enforcement arrival to the incident, employees need to be trained mentally and physically to cope with an active shooter situation (OSHA, 2019d). DHS has developed a protocol for dealing with an active shooter: https://www.dhs.gov/xlibrary/assets/active_shooter_booklet.pdf

Legislation

The American Nurses Association (ANA, 2015) developed a Position Statement on Incivility, Bullying, and Workplace Violence. Position statements by the (Professional Issues Panel on Incivility, Bullying, and Workplace Violence 2015) include:

- The nursing profession will not tolerate violence of any kind from any source.
- Nurses and employers must collaborate to create a culture of respect.
- The adoption of evidence-based strategies that prevent and mitigate incivility, bullying, and workplace violence; and promote health, safety, and wellness and optimal outcomes in health care.
- The strategies employed are listed and categorized by primary, secondary, and tertiary prevention.
- The statement is relevant for all health care professionals and stakeholders, not exclusively to nurses.

Lawmakers have taken steps to protect health care workers from violence in the workplace. The US House of Representatives proposed the *Healthcare Workplace Violence Prevention Act* in March 2018 titled H.R. 5223. The bill would have guided OSHA to develop a criterion that required and encouraged health care organizations to develop workplace violence prevention plans. Although the bill did not move forward, it was reintroduced in February 2019 as H.R. 1309. The current bill "requires the Department of Labor to address workplace violence in the healthcare and social service sectors" (Henkel, 2019). This bill will encourage employees to speak up, decreasing fear of retaliation as they would be protected from such acts. On November 21, 2019 the

BOX 20.3 Protocol for Dealing with an Active Shooter

Be Informed
- Sign up for an active shooter training.
- If you see something, say something to an authority right away.
- Sign up to receive local emergency alerts and register your work and personal contact information with any work sponsored alert system.
- Be aware of your environment and any possible dangers.

Make a Plan
- Make a plan with your family, and ensure everyone knows what they would do, if confronted with an active shooter.
- Look for the two nearest exits anywhere you go, have an escape path in mind, and identify places you could hide.
- Understand the plans for individuals with disabilities or other access and functional needs.

During
RUN and escape, if possible
- Getting away from the shooter or shooters is the top priority.
- Leave your belongings behind and get away.
- Help others escape, if possible, but evacuate regardless of whether others agree to follow.
- Warn and prevent individuals from entering an area where the active shooter may be.
- Call 911 when you are safe, and describe shooter, location, and weapons.

HIDE, if escape is not possible
- Get out of the shooter's view and stay very quiet.
- Silence all electronic devices and make sure they won't vibrate.
- Lock and block doors, close blinds, and turn off lights.
- Don't hide in groups—spread out along walls or hide separately to make it more difficult for the shooter.
- Try to communicate with police silently. Use text message or social media to tag your location, or put a sign in a window.
- Stay in place until law enforcement gives you the all clear.
- Your hiding place should be out of the shooter's view and provide protection if shots are fired in your direction.

FIGHT as an absolute last resort
- Commit to your actions and act as aggressively as possible against the shooter.
- Recruit others to ambush the shooter with makeshift weapons like chairs, fire extinguishers, scissors, books, etc.
- Be prepared to cause severe or lethal injury to the shooter.
- Throw items and improvise weapons to distract and disarm the shooter.

After
- Keep hands visible and empty.
- Know that law enforcement's first task is to end the incident, and they may have to pass injured along the way.
- Officers may be armed with rifles, shotguns, and/or handguns and may use pepper spray or tear gas to control the situation.
- Officers will shout commands and may push individuals to the ground for their safety.
- Follow law enforcement instructions and evacuate in the direction they come from, unless otherwise instructed.
- Take care of yourself first, and then you may be able to help the wounded before first responders arrive.
- If the injured are in immediate danger, help get them to safety.
- While you wait for first responders to arrive, provide first aid. Apply direct pressure to wounded areas and use tourniquets if you have been trained to do so.
- Turn wounded people onto their sides if they are unconscious and keep them warm.
- Consider seeking professional help for you and your family to cope with the long-term effects of the trauma.

Source: Department of Homeland Security (DHS). (2020). *Active shooter*. https://www.ready.gov/active-shooter.

bill passed the House with a 251–158 vote (Congress. Gov, 2019–2020). H.R. 1309 remains in the House as of this publication. California has the most thorough legislation affecting health care workers. Beginning April 2017, senate bill 1299 required hospitals to create, implement, and educate employees on comprehensive workplace violence prevention plans (Henkel, 2019).

Bullying Prevention

Eradicating bullying is an enormous undertaking. Solutions can happen simultaneously, and each takes effort, patience, dedication, and time. The following are recommendations for leaders: (1) acknowledge bullying is occurring then establish a consistent process to collaboratively examine and manage nurse bullying so that staff can work in a healthier workplace, (2) C-suite executives should collaborate with staff and human resources to enforce a "No Tolerance" or code of conduct policy, and (3) behaviors of bullying and incivility should be clearly delineated in policies, and perpetrators are to be held accountable for their behavior and take responsibility for their actions by making amends to those affected, (4) create a reporting system that prevents retaliation, (5) encourage staff to speak when bullying actions are witnessed without fear of retribution, and (6) provide awareness, education, and training.

Organizations should develop workplace bullying policies and guidelines as directed by TJC, NIOSH, and OSHA. Collaborating with risk management, human resources, employee health, leaders, and educators would be advisable to encourage staff to report bullying conduct through an incident reporting system for tracking and trending. The language should be clear and concise with a strong message on consequences when policies are not followed; how to report bullying; and how to appropriately document the event, investigate, and follow-up. Employees need to be provided psychological safety for reporting bullying. Bullying goes under-reported for fear of retaliation or that nothing will be done about it. Leaders have a great opportunity to change a negative work environment by promoting a culture of civility through their own behavior. When leaders do nothing, this sends a negative message to employees that uncivil behavior is condoned. Inaction will make employees feel that they cannot trust their leaders to uphold a culture of safety and well-being. Leaders must support employees by reinforcing the importance of speaking up. Management of this population and related

destructive behaviors begins with awareness and education. Education is key for addressing workplace bullying given the current prevalence.

Cognitive rehearsing (CR) described by Longo (2017) allows staff to effectively practice communication to recognize and respond to bullying behavior in the workplace. CR is reported to decrease toxic work environments, create a healthy workplace, and improve staff satisfaction (Longo, 2017). CR decreases the fear of dealing with perpetrators who are verbally condescending, insulting, and intimidating. It cultivates a nurse's confidence by identifying a bully and mentally preparing for when they are confronted with bullying behaviors. In a study conducted by Razzi and Bianchi (2019) with nurses in a community hospital, it was identified that the nurses felt more empowered to confront an uncivil situation through the CR education and training. When nurses are given techniques to face a bully and stop destructive behavior, it minimizes the probability of a perpetrator targeting others.

Taking into consideration the universal nursing shortage, attempts need to be made to safeguard seasoned and newly licensed professional nurses to clinical practice by encouraging bully-free conditions, aiding their positions in the workforce. To counter the culture of bullying in their work environments, organizations need to (1) determine what types of bullying are occurring, (2) endorse training, continuing education, and awareness of what bullying is and the characteristics of the perpetrators of bullying, (3) respond to signs of bullying, (4) identify staff in jeopardy for other emotional or performance issues, and (5) develop the skills needed to create safe workplaces to provide early interventions and detection of risky behaviors by perpetrators. It would be advantageous to identify work units at high risk, determine what types of bullying are occurring, and identify what kind of education is needed to increase a healthier work environment.

Legal Implications

Bullying is legal in every US state. To counteract this, nearly 30 states and two territories have introduced some version of the Healthy Workplace Bill (HWB) on antibullying (Healthy Workplace Bill, 2019; Namie, 2019). Fig. 20.3 illustrates those states with an antibullying bill.

"Bullying potentially violates the law if it is proven that the bullying falls within the clearly defined terms of

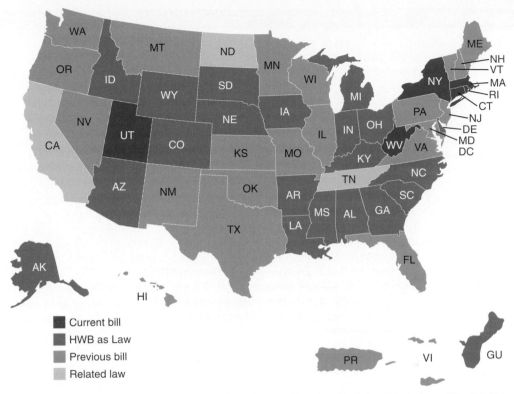

Fig. 20.3 Healthy Workplace Bill Locations, 2019. Source: Healthy Workplace Bill. (2019). *Healthy workplace campaign*.https://healthyworkplacebill.org/.

the legislation" (Pelletier, 2015, p. 59). Basic provisions of the model HWB legislation, developed and introduced by David Yamada in 2000, include a clear definition of an "abusive work environment." These bills offer a way to obtain legal compensation for being exposed to a toxic work environment. Employees would be allowed to prosecute the bully as an individual and hold the employer answerable to a cruel work environment and compensation for lost wages and benefits, forcing the employer to make changes to institutional processes (HWB, 2019).

CONCLUSION

Stamping out bullying will create a healthier, happier, more satisfying, and positive workplace for all employees and patients; decrease the risk of harm to patients; and shield seasoned and newly licensed nurses to practice under safe conditions to avoid needless distractions of being bullied.

Workplace bullying and violence add stress factors to an employee's longevity in their current work environment. Addressing bullying reduces the risk of losing veteran bedside nurses, reduces the financial impact on organizations, reduces the risk of increasing hospital-acquired infections, and most importantly places perpetrators accountable for their pathological and unforgivable behavior. Regardless of whether an employee enjoys their work or not, the income provides families with housing, food on the table, transportation, and increased access to health care.

The struggle to come to work every day in a hostile environment, being psychologically assaulted, is agonizing. Nurse bullying increases the threat of losing skilled and experienced bedside nurses, decreases intent to stay in the organization and nursing, and increases patients at risk for harm. Everyone has a right to work in a bully-free environment. Therefore taking actions to expose and stop workplace bullying is imperative.

RESEARCH NOTE

Source
(Bambi, S., Guazzini, A., Piredda, M., Lucchini, A., De Marinis, M., & Rasero, L. 2019). Negative interactions among nurses: An explorative study on lateral violence and bullying in nursing work settings. *Journal of Nursing Management, 27*(4), 749–757.

Purpose
Lateral violence and bullying have an effect on nurses' professional and health status. The purpose of this research was to investigate prevalence and risk factors of lateral violence and bullying among Italian nurse peers in different work settings, both inside and outside hospitals.

Discussion
Data were collected via a web survey using the 17-item "Negative Interactions Among Nurses Questionnaire" and a cross-sectional method. Emails were sent to 5009 nurses in three Tuscan public health care institutions. The response rate was 18.6% (*n* = 930). Twenty-six respondents were removed as they reported working with no peer colleagues. Negative interactions were experienced by 35.8% (*n* = 324), 42.3% (*n* = 137) of whom were bullied, with intensity being moderate and wide variability of prevalence. Psychophysical consequences of negative interactions were reported by 59% (*n* = 191). Victims who thought of leaving nursing were 21.9% (*n* = 71).

The main interventions implemented to confront these problems were sensitizing nurses, managers and administrators; prevention education events; acquisition of communication and conflict management skills; zero tolerance strategies; and codes of conduct that explicitly condemn unacceptable behaviors. However, there is no evidence of effectiveness for many of these interventions.

Application to Practice
Of note is that lateral violence and bullying among nurses were consistently present in all studied settings. Nurse managers could play a crucial role in preventing negative interactions among nurses. Strategies could include continuing education programs to promote awareness of this problem, implementation of an anonymous reporting system for bullying, introduction of occupational psychologists in wards with larger numbers of reported negative interactions and bullying, and increasing changes in staff composition within shifts.

The results suggest the need for an important cultural change by increasing the awareness of lateral violence and bullying among peers, which could be maintained through continuing education programs for nurses employed in all institutions and positive leadership by head nurses to promote healthy work environments with lower conflicts and psychosomatic complaints among nurses. In parallel, nurse managers need to monitor the work climate to break the occurrence of lateral violence and its escalation towards bullying.

CASE STUDY

Kelly, nurse manager (NM) of 15 years, oversees a busy 28-bed solid organ transplant unit in a large city hospital. Patients who have end-stage kidney failure get transported there to the dialysis unit for treatment. The transplant nurses needed to get clarity on whether nurses can administer antibiotics to patients who are receiving dialysis. Kelly reached out via email to Nurse Charlie, who had a long history with the dialysis nursing practice at this institution, to inquire when and if nurses can initiate orders for antibiotics in dialysis. Kelly wanted to make sure she understood some of the background history of what nurses in dialysis can and cannot do in regard to initiating orders that originated from the transplant team versus a nephrologist, so that she had some background information prior to then contacting Michael, NM of the dialysis unit. When Charlie replied to the email, he included Michael the dialysis NM and Marge, the nurse administrator, and the charge nurse in the dialysis unit. Michael noted that a patient being treated in dialysis is technically under the care of the nephrologist. This was new knowledge for Kelly. Dialysis nurses are not permitted to administer any medication to patients unless ordered by the nephrologist. If medication must be administered, the primary physician would need to contact the nephrologist. Kelly shared this information with her nursing staff.

CASE STUDY—cont'd

That same day nurse administrator Marge emailed Kelly and Kelly's nurse administrator regarding the recent inquiry. She accused Kelly of purposely going around Michael, the dialysis NM, to make him look bad. Kelly personally called Marge to explain that was not her intent. Kelly did not have a strong background in dialysis practice and was seeking information. Nurse Charlie was a historian regarding the dialysis unit. Kelly thought he would be a great resource to understand policies and procedures in that area. Once she got the information she needed, it may not have been necessary to reach out to NM Michael to report any potential delays of medication administration by his nurses. Marge insisted that Kelly purposely had malicious intent. That call led to an immediate meeting with Kelly's administrator, Allison. Allison accused Kelly of blindsiding Michael and purposely avoiding him, so he looked bad to his subordinates. Kelly sunk into the office chair in disbelief. Kelly was given a verbal warning. Allison began spreading rumors about Kelly to her peers and colleagues regarding her lack of self-awareness, poor teamwork, unprofessionalism, and sabotaging Michael's stellar reputation. Kelly did not know what to do. She was accused of things that were false. This caused her peers to avoid her, she often sat alone, and was removed from two committees.

At a meeting a few days later, she saw Michael. She decided to apologize for any misunderstanding regarding the inquiry she made about medication administration. Michael looked confused. Kelly shared that she was under the impression she had purposely made him look bad. He assured Kelly that was absolutely false. Michael was supportive about Kelly reaching out to Charlie and was not offended in the least.

Kelly tried to make every effort to clear the air about this matter. It weighed heavy on her and negatively impacted her reputation and working relationship with her peers. Kelly contacted administrators Allison and Marge. She

shared the positive conversation she had with Michael. Marge thanked her for the update. Allison, on the other hand, wrote Kelly up for insubordination. Kelly was clearly being bullied by her administrator. Allison was being completely unreasonable; she told Kelly that Kelly would not be successful in this organization if she had anything to do with it. Kelly stated that she would have no choice but file a grievance with human resources (HR) to settle this matter. Allison said, "Good luck, they won't believe you over me."

Kelly did go to HR, and Allison was correct in that they did not believe her. Their comment was "if you don't like the way this played out, this organization may not be the right place for you." Kelly did some research on this type of behavior. She was experiencing isolation, gaslighting, false accusations, emotional abuse, professional sabotage, and intimidation. Kelly felt alone, depressed, and defeated. She went onto social media and found several bullying support groups that provided her with good information on how to cope with workplace bullying. Those resources led to others. All these resources gave her the needed strength to understand bullies and why and how they target certain types of people as their victim. As Kelly gained strength and confidence from information and supportive colleagues, she took positive and affirming steps to diminish the effects of bullying and to better counter negative behaviors at work.

1. How would you feel if you were Kelly?
2. Would you have done anything differently in this situation?
3. Having support is important to survive bullying. What other resources would you have used and why?
4. If you were a witness to this type of bullying, how would you provide Kelly support? Would you too isolate yourself from her for fear of being a target?
5. What have you identified as the characteristics of the bully and target?

▍CRITICAL THINKING EXERCISE

Two East evening shift has been having constant turnover. The director Shelly was concerned since there was a need for continuity on the Dedicated Diabetes Care Unit. Patients on that unit would typically be readmitted for diabetic ketoacidosis or infections.

When Shelly attended a conference she met Beth, a Certified Diabetes Educator. She convinced Beth to interview to ensure that there was an experienced person

to hire to reduce the constant turnover that was very concerning to her. Beth had worked for an Outpatient Diabetes Setting for 10 years and was very excited about the new role.

During her orientation, she felt highly supported and provided her preceptor with tips to better manage acute patients. After the orientation, Beth was assigned to the 3–11 shift. On her first 3–11 shift the other nurses seemed very reserved. During the break time, Beth felt isolated from the other nurses. She felt that she was being excluded. At times, she thought it may be her imagination, but it continued, and she observed it happening with selected people on the unit. After work she would return home and feel anxious at bedtime.

Beth decided she would speak to Shelly about the hostility she was experiencing. She scheduled an appointment with Shelly and brought a list of her experiences and that of her peers.

1. If you were Shelly, what additional information would you want from Beth?
2. Should Shelly take Beth's word for the situation?
3. As a leader, what is the first action you would take?
4. What is the evidence base for Shelly's leadership actions?
5. How can Shelly track turnover after she takes action?

REFERENCES

American Nurses Association (ANA). (2015). *Incivility, bullying, and workplace violence: ANA position statement.* https://www.nursingworld.org/practice-policy/nursing-excellence/official-position-statements/id/incivility-bullying-and-workplace-violence/.

American Psychiatric Association Foundation. (2020). *Bullying.* http://workplacementalhealth.org/Mental-Health-Topics/Bullying.

American Psychological Association (APA). (2020). *Violence.* https://www.apa.org/topics/violence/index.

Arnetz, J., Hamblin, L. E., Sudan, S., & Arnetz, B. (2018). Organizational determinants of workplace violence against hospital workers. *Journal of Occupational and Environmental Medicine*, 60(8), 693–699. https://doi.org/10.1097/JOM.0000000000001345.

Bambi, S., Guazzini, A., Piredda, M., Lucchini, A., De Marinis, M., & Rasero, L. (2019). Negative interactions among nurses: An explorative study on lateral violence and bullying in nursing work settings. *Journal of Nursing Management*, 27(4), 749–757.

Bureau of Labor Statistics (BLS). (2019a). *Census of Fatal Occupational Injuries (CFOI) for 2018,* Bureau of Labor Statistics Injuries, Illnesses, and Fatalities. https://www.bls.gov/iif/oshcfoi1.htm#rates.

Bureau of Labor Statistics. (2019b). *Survey of Occupational Injuries and Illnesses (SOII) for 2018.* Bureau of Labor Statistics Injuries, Illnesses, and Fatalities. https://www.bls.gov/respondents/iif/.

Ciocco, M. (2018). *Fast facts on combating nurse bullying, incivility and workplace violence.* New York: Springer.

Congress.Gov, 116th Cong. (2019–2020). *H.R.1309—Workplace Violence Prevention for Health Care and Social Service Workers Act.* https://www.congress.gov/bill/116th-congress/house-bill/1309/actions?KWICView=false.

Department of Homeland Security. (2020). *Active shooter.* https://www.ready.gov/active-shooter.

Glambeck, M., Skogstad, A., & Einarsen, S. (2018). Workplace bullying, the development of job insecurity and the role of laissez-faire leadership: A two-wave moderated mediation study. *Work and Stress: An International Journal of Work, Health & Organisations*, 32(3), 1–16. https://doi.org/10.1080/02678373.2018.1427815.

Healthy Workplace Bill. (2019). *Healthy workplace campaign.* https://healthyworkplacebill.org/.

Henkel, S. (2019). *Threat assessment strategies to mitigate violence in healthcare.* IAHSS Foundation. https://iahssf.org/assets/IAHSS-Foundation-Threat-Assessment-Strategies-to-Mitigate-Violence-in-Healthcare.pdf.

Longo, J. (2017). Cognitive rehearsal. Learn a strategy for addressing incivility and bullying in nursing. *American Nurse Today*, 12(8), 41–44. https://www.americannursetoday.com/cognitive-rehearsal/.

Namie, G. (2017). *2017 WBI US Workplace Bullying Survey.* Workplace Bullying Institute. http://www.workplacebullying.org/wbiresearch/wbi-2017-survey/.

Namie, G., (2019). *WBI frequently asked questions.* https://www.workplacebullying.org/faq/#14.

National Institute for Occupational Safety and Health (NIOSH) Centers for Disease Control and Prevention, US Department of Health and Human Services. (2013). *Workplace violence prevention for nurses*: DHHS, NIOSH Publication. No. 2013–155. https://www.cdc.gov/niosh/topics/violence/training_nurses.html.

National Institute for Occupational Safety and Health (NIOSH) Centers for Disease Control and Prevention, US Department of Health and Human Services. (2015). *Notable milestones in NIOSH history.* https://www.cdc.gov/niosh/timeline.html.

National Institute of Occupational Safety and Health (NIOSH). (2019). *Occupational violence.* https://www.cdc.gov/niosh/topics/violence/default.html.

National Safety Council (NSC). (2019). *Assaults fourth leading cause of workplace deaths.* https://www.nsc.org/work-safety/safety-topics/workplace-violence.

Occupational Safety and Health Administration (OSHA). (2015a). *Preventing workplace violence: A roadmap for healthcare facilities.* https://www.osha.gov/Publications/OSHA3827.pdf.

Occupational Safety and Health Administration (OSHA). (2015b). *Workplace violence in healthcare.* https://www.osha.gov/Publications/OSHA3826.pdf.

Occupational Safety and Health Administration (OSHA). (2015c). *Guidelines for preventing workplace violence,* pp. 6–7. https://m.afscme.org/issues/health-safety/resources/document/osha3148.pdf.

Occupational Safety and Health Administration (OSHA). (2019d). *Emergency preparedness and response: Getting started.* https://www.osha.gov/SLTC/emergencypreparedness/gettingstarted_evacuation.html.

Pelletier, P. (2015). *Workplace bullying: It's just bad for business* (p. 54). Vancouver, CA: Diversity Publishing.

Professional Issues Panel on Incivility, Bullying, and Workplace Violence. (2015). *Incivility, bullying, and workplace violence position statement.* http://www.nursingworld.org/DocumentVault/Position-Statements/Practice/Position-Statement-on-Incivility-Bullying-and-Workplace-Violence.pdf.

Razzi, C., & Bianchi, A. (2019). Incivility in nursing: Implementing a quality improvement program utilizing cognitive rehearsal training. *Nursing Forum, 54*(4), 526–536. https://doi.org/10.1111/nuf.12366.

Spader, C., (2019). *2019 Nursing Trends and Salary Survey results.* https://www.myamericannurse.com/2019-nursing-trends-and-salary-survey-results/.

The Joint Commission (TJC). (2016). *Quick Safety Issue 24: Bullying has no place in health care.* https://www.jointcommission.org/-/media/tjc/documents/newsletters/quick_safety_issue_24_june_2016pdf.pdf.

The Joint Commission (TJC). (2019a). *Sentinel Event Alert 45: Preventing violence in the health care setting.* https://www.jointcommission.org/resources/patient-safety-topics/sentinel-event/sentinel-event-alert-newsletters/sentinel-event-alert-issue-45-preventing-violence-in-the-health-care-setting/.

The Joint Commission (TJC). (2019b). *Quick Safety Issue 47: De-escalation in health care.* https://www.jointcommission.org/resources/news-and-multimedia/newsletters/newsletters/quick-safety/quick-safety-47-deescalation-in-health-care/.

The Joint Commission (TJC). (2020a). *Resources for consumers.* https://www.jointcommission.org/resources/for-consumers/.

The Joint Commission (TJC). (2020b). *Sentinel event alert and quick safety newsletters.* https://www.jointcommission.org/resources/patient-safety-topics/workplace-violence-prevention/sentinel-event-alert-and-quick-safety-newsletters/.

Thompson, R. (2019). *Enough! Eradicate bullying &incivility in healthcare: Strategies for front line leaders* (p. 25). United States of America: Incredible Messages Press.

World Health Organization (WHO). (2020). Violence against healthcare workers. https://www.who.int/violence_injury_prevention/violence/workplace/en/.

21

Nursing Workforce Staffing and Management

Therese A. Fitzpatrick

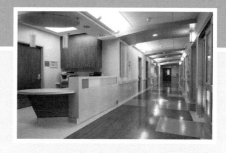

 http://evolve.elsevier.com/Huber/leadership

Staffing and scheduling are perennial concerns for nurses. Nursing is essential in the delivery of health care to society. According to the Gallup organization, for the past 18 consecutive years more than four in five Americans (84%) rated the nursing profession's honesty and ethical standards as very high or high, earning nurses the top spot among a diverse list of professionals (Brenan, 2018; Thew, 2020) The American Nurses Association's (ANA) *Nursing's Social Policy Statement* reflects the societal contract for the provision of safe and quality nursing care and services for all people in every health care setting (ANA, 2010). Therefore, staffing management is a critical contributor to achieving the societal contract. Staffing management is one of the most crucial yet highly complex and time-consuming activities for nurses and nurse leaders at every level of the health care organization today.

Although nursing's goals remain focused on providing patients the right nursing resources to achieve the best clinical outcomes for a reasonable cost, the environment in which leaders contend has becoming increasingly complex and chaotic. Evolving payment reform initiatives such as value-based care, bundled payments, and various shared savings programs all consider the quality and efficiency of services delivered to patients, both in the inpatient and outpatient settings. Although the notion of value is still being defined by the Centers for Medicare & Medicaid Services (CMS) and various professional organizations, generally it is defined as the quality of care (numerator) divided by the cost of care (denominator) or stated simply, patient health outcomes achieved by dollar spent (Shi & Singh, 2019). These developments in payment methods will continue to place the utilization of all resources, both labor (including nursing) and non-labor under significant scrutiny and pricing pressure.

The seminal work of Aydelotte (1973) stated that the aim of staffing is to provide, at a reasonable cost, a standard of nursing care acceptable to its clientele and the nursing staff serving it. This continues and remains as a critical issue affecting the quality, safety, and cost of health care (Aiken et al., 2002, 2003, 2014, 2016; Blegen et al., 1998; Kane et al., 2007a,b; Litvak et al., 2005; Mensik, 2014; Needleman et al., 2002, 2006, 2011; Unruh, 2008).

Emerging knowledge suggests that we begin to examine staffing as a complex adaptive system. Clancy (2007) posited that as organizations evolve, they become more complex over time, which means the traditional methods to measure and manage these complex systems must also evolve. By their very nature, complex systems are a dynamic network of many elements acting in parallel, and constantly acting and reacting to what other agents are doing. The planning and deployment of nursing resources is an example of such a complex system and includes the need to predict demand, synchronize complex work rules, control costs, and manage fluctuating labor markets while simultaneously being mindful of staff's personal preferences.

What is needed is the means to measure and manage the confluence of competing and dynamic interests using a system of staffing influenced by a changing external environment, data, many interacting agents (work rules, work load, work flow, and financial imperatives), and individual factors such as schedules, personal preferences, communications, and policies. These forces all influence how one staffs optimally (Gavigan et al., 2016). In addition, the nursing workforce is undergoing transformation and is being affected by generational differences, diversity, new lifestyles, family lives, cultural differences, technological skills, and the need for greater integration of work life into personal life. These traditions, emerging knowledge, and workforce transformations call for the profession of nursing to fulfill its societal contract and envision staffing methodologies to inform the future (Flanders & Carr, 2016; Joseph & Fowler, 2016; National Council of State Boards of Nursing [NCSBN], 2016).

The major goal of staffing management is to provide the right number of nursing staff with the right qualifications to deliver safe, high-quality, and cost-effective nursing care to a group of patients and their families as evidenced by positive clinical outcomes, satisfaction with care, and progression across the care continuum (Eck Birmingham, 2010). Additionally, in an effort to fulfill the responsibilities as leaders in the creation of innovative systems and processes of care and as full participants in the governance of our organizations, nursing resource allocation needs to also reflect the critical activities that support direct care as well as our professional development. The ANA (2016a) noted that nurses are the largest clinical subgroup in hospitals and a common target for cost containment by reducing nursing hours. However, "appropriate safe nurse staffing and skill mix levels are essential to optimize quality of care" (ANA, 2016a), and this determination is challenging yet essential.

Staffing management is one of the most critical yet highly complex and time-consuming activities for nurse leaders at every level of the health care organization. How well or poorly nursing leaders execute staff management affects the safety and quality of patient care including minimizing complications and unnecessary readmissions, the financial results, and organizational outcomes, such as job satisfaction and retention of registered nurses (RNs). The purpose of this chapter is to assist students, nurses, and nursing leaders at all levels to understand the complex issues associated with staffing management in patient care. A framework for staffing management is presented, and critical components of the staffing management plan are described. New evidence that fosters an understanding of just-in-time service delivery, big data analytics, technology, and algorithmically driven applications are presented for optimal and effective staffing.

DEFINITIONS

Staffing terminology in nursing is multifaceted and often confusing, with a specific set of terms used.

Admissions, discharges, and transfers (ADT): ADT refers to the patients who are admitted, discharged, and transferred. The ADT factor has also been referred to as a churn or turnover of patients. ADT is associated with increased care or workload to meet the standard of care for the patient and with safe and effective RN-to-RN communication or handoff regarding the patient's condition and plan of care. The movement of patients in, out, or between units has a significant impact on scheduling and assignment of clinical resources because this is time-consuming work.

Average daily census (ACD): The average number of inpatients on any given day, calculated by dividing the number of patients cared for per day over a certain period by the number of days in a period is the ADC. It may be an actual ADC or a budgeted (anticipated) ADC. It is important to note when creating a budget or staffing plan for a unit that there may be additional categories or classification of patients cared for on an inpatient unit and that volume must be accounted for in the plan. For example, patients in an outpatient, observation, or phase 2 recovery status may be placed on an inpatient unit. For departments outside of acute care the average workload may be measured in other types of mathematical units such as surgical minutes in the operating room, or average daily visits (ADV) in ambulatory settings or emergency departments. It is important to note that emergency department patients waiting for an inpatient bed in order to be admitted or transferred still need to be included in the emergency department's workload.

Average length of stay (ALOS): ALOS is the average number of days each patient is in the hospital. It is determined by dividing the total number of patient days by the total number of admissions (Finkler et al., 2013; Fitzpatrick & Brooks, 2010). Patient and organizational needs are evolving based on improved care models, technology, advanced pharmacology, and payer mandates. As a result, lengths of stay are significantly decreasing. Therefore, encounters with a hospital, whether inpatient or outpatient, may be measured in hours rather than days.

Human resources staffing strategy: This is process that determines human resource needs; links to the strategic plan, recruits, selects, and retains qualified applicants; and meets the needs of the organization by ensuring that there is appropriate, sufficient, qualified, and competent staff. The human resource strategy also supports professional development and succession planning processes.

Nurse staffing: Nurse staffing refers to the process of identifying and allocating nursing staff on a shift to a patient care area. It typically is a daily operations function. "Appropriate nurse staffing is a match of registered nurse expertise with the needs of the recipient of nursing care services in the context of the practice setting and situation. The provision of appropriate nurse staffing is necessary to reach safe, quality outcomes; it is achieved by dynamic, multifaceted decision-making processes that must take into account a wide range of variables" (ANA, 2012, p. 6). The geography of a nursing unit may also impact staffing. Examples include blind spots, hallway separations, or sheer size. Any of these limitations may need to be mitigated by adjusting staffing.

Nurse staffing management plan: This is a structured approach to the process of identifying and allocating unit-based personnel resources to optimize care needs, quality outcomes, and effectiveness.

Nursing direct-care hours: Direct-care hours are the number of nursing staff hours that are assigned to provide direct care to a patient or groups of patients for a specified period; the most common direct-care staff include the RN, licensed practical nurse (LPN)/licensed vocational nurse (LVN), and unlicensed assistive personnel (UAP). The hours are typically calculated per patient day or nursing hours per patient day (NHPPD).

Nursing indirect-care hours: Indirect-care hours are the number of staff hours that are assigned to complete organization business such as performance improvement activities, staff development, committee work, or shared governance participation. Indirect-care hours may also include nurses in support roles such as preceptors that support either the direct-care staff or the business of the organization or department.

Nurse-to-patient ratio: The RN-to-patient ratio reflects the actual patient care assignment, model of care, or a state-mandated regulatory requirement for an RN-to-patient assignment. The number of RNs assigned to care for a certain number of patients is stated as a ratio. For example, 1:2 is a common ratio for one RN to care for two patients in an intensive care unit (ICU) and may be changed based on the condition of the patients.

Nursing workload: Nursing workload is the patient care plus non-patient care activities (direct and indirect) performed by a nurse and includes the time, complexity of skill mix, patient dependency, and severity of illness (intensity in terms of effort required) of the work a nurse performs within a given period (Morris et al., 2007). It is typically measured by units of service. For most inpatient departments care requirements are defined as hours per patient day (HPPD). When multiplied by the expected patient volume, the total number of care hours is determined and used to create a personnel budget. In the operating room (OR) surgical minutes or numbers of cases drive the workload calculation; in ambulatory areas such as the emergency room, an hours per patient visit (HPPV) calculation is used as the measure of the workload.

Optimizing a staffing strategy: The planning of staffing is predicated on predictions of the future state of a system and is highly dependent on describing its current state. The ability to analyze demand is a powerful means to describe and understand the behavior of the system, and the results of these analyses form the basis of an optimal strategy. This requires an understanding of a variety of data, the interactions and dependencies of those data elements, statistical analysis, and the quantification of patient need, specifically acuity. Mathematical optimization produces the best result or option given the myriad of competing factors.

Innovative organizations are now beginning to consider multidisciplinary, patient-needs driven, unit-based care models. For example, it may be more effective and efficient to add physical therapists to a direct care team on an orthopedic unit or include a respiratory therapist in a critical care team. As a result, the measurement of direct care hours beyond just nursing will need to evolve as well.

Scheduling: Scheduling is the process of determining a set number and type of staff for a future time period by assigning individual personnel to work specific hours, days, or shifts and in a specific unit or area over a specified period of time.

Skill level: Skill level is a function of education and competency for the job. In nursing, it is determined by the licensure (e.g., RN, LPN, LVN) or certification (e.g., UAP, NA) of a staff member.

Skill mix: Skill mix is the range of types and levels of ability and preparation of the workforce. In nursing it is the proportion of direct-care RNs to total direct-care nursing staff expressed as a percentage of RNs to total nursing staff. For example, a medical surgical patient care unit may have a skill mix of 60% RNs and 40% UAP. A skill mix ratio is typically budgeted for at the patient care unit level but must also be examined at the shift level during the scheduling process. The determination of an appropriate skill mix requires the understanding and examination of the specific care requirements of a group of patients and a responsible determination of those activities that can be safely delegated to UAP or other care providers. Those elements of care that may be delegated are often outlined in the State's Nursing Practice Act.

Staffing is composed of four distinct and interdependent processes, including (1) budgeting, (2) scheduling, (3) deployment, and (4) assignment making. Box 21.1

BOX 21.1 Definitions of Staffing Processes

1. **Budgeting:** A formal plan established by leaders that compares expected revenues with expenses. It requires an understanding of the expected demand for care by patient type, specific care requirements, anticipated cost of that care, and specific human resources required to provide that care, including the appropriate mix of staff.
2. **Scheduling:** The procedural plan to inform nurses and other providers of the days and hours/shifts when they are expected to work. Schedules are typically created several weeks or months in advance and reflect the variety of work rules determined by the organization, department, or as designated in a collective bargaining agreement. Examples of work rules are number of consecutive shifts permitted, weekend rotations, and shift length. Schedules may be created using advanced technology applications that allow the staff remote access to the schedule, standard spreadsheet applications, or even paper-based in smaller departments or organizations such as surgical centers.
3. **Deployment:** After the schedule has been created, the immediate or real time allocation of personnel to a department is called deployment. This process typically occurs immediately prior to the start of a shift when demand is reassessed, the numbers and types of scheduled resources assessed, staff is reassigned, or additional staff are assigned based on patient requirements or to supplement scheduled staff. This process may also include the assignment of nurses in a float pool or other flexible resources.
4. **Assignment:** The process by which a department leader allocates the right care giver, with the right competencies, at the right time to a specific patient or group of patients based on clinical requirements. Modifications to assignments may occur throughout the course of a shift based on dynamic patient needs.

---

displays these definitions. In the discussion of staffing, it is important to specify which subprocess is the topic of focus. For example, if a leader determines that a department is understaffed, is the root cause a budget that does not reflect the actual demand within the department, whether insufficient resources were scheduled for a particular day, whether there was a lack of adequate backfill to accommodate a sick call, or was an assignment created that did not reflect the actual care requirements for a specific group of patients. Not unlike correcting a clinical misstep, isolating the root cause of a problem is required before an appropriate intervention can be deployed.

Staffing effectiveness: An evaluation of the effect of nurse staffing on clinical quality and patient, financial, organizational, and professional nursing outcomes.

Staffing pattern: A staffing pattern lists the total number of direct-care staff by skill level scheduled for each day and each shift. For example, for a 12-hour day shift for a pediatric unit on Mondays, there may be six RNs and two UAP for direct care. An additional RN assigned to care for children being admitted or discharged may be scheduled from 3 to 6 pm, during this peak time where children are returning from the OR or going home.

BACKGROUND

Staffing strategies reflect the organization's mission, annual strategic goals, and service line strategies and are executed to meet the staffing management plan of an organization. In hospitals, chief nursing officers are accountable to establish and translate staffing management strategies for the overall patient care areas. The nurse manager who is accountable for a patient care unit or area executes staffing management strategies to yield an optimal health experience and clinical outcomes for patients and their families; a healthy, satisfying work environment; and cost-effective staffing model for the organization. Nursing leaders at all levels are challenged to fairly balance staffing management and adopt technologies that provide the real-time tools to execute, measure, and achieve desired outcomes. Direct-care nurses are involved in the responsibility for coverage of patient care needs, determining patient acuity and intensity, and making patient assignments.

Direct care nurses are increasingly called to participate in the creation of staffing strategies. This strategic work may happen through involvement in professional shared governance committees, organizational advisory panels, or even through state mandated committees. For example, as an alternative to state mandated staffing ratios, the state of Illinois in 2007 passed the Nurse Staffing by Acuity Law (Public Act 09509491). This legislation requires every hospital within the state to create a Nursing Care Committee with 50% of its membership to be composed of staff nurses. These groups are charged with reviewing staffing plans and providing feedback for the selection, implementation, and evaluation of staffing levels (Fitzpatrick et al., 2013). This suggests the importance of staff nurses understanding the science of budgeting; the quantification of clinical requirements; and the creation, execution, and evaluation of staffing plans. These types of committees or panels give staff an important seat at the table along with operational and finance executives in creating and evaluating staffing plans. This requires that nurses develop the vocabulary and the skills to be able to communicate the impact of various staffing strategies on clinical outcomes when conversing with key decision makers.

FRAMEWORK FOR STAFFING MANAGEMENT

Nurse staffing can be determined in multiple ways. The three main models of nurse staffing are (1) budget based: nurse staff are allocated according to NHPPD, which is a financial metric; (2) nurse–patient ratio: this is the number of nurses per number of patients or patient days, which is a mathematical workload balancing; and (3) patient acuity (or intensity) based. Patient characteristics are used to determine staffing needs, which is a determination of the need for care and not based on raw numbers of patients (Mensik, 2014). Staffing management is complex and challenging because of the numerous dependencies and interrelated organizational processes. A conceptual framework provides logic and order to complex processes for administrators and scientists to consider (Edwardson, 2007). A conceptual framework for staffing management is proposed and illustrated in Fig. 21.1.

This conceptual framework is adapted from Donabedian's (1966) framework for the evaluation of quality of care, relating various structures (e.g., hospital characteristics) that affect various processes (e.g.,

actual staffing) and subsequently influence various outcomes (e.g., patient quality, patient satisfaction, and staff satisfaction). Multiple staffing studies have adapted this framework to organize the variables of interest (Edwardson, 2007; Kane et al., 2007a,b; Mark et al., 2007). In the proposed framework, structures represent the various nursing strategies—both internal and external to the organization—that directly influence an organization's ability to effectively manage processes for staffing. The processes are a series of defined stages with outputs that directly affect subsequent stages of staffing. Finally, the outcomes of staffing management are multidimensional and measured in terms of organizational outcomes including patient, fiscal, and staff outcomes. The staffing management framework is not intended to address all possible variables, but instead is intended to provide a guide for nursing leaders to assess staffing management in their organizations.

STRATEGIES INFLUENCING STAFFING MANAGEMENT

It is important for all nursing leaders to remain current on both the internal and external influences affecting staffing management. Some major influences are (1) professional resources and recommendations, (2) patient acuity and intensity, (3) nursing care delivery models, (4) The Joint Commission (TJC) and other regulatory agencies' regulations, (5) local state legislation, and (6) nurse union agreements.

American Nurses Association's Principles for Nurse Staffing

The ANA is the professional organization that speaks for the profession of nursing and develops and maintains scope and standards of practice and ethics. ANA has published guiding documents that serve as resources to understand the complex staffing issues associated with creating a nursing unit schedule, preparing an organization-wide staffing plan, or meeting staffing legislation. *ANA's Principles for Nurse Staffing* (ANA, 2012) identified the major elements needed for achieving optimal nurse staffing. The document first defines appropriate nurse staffing and presents the core components of nurse staffing. It then groups the principles into five areas: (1) the health care consumer, (2) RNs and other staff,

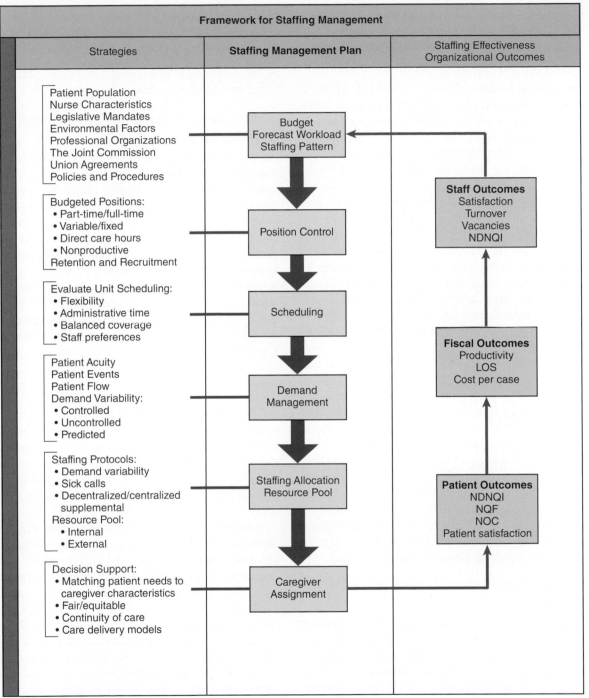

Fig. 21.1 Framework for staffing management. *LOS,* Length of stay; *NDNQI,* National Database of Nursing Quality Indicators; *NOC,* nursing outcomes classification; *NQF,* National Quality Forum.

(3) organization and workplace culture, (4) the practice environment, and (5) staffing evaluation. ANA emphasized their use of evidence to drive the development of the principles, which serve as guidelines for RN staffing solutions.

In its second edition, ANA (2012) noted that since the initial publication of the original *Principles for Nurse Staffing,* the evidence has grown supporting the link between adequate nurse staffing and better patient outcomes. Under principles related to the practice environment, ANA (2012, p. 10) stated, "Registered nurses should be provided a professional nursing practice environment in which they have control over nursing practice and autonomy in their workplace," and "routine mandatory overtime is an unacceptable solution to achieve appropriate nurse staffing. Policies on length of shifts; management of meal and rest periods; and overtime should be in place to ensure the health and stamina of nurses and prevent fatigue-related errors." This is an area where staff can provide valuable input as their insights and experience will assure that staffing plans are practical, implementable, and achieve desired clinical outcomes.

ANA's *Principles for Nurse Staffing* (ANA, 2012) has been augmented by ANA's advocacy for the proposed Registered Nurse Safe Staffing Act, which would require Medicare-participating hospitals to establish and publicly report unit-by-unit staffing plans. These plans would establish adjustable minimum numbers of RNs; have input from RNs; be based on patient numbers and variable intensity of care needed; consider elements such as education, training, and experience levels of RNs and staffing recommendations from professional organizations; ensure RNs are not forced to float to areas where they have no experience; have whistleblower protections; and require public reporting (ANA, n.d.).

American Organization for Nursing Leadership

The American Organization for Nursing Leadership (AONL, formerly called American Organization of Nurse executives, AONE), a subsidiary of the American Hospital Association, is a national organization whose mission is to represent nurse leaders. This key leadership group published *Staffing Management and Methods: Tools and Techniques for Nurse Leaders* (AONE, 2000), which presents an introduction to evolving staffing measures. It has a chapter dedicated to staffing management approaches in each of four hospital types: the large academic medical center, an integrated health care system, a small community hospital, and a rural hospital setting. The final chapter discusses how various innovations in information systems support nurse staffing. AONL continues to be involved in advocacy, policy, and issues around nurse staffing.

Staffing Recommendations by Professional Organizations

Adoption of staffing recommendations in clinical settings by relevant professional organizations is endorsed in the *Principles of Nurse Staffing* (ANA, 2012) and frequently seen written into staffing plans. Nursing leaders in specialty practice need to encourage identification and discussion of the position statement or guidelines promulgated by the relevant specialty professional organization during the annual staffing plan review. Several professional nursing specialty organizations have published position statements for nurse staffing to offer evidence-based guidelines for specialty practice. For example, the National Association of Neonatal Nurses (2014) has a staffing position statement. Recommended staffing ratios are also described in the *Guidelines for Perinatal Care* (American Academy of Pediatrics [AAP] and the American College of Obstetricians and Gynecologists [ACOG], 2012). The ratios delineate care provided for women and newborns in the antepartum, intrapartum, and postpartum settings, as well as the newborn nursery. The Association of Women's Health, Obstetric and Neonatal Nurses (AWHONN, 2010) described the specific staffing recommendations for women in the various stages of normal labor and labor with complications.

Similarly, the Association of Perioperative Registered Nurses (AORN, 2014) has a position paper addressing key staffing issues in the OR, and the Emergency Nurses Association (ENA, 2015) has published recommendations for staffing in emergency departments. The American Academy of Ambulatory Care Nursing (AAACN, 2005) published an annotated bibliography summarizing the ambulatory nurse staffing literature. Although they do not offer a position paper or guidelines, research continues in staffing models in ambulatory care, where staffing needs to be highly related to the problems, complexity, and needs of patient populations (Haas et al., 2016).

Patient Acuity and Nursing Intensity

Patient acuity is a concept commonly referenced but without specificity or consistency (Habesevich, 2012).

In a concept analysis, Brennan and Daly (2008) defined acuity as the severity of the physical and psychological status of the patient, while the intensity attribute of acuity indicates the nursing care needs and the corresponding workload required. Essentially, patient acuity is a measure of the severity of illness of the patient, whereas nursing intensity is the number of nursing hours with associated costs and total time and staff mix of nursing personnel resources consumed by an individual patient during the episode of care under review (Thompson & Diers, 1985; Welton & Dismuke, 2008). According to Unruh and Fottler (2004), estimation of staffing should be considered based on work intensity. The authors defined two indicators for nurse intensity: patient acuity and patient turnover. Because nursing accounts for the highest expenditures in hospitals, Welton and Dismuke (2008) called for a nursing billing model. A billing model based on the intensity of care allows appropriate reimbursement and thus allows for appropriate staffing and a way to capture the direct value of nursing. Despite changes in health care reimbursement structures, nurses still need to demonstrate value, which is determined by a fair and accurate method that shows nurses' work.

Patient classification systems aimed at adjusting staffing for acuity have been plagued with an inability to accurately and reliably measure patient care variability. Further, they have lacked organizational credibility and added documentation burden to the direct-care nurse. The Health Information Technology for Economic and Clinical Health (HITECH) Act, enacted as part of the American Recovery and Reinvestment Act of 2009, was signed into law on February 17, 2009, to promote the adoption and meaningful use of health information technology. This health care reform and meaningful use legislation has catapulted the advancement of health information technology into widespread adoption of electronic medical records (EMR) in the United States (http://www.hipaasurvivalguide.com/hitech-act-summary.php). These advances additionally offer nursing leaders technologies that leverage the automated patient assessment information entered in the patient EMR by nurses to generate accurate measurements of patient acuity (Eck Birmingham et al., 2011). The electronic patient assessment information is translated not only into workload information at the patient level but also standardized outcomes of care that may assist the nurse and care team in tracking patient progression to the Medicare Severity Diagnosis Related Groups (MS-DRGs) and length of stay (LOS) (Eck Birmingham,

2010). The objective patient acuity information generated as a by-product of routine clinical documentation allows frontline charge nurses to make informed patient care assignment decisions. From the chief nurse's perspective, new acuity technologies help build the business case for acuity-adjusted staffing for both improved quality and cost outcomes (Dent & Bradshaw, 2012).

There are three basic types of patient classification/acuity measurement (PCAS) methodologies, each predicated on a different philosophical assumption. Each type defines nursing care and the fluctuations in that care and connects to or informs the staffing and scheduling systems. Box 21.2 describes these three types of PCAS methods.

BOX 21.2 Three Types of PCAS Methods

Prototype Tools

This methodology generally describes different patient care levels in terms of subject categories of *minimum, moderate, or maximum* care requirements. When classifying a patient, the nurse subjectively compares their assessment of the patient's needs to prototypical vignettes describing patients with similar care needs. Often these systems do not accommodate the rapidly changing needs of a patient throughout the day.

Summative Task Tools

These measures are task and frequency based and are predicated on the assumption that care requirements are best expressed through a series of observable activities. Each task is assigned a time-based weight and points are added, converted to hours, and eventually computed to nurses required per shift. A task-based methodology presumes each task is discrete and often not reflective of the critical thinking upon which a task is based. A nurse may be performing multiple assessments along with a specific task making it difficult to quantify. The reality of clinical practice is frequent multi-tasking.

Care Interaction Tools

This approach to acuity measurement presumes that care is more complex than simply a series of tasks but rather is a combination of qualitative and quantitative attributes. Using professional judgment, the interaction between various subjective and objective critical predictors of care, such as the type, frequency, duration, and complexity of care requirements, are documented. This system accepts that patient care is greater than the sum of its parts (American Nurses Association, 2020).

Nursing Care Delivery Models

Nursing care delivery models significantly influence staffing management. Care delivery models are the operational mechanisms by which care is actually provided to patients and families. Specific nursing care delivery models are discussed in Chapter 15.

Person (2004) described the four fundamental elements of any nursing care delivery model as follows: (1) nurse/patient relationship and decision-making, (2) work allocation and patient assignments, (3) communication among members of the health team, and (4) management of the unit or environment of care. Translating the nursing care delivery model's elements and inherent values to staffing management is a key role for nursing leaders. One common element among care models is the value of the nurse and patient/family relationship. Patient assignment technology offers charge nurses access to real-time data in order to match the right nurse (i.e., competency, expertise) with the right patient and provide continuity of care during an episode of care. A second common trend is the evolving role of the charge nurse as a hospital's frontline leader with responsibility to coordinate patient flow with expert communication among health care team members as well as serving as a key resource and expert advisor to staff and the interdisciplinary care team.

Increasingly a charge nurse is appointed as a resource, managing patient flow and supporting novice nurses, and thus does not always assume a direct-care assignment. In this role, the charge nurse works closely with patient placement or transfer centers in managing efficient throughput as well as with central staffing or resource centers to assure adequate resources to provide safe and effective care. In large health care systems, these command centers may manage patient flow across multiple organizations. The charge nurse may also coordinate communication with the interdisciplinary team, including facilitation of discharges and post-acute care.

Three nursing care delivery models of relationship-based care (RBC) influence staffing management: the synergy model, case management, and the clinical nurse leader (CNL). RBC is a common model used in care delivery (Koloroutis, 2004) that supports achieving recognition by the Magnet Recognition Program® (Guanci & Felgen, 2016).

The Synergy Model for Patient Care was developed by the American Association of Critical-Care Nurses (2016) and is a patient-centered model focused on the needs of the patient, the competencies of the nurse, and the synergy created when the needs and competencies match. Synergy—or optimum patient outcomes—results when the needs and characteristics of the patient and clinical unit or system are matched with a nurse's competencies. Patient assignment technology may assist in defining—and thereby aligning—patient needs with the nurse's abilities, a concept that is central to the model.

Case management is defined by the Case Management Society of America (CMSA) as "a collaborative process of assessment, planning, facilitation, care coordination, evaluation, and advocacy for options and services to meet an individual's and family's comprehensive health needs through communication and available resources to promote quality, cost-effective outcomes" (CMSA, 2016). Case management can be coupled with demand management to best coordinate care and resources to achieve positive patient outcomes, transitions of care coordination, and hospital reimbursement (Pickard & Warner, 2007).

Complementing these models, the American Association of Colleges of Nursing (AACN, 2007) has introduced a new professional nurse role, the clinical nurse leader (CNL), in current care delivery models. The CNL role integrates various aspects of previous roles in nursing, such as the case manager and clinical nurse specialist. The CNL vision statement notes that the CNL champions innovations to improve patient outcomes, ensure quality care, and reduce health care costs. The CNL leads this effort to enhance patient care. The CNL is an advocate for putting best practices into action (AACN, 2007). CNLs are master's prepared and are being used at the unit level to provide knowledge, clinical expertise, and skill in evidence-based practice implementation.

Nursing leaders often utilize other resources in the creation of their staffing plans, most frequently benchmarks, whereby they can compare themselves to other organizations and units with similar characteristics and patient types to determine how like organizations are staffed. The National Database of Nursing Quality Indicators (NDNQI), which was acquired by the Press Ganey organization in 2014, is a popular resource. NDNQI was founded by the ANA in 2001 and had been managed by the University of Kansas School of Nursing. The NDNQI database is utilized by 2000 hospitals nationwide, and participation is a requirement for Magnet designation. On a monthly basis, participants submit to the database nurse-sensitive quality data as well as financial and staffing related data such as hours per patient day, skill mix, direct and indirect care hours, direct care responsibilities, and contract labor utilization. Organizations are then able to extract robust comparative data to assist in planning staffing strategy, developing budgets, and as a periodic performance monitor (NDNQI, 2011).

The staffing management plan should reflect the values and roles established in the care delivery model that will ultimately influence patient and organizational outcomes. Both the care delivery model and staffing plan within the context of patient populations in the health care organization are critical to the overall annual strategic plan for nursing.

Systemic changes in the national health care system, including evolving payer schemes as well as dynamic market forces, require that nurses continue to innovate new models of care. There are significant efforts underway in hospitals and health care systems and within professional organizations to leverage the full interdisciplinary team to create systems and processes of care that are more efficient and cost effective. There is recognition that inpatient utilization will continue to decline as ambulatory care becomes increasingly sophisticated. The health care industry now finds itself in competition with new entrants into the health care market, including large employers and technology companies with significant resources. These organizations have created an Internet-savvy consumer market expecting real-time, 24/7 convenience, and coordination of services. Nurses will need to leverage creativity to respond to and lead model of care innovative efforts.

The Joint Commission Staffing Regulation

Private regulatory agencies such as TJC are widely used by hospitals today to conduct external reviews for quality of care and patient safety. TJC standards include the human resources function of verifying that nurses are qualified and competent to ensure that the hospital determines the qualifications and competencies for staff positions based on its mission, populations, care, treatment, and services. Hospitals must also provide the right number of competent staff members to meet the patients' needs (TJC, 2016). TJC human resource standards clearly outline the complex requirements

associated with staffing management and include, but are not limited to, the adequacy of staff numbers, mix of staff levels, licensure, education, certification, experience, and continuing education.

Det Norske Veritas (DNV) Staffing Regulation

Several health care organizations are now utilizing Det Norske Veritas (DNV) as their external consultancy to help provide regulatory oversight in assuring there are systems and processes in place to provide safe, quality care as well as ensuring general safety for staff and visitors. Not unlike other regulatory organizations, DNV, which has been awarded deemed status by CMS, has developed written standards and interpretative guidelines and conducts periodic onsite inspections. Their standard related to Nursing Services requires a plan to assure adequate staffing with qualified personnel and further requires a periodic assessment of skill mix and nurse to patient ratios that deliver safe and effective care that meets service users' physical, emotional, and social needs (DNV, 2019).

Collective Bargaining Agreements and Staffing Management

Provisions in the ANA Code of Ethics articulate the rights of nurses to address work conditions through collective action (ANA, 2015a). The two largest nursing and health care unions are (1) National Nurses United, a branch of the ANA; and (2) the Service Employees International Union (SEIU) District 1199. Nursing unions are organizations that represent nurses for the purpose of collective bargaining, which has been defined as "the performance of the mutual obligations of the employer and the representative of the employees to meet at reasonable times and confer in good faith with respect to wages, hours, and other terms and conditions of employment ... such obligation does not compel either party to agree to a proposal or require the making of a concession" (National Labor Relations Board, 2016, Section 8b, paragraph 7d).

In nursing, there is a process of negotiation between the health care employer and the union representatives of nurse employees to reach a written agreement regarding certain terms of employment. The mandatory terms of employment vary widely, but they include subjects such as, but not limited to, wages, hours, overtime, low census call-off procedures, recall, floating, use of UAP, seniority, sick leave, discharges, and leaves of absence.

The National Labor Relations Board has legislated these as mandatory subjects of bargaining, stating that issues related to wages, hours, and other conditions of employment, when introduced into negotiations, must be bargained (Fried & Fottler, 2008; NLRB, 2020) These employment subjects have significant implications for staffing management and vary in their specificity regarding nurse staffing and scheduling.

Nursing leaders working in settings with collective bargaining units need to have detailed knowledge of the relevant contractual implications for staffing management and incorporate them into the staffing technologies for compliance monitoring. Collective bargaining environments are compatible with professional nursing practice. Porter (2010) described a successful model of professional practice labor partnerships. Lawson et al. (2011) described a program to recognize nurse professional growth and development and its implementation in a collective bargaining environment.

LEADERSHIP AND MANAGEMENT IMPLICATIONS

Legislative Impact on Staffing Management

Evidence has accumulated over the years to indicate that low nurse staffing levels have an adverse effect on patient outcomes and that there is an association between higher levels of experienced RN staffing and lower rates of adverse patient outcomes (ANA, 2016b). This is seen, for example, in the work of Kane et al. (2007a,b) and multiple studies by Aiken et al. (e.g., Aiken et al., 2002, 2003, 2007, 2014, 2016). At issue are safety, attainment of outcomes, and patient and nurse satisfaction.

Nurse dissatisfaction and concern for adequate staffing to provide quality nursing care to patients and their families arose from hospital cost-reduction initiatives throughout the 1990s. Armed with quality-of-care concerns, nurses began to organize and craft proposed staffing legislation in many states. The historical context that led to quality-of-care concerns continues to affect legislation today. Throughout the 1990s, hospital administrators relied on consultants to implement work redesign to promote patient-focused care as a method of cost reduction. The central labor reduction approach in patient-focused care was reducing the number of RNs and increasing the number of UAP. This approach for decreasing nursing RN skill mix was implemented in a "one size fits all" approach across organizations and often lacked evaluation of the skill mix change and other changes on the quality of care and nurse job satisfaction and retention (Norrish & Rundall, 2001). This was most apparent in California, where a leaner RN skill mix was tried by Kaiser Permanente Northern California in the early 1990s. Skill mix was reduced from 55% RNs to 30% RNs in 1995 (Robertson & Samuelson, 1996). The changes in skill mix led to widespread real and perceived increases in RN workload, patient safety concerns, and nurse and consumer complaints (Norrish & Rundall, 2001; Seago et al., 2003). This is partially because the workload element of supervision responsibility of the RN for UAP was not accounted.

Despite patient complaints and reports of nurse dissatisfaction, little was done until 1999. Only then did the California legislature pass Assembly Bill 394 (AB 394) to mandate minimum nurse staffing ratios and acuity-adjusted staffing. The mandating of minimum nurse-to-patient ratios legislated in California ignited great debate, controversy, and study. Nurse scientists and policy experts have presented compelling arguments against mandated ratios and note that local nursing leaders are in the best position to determine the actual staffing required by the patient population (Clarke, 2005). However, the bold action of the California state legislative mandate stimulated focused attention on addressing nurse staffing issues.

Since the late 1990s, state legislation regarding nurse staffing issues has been commonplace, and 14 states have various regulations (ANA, 2016b). There are three general models of state staffing laws: (1) require a nurse-driven staffing committee to create staffing plans, (2) mandate specific nurse-to-patient ratios (California is the only one, but Massachusetts passed a law specific to intensive care units), or (3) require disclosure of staffing levels to the public and/or a regulatory body (ANA, 2016b). ANA supports the first model (nurse-driven staffing plans). Primary areas of focus for state legislation include limiting or precluding mandatory overtime, requiring staffing committees with direct-care nurse input, whistleblower protection, mandated public access to staffing information, and a requirement that implementation of patient acuity methodologies must adjust for staffing workload. State nurse staffing legislation has a significant impact on staffing management through regulation. The economic downturn in 2008 following the end of the George W. Bush administration shifted political attention to jobs and the economy and stalled further legislative nurse staffing mandates. However, the reductions in nursing budgets and challenges of the nurse shortage have resulted in fewer nurses and longer hours of work under the burden of care for sicker patients. The result is compromised care and exacerbation of the nurse shortage due to the environment of care. ANA (2015b) urged passage of the Registered Nurse Safe Staffing Act (H.R. 2083/S. 1132), national legislation to require all Medicare-participating hospitals to establish RN staffing plans using a committee.

THE STAFFING MANAGEMENT PLAN

The staffing management plan provides the structured processes to identify patient needs and then to deliver the staff resources as efficiently and effectively as possible. An effective plan first focuses on stabilizing the unit core staffing. In many organizations the staffing management plan also includes the creation of a float pool or flexible team of nurses available for deployment to cover various leaves, unscheduled absences, vacations, or an unanticipated surge in demand. This ability to augment core staffing requires a robust orientation and training infrastructure to assure that these nurses possess the competencies required to work on multiple units.

A staffing pattern, or core coverage, is determined through a forecasted workload and a recommended care standard (e.g., HPPD). Hiring to the associated position complement and developing balanced and filled schedules without holes are essential building blocks for efficient and cost-effective daily resource allocation. This also allows nurses to have predictable schedules to support work life balance. Balanced and complete schedules also enable leaders to more effectively manage the unit's finances.

Daily staffing allocation requires managing a variable staffing plan, measuring and predicting demand, and then providing balanced workload assignments to ensure that the correct caregivers are best matched to patient needs (ANA, 2012). A successful staffing management plan incorporates the policies of the organization, patient care unit, and nurse population including union and contracting affiliations. Kane and colleagues (2007a,b) suggested that nurse staffing policies should address both patient care units and organizations, such as shift rotation, overtime, full-time/part-time mix, and weekend staffing. The traditional emphasis in staffing planning has been on hospital settings. However, with shifts to primary care as the predominant site of care delivery, staffing planning is equally critical there and in all settings where nurses practice.

Forecasted Workload and Staffing Pattern (Core Coverage)

Forecasting nursing workload for each patient care area is typically carried out at least once a year and as part of the annual budgeting process or when the patient characteristics, services, and/or volume changes. The amount of work performed by a unit is referred to as its workload, and *workload* volume is measured in terms of units of service. The unit of service is specific to the type of unit, such as the number of patients, patient days, deliveries, clinic or home visits, treatments, encounters, or procedures.

Not long ago, demand forecasting, or deciding on the units of service to anticipate during the next budget cycle, was primarily focused on the current year's performance coupled with an educated guess of what the following year might hold. More sophisticated organizations examined local market trends, refreshed strategic plans, and met with key providers for their opinions.

In the contemporary health care organization, however, teams of data scientists can harness significant computational and mathematical power to analyze large data sets to more accurately predict future demand, resources requirements, and create sophisticated scenario models of financial performance. The term *big data* does not just refer to large data sets. Big data is characterized by three V's: velocity, meaning acquisition of the data is rapid; variety, meaning that there are many data types used, and volume, meaning there is a vast amount of information. Some authors suggest a fourth V that is veracity, or that data are correct and error free, as well as a fifth V of value (Rambur & Fitzpatrick, 2017, Roski, Bo-Linn & Andrews, 2014 & Rubenfire, 2017).

Fig. 21.2 describes the evolution of big data analysis. Although these types of analyses continue to evolve, they are becoming increasingly more refined. Nurse executives, in partnership with interdisciplinary teams of data scientists, mathematicians, and operations research scientists, are optimizing operational performance and developing innovative staffing models, often through the use of management simulation models that can be shared with staff for their valuable input.

Exhibit A: Evolution of Reporting to Optimization

Through Operations Research we can understand and predict how your clinical labor management system "behaves" and quantitatively fix the associated operational problems and offer the best solutions possible.

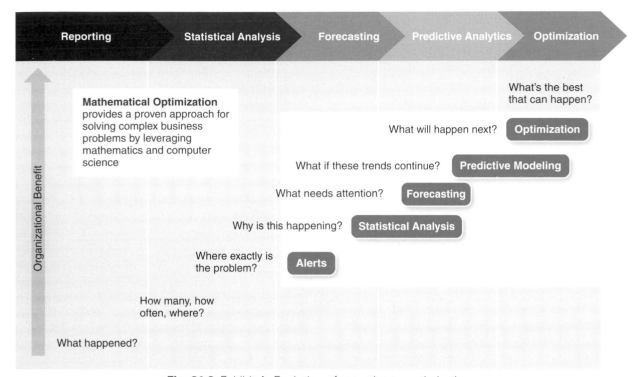

Fig. 21.2 Exhibit A: Evolution of reporting to optimization.

Staffing planners often presume patient demand patterns are somewhat random and, as a result, often plan staffing for "what if" scenarios. By analyzing big data sets that contain multiple years of patient census data at the hourly level, seasonal, daily, and even hourly patterns emerge. This allows staffing plans to go from "what if" to "what's best." These advanced computational methods simultaneously consider multiple and often disparate variables such as staffing to demand while accommodating work rules such as weekend requirements or shift lengths.

Once the unit of service is determined, the number of units of service that will be provided in the coming year must be forecasted. Total patient days are commonly used in inpatient hospital areas. This is calculated by multiplying the ALOS and the ADC. The workload standard commonly used is NHPPD, although the validity of this measure is disputed. In outpatient settings, balanced workload, patient waiting times, and staff overtime are measures used. There are intensity/acuity tools

in ambulatory settings to establish appropriate staffing levels (Liang & Turkcan, 2016).

However, not all patients require the same number of care hours, and the total number of patient days may be inadequate for planning purposes. Finkler and colleagues (2013) suggested using adjusted units of service. For example, a nursing unit can be adjusted using a system for classifying patients, such as a patient acuity system, based on the resources each classification category is expected to use. Segregating patients into acuity classifications allows the staffing pattern to be developed based on the resource requirements of the specific mix of patients forecasted for the unit. Similar calculations can be made in ambulatory and primary care by using a method to classify patients into different categories to estimate the average resource required for patients in each category (Finkler et al., 2013).

Nursing's work is complex and measuring nursing care requires sophisticated methods. Malloch (2015) presented a nursing workforce staffing model that aimed for accurate and reliable determination of the required time for care needs aligned with the appropriate nurse competencies and available time. Clear identification of care needs leads to required staff for nurse interventions, which leads to a matching process and then to value-based outcomes. High variability and intensity (or acuity) are complex patient scheduling and nurse assignment factors in clinic settings (Liang & Turkcan, 2016).

In addition to workload adjustment based on acuity, patient turnover on the unit is an important factor in patient care workload measurement. Reduced LOS in hospitals or higher patient turnover require intensive periods of higher resources for patient admissions, transfer, discharge, and other 1:1 activities that will affect overall workload, such as when the RN accompanies an unstable patient off the unit for a test or procedure.

Outside of state-mandated nurse staffing ratios, there is no one gold care standard or recommended process to determine nursing workload. Inconsistent operational definitions and methods of measuring care have been a challenge both for benchmarking resources across organizations and for research analysis related to adequate nursing care (Kane et al., 2007a,b). Therefore, each organization must document and provide rationale regarding how staffing standards are determined within each patient care area. Once the annual workload is forecasted, the skill mix required on each shift is determined.

There are two general staffing methods: (1) with *fixed staffing*, staffing is built around a fixed projected maximum workload requirement, and the staffing pattern is based on maximum workload conditions; (2) with *variable staffing*, units are staffed below maximum workload conditions and staff is then supplemented when needed. An effective staffing pattern requires clear definitions for productive time, non-patient care or "nonproductive" time (i.e., benefits time, work for the organization, knowledge-related projects), worked time, paid full-time equivalents (FTEs), and hours per unit of service. In addition, staff roles must be clearly defined as to whether they are fixed or variable. The necessary number of FTEs to yield the desired care standard for the forecasted number of patients in each department must be calculated. In addition, the number of FTEs to replace staff members when they use non-patient care,

---

BOX 21.3   Variable Staff Calculation

- 2080 paid hours per full-time equivalent (FTE)
- 80% productive hours to total paid hours
- 2080 × 0.8 = 1664 productive hours per FTE
- 71,830 care hours ÷ 1664 = 43.17 FTEs
- 71,830 care hours ÷ 365 days per year = 197 hours of care per day
- 197 hours of care per day ÷ 8-hour shifts = 24.6 person shifts

---

such as benefit time, must be accounted for in the model. Finkler and colleagues (2013) described the method for calculating a staffing pattern as follows:

1. Determine the number of paid hours per FTE.
2. Determine the percentage of productive hours to total paid hours.
3. Multiply the number of paid hours per FTE by the percentage of productive hours to find the number of productive hours per FTE.
4. Divide the required care hours by productive hours per FTE to find the required number of FTEs.
5. Divide the required care hours by the number of days per year that the unit has patients to find care hours/day.
6. Divide that result by hours per shift to find the number of person shifts needed per working day.
7. Assign staff by employee type and among required shifts per day.

Box 21.3 refers to an example of variable staff calculation. Table 21.1 provides a sample staffing pattern that includes the final step of allocating total FTEs across shifts and by skill mix. In many patient care areas, the staffing pattern may be different by day of week. For example, a post-surgical unit may have a lower patient census on weekends because of the lack of a surgical schedule, thus a different staffing pattern may apply (McKinley & Cavouras, 2000).

Mathematical Staffing Optimization: The Next Evolution of Staffing Science

As organizational capabilities around big data analysis evolve, approaches to predicting workload and planning staffing have become increasingly sophisticated and precise. Utilizing averages such as a department's average daily census, typically marked at midnight, in budget

TABLE 21.1   Sample Staffing Pattern for a Wednesday for a Medical Surgical Unit (39 Beds)

Staff Type	7 am–7 pm Shift	7 pm–7 am Shift	Skill Mix	Total
Fixed 8-hour day staff				
Nurse manager	1			1
Nurse educator—shared	0.5			0.5
Lactation specialist	1			1
Variable staff				
Charge nurse	1*			1
RN	8	7	75% RN	15.0
LPN/LVN	0	1	5% LPN	1
UAP	2	2	20% UAP	4
HUC	1	1		2

*Charge nurse on day shift without a direct-care assignment.
HUC, Health unit coordinator; LPN/LVN, licensed practical nurse/licensed vocational nurse; RN, registered nurse; UAP, unlicensed assistive personnel.

and staffing calculations is imprecise and often leads to either significant over- or understaffing.

"Approaches that use advanced and predictive analytics to anticipate customer demand and proactively improve productivity are now common in grocery stores, automotive plants, and even professional sports to solve common yet seemingly unsolvable problems. While nascent in healthcare, productivity approaches that leverage data to predict volume and other clinical challenges have the potential to make redesigning patient care and safety, managing hospital throughput, and improving clinician and patient satisfaction more science and less art. This data-driven approach also helps align and embed workforce optimization and planning with overall hospital strategic and operational planning" (Fitzpatrick et al., 2018, p. 3).

The midnight census has long been the cornerstone for determining how many nurses are needed for each shift, applying the number of patients on the unit at midnight for the entire 24-hour period. This measure is then lined up to the nursing unit's target for HPPD to determine the minimum number of nurses needed on the unit at any given time. The dynamic ADT activity experienced throughout the course of a day cannot be accurately represented by a midnight census.

When the logic of this exercise is examined, flaws emerge. How does the unit adjust to variations in patient demand throughout the day, and how do we know the census at midnight is not the lowest point of the day when applying it as an average? Given these caveats, potential understaffing or overstaffing is likely. Fig. 21.3 illustrates this "flaw of averages" on a surgical unit that has budgeted staffing based on an ACD of 25. As these data demonstrate, adjustments to staffing are required to accommodate actual demand, meaning that staff are sent home on Tuesday and costly premium labor such as overtime may be required on Thursdays (Fitzpatrick et al., 2018).

Big data analysis allows a view of demand data or patient census at the hourly level over the course of several years by extracting data directly from the electronic medical record (EMR). Understanding the census on a surgical unit at 2 pm on Tuesdays or 8 pm on Wednesdays over the course of several years provides valuable insight not only for staffing but will also inform multiple other operational processes such as surgical throughput, surgeon block scheduling, the delivery of supplies to the unit, and OR utilization, to name a few. This valuable census data, when combined with acuity data, will produce schedules that are significantly more accurate and predictable, requiring less

Exhibit B: Average Daily Census

Example

Tuesday and Thursday have the same **average demand** of 25, but Tuesday fluctuates between **18 and 32**, whereas Thursday fluctuates only between **22 and 28**. What is the "right" level of staffing?

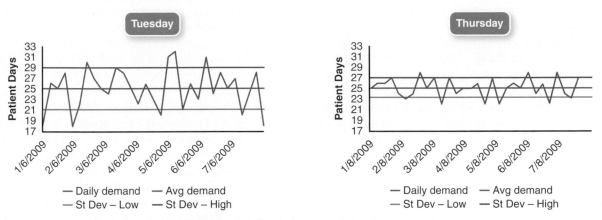

Fig. 21.3 Exhibit B: Average daily census.

last-minute adjustment. Seasonal, monthly, weekly, and daily demand patterns emerge that can provide the basis for aligning schedules and staffing patterns with demand. For example, in areas of the country impacted by seasonal weather patterns that may increase inpatient utilization, staffing can be adjusted upward to assure appropriate nurse availability.

How Does Optimization Work?

Optimization modeling based on linear programming is a computational methodology that not only solves this difficult problem with a single solution but also provides the *best* solution from a myriad of possibilities—often millions of possible solutions. The process of modeling is best described as mathematically representing every nuance or constraint and variable in the scheduling process, including demand, staffing models, and the quantification of every work rule.

To mathematically represent the staffing business problem, the optimization model illustrated in Fig. 21.4 includes the following:

- The business objectives, including the staffing model or desired ratio minimizing overall cost (best coverage at the lowest cost);

Exhibit C: What is optimization?

Optimization takes decision making from **what-if** to **what-is-best** solutions by applying sophisticated modeling to produce a staffing strategy **optimized** to **best coverage at the lowest cost**, while accommodating unique organizational and staff needs

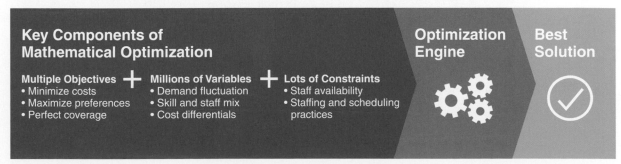

Fig. 21.4 Exhibit C: What is optimization?

- The decision variables such as skill mix, demand fluctuations, and the various costs of the staff (full time, part time, flexible staff);
- The business constraints such as staff availability, time off requirements, and various work rules or scheduling practices.

When conceptualizing this model, it is helpful to envision a giant Rubik's Cube, whereby every small square on the cube represents a distinct demand value or an individual work rule, practice, or process. The model is then dropped into a solver that essentially arranges the cube to produce the *best* answer for the business objective. For example, if a nurse could work no more than three consecutive 12-hour shifts, needed to be scheduled every other weekend, and needed to be paid overtime for hours over 40 each week, what is the optimal size and configuration of the position roster for this unit? Imagine the complexity of calculating this when considering the hourly demand patterns (Fitzpatrick, 2014; Fitzpatrick & Brooks, 2010; Gavigan et al., 2016).

When optimizing staffing, however, demand is only one of the myriad of complex variables that need to be considered. Work rules, policies, or terms within a labor contract also play a significant role in determining accurate staffing. Fig. 21.5 illustrates the significant impact of just the one work rule of weekend requirements. In this simple example, two nurses need to be scheduled for each day of the week. In the "every third weekend" example, in order to provide two nurses per day, two full-time (0.9) nurses are required in addition to four part-time (0.6) nurses. This model requires a total of six employees. By contrast, when the staff works every second weekend, four full-time (0.9) and only one part-time (0.6) nurses are required. During a period of nursing shortages, or if there are other prevailing market conditions, it is extremely important that the implications of various work rules are quantified as they relate to staffing plans as well as the overall staffing strategy (Brian J. Cole, personal communication, July 17, 2019).

Exhibit D: Weekend Pattern Work Rule Overview

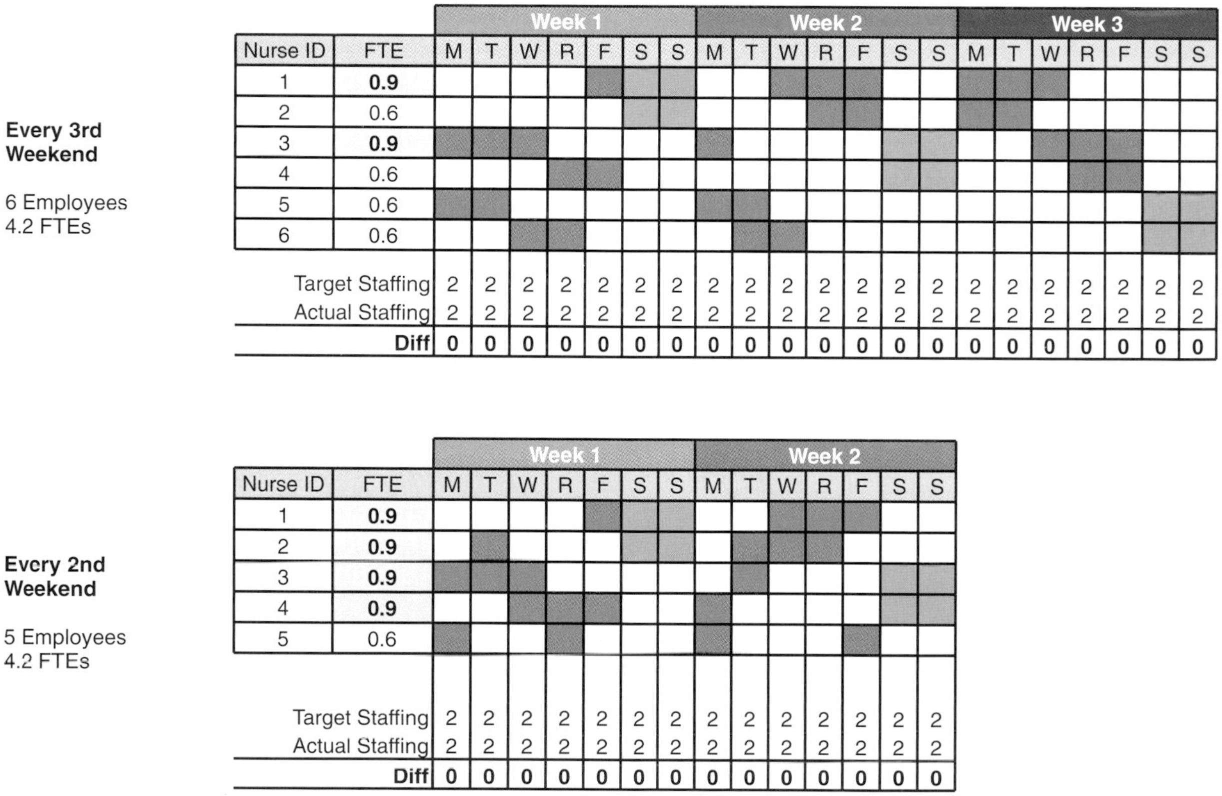

Fig. 21.5 Exhibit D: Weekend pattern work rule overview.

Exhibit E: Weekend Pattern FTE Impact (Sample of Large Academic Medical Center)

The **Every 2nd Weekend Model** requires **794 Total Employees**, with **total Core FTEs of 685.5**
The **Every 3rd Weekend Model** requires **933 Total Employees**, with **total Core FTEs of 678.3**

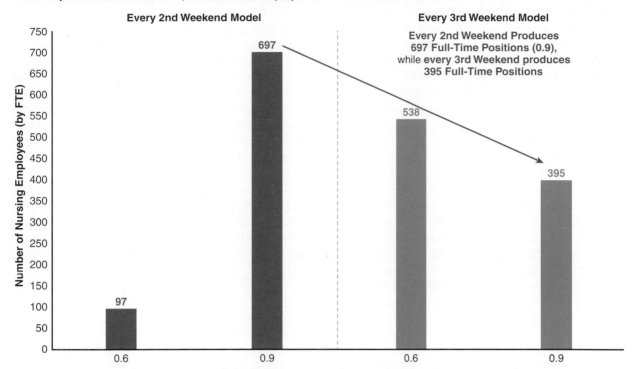

Fig. 21.6 Exhibit E: Weekend pattern FTE impact (sample of large academic medical center). *FTE,* full time equivalent.

Fig. 21.6 is another poignant example of the impact of various work rules on the overall staffing strategy. As illustrated, the weekend requirement changes the need for full-time (0.9) nurses by almost half. If this hospital were in a market where there were significantly more nurses preferring full-time employment, there would be negative consequences for their recruitment strategy (Brian J. Cole, personal communication, February 25, 2019).

More precise modeling of staffing to actual demand helps health care organizations meet staffing and scheduling challenges. Organizations using this scientific approach have seen significant improvement in their ability to have the appropriate nursing resources available when required, reduced staffing costs and demonstrating an improvement in staff satisfaction with the scheduling process. Using these big data analyses provides the evidence required to continue to innovate around staffing strategies, recognizing the complexity of this leadership responsibility.

Position Control

Irrespective of the methodology utilized to create a staffing strategy, once the staffing pattern for each unit has been established, the next step for safe staffing coverage is to provide a structured measurement and evaluation of position control. Future schedule coverage and adequate staffing first require that unit staff are available to work the needed shifts. Therefore, the hours of care requirement on a unit must be converted to the correct number of FTE positions. Position control, which can be thought of as the means to operationalize a budget, is the process of providing and measuring the correct FTE, or complement, to adequately staff a given area. Full-time and part-time mix, shift lengths, weekend commitments, and available contingency, or flex staff, are components to be analyzed to produce the ideal complement. The correct complement of full-time and part-time employees requires an understanding of the institution's non-patient care time and other budgeted activities (e.g., new staff orientation, continuing education) that are not included in the direct patient care hours required for the staffing pattern. An ideal measure of nursing staff adequacy considers intensity. A staffing adequacy measure needs to indicate the volume of nurses of a certain skill level needed for a given volume of patients and the given intensity of nursing care required for those patients.

Once position control is established to support the staffing patterns, vacancy and turnover rates need to be managed. A strategy for developing a recruitment pipeline and covering future vacant positions needs to be identified to prevent the use of costly, last-minute staff resources. For example, one organization reported actual cost savings by over-recruiting by 1.0 FTE in the ICU area, which resulted in lower use of more expensive contingency and external staff resources (Cipriano & Cutruzzula, 2007). With fiscal and human resources support, managers need to recruit and retain the FTE complement of the full-time and part-time mix needed for each staffing level. This will then increase the available resource pool to respond to higher-than-budgeted patient volume. Filled positions are the foundation for adequate, balanced work schedules.

Scheduling

Best practice for scheduling is a system that is automated, provides data-driven targets for core coverage, and engages staff members to participate in working specific shifts, hours, and days in their clinical area. The schedule typically spans a period of 4 to 6 weeks into the future. Staff members are usually hired by the organization with a commitment to work a number and type of hours (e.g., 36 hours, rotating day and night shifts). Balanced, flexible, and predictable work schedules are powerful human resource strategies for recruitment and retention, because, for nurses, choice over work schedules is one of the most important aspects of a healthy work environment (MacPhee & Borra, 2012). There is some controversy over the advantages of flexible self-scheduling versus fixed scheduling. Koning (2014) advocated for the freedom to organize shifts worked around nonwork commitments using self-scheduling; Kullberg and colleagues (2016) advocated for fixed scheduling because it lowered overtime. Whether utilizing a fixed or variable approach, creating predictability around schedules is of great benefit to the nurse in planning personal time as well as for the manager to assure adequate qualified resources for the unit.

An assessment of scheduling procedures should include the manager's role and time spent in scheduling. A recent strategy to better align the nurse manager's role to the accountabilities of the role included providing support through technology, staffing office assistants, and having staff members on scheduling committees. The manager's role is accountable for the oversight of the scheduling process, approval of the final complete schedule, and to assure that the schedule aligns with the budget. The final schedule then needs to be accessible electronically to all staff members, whether at work or remotely from home or on their cell phone. Maintaining a consistent annual schedule of the precise dates for each scheduling request period and for when the final schedule is available is a best practice for staff satisfaction and work–life balance. The managerial role shifts from time-consuming scheduling tasks to a role approving a complete schedule that meets the guidelines of the organization and *ANA's Principles for Nurse Staffing* (ANA, 2012).

The definition or perception of a "complete" schedule is likely as variable as nursing staff member satisfaction with staffing. Direct-care nurses, however, expect when a schedule is electronically submitted to their home computer or cell phone that is it complete. Specifically, the staff expects that RNs, LPNs/LVNs, UAP, unit secretaries, and key staff are scheduled to their target number for every shift of the schedule. Sharing the patient census and acuity trends by month, day of week, and time of day with the staff will foster mutual understanding in how targets are established. Dialogue about nurse staffing for patient care is credible when it is data driven. Direct-care nurses expect that there will be a clinical expert on every shift and that new graduates are distributed across shifts with their preceptors. These are a few examples of how nursing leaders at all levels may engage staff to develop value statements and data-driven guidelines that serve to explicitly and transparently articulate the organization's scheduling process. Many scheduling committees have developed such documents to reflect values such as a shared commitment to safe and excellent nursing care for all patients and families, support for staff members' pursuit of education leading to a bachelor of science in nursing, fairness in scheduling the major holidays (e.g., Thanksgiving, Christmas, and New Year), fiscal stewardship to not pre-schedule overtime, guidelines for numbers of staff vacations at one time by role, clarity in self-service dates for scheduling and communication, fatigue management guidelines, and a fair on-call schedule.

Demand Management

Demand management as a discipline focuses on (1) measuring, predicting, and understanding demand for an institution's products and services; (2) deploying resources and management to ensure that demand is met in the way the consumer's wants and needs are satisfied; and (3) directing demand as feasible to optimize patient placement, workload, and throughput, along with operational needs. For hospitals, a key component of the "product and service" equation is high-quality, safe patient care, with the goal of having the patient leave the hospital with the best care experience, in the shortest amount of time and at the lowest cost care (Pickard & Warner, 2007). McDonough (2013) described an evidence-based optimum staffing method based on patient demand with a focus on work activities. Time observations determined nursing work activities and were then matched to patient demand by hour of day and day of the week.

An often-overlooked strategy for creating predictable and cost-effective staffing is the need to staff according to real-time patient information or to make staffing decisions that facilitate individual patients moving through their stay as quickly as possible with high-quality, safe care (throughput or patient flow initiatives). Because most staffing plans staff to average forecasted care levels, periods of higher patient volume and/or acuity levels or peaks may create serious stressors for both patients and nurses. Severe stress occurs with sustained peaks of volume or acuity. Litvak and colleagues (2005) described the following three types of stress intrinsic to daily operations:

- Flow stress, representing the rapid rate of patients presenting for hospital care
- Clinical stress, which is expressed in the variability in type and severity of disease
- Stress caused by competing responsibilities of health care providers.

System stress introduced by demand for nurses to care for more or sicker patients has been shown to be a leading cause of adverse patient outcomes (Litvak et al., 2005). When variability is minimized and/or better predicted, a hospital has greater resources for the remaining patient-driven peaks in demand over which it has no control. Effective staffing requires an assessment of

demand variability or the required hourly nursing care for each day on each unit. Ways to control variability (and hence decrease peaks and valleys) include better planning for scheduled events such as elective OR procedures, physician vacations or major conferences, seasonal variations, integration to patient flow and bed management systems, better control over bed assignments based on current unit workload, and improved planning for discharges—all of which decrease the demand and stress for nursing resources.

Computer technologies and big data analysis that continuously track and predict demand assist managers with variability analysis and prospective planning for predicted variability. These data support managerial decisions for non-traditional shorter shifts for the care areas that have high requirements at select predictable portions of the day. Predictive modeling can forecast unplanned patient and staff events, such as admissions by day of week and unplanned sick calls. These data are also helpful in understanding patient movement through the system, including inter-institutional transfers in large health systems.

Several examples driven by data include higher cesarean section rates in a labor and delivery unit may necessitate two RNs in the OR; infant births that are higher in the evening than during the day may require a shift of resources from days to evenings; or late-afternoon patient transfers from the recovery room after neurosurgery on Tuesdays and Thursdays may require an increase in RN staff for those days and specific hours in a neurosurgical ICU.

Pickard and Warner (2007) outlined the essential components for effective demand management as the following 10 principles:

1. Being based on patient outcomes (how well they are progressing)
2. Being focused on the individual patient
3. Incorporating progress goals for each patient throughout their stay with which actual progress may be compared
4. Continuously measuring progress in real time so that decisions can be made as the patient's needs change (rather than once a shift or once a day, which inherently bases decisions on information that is typically 8 to 16 hours old)
5. Being projected into the near future (several days ahead) to allow time for optimal staffing decisions to be made while there is still time for numerous

choices among available caregivers and cost-effective options

6. Being able to be embedded in a decision support system

7. Being acceptable to all stakeholders, especially administration and finance, to avoid organizational polarity

8. Producing a need for care in terms of not only quantity and skill but also the caregiver attributes necessary to provide optimal care for the patient

9. Using outcomes-driven acuity system based on an established taxonomy for assessing and documenting patient care on outcomes

10. Incorporating all presently and planned electronically available data to reduce nursing time in data gathering and provide as much real-time, valid data as possible

"Incorporating these elements is not a simple task but doing so offers significant advantages and benefits. By focusing on the individual patient, with individual outcome progress goals for each patient, hospitals can achieve results not previously addressed with traditional models" (Pickard & Warner, 2007, p. 31). In addition, this allows organizations to be informed and responsive when a select population of patients typically cared for in one location is housed in a new location. These results include (1) best-practice staffing protocols based on what is called "true (outcomes-oriented) demand" and the optimal staffing levels to move a patient through each phase of their stay as quickly as possible, (2) early identification of patients who are not moving through their hospital stay as planned, and (3) improved near-term projection and prediction of staffing needs. These data are a vital part of service line management, which may include various venues of care, both inpatient as well as ambulatory.

Staffing Allocation and Resource Pool

Even with the best planning and most accurate prediction of supply and demand, uncontrolled events such as unexpected high demand and sick calls are intrinsic to the health care environment and overall personnel management. Key to effective staffing are protocols and processes for daily staffing decision support that are aligned with a budget-sensitive variable staffing plan. In a decentralized model, individual department managers and directors are responsible for daily staffing allocation. Units with decentralized staffing are typically units

in which volume and/or acuity may be most unpredictable and the nursing competencies are unique to that area (e.g., emergency department, labor and delivery, critical care). However, a decentralized model places a higher level of staffing responsibility on managers, which may take them away from other more strategic responsibilities.

In contrast, centralized staffing is filtered through a central staffing office, which maintains responsibility for ensuring adequate staffing for multiple units or for multiple hospitals or business units in larger systems. Centralized staffing offers the benefit of being able to view supply and demand from an enterprise perspective. With patient acuity, nursing competencies, and available staff viewed across multiple units, staffing resources can be optimized by increasing staff in one area and reducing staff in another to accommodate variable patient demand. Staffing protocols for obtaining supplemental staff can be standardized, such as procedures for using internal staff, per diems, and external sources (e.g., travelers and agency). The staffing office can relieve nurse managers and/or charges nurses of the time-consuming administrative task of responding to sick calls and obtaining supplemental staff. In addition, the central staffing office provides a command center with protocols and information to manage disasters in which staff must be quickly obtained and deployed.

The downside to relying solely on a centralized staffing office is that it can become too remote from the unit, thus losing some of the intelligence that may be considered when making staffing decisions (Lauw & Gares, 2005). Policies and procedures clearly define the roles and responsibilities and communication among areas. But as with any of these staffing models, the key to eliminating chaotic, last-minute staffing decisions is to adopt predictive tools and move more of the staffing decisions to the near future or the next 2 to 4 days (Pickard & Warner, 2007). Assessment and analysis of staffing needs in the near future provide more available options, including more competent staff, at optimal costs.

Computerized staffing systems play a pivotal role in providing what is described as a "single version of the truth" and offering decision support such as staffing variances across units, workload indicators, employee competencies, and decision costs. Many of these systems interface with time and attendance systems and therefore provide various productivity reports, dashboards, or other performance metrics required by managers.

Information for staffing decisions must be readily available and accurate. Staffing systems serve as a communication tool for all staffing "stakeholders," including employees, unit managers, centralized staffing office, and executives. Staffing systems also offer automated open-shift management, which posts open shifts electronically to qualified staff. Protocols direct which personnel are the best qualified and the most cost effective to fill needed shifts. The staffing system measures and reports the staffing management performance at both unit and organization levels, providing staffing effectiveness data for the organization.

Access to nurses outside the unit to cover transient shortages is critical to meet last-minute, unplanned nurse shortages, such as sick calls, and high patient demand. Supplemental staffing resources—frequently referred to as the *staffing pool*—are defined as a group of nurses who supplement the core unit staffing. This includes per diem nurses, float pool nurses, part-time nurses desiring additional hours, seasonal nurses, agency nurses, and traveling nurses. The scope of clinical competency, pay rates, and contractual arrangements varies among these internal and external pools of nurses as well. For example, select nurses may be competent to work on all of the adult medical–surgical units, whereas other specialty nurses may be competent to work in several areas, such as perioperative practice sites, or only one area, such as labor and delivery, the emergency department, or the dialysis unit.

Supplemental staffing resource guidelines need to be established to direct the use of additional resources detailing the data for decision-making and algorithms for staffing. These guidelines are designed to prevent depletion of supplemental resources for core staff coverage and instead to reserve them for unexpected intervals of high acuity or transient shortages. For example, a guideline may direct the use of a part-time nurse who has signed up to work extra shifts to fill a sick call, then to use a supplemental float pool nurse, and finally to use an external agency nurse if previous resources are unavailable. The option for overtime is also a consideration based on policy regarding the fatigue associated with excessive hours in a day or days worked in a row and cost. The costs associated with each resource progression are then inherently built into the staffing decision model. Additional strategies for covering long-term family medical leaves are also needed to meet core coverage. Strategies for covering these longer-term shortages are critical, otherwise a manager is depleting the resource pools intended for last-minute and transient shortages.

Operational metrics for the supplemental resource pool are not only defined for daily staffing allocation but also may be defined during the scheduling stage. The operational total nurse vacancy rate for scheduling purposes is defined as all budgeted nurse positions that are vacant during the scheduling period, including the unfilled or vacant positions and positions for which nurses are on short-term or long-term leaves of absence (e.g., Family and Medical Leave Act [FMLA], workers' compensation). For example, if a unit has an operational RN vacancy rate of 5% to 10%, it may be approved to cover the shortage with part-time nurses working additional shifts and possibly overtime but would not be approved for agency nurses. Alternatively, a unit with a 22% operational RN vacancy rate may be approved for longer-term contracted higher labor expense (e.g., travelers). Defining operational vacancy rates and incremental resource actions are important aspects of consistently managing staff shortages and ensuring a standard of care delivery. As such, protocols driven by operational vacancy rates generate consistency in how higher labor costs are aligned with the greatest need. In addition, wages, benefits, transfers, and work policies of supplemental internal float pools should be carefully designed so that the stability of unit-based core nursing staff is not compromised.

Fitzpatrick and Brooks (2010) and Gavigan and colleagues (2016) called for the optimization of human capital as a staffing consideration. These authors believe that there is a need to build a scaffolding structure to allow for optimal mathematical optimization for best staffing solutions. Box 21.4 lists criteria to optimize modeling of staffing for best solutions.

BOX 21.4 Criteria for Optimization of Staffing

1. Multiple objectives
   +
2. Variables
   +
3. Constraints

Optimization Modeling for Best Solutions

From Fitzpatrick, T., & Brooks, B. (2010). The nurse leader as logistician: Optimizing human capital. *Journal of Nursing Administration, 40* (2), 69–74.

Patient Assignments

Nurse managers are responsible not only for forthcoming schedules and immediate staffing but also for ensuring that the patient care assignments reflect appropriate use of personnel considering scope of practice, competencies, patient needs, and complexity of care. Patient assignment in hospitals is defined as the task of assigning the scheduled staff to specific patients for the shift duration. Nurse managers in hospitals typically delegate assignment making to the charge nurse in the patient care area. The charge nurse is responsible for matching the qualified caregivers to meet the patients' needs and for providing a balanced workload across caregivers. Often the nursing care delivery model articulates the value of nurse-to-patient continuity across time. A balanced workload enables nurses to provide reasonable equity in nursing care delivery to patients and their families. In addition, the staff members expect the charge nurse to create equitable assignments as a valued measure of fairness in workload distribution. Many organizations require an annual charge nurse competency review and peer feedback demonstrating effective assignment making.

In the staffing management framework, the patient assignment is the point at which individual patients are linked with individual nurses. Welton (2010) identified this as a critical new level of analysis to examine the relationship between staffing and clinical quality and cost that may better inform operational decision-making.

ORGANIZATIONAL OUTCOMES

Staffing Effectiveness

ANA says that identifying and maintaining the appropriate number and mix of nursing staff are central to the provision of quality care (ANA, 2016b). Optimal nurse staffing is fiscally responsible and appropriate to patients' needs. Hospital organizations examine the relationships between staffing and nurse-sensitive outcomes to meet TJC staffing effectiveness requirements showing that there is the appropriate number, competency, and skill mix of staff in relation to the provision of needed care and treatment. However, staffing for effectiveness, including cost effectiveness, is highly complex and a critical issue for nurse leaders.

The Staffing Evidence on Quality

The link between nurse staffing and quality of care is evidence based and long-standing. Better RN staffing has been shown to reduce patient mortality, enhance outcomes, and improve nurse satisfaction (Mensik, 2014). Over a decade of rigorous studies and a summary of current research conducted by the Ruckelshaus Center at the University of Washington concluded that "fewer patients per nurse or more NHPPD is associated with fewer adverse outcomes—in particular mortality, failure to rescue, and some specific adverse events among surgical patients" (Mitchell, 2008, p. 30). Comprehensive reviews of staffing evidence and sentinel works are available (Aiken et al., 2002, 2003, 2014; Blegen et al., 1998; Needleman et al., 2002, 2006, 2011; Unruh, 2008). These studies and a meta-analysis by Kane and colleagues (2007a,b) demonstrated the strong evidence linking inadequate staffing with adverse events and failure to rescue. Frith and colleagues (2010) found that higher RN staffing was associated with a reduced LOS among community hospitals. These findings suggest the direct fiscal impact that nurses have on hospital margin today (Bogue, 2012). A body of research over at least the past decade has shown that sufficient nurse staffing levels and favorable work environments function to facilitate nurses' effectiveness as a surveillance system. Sufficient numbers of RNs are necessary to manage complex patient care needs and identify and intervene when something goes wrong (McHugh et al., 2016). Because research continues to confirm the many associations of nurse staffing with outcomes, innovative and technology-based strategies are being employed to more precisely manage staffing for quality outcomes.

Hospitals routinely employ supplemental nurses to provide additional resources to cover transient shortages. However, little is known about this nurse workforce and its relationship to quality of care. Aiken and colleagues (2007) examined the characteristics of supplemental nurses and the relationships of the supplemental staff to nurse outcomes and adverse events. Their findings suggested that widely held negative perceptions of temporary nurses may be unfounded. However, the effect on the organization's culture is unknown but suspected to be disruptive. The employment patterns of nurses and their effect on cost and quality is an important area needing further study.

Nurse leaders at all levels are called to action to incorporate relevant scientific findings in staffing administrative policy and practice and to lead the evaluation of all innovations in care delivery. Balancing these decisions with organizational fiscal constraints and conducting cost-effectiveness analyses are the current challenges for organizations and nurse leaders.

CURRENT ISSUES AND TRENDS

There is an increasing call to use technology and innovate with scheduling. Fitzpatrick (2015) suggested nurses reflect on the airline industry and how they have managed to coordinate flights, maintenance, staggering across different time zones, and weather conditions. These industries use logistics science and a form of mathematical modeling called optimization to solve scheduling problems. Logistic science offers new insights in planning and deployment of clinical workers because it recognizes the complexities and interconnectedness of the systems and processes involved in scheduling and deploying nurses (Joseph & Fowler, 2016).

Fitzpatrick (2015) illustrated how the field of nursing has started to transition from standardized, computerized scheduling to the use of sophisticated, algorithmically driven applications like how the airline industry used logistics science and a form of mathematical modeling called optimization to solve scheduling problems. To ensure optimization of staffing modeling, the author calls for three key variables: (1) business objectives such as staffing costs and ensuring adequate coverage, (2) decision variables such as skill mix and cost differences, and (3) business constraints such as vacancy rates, work rules (e.g., weekend requirement), and cultural issues such as being off for Mother's Day. The use of optimization can move decision-making from "what-if" to "what is the best" solution. When all these factors are considered, there is more precise modeling of staffing to actual demands, allowing health care organizations to meet staffing and scheduling challenges. Additionally, the process of optimization cuts the time spent on scheduling by 50%. Nurse leaders need to reflect on how they have mastered modeling with care processes such as medication administration and use that experience as a requisite to optimize problems with staffing and scheduling (Fitzpatrick, 2015).

In the quest to validate nursing's value, the next two discussions illustrate good examples of how the appropriate data can guide administrators with appropriate decision-making for staffing. Pappas and colleagues (2015) called for greater precision with staffing. The authors demonstrated that approaches to minimize patient risks are needed to avoid unwanted clinical and subsequent negative financial outcome. The authors advocated for staffing models that are based on unit-specific data that incorporate the nurse's view of the amount of surveillance to prevent hospital-acquired harm and the associated costs.

Pruinelli and colleagues (2016) stated that the emergence of Big Data for data analytics is poised to influence the value of nurses' work. Their recent article advocates for the use of the nursing management minimum data set (NMMDS) in conjunction with staffing systems in electronic health systems. The NMMDS is an evidence-based tool that defines and measures the context of care within and across all enterprise settings. Use of the NMMDS provides data about variables affecting the delivery of timely, cost-effective care. This knowledge is critical to maintain clinical and operational excellence. The authors advocated for integration of data from multiple sources because this helps nurse leaders to balance workloads, thus improving patient outcomes and nurse satisfaction. Technology that integrates elements of the NMMDS for staffing or other complex management decisions can return valuable hours to the nurse leaders. This is the emergence of Big Data for data analytics.

A health care system in Oregon underwent a transformation to define and implement staffing and scheduling by using software to optimize scheduling. The criteria included a simple and easy-to-use network, remote and mobile access, integration of personal calendars, and time and attendance. Intelligence included definitions, predictive staffing, acuity-based scheduling, and patient acuity. Customization included staffing based on skill mix, with customization of reports, shifts, and dashboards. Bonus features were ease of build, maintenance, upgrades, and successful integration.

The Magnet Recognition Program® continues to be a driver of current staffing trends. For more than 20 years, Magnet designation has been associated with healthier work environments (better staffing—excluding California, where there is a state-mandated ratio; lower burnout; lower turnover; and improved RN–MD collaboration) (Kelly et al., 2011) and higher-quality patient care. Achieving Magnet designation has been increasingly associated with quality. It is now incorporated in the scoring for *U.S. News & World Report's* Best Hospitals in America Honor Roll and earns full credit for Safe Practice Standard #9 Nursing Workforce in the Leapfrog Hospital Survey, which scores hospitals on their commitment to staffing with highly trained nurses. A number of the hospital financial credit rating agencies utilize Magnet designation in their evaluation of an organization's operating performance.

Given the advent of value-based purchasing (VBP) and the CMS provision 1533-F, health care leaders have been incentivized to focus on improving care processes. CMS provides health care coverage for 80 million Americans via Medicaid, Medicare, and state children's programs and represents the largest payer in the world, administering more than $800 billion in benefits annually. Many of the clinical processes and patient satisfaction measures under VBP are directly affected by the quality and quantity of nursing care, and the outcomes will have a significant impact on the key metrics that will drive hospital reimbursements (Bogue, 2012).

Since CMS provision 1533-F became effective on October 1, 2008, hospitals are not being reimbursed for hospital-acquired conditions (HACs). These are conditions such as skin pressure ulcers, urinary tract infections, ventilator-acquired pneumonia, and falls with injury that occurred within the hospital stay and were not present on admission (POA). Among the 14 HACs in the provision, at least nine of the conditions are sensitive to nursing care intervention. Thus, hospitals have new financial incentives to support both nursing education and appropriate staffing to prevent HACs, reduce costs, and increase reimbursement. In addition, the Patient Protection and Affordable Care Act (ACA) mandates 2% of hospitals' Medicare payment will be at risk under value-based payments in 2017. Penalties for certain 30-day admissions began in 2012. The LOS and readmissions financial penalties are the most compelling incentives for hospitals to support the appropriate amount of nursing care that is of high quality because of the known positive effect of nursing care and coordination on patients' transitions of care and acute care LOS (Frith et al., 2010). The nurse's inherent role in discharge planning with the interdisciplinary team, linkages to community services, and effective medication, symptom, and disease management teaching in all care settings is becoming increasingly important to organizational outcomes.

There are national policy initiatives to identify and make visible nursing care in the US health care reimbursement system. It has long been known that nursing care historically has been bundled within the "room and board" hospital charges, which do not capture the variability in nursing care costs. Given the variability in nursing care intensity and cost of nurse staffing, this traditional costing system has resulted in cost compression and distortion in the inpatient prospective payment system (Dalton, 2007). A proposed solution separates nursing care from the room and board charges and accounts for this care as a variable, direct cost within the billing system based on actual nursing time delivered to patients (Welton & Harris, 2007; Welton et al., 2006). Finkler and colleagues (2013) describe this as nursing as a revenue center and explain the use of variable billing. Even in a bundled payment system, nurses need both cost and productivity data to better manage care for both efficiency and effectiveness. Welton (2010) suggested a new value-based nursing care model, including (1) allocating nursing cost and intensity to each patient, (2) new metrics that link nursing-specific outcomes to individual patients, and (3) moving the focus from staffing to the assignment of caregivers to individual patients. Simpson (2012) further called to action the adoption of technology at the point of care to achieve value-based nursing care.

These current issues in health care policy raise the visibility and importance of nursing care in society and create a climate to advocate for safe, cost-effective, high-quality nursing care for all. Current issues and trends in staffing and scheduling demonstrate that nursing has transformed its thinking and approaches based on the evolving science of systems theory, technology, advanced mathematics, and logistics science—as well as human capital and social theory—to optimize its staffing needs.

RESEARCH NOTE

Purpose

The Affordable Care Act's Readmission Reduction Program penalizes hospitals based on excess readmission rates among Medicare beneficiaries. Many evidence-based interventions that reduce readmissions are grounded in the fundamentals of basic nursing care. Hospitals with higher nurse staffing had 25% lower odds of being penalized compared with similar hospitals with lower staffing.

Discussion

Effective October 2012, the Centers for Medicare & Medicaid Services (CMS) implemented a policy under the Affordable Care Act intended to curb the estimated $15 billion Medicare spends annually on preventable readmissions. The logic behind the Hospital Readmissions Reduction Program (HRRP) is that hospitals can reduce readmissions by implementing evidence-based practice standards of care, specifically focused on single disease-based populations such as heart failure. Many of these interventions, known to reduce complications and readmissions, such as discharge planning, care coordination, and patient education are clearly within the scope and responsibility of nursing. Further evidence suggests that hospitals that staff for manageable nurse workloads have lower readmission rates.

These researchers studied the impact of nurse staffing on readmission penalties by analyzing the CMS HRRP data for fiscal year 2012 and compared these data to nurse staffing as reported in the American Hospital Association (AHA) Annual Survey for the same time period. Staffing was measured as the ratio of registered nurse hours per adjusted patient day. Full time equivalent registered nurse staffing was multiplied by 1768 and divided by adjusted patient days to determine average hours per adjusted patient day.

Adjusting readmissions for other factors such as racial, ethnic, and socioeconomic factors, the researchers observed a significant and consistent difference in readmission penalties when nurse staffing levels were higher. In fact, their estimates suggest that each additional nurse hour per adjusted patient day was associated with 10% lower odds of being penalized.

Application to Practice

This important work adds to the growing literature that describes the implications of nurse staffing on multiple clinical outcomes including surgical complications, falls, and hospital acquired infections, to name a few. Understanding how to define adequate staffing by patient type continues to be a challenge, however, yet the ramifications of not doing so create significance consequences for individual patients and the financial health of organizations generally. The mechanism by which better staffing affects readmissions is multifactorial considering the presence of and need for nursing care across the duration of patients' hospitalizations. Nurses are responsible for the core processes that have been widely associated with readmissions: discharge planning, patient and family education, complication surveillance and intervention, knowledge assessment, and care coordination. By focusing on a system factor such as nurse staffing, leaders may be able to address multiple quality issues while reducing their likelihood of penalties for readmissions. Policy makers also may be able to gain traction on complications and attendant costs through policy that creates a care environment sufficiently staffed and resourced to allow nurses to do their important work more effectively.

NEXT-GENERATION NCLEX® EXAMINATION-STYLE CASE STUDY

Nurse Manager Dan's budget has been cut and is projected to have increasing cuts over the next two years due to COVID-19 implications. He made the decision to not hire new employees and use the existing employees to cover staffing needs. Employees on his unit are feeling overworked. Many employees are being asked to do mandatory overtime without adequate compensation. Dan's director was told by human resources that employees are feeling overwhelmed with the increasing staffing demands without adequate compensation. The director pulls Dan's non- salary YTD expense report to examine where opportunities may exist to reallocate funds towards staffing.

NEXT-GENERATION NCLEX® EXAMINATION-STYLE CASE STUDY—cont'd

Question

Utilizing the non-salary expense report, the director makes the recommendation for Dan to redirect dollars from some itemized items in the budget. Dan decides to redirect budgetary dollars. Which indicate an effective strategy to fund staffing? **Select all that apply.**

1. Redirect dollars from food service to staffing
2. Redirect dollars from equipment rental to staffing
3. Redirect dollars from departmental supplies to staffing
4. Redirect dollars from travel to staffing
5. Redirect dollars from other expenses to staffing

YTD Non-Salary Expense Report

Non-salary expense	Actual	Budget	Var%	Prior
Purchase Professional	350	0	0.0%	0
Patient Nonchargeable (e.g., Kleenex, bath wipes, deodorant)	100,655	60,656	(65.0%)	59,999
Drugs	0	178	100.0%	0
Food service	6,252	4,200	(48.0)%	4,736
Medical supplies	0	449	100.0%	0
Department Supplies	8,668	8,546	(1.4)%	5,429
Forms and access to databases	1,025	1,255	18.3%	1,204
Minor equipment (e.g., vital signs machine, I.V. vein finder)	0	1,080	100%	0
Equipment Rental (e.g., wound VAC, low bed, bariatric bed)	6,148	6,800	9.5%	1,529
Publications	350	50	(600)%	44
Dues and Memberships	0	8	100%	0
Travel	567	1,058	46.4%	1,325
Other Expenses (e.g., outside catering, holiday parties, recognition trophies)	0	8000	100%	3,000
Total Non-salary expenses	124,015	92,280	34.3%	77,266

CRITICAL THINKING EXCERCISE

Gizelle Guadalupe is a new manager on the busiest medical and surgical unit in a tertiary hospital. There are 39 beds on 9 Tower, which has a high volume of diabetic and other patients with multisystemic clinical conditions requiring complex care planning. She is excited to improve the quality and outcomes on this unit. During her interview, she learned that under the previous leadership the quality was deteriorating, as reflected in the Hospital Consumer Assessment of Healthcare Providers and Systems (HCHAPS) scores, staff absenteeism, and increasing turnover rates. It was costing the unit between $42,000 to $65,000 to replace a nurse, including the cost of recruitment and temporarily filling the vacancy at premium labor costs, as well as the immeasurable costs to quality outcomes.

While making rounds, Manager Guadalupe observed complaints about missed nursing care from all shifts and decided to make staff accountable for ensuring that patient care is completed. She asked a Clinical Nurse Leader (CNL) to monitor the types of patient care activities that were being omitted. After 1 week, the CNL stated that it was difficult to make that determination because everyone had a different opinion on which interventions were being omitted. Additionally, she reported that staffing was an issue. The manager's initial response was, "What's wrong with staffing? Why would you blame staffing for omissions in patient care?"

1. Based on documented evidence in the literature, does staffing and resource allocation play a role in clinical outcomes, including the omission of various elements of patient care?
2. What types of quantitative data would you look at to determine if indeed nursing care was inadvertently being omitted? Additionally, what types of analyses would you perform to understand the root cause of missed care?
3. What questions could you pose to frontline nurses to understand how their staffing experience related to missed care?
4. Whom will you engage institutionally to understand the issue fully? Why them?
5. Which qualitative data elements may be required to build a case for staffing and missed nursing care?
6. What ideas would you propose to administration to reverse the financial effects and improve HCHAPS scores?
7. Presuming you receive support to implement your ideas, how would you measure and monitor the outcomes of your plans?

REFERENCES

Aiken, L. H., Clarke, S. P., Cheung, R. B., Sloane, D. M., & Silber, J. H. (2003). Educational levels of hospital nurses and surgical patient mortality. *Journal of the American Medical Association, 290*(12), 1617–1623.

Aiken, L. H., Clarke, S. P., Sloane, D. M., Sochalski, J., & Silber, J. H. (2002). Hospital nurse staffing and patient mortality, nurse burnout, and job dissatisfaction. *Journal of the American Medical Association, 288*(16), 1987–1993.

Aiken L. H., Sloane D. M., Bruyneel L., Van den Heede K., Griffiths P., Busse R., et al. (2014). Nurse staffing and education and hospital mortality in nine European countries: A retrospective observational study. *Lancet, 383*(9931), 1824–1830.

Aiken L. H., Sloane D. M., Griffiths P., Rafferty A. M., Bruyneel L., McHugh M., et al. (2016). Nursing skill mix in European hospitals: Cross-sectional study of the association with mortality, patient ratings, and quality of care. *BMJ Quality & Safety*, 1–10. http://qualitysafety.bmj.com/content/early/2016/11/03/bmjqs-2016-005567.full.pdf+html.

Aiken, L. H., Xue, Y., Clarke, S. P., & Sloane, D. M. (2007). Supplemental nurse staffing in hospitals and quality of care. *Journal of Nursing Administration, 37*(7–8), 335–342.

American Academy of Ambulatory Care Nursing (AAACN). (2005). *Ambulatory care nurse staffing: An annotated bibliography*. Author.

American Academy of Pediatrics (AAP) and the American College of Obstetricians and Gynecologists (ACOG). (2012). *Guidelines for perinatal care* (7th ed.). March of Dimes.

American Association of Colleges of Nursing (AACN). (2007). *White paper on the education and role of the clinical nurse leader*. Author.

American Association of Critical-Care Nurses. (2016). *AACN synergy model for patient care*. http://www.aacn.org/wd/certifications/content/synmodel.pcms?menu=certification.

American Nurses Association (ANA). (n.d.). *Safe staffing: The registered nurse safe staffing act HR 876/S.58*. http://www.nursingworld.org/SafeStaffingFactsheet.aspx.

American Nurses Association (ANA). (2010). *Nursing's social policy statement: The essence of the profession* (3rd ed.). Author.

American Nurses Association (ANA). (2012). *ANA's principles for nurse staffing* (2nd ed..) Author.

American Nurses Association (ANA). (2015a). *Code of ethics for nurses with interpretive statements*. Author.

American Nurses Association (ANA). (2015b). *The registered nurse safe staffing act HR2083/S.1132*. https://www.nursingworld.org/news/news-releases/2018/ana-applauds-nurse-staffing-legislation/.

American Nurses Association (ANA). (2016a). *Nurse staffing*. https://www.nursingworld.org/practice-policy/nurse-staffing/.

American Nurses Association (ANA). (2016b). *Nurse Staffing*. https://www.nursingworld.org/practice-policy/nurse-staffing/nurse-staffing-advocacy/.

American Nurses Association (2020). *Patient Acuity/Classification Systems (PCAS)*. https://www.nursingworld.org/practice-policy/nurse-staffing/workforce-management-pcas.

American Organization of Nurse Executives (AONE). (2000). *Staffing management and methods: Tools and techniques for nurse leaders*. Author.

Association of Perioperative Registered Nurses (AORN). (2014). *AORN position statement on perioperative safe staffing and on-call practices*. Author. https://www.aorn.org/guidelines/clinical-resources/position-statements.

Association of Women's Health, Obstetric and Neonatal Nurses (AWHONN). (2010). *Guidelines for professional registered nurse staffing for perinatal units*. Author.

Aydelotte, M. K.. *Nurse staffing methodology: A review and critique of selected literature*. US Department of Health,

Education and Welfare, Division of Nursing. Publication No. (NIH) (1973) Government Printing Office pp. 73–433.

Blegen, M. A, Goode, C. J., & Reed, L. (1998). Nurse staffing and patient outcomes. *Nursing Research, 47*(1), 43–50.

Bogue, R. J. (2012, May 29). Nurses: Key to making or breaking your future margin. *Hospitals and Health Networks*.

Brenan, M. (2018, December 20). Nurses again outpace other professions for honesty, ethics. *Gallup*. https://news.gallup.com/poll/245597/nurses-again-outpace-professions-honesty-ethics.aspx.

Brennan, C. W., & Daly, B. J. (2008). Patient acuity: a concept analysis. *Journal of Advanced Nursing, 65*(5), 1114–1126.

Case Management Society of America (CMSA). (2016). *What is a case manager?* Little Rock, AR: Author. http://www.cmsa.org/Home/CMSA/WhatisaCaseManager/tabid/224/Default.aspx.

Cipriano, P., & Cutruzzula, J. (2007). Over-recruiting: Breaking the short staffing and turnover cycle. *Nurse Leader, 5*(6), 28–32.

Clancy, T. R. (2007). Planning: what we can learn from complex systems science. *Journal of Nursing Administration, 37*(1), 436–439.

Clancy, T. R. (2007). Organizing: new ways to harness complexity. *Journal of Nursing Administration, 37*(12), 534–536.

Clarke, S. P. (2005). The policy implications of staffing-outcomes research. *Journal of Nursing Administration, 35*(1), 17–19.

Dalton, K. (2007). *A study of charge compression in calculating DRG relative weights*. Centers for Medicaid & Medicare Services (CMS): Contract no. 500-00-0024-TO18 Baltimore, MD: CMS.

Dent, R. L., & Bradshaw, P. (2012). Building the business case for acuity-based staffing. *Nurse Leader, 10*(2), 26–28.

DNV. (2019). *DNV GL- Healthcare NIAHO accreditation requirements, interpretive guidelines and surveyor guidance*. https://www.dnvgl.us/assurance/healthcare/standards/niaho-ac-dl.html.

Donabedian, A. (1966). Evaluating the quality of medical care. *Milbank Memorial Fund Quarterly, 44*(3), 166–206.

Eck Birmingham, S. (2010). Evidenced-based staffing: The next step. *Nurse Leader, 8*(3), 24–26, 35.

Eck Birmingham, S., Nell, K., & Abe, N. (2011). Determining staffing needs based on patient outcomes vs. patient interventions. In P. Cowan, & S. Moorhead (Eds.), *Current issues in nursing* (8th ed., pp. 391–404): Mosby Elsevier.

Edwardson, S. (2007). Conceptual frameworks used in funded nursing health services research projects. *Nursing Economics, 25*(4), 222–227.

Emergency Nurses Association (ENA). (2015). *Staffing and productivity in the emergency care setting*. https://www.ena.org/docs/default-source/resource-library/practice-resources/position-statements/staffingandproductivityemergencydepartment.pdf?sfvrsn=c57dcf13_8.

Finkler, S. A., Jones, C. B., & Kovner, C. T. (2013). *Financial management for nurse managers and executives* (4th ed.). Saunders.

Fitzpatrick, T. A. (2014). Does the package delivery industry hold the answer to our scheduling problems? *American Nurse Today, 9*(3), 48–54.

Fitzpatrick, T., & Brooks, B. (2010). The nurse leader as logistician: Optimizing human capital. *Journal of Nursing Administration, 40*(2), 69–74.

Fitzpatrick, T., Goetz, K., & Cole, B. (2018). Advanced analytics must drive the next round of productivity initiatives. *Healthcare Cost Containment (Newsletter of the Healthcare Financial Management Association)*, 1–4.

Fitzpatrick, T., Anen, T., & Martinez-Soto, E. (2013). Nurse staffing: The Illinois experience. *Nursing Economics, 31*(5), 221–229.

Fitzpatrick, T. (2015, June 24). *Clinical labor optimization: Managing supply and demand in a dynamic environment*. International webinar innovations for advancing nursing administration [Webinar]..

Fitzpatrick, T. A., & Brooks, B. A. (2010). The nurse leader as a logistician: Optimizing human capital. *Journal of Nursing Administration, 40*(2), 69–74.

Flanders, K., & Carr, D. (2016). Staffing by acuity: Building a bridge to support nursing effectiveness. *Voice of Nursing Leadership, 14*(5), 12–14.

Fried, B. J., & Fottler, M. D. (2008). *Human resources in healthcare*: Health Administration Press.

Frith K., Anderson F., Caspers B., Tseng F., Sanford K., Hoyt N., et al. (2010). Effects of nurse staffing on hospital-acquired conditions and length of stay in community hospitals. *Quality Management in Health Care, 19*(2), 147–155.

Gavigan, M., Fitzpatrick, T., & Miserendino, C. Effective staffing takes a village: Creating the staffing ecosystem. *Nursing Economics, 34*(2), 58–65.

Gavigan, M., Fitzpatrick, T. A., & Miserendino, C. (2016). Effective staffing takes a village: Creating the staffing ecosystem. *Nursing Economics, 34*(2), 58–65.

Guanci, G., & Felgen, J. (2016). How relationship-based care supports the Magnet journey. *Nursing Management, 47*(1), 9–12.

Haas, S. A., Vlasses, F., & Havey, J. (2016). Developing staffing models to support population health management and quality outcomes in ambulatory care settings. *Nursing Economics, 34*(3), 126–133.

Habasevich, B. (2012, July 26). *Re: Defining acuity* [Online forum blog]. https://www.mediware.com/rehabilitation/blog/defining-acuity/.

Joseph, M. L., & Fowler, D. (2016). Innovating traditional nursing administration challenges. *Journal of Nursing Administration, 46*(3), 120–121.

Kane, R., Shamliyan, T., Mueller, C., Duval, S., & Wilt, T. (2007a). *Nurse staffing and quality of patient care.* US Department of Health and Human Services AHRQ Publication No. 07-E005. Author.

Kane, R., Shamliyan, T., Mueller, C., Duval, S., & Wilt, T. (2007b). The association of registered nurse staffing levels and patient outcomes. *Medical Care, 45*(12), 1195–1204.

Kelly, L. A., McHugh, M. D., & Aiken, L. H. (2011). Nurse outcomes in Magnet and non-Magnet hospitals. *Journal of Nursing Administration, 41*(10), 428–433.

Koloroutis, M. (Ed.). (2004). *Relationship-based care: A model for transforming practice.* Creative Health Care Management.

Koning, C. (2014). Does self-scheduling increase nurses' job satisfaction? An integrative literature review. *Nursing Management, 21*(6), 24–28.

Kullberg, A., Bergenmar, M., & Sharp, L. (2016). Changed nursing scheduling for improved safety culture and working conditions-patients' and nurses' perspectives. *Journal of Nursing Management, 24*(4), 524–532.

Lauw, C., & Gares, D. (2005). Resource management: What's right for you. *Nursing Management, 36*(12), 46–49.

Lawson, L. D., Miles, K. S., Vallish, R. O., & Jenkins, S. A. (2011). Recognizing nursing professional growth and development in a collective bargaining environment. *Journal of Nursing Administration, 41*(5), 197–200.

Liang, B., & Turkcan, A. (2016). Acuity-based nurse assignment and patient scheduling in oncology clinics. *Health Care Management Science, 19*(3), 207–226.

Litvak, E., Buerhaus, P., Davidoff, F., Long, M., McManus, M., & Berwick, D. (2005). Managing unnecessary variability in patient demand to reduce nursing stress and improve patient safety. *Journal on Quality and Patient Safety, 31*(6), 330–338.

MacPhee, M., & Borra, L. S. (2012). *Flexible work practices in nursing.* International Council of Nurses.

Malloch, K. (2015). Measurement of nursing's complex health care work: Evolution of the science for determining the required staffing for safe and effective patient care. *Nursing Economics, 33*(1), 20–25.

Mark, B. A., Harless, D. W., & Berman, W. F. (2007). Nurse staffing and adverse events in hospitalized children. *Policy, Politics, and Nursing Practice, 8*(2), 83–92.

McDonough, K. S. (2013). Development of the McDonough Optimum Staffing Method: Evidence-driven recommendations based on patient demand. *Virginia Nurses Today, 21*(2), 8–11.

McHugh M. D., Rochman M. F., Sloane D. M., Berg R. A., Mancini M. E., Nadkarni V. M., et al. (2016). Better nurse staffing and nurse work environments associated with increased survival of in-hospital cardiac arrest patients. *Medical Care, 54*(1), 74–80.

McKinley, J., & Cavouras, C. (2000). Evolving staffing measures. In American Organization of Nurse Executives (AONE). *Staffing management and methods: Tools and techniques for nurse leaders,* 1–33. Jossey-Bass.

Mensik, J. (2014). What every nurse should know about staffing. *American Nurse Today, 9*(2), 1–11.

Mitchell, P. (2008). *Nurse staffing—A summary of current research, opinion and policy* (pp. 1–37). The William D. Ruckelshaus Center.

Morris, R., MacNeela, P., Scott, A., Treacy, P., & Hyde, A. (2007). Reconsidering the conceptualization of nursing workload: Literature review. *Journal of Advanced Nursing, 57*(5), 463–471.

National Association of Neonatal Nurses (NANN). (2014). *RN staffing in the neonatal intensive care unit.* NANN Position Statement No. 3061. Author.

National Council of State Boards of Nursing (NCSBN). (2016). A changing environment: 2016 NCSBN environmental scan national council. *Journal of Nursing Regulation, 6*(4), 4–37.

National Database of Nursing Quality Indicators version 9.3. (August 2011). Kansas City: University of Kansas School of Nursing.

National Labor Relations Board (NLRB). (2016). *National Labor Relations Act.* Author. https://www.nlrb.gov/how-we-work/national-labor-relations-act.

National Labor Relations Board. (2020). Bargaining in good faith with employees' union representative (Section 8 (d) & 8 (a)(5). https://www.nlrb.gov/rights-we-protect/whats-law/employers/bargaining-good-faith-employees-union-representative-section.

Needleman, J., Buerhaus, P., Mattke, S., Stewart, M., & Zelevinski, K. (2002). Nurse-staffing levels and the quality of care in hospitals. *New England Journal of Medicine, 346*(22), 1715–1722.

Needleman, J., Buerhaus, P., Pankratz, S., Leibson, C., Stevens, S., & Harris, M. (2011). Nurse staffing and inpatient hospital mortality. *New England Journal of Medicine, 364*(11), 1037–1045.

Needleman, J., Buerhaus, P. I., Stewart, M., Zelevinsky, K., & Mattke, S. (2006). Nurse staffing in hospitals: Is there a business case for quality. *Health Affairs, 25*(1), 204–211.

Norrish, B. R., & Rundall, T. G. (2001). Hospital restructuring and the work of registered nurses. *Milbank Quarterly, 79*(1), 55–79.

Pappas, S., Davidson, N., Woodard, J., Davis, J., & Welton, J. (2015). Risk-adjusted staffing to improve patient value. *Nursing Economics, 33*(2), 72–87.

Person, C. (2004). Patient care delivery. In M. Koloroutis (Ed.), *Relationship-based care: A model for transforming practice* (pp. 159–182). Creative Health Care Management.

Pickard, B., & Warner, M. (2007). Demand management: A methodology for outcomes-driven staffing and patient flow management. *Nurse Leader, 5*(2), 30–34.

Porter, C. (2010). A nursing labor management partnership model. *Journal of Nursing Administration, 40*(6), 272–276.

Pruinelli, L., Delaney, C., Garcia, A., Caspers, B., & Westra, B. L. (2016). Nursing management minimum dataset: Cost effective tool to demonstrate the value of nurse staffing in the Big Data science era. *Nursing Economics, 34*(2), 66–89.

Rambur, B., & Fitzpatrick, T. (2017). A plea to nurse educators: Incorporate big data use as a foundational skill for undergraduate and graduate nurses. *Journal of Professional Nursing, 34*(3), 176–181.

Robertson, R., & Samuelson, C. (1996). Should nurse patient ratios be legislated? Pros and cons. *Georgia Nursing, 56*(5), 2.

Roski, J., Bo-Linn, G., & Andrews, T. (2014). Creating value in healthcare through big data: Opportunities and policy implications. *Health Affairs, 33*(7), 1115–1122.

Rubenfire, A. (2017). Understanding value at the crossroads of cost and outcomes. *ModernHealthcare. http://www.moderhealthcare.com/article/20170601/ SPONSORED/170609999.*

Seago, J. A., Spetz, J., Coffman, J., Rosenoff, E., & O'Neil, E. (2003). Minimum staffing ratios: The California workforce initiative survey. *Nursing Economics, 21*(2), 65–70.

Shi, L., & Singh, D. (2019). *Essentials of the U.S. health care system.* Burlington, MA: Jones & Bartlett.

Simpson, R. (2012). Technology enables value-base nursing care. *Nursing Administration Quarterly, 36*(1), 85–87.

The Joint Commission (TJC). (2016). *Joint Commission FAQ page.* Author. https://www.jointcommission.org/about/ jointcommissionfaqs.aspx.

Thew, J. (2020, January 9). *Nursing tops Gallup's most honest and ethical professions list.* https://www. healthleadersmedia.com/nursing/nursing-tops-gallups- most-honest-and-ethical-professions-list.

Thompson, J. D., & Diers, D. (1985). DRGs and nursing intensity. *Nursing & Health Care, 6*(8), 434–439.

Unruh, L. (2008). Nurse staffing: Patient, nurse, financial outcomes. *American Journal of Nursing, 108*(1), 62–71.

Unruh, L., & Fottler, M. D. (2004, June). *Patient turnover and nursing staff adequacy,* Paper presented at Academy Health Annual Research Meeting.

Welton, J. M. (2010). Value-based nursing care. *Journal of Nursing Administration, 40*(10), 399–401.

Welton, J. M., & Dismuke, C. E. (2008). Testing an inpatient nursing intensity billing model. *Policy, Politics, & Nursing Practice, 9*(2), 103–111.

Welton, J. M., & Harris, K. (2007). Hospital billing and reimbursement: Charging for inpatient nursing care. *Journal of Nursing Administration, 30*(6), 309–315.

Welton, J. M., Zone-Smith, L., & Fischer, M. H. (2006). Adjustment of inpatient care reimbursement for nursing intensity. *Policy, Politics, & Nursing Practice, 7*(4), 270–280.

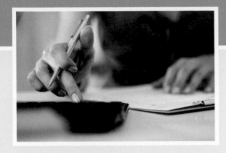

22

Budgeting, Productivity, and Costing Out Nursing

Linda B. Talley, Diane H. Thorgrimson

ⓔ http://evolve.elsevier.com/Huber/leadership

National Health Expenditures (NHEs) are a measure of spending for health care in the United States. In 1998 NHEs exceeded $1 trillion for the first time. By 2027, NHEs are projected to increase to $6 trillion. Considered from another perspective, by 2027, this level of health care spending will exceed Gross Domestic Product (GDP) (the value of all the goods and services produced in the US in 1 year) growth by 0.8 percentage points, representing 19.4% of the GDP. In 2014 NHEs represented 17.5% of the GDP. Health care spending is projected to increase at a rate of 5.8% per year for the next 10 years (Centers for Medicare & Medicaid Services [CMS], 2019). Projections for insured and Medicare enrollment growth used to forecast the above expenditure increases do not include potential changes to federal health care legislation that may significantly increase the percentage of insured individuals in the United States.

Under a new rule of the Patient Protection and Affordable Care Act, which was signed into law March 2010, effective January 1, 2019, CMS required all hospitals to post prices on line in efforts to provide patients more cost information related to their health care (Gander, 2018). Price categories for posting include stays, procedures, services, drugs, and supplies. Given the complexities of health care billing and reimbursement, this transparency of pricing may not immediately drive down costs. Consumers of health care have multiple avenues to explore related to health care pricing and providers before making knowledgeable and significant changes to their practices (Viviano, 2019). From a provider perspective, this new transparency highlights the importance of nursing staff at all levels in identifying and understanding health care costs and cost drivers.

The magnitude of these expenditure increases—along with the changes in practice related to the Affordable Care Act—emphasizes that nurses, as members of the largest health care profession, need to understand the implications of these data for clinical practice. Understanding budgeting, productivity, and costing out nursing and relating that knowledge to the management of professional nursing is a leadership skill that will serve the nursing profession in an era of accelerating health care expenditures.

BACKGROUND

Staff nurses, new and experienced, may not recognize their important role in identifying and managing budgeted resources for patient care and the related outcomes to patient and staff satisfaction. Through transformational leadership a staff nurse can contribute to changes in patient care and financial practices and innovations across the organization. This transformative work places the staff nurse "at the table" where discussions focusing on the responsible management of financial resources address, but are not limited to, patient care, patient acuity, patient flow, workforce measures, workforce productivity, staff training, and supplies. As nurses across an organization improve their individual and collective knowledge of health care financial management to guide their decision making, outcomes related to resource allocation, patient care, and staff satisfaction will be achieved (Nurses First Solutions, 2018).

Budgeting is a major aspect of an organization's or unit's planning processes. A budget is a plan that is specified in dollar amounts. This plan becomes a guiding framework for organizational activities. It conveys management's intentions and financial expectations regarding revenues and expenditures. An organization-level budget compares expected revenues with expected expenses to forecast profit (margin) or loss (deficit). Budgeting is a cyclical process of planning, implementing, and evaluating.

Budgets are designed to be planning documents, but one often hears the statement "we don't have the budget for that" or "the budget won't allow it." It is crucial to understand that the budget is a tool created by humans. To be useful, it must be flexible and have processes in place to modify it when necessary. Individuals and organizations should not become so constrained by the approved budget that they hesitate to take appropriate actions or make appropriate decisions that vary from, or were unanticipated in, the budget process.

DEFINITIONS

A **budget** is defined as a written financial plan aimed at controlling the allocation of resources. It functions as both a planning instrument and an evaluation tool useful for financial management. A budget is used to manage programs, plan for goal accomplishment, measure change, and control costs.

Expenses are defined as the costs or prices of activities undertaken in the organization's operations.

Income (or profit) is the excess of revenues over expenses, or revenues minus expenses.

Revenue is defined as income or amounts owed for purchased services or goods. *Total operating expenses* are the result of summing the costs of all resources (e.g., labor, patient consumable supplies, small medical equipment, utilities, office supplies, and other related miscellaneous fees and materials) used to produce services.

Total operating revenues are the result of multiplying the volume of services provided by the charges (rate) for the services.

A **variance** is the difference between the budgeted and the actual amounts. A variance may be favorable or unfavorable relative to the budget amount. A budget developed to provide resources for direct patient care, such as nursing budgets, will use actual volumes (units of service) to interpret favorable or unfavorable variances.

There are three main types of organizational budgets, as follows:

1. *Capital budget:* This budget is the plan for the purchase of major equipment or assets. Each organization will define its own capital dollar threshold limits.
2. *Operating budget:* The operating budget is the annual plan for the unit's or organization's daily functioning revenue and expenses for a single year. For nursing units, this is a plan that lays out what it is going to cost to run the unit in the coming year. It includes such things as consumable and non-consumable supplies, small medical equipment, telephones, postage, paper, personal electronic devices for staff, printers, and copy machines. In addition, there may be a cost allocation for such things as heat, light, and housekeeping. Inflation projections for goods need to be factored into each year's budget.
3. *Personnel budget:* This is the staffing budget of the cost center (department or unit). It may be developed as part of the operating budget, or it may stand alone. Personnel budgets must include expenses related to productive and nonproductive time as well as projected replacement time. Use of premium pay—to include, but not be limited to, overtime and shift differential—is to be included in all personnel budgets. A good personnel budget contains fiscal resources to flex up staffing during periods of high inpatient census and/or patient volumes.

THE BUDGET PROCESS

Each institution establishes standard budgetary formats and processes. Because employees of a cost center will have to implement the budget decision, it is imperative that they have input in the process. This is often done in staff meetings where the manager uses the opportunity to teach about the process, present financial and volume data, and solicit staff input. Nursing and administrative leadership rounds also provide a forum for staff nurses to share their observations and recommendations regarding the many factors that affect resource use related to direct patient care on their unit and/or across the organization. Such factors may include quality and safety concerns, patient acuity, volumes, staffing, patient throughput, average length of stay, and patient experience.

The annual budgeting cycle process is complex and requires the completion of several related documents. It may be compared with income tax preparation, where an individual gathers all the necessary data and receipts, completes all of the required forms, and submits them to the Internal Revenue Service. Like tax preparation, the budget process may require multiple revisions.

A typical budget process follows the priorities identified in the organization's strategic plan and supports the organization's mission and vision. This is done to ensure that resources are appropriately aligned with key organizational initiatives. The budget process consists of three periods:

1. *Preparation:* As a beginning point, the manager reviews the organization's strategic plan and the last year's budget for the cost center (including budget and current year projected). The strategic plan will aid in writing budget justifications and links requests to organizational priorities. The prior year's budget for the cost center will help the manager to identify volume projections and changes in the past year and potential changes in the coming year. In concert with nursing leadership, the organization's finance staff and other members of the leadership team will often establish the next year's budgeted volumes through analysis of relative internal and external environmental factors and activity. Such analysis includes input from key departments such as strategy, managed care, case management, and reimbursement. Hospitals that employ physicians will also include physicians in budget volume projection work. In the hospital, patient days and adjusted patient days are the usual volume measurement. For example, if the manager of a surgical unit knows that two general surgeons are being recruited to the organization, it is reasonable to project an increase in patient days. With a review of the previous year's data, an informed projection can be made about the increase that can be anticipated. Similarly, the manager may be aware of factors that will decrease the volume of patient days, such as a new hospital being built nearby. In ambulatory care, the volume unit of measurement is clinic visits. If a new nurse practitioner (NP) is being hired, how will that affect the volume of visits projected? Volume measurements, or units of service, are determined by the type of service provided. For example, in the operating room (OR), budgets are based on resources required for OR minutes; in an outpatient setting, budgets are based on resources required for a patient visit.

2. *Completing the forms:* Typically, the manager will have access to sophisticated budget software for use in preparing the cost center budget. The software includes embedded formulas that compute differential pay, premium pay, productivity, and other summary statistics, thereby reducing human error and promoting consistency across the organization. Firm due dates are assigned for the completion of this first draft of the budget. Typically, a margin target is assigned to each cost center to guide managers in preparing their first draft. The finance department then "rolls up" the unit budget into the organizational budget.

3. *Revise and resubmit:* As budget documents go through review by senior management, requests tend to exceed the available resources. This necessitates review, adjustment, and appeal. This is when competition for available resources enters the process. Managers may be asked to reduce their unit budget by a dollar percentage, leaving the question of where to cut as the manager's decision. At other times, a manager may be directed to reduce the personnel budget by a number of full-time equivalents (FTEs), thereby reducing labor expenses and addressing productivity. This is the point at which the nurse manager needs to skillfully advocate for patient care to ensure safety and quality.

The nurse manager's knowledge of clinical care processes may be in conflict with directives of a financial administrator who lacks clinical expertise. This is when nurses need to be prepared to "speak finance" to effectively respond to budget challenges. The nurse manager must be able to speak to the variable needs of a patient care budget, for example, the ability to flex up direct-care nursing (variable) staff when patient volumes surge and/or patient acuity increases and the ability to flex down nursing staff when patient volumes and acuity decrease. The nurse manager needs to be sure that budgets include adequate expenses for reasonable productive and non-patient care paid hours for all staff. Non-patient care hours include sick, vacation, holiday, family leave, jury duty, and other types of leave as well as time spent away from the patient care area in education programs or working on administrative assignments and meetings. Failure to ensure that non-patient care labor expenses are budgeted appropriately will lead to a budget bust as well as staffing difficulties and other issues related to patient care, patient outcomes, patient experience, and employee relations.

An often-overlooked aspect of the labor budget is anticipated turnover. Turnover will typically generate additional labor expenses through replacement of exiting staff with premium pay labor. In addition, expenses related to training new staff can extend through several months to a year. To this end, those areas that experience significant turnover need to focus on staying ahead of the turnover through an "over-hired" or "rightsizing" strategy. There may be multiple iterations of budget drafts before the final budget is approved.

Capital Budget Development

Capital budget preparation is usually the first step in the annual budget cycle. The organization will define a capital expense in terms of a dollar amount and the anticipated life span of the purchase. For example, capital expenditures may be "items costing over $10,000 and having a life span of 5 years." Items of this magnitude are not placed in the operating budget.

The specific process used to create a capital budget will vary from organization to organization, but most organizations require extensive background material to support capital budget requests. The background or supporting material required will probably include vendor quotes for costs of purchase, installation, staff education and training, and a justification or explanation of the reasons that the capital expenditure is needed. The justification must relate the expenditure to the organization's strategic goals or objective. For capital construction projects, architectural plans, regulatory considerations, and other supporting materials may also be required as part of the capital budget preparation process.

After each unit submits the capital expenditure list to the finance department, a compiled list is generated and typically prioritized by senior management. This is a period of intense negotiation. Given that there are rarely enough financial and/or labor resources to meet all of the requests, difficult decisions must be made.

Operating Budget Development

The *operating* budget covers a specific period, called a *fiscal year*. The fiscal year may begin July 1, may correspond to the calendar year beginning January 1, or may follow the federal government year that starts on October 1. Regardless of the fiscal year start date, the operating budget is the budget plan for day-to-day service delivery operations. It has at least two parts: the labor budget and the expense budget for costs other than labor. Expense budgets typically include consumable and non-consumable patient supplies, office supplies, pharmacy, and nutrition expenses. Use of budget software easily allows for the sharing of information regarding historical or trend data, expenses, and revenues. Typically, the revenue associated with a nursing unit reflects charges for room and board services. Room and board charges represent a bundling of hospital expenses related to patient care that are not individually billed elsewhere. Such expenses may include nursing and non-nursing labor, utilities, housekeeping, linen, and miscellaneous administrative services. All nursing service areas will adopt a unit of service measure that reflects the type of service provided. Inpatient nursing units measure patient volumes in the form of daily room and board charges or observation hourly charges. The OR measures volumes in terms of OR minutes, and ambulatory settings measure volume in terms of patient visits. Use of units of service measures comes into play when productivity analyses are conducted for budgeting, trending, benchmarking, regulatory reporting, and other purposes. The nurse manager who conducts his or her budget performance analysis referencing units of service can better represent their budget performance to hospital administration and finance. An astute manager will look for multiple ways to interpret budget performance.

The specific process used to develop operating budgets will vary considerably from one organization to another. The nurse manager's and/or nurse executive's role in developing operating budgets for nursing units and services will typically include input on or determination of volume projections, development of associated expense projections (including supplies, equipment, and salary/labor expenses), and some form of revenue projection. Many organizations develop and disseminate a set of budget assumptions that are to be used by managers and leaders in developing the operating budget. These assumptions may include such items as pre-established increases in labor or salary expenses based on contractual obligations, adjustments that must be made based on economic forecasts for supply charge changes (e.g., increased utility rates, increased cost of pharmaceuticals), or factors that will affect patient volume, such as the addition of a new service line. The nurse manager who can share benchmark comparisons, both internal and external, demonstrates greater knowledge of the impact of required resources throughout the budget process.

Projected Volume

The foundation of the development of the operating budget at the unit level is based on the projected volume of work for the coming year. The workload aspect often is measured in units of service. Key units of service need to be identified, the number of units predicted, and related expenses and staffing calculated accordingly. Activity reports such as historical census and average length of stay identify trends related to volume of activity. The unit of service often needs to be adjusted to the case or patient mix, which is a proxy for severity of illness or need (Jones et al., 2019). Given that a budget is a plan prepared several months before implementation, budget assumptions can be proven wrong throughout the budget year. In this event, budget variances—the measure between actual and budget—are often demonstrated. The successful nurse manager will know when and why budget assumptions have been incorrect and can speak to the related impact and possible adjustments required for the current and or following budget year.

Tables 22.1 and 22.2 show sample volume budget flow sheets. Historical trend data are needed (e.g., occupancy percentages by time frames such as weekly or monthly) to determine growth projections and any impact of seasonality. Table 22.1 displays volume changes on Unit X by month for 1 fiscal year, with variances clearly

TABLE 22.1 Volume Budget Flow Sheet
Fiscal Year Y; Volumes for Unit X

Month	Patient Days Budgeted	Patient Days Actual	Variance	% Variance
July	650	667	17	2.6%
August	668	652	−16	−2.4%
September	652	680	28	4.3%
October	667	692	25	3.7%
November	700	665	−35	−5.0%
December	752	721	−31	−4.1%
January	691	682	−9	−1.3%
February	683	692	9	1.3%
March	667	671	4	0.6%
April	665	652	−13	−2.0%
May	667	674	7	1.0%
June	673	685	12	1.8%
TOTAL	**8135**	**8133**	**22**	**0.0%**

TABLE 22.2 Volume Budget Flow Sheet
Fiscal Year Trends; Volumes for Unit X

Fiscal Year	Patient Days Budgeted	Patient Days Actual	Variance	% Variance
FY A	8021	8650	629	7.8%
FY B	8210	8689	479	5.8%
FY C	7658	7789	131	1.7%
FY D	7432	7652	220	3.0%
TOTAL	**31,321**	**32,780**	**1459**	**4.7%**

demonstrated. Table 22.2 shows volume changes on Unit X over 4 fiscal years, with variances rolled up to yearly values for comparison purposes. The volume of services delivered for a year may be expressed as patient days, visits, procedures, or other units of service. Effects on volume are environmental effects such as reimbursement changes, new programs, process improvements, new technology, and marketing. If volume projections depend on another service or department, it is important for the two departments to communicate closely so that similar assumptions are used in establishing volume projections.

Staffing Calculation

Once the volume projection has been completed, the manager can determine the *personnel services* (or *staffing/labor budget*) portion of the expense budget. Calculation of staffing in a variable environment is complex and given that staffing expenses generally are the largest portion of the nursing operating budget, nurse managers and nurse executives need to have a consistent and well-defined approach to estimating staffing expenses. The methodology and/or terminology used will likely vary from organization to organization.

Rundio (2016) described the following method that may be used to estimate staffing expenses. For inpatient nursing units, the first step in budgeting variable staffing expenses is to know the number of planned patient days. This number can be presented on an annual basis or daily basis, known as average daily census (ADC). The next step is to determine the number of required hours, by discipline, for each patient day. For instance, based on projected patient acuity for Unit X, it is determined that each patient will require an average of 9.0 direct nursing care hours each day. This is stated as 9.0 direct registered nurse (RN) hours per patient day (HPPD). Note that this is a calculated average, not actual needs. To determine the number of FTEs required on Unit X, the nurse manager will multiply 9 hours by the projected number of patient days (8021) and find that 72,189 hours of direct RN care are required for patient care. Dividing the 72,189 hours by 2080 hours (1 FTE), the nurse manager will conclude that 34.71 direct-care RN FTEs are required to deliver safe patient care. The unit manager will next add in nonproductive time to determine the number of required budgeted RNs for Unit X. Should the manager determine that nonproductive time equals 13% per each RN FTE, the total number of "replacement" RNs equals 4.51 FTEs. Therefore, Unit X needs to budget for a total of 39.22 RN FTEs for direct patient care.

Salary Calculations

Table 22.3 displays a sample budget expense sheet for salaries based on the total unit. Similar tables can be created for subgroups, such as direct-care RNs. Table 22.4 demonstrates how personnel budgets might be displayed. Salary increases might also be included as another column. These are examples to show how data might easily be displayed as a report. Today's sophisticated budget software has reduced the effort once required for these calculations. The software will calculate salary expenses in an expeditious manner, working from historical data related to pay rates, use of premium pay,

TABLE 22.4   Personnel Budget Flow Sheet

Fiscal Year Y; Personnel Budget for Unit X

Position	FTE	Average Hourly Rate	Annual Salary
Unit Manager	1.0	40.00	83,200
Direct-Care RN	22.3	37.00	1,716,208
RN Education	1.0	34.00	70,720
Patient Care Tech	4.7	19.00	185,744
Unit Clerk	5.2	17.00	183,872
	34.2	31.49	2,239,744

FTE, Full-time equivalent; *RN*, registered nurse.

and differentials. Table 22.5 demonstrates the percentage variance when measuring actual staffing against target staffing, developed by multiplying budgeted HPPD against actual census.

Supply and Revenue Budgets

Supply budgets are a major component of the operating budget. Similar to labor, many supply items are variable (the amount used will vary based on the volume of service provided). Other supply costs are fixed and will be incurred at the same level no matter the volume of service that is provided. Items such as office supplies, intravenous (IV) solutions, instruments, linens, gloves and other personal protective equipment, medical/surgical supplies, and drugs are examples of supplies that would vary with a higher volume of patient days. Leases, maintenance contracts, staff education funds for travel to conferences or meetings, and books and subscriptions are all examples of supply items that would not vary with a higher volume of patient days. Dollar amounts are assigned based on historical projections and any known or anticipated adjustments resulting from inflation, contractual increases, or other factors as specified in the organization's budgetary assumptions. The operating budget will also need to include expenses for overhead, depreciation, utilities, telecommunications services, and other related facility expenses. Finance will typically guide nurse managers in budgeting for these overhead expenses.

Revenue budgets are based on a set of calculations that determine expected receipts that will result from charging patients and payers for services. Nursing services are often not viewed as revenue-generating

TABLE 22.3   Budgeted Salary Expense Flow Sheet

Salaries and Wages: Unit X for Fiscal Year Y

	Budget	Actual	Variance	% Variance
Regular				
Overtime				
Differential				
Holiday				
Vacation				
Sick				
Education				
Administrative				
Other				
TOTAL				

TABLE 22.5 Measures of Productivity

Fiscal Year Y; Productivity for Unit X

	Budget	Actual	Variance	% Variance
Total productive hours/patient day	12.2	13.1	0.9	−7.4%
Total productive direct-care RN hours/patient day	9.0	9.2	0.2	−2.2%
Salaries and wages/patient day	621.2	643.2	21.9	−3.5%
Contract hours/day	12.0	36.0	24.0	−200.0%
Contract expenses/day	600.0	1980.0	1380.0	−230.0%
Total supplies/patient day	32.0	35.3	3.3	−10.3%

RN, registered nurse.

departments, but in many organizations the patient days and related charges are used as a proxy for revenue. Revenue projections are based on volume projections. Factors such as payer mix and contractual rates will affect the overall revenue that is received. Contractual allowances (discounts), bad debt, and indigent care all become reductions of gross revenue and generally are not under the nurse manager's control (Jones et al., 2019).

TRACKING AND MONITORING OF BUDGETS

The budget process is continual. It is not an event that occurs once a year and then ends until the next budget development process begins. Although "formal" budget development may occur once a year, the budget sets the stage for ongoing monitoring and evaluation of the organization's financial performance related to the budget projection (plan) as well as external benchmarking. Regular budget analyses (e.g., quarterly or monthly) are used for monitoring, feedback, and managerial control. The variance (difference) between budgeted and actual revenue and expenses is determined to identify problem areas, enhance control, and ensure timely adjustments. Variances between actual and budgeted (planned) performance need to be analyzed to determine the cause so that nurses and managers can take the appropriate action. Variances can be favorable or unfavorable. Most organizations now use electronic reporting formats that automatically calculate variance rates, but it is important that nurses understand the reasons for the variances. Variances can result from a single cause (e.g., volume of patients or a rate change such as salary, usage, or price) or from a combination of causes.

Nurse executives often require nurse managers to document their analysis of budget variances on a monthly basis. Many nurse managers also find it is useful to share variance reports and the reasons for budget variances at unit meetings with their nursing staff. If, for example, the overtime was 4% over the budget rate, staff can engage in discussing the reasons for this expense and perhaps how it may be managed differently in the future. It may be that acuity was very high or that there were sick calls that required nurses to "work short," resulting in overtime. This will enhance the nursing staff's awareness of the unit's financial performance. Engaging unit staff in discussions about the unit's financial performance will also provide nursing staff the opportunity to suggest cost-saving strategies to control costs at the unit level. Some managers post and present unit financial data monthly. This way, all nurses and staff better understand and can be a part of generating solutions to financial issues. Use of a dashboard tool to review monthly financial performance measures is helpful to the manager and staff. In addition to tracking of expenses and revenues, related workforce measures such as premium pay, vacancy rate, turnover, and absenteeism assist the manager in telling their story. Working together as a team, nurse managers can better understand and guide activities that influence budget development and fiscal performance.

LEADERSHIP AND MANAGEMENT IMPLICATIONS

Nursing services make up the single largest aggregate expense in most health care organizations because they represent a large personnel component and control a large share of supplies and equipment. This is both an advantage and a vulnerability. It is a strength and advantage because nurses clearly manage the organization and system, especially at the operational unit level. With powerful and accurate data and analysis support, unit-level management becomes effective and efficient. However, many organizations simply do not provide a nurse-friendly support structure.

It is a vulnerability to be the largest aggregate expense because quick, short-term economic gains can be made by ratcheting down resources allocated to nursing services. This often occurs at the expense of strategy, long-term gains, staff satisfaction, group cohesion, patient experience, quality, and safety. Because health care generally faces strict fiscal constraints, both staff nurses and nurse managers need to be knowledgeable and skilled in anticipating financial fluctuations and trends and in making bold decisions based on rapid analysis of information. Staff nurses often will be handling day-to-day budgetary decisions; thus they must be aware of the unit's budget, the financial status of the unit and the organization, and the impact of their decisions about supply and resource (staff) utilization on the financial performance of the unit. Nurse leaders are more involved with strategic or long-range financial planning and decision making, but they may track unit productivity carefully.

The budgeting process requires a broad range of leadership and management skills. Resources are limited. This fact is difficult for some nurses, especially if they believe they should be able to do everything for every patient under every circumstance. Some professionals think that their job is to provide the maximum quantity and quality of service and that cost consciousness should not be a concern of direct-care providers. Nurses are familiar with managing clinical care delivery. These skills can be transferred to the management of money as a necessary component of providing care. However, the management of any scarce resource such as money includes balancing competing interests and making difficult decisions.

Leadership is involved in influencing others to achieve the group's goals within the constraints of scarce resources. Leaders need to be actively involved in setting the vision for how to accomplish goals through budget planning. Ethical considerations such as fairness, transparency, and reasonable targets are part of leadership decision making. Leaders can influence employee morale and organizational culture through role modeling and the decision-making process. Organizational culture can be engaged to diminish negative aspects of budgeting and financial management. There is an opportunity for innovation to occur in a way that eases financial pressures. For example, with the use of data, a better schedule may be devised that deploys the same RN and assistive personnel in a new configuration that better addresses peaks and flows and the needs of patients for nursing care.

Fiscal Responsibility for Clinical Practice

Continuous change in the health care delivery and reimbursement systems has created a challenge to controlling costs while continually improving the quality of care. The programs of the Affordable Care Act, designed to improve patient care quality and control costs, utilize the expanding transformative leadership role of the staff nurse and nurse executive to guide changes in health care practice and fiscal responsibility. Today's nurse is positioned to lead fiscal responsibility and innovation through a unique skill set that includes expertise in wellness, population care, patient-centered care, care coordination, data analytics, and quality improvement (Salmond & Echevarria, 2017).

Being fiscally responsible means that the nurse manager makes responsible resource allocation decisions. Some decisions a nurse manager might need to make include the following:

- Staff time: Are there sufficient budgeted HPPD to provide quality care?
- Staff assignments: Which member of the patient care team can care for the patient in a cost-effective manner?
- Discharge planning: Is there a process in place to avoid delays in discharges to nursing homes?
- Costs of human resources: How can you evaluate workforce metrics and track the impact of turnover, onboarding, and orientation as related to the budget?
- Professional growth and development: How do you support continual growth and professional development of nursing staff across the continuum in equitable and diverse ways?

There are also multiple opportunities for staff nurse nurses to demonstrate fiscal responsibility. For a client with poor skin integrity, perhaps the most expensive tape should be used because the tape needs to stick and be waterproof. However, in a routine situation, can a lower-cost item be substituted with equal results? Nurses cannot help reduce costs unless they know the per-item cost of the supplies they use, and then use this information to evaluate substitutions. Even small cost reductions can be significant if they are applied to high-volume items. Immediately apparent is the costliness of inappropriate use of items (e.g., wiping up spills with a sterile pad; opening a sterile pack in the OR "to be ready just in case" or to use only one of the instruments). Convenience versus cost trade-off must be considered (e.g., bag baths may be convenient or necessary in a staffing shortage but are an expensive supply cost).

Evaluation of Budget Expenditures

The public is becoming increasingly knowledgeable regarding the quality and safety of health care. Health care consumers and payers expect that money for new initiatives will result in added value in terms of improved quality, safety of care, and patient experience. Business plans must include specific metrics that will be used to measure the impact of expenditures on clinical outcomes, quality, safety, and patient experience, as well as on cost. Metrics should specify the impact on nurse-sensitive indicators when feasible to further validate the significant role that nurses play in improving the health status of patients.

Costing Out Nursing Services

Accurately determining the costs of providing nursing service is an important budgetary function. Nurses need to know their costs to plan better and negotiate more effectively. Nursing has historically been seen as a cost center but not a revenue generator. One strategy proposed to compensate for nursing's revenue disparity was to cost out nursing services. This idea became popular for a while but lost attraction as capitated reimbursement systems gained prominence. With a "per member per month" flat payment structure, many felt that efforts to cost out for purposes of charging a fee for service were useless. Therefore, costing out nursing services was abandoned by some. However, the unintended consequence was that the value of knowing precisely what it costs to deliver nursing services was lost.

Costing out nursing services is defined as the determination of the costs of the services provided by nurses. By identifying the specific costs related to the delivery of

nursing care to each client, nurses have data to identify the actual amount of services received. In reviews of the literature related to costing out nursing services, a variety of variables were examined, such as length of stay, nursing care costs, direct-care costs, patient acuity, and diagnosis-related group (DRG) reimbursements. Analyses of cost data continue to expand in correlation with increasing sophistication of related software products. Understanding costs through data and measurements allows leaders to achieve improved productivity for both variable and fixed expenses. Today's sophisticated software products provide data that ultimately links costs to patient acuity, scheduling and staffing, volumes, supply management, workforce management, care delivery decisions, and other benchmarking metrics (Bannow, 2019).

The process of costing out nursing services provides data for productivity comparisons. Activity-based costing (ABC) is one approach to service costing that may be useful in multiple settings. The key advantage of ABC is that it reflects what it costs to provide services and identifies why costs were incurred. The first step in ABC is to identify all the cost drivers associated with a specific service. For example, if the service is a preschool physical examination provided by a nurse practitioner, here are some potential costs associated with the service:

- Nursing assistant (NA): 5 minutes to room the patient and 5 minutes to clean the room after the visit. The NA is paid $15 per hour with a 35% benefit rate and works 52 weeks per year, 40 hours per week. The cost of the NA time is $31,200 + $10,920 = $42,120/2080 (number of hours in a year), for an hourly cost of $20.25, or $20.25/60, $0.3375 per minute or $1.69 cost per visit.
- One-half hour of NP time: The nurse is paid $86,000 per year and associated benefits at 35% ($30,100); the NP works 52 weeks (40 hours per week) per year. The cost of the time of the NP is ($116,100/2080) = $55.86 cost per hour or $27.91 cost per NP time.
- All other costs are identified in the same manner: equipment, such as stethoscope, tongue depressor, and linens on examination table; cost of electronic health record (EHR); costs of a billing clerk.

Once this process is completed, the costs are aggregated, yielding what it costs to provide one unit of one nursing service—providing a preschool physical examination. The next step is to assign activities to cost centers, service lines, or programs. In the previous example, the cost of the service may be placed in a pediatric wellchild clinic program.

A more sophisticated and rapidly expanding approach to collecting nursing's cost data is using *acuity*, or patient classification systems. The premise is that nursing care needs to be based on patients' actual needs for care, not on historical allocation of nursing time. *Acuity* is defined as a measure of the severity of illness of an individual patient or the aggregate patient population on a unit. The acuity of patients has increased dramatically in the past 10 to 15 years. Formerly, patients were admitted for diagnostic tests and for additional preparation before surgery. They typically remained in the hospital until they were able to care for themselves, often through a lengthy convalescence. A nurse was able to provide care to larger numbers of these patients because they required less care, assessment, and monitoring. Today, these patients are receiving care in other settings and only very ill patients remain in the hospital. Utilization review experts have stated that the only reason a patient is in the hospital is because they need monitoring and assessment by an RN. If these skills are not needed, patients can probably be safely cared for in a less expensive setting. The increased acuity seen today decreases the number of patients for whom a nurse may safely provide care. This results in what might look like (on paper) a decrease in productivity. Any measure of the productivity of nursing staff that does not consider the acuity level of patients is seriously flawed and would probably result in a gross underestimation of the output. Nurse executives reflect that patient acuity increases year after year, creating increased demand for additional direct-care RNs.

Many of the classifications share a similar approach to the determination of the workload based on the required hours of nursing care. This is intuitively attractive because it can be assumed that a ventilator-dependent patient in an intensive care unit (ICU) will require more care than a patient who has had a total knee replacement. If the nurse manager uses a classification system whereby, for example, type 1 patients receive 2 to 4 hours of nursing care per day and type 2 patients receive 5 to 8 hours per day, these data can be used in constructing a personnel budget when it is linked to the volume indicator of patient days. If the nurse manager predicts that the unit will provide 800 days of type 1 patients, this information can be used to predict the staffing requirements for that patient group. Multiple commercial patient classifications systems are available

for purchase. Some involve entering nurse-collected patient data in a software program, yet increasingly this information can be extracted from electronic medical records to calculate objective scores for acuity. One caveat to this process is that, when used to create staffing ratios, the judgment of an expert nurse clinician must override an empirical system and be based on patients' needs in real time.

Various approaches are used to determine this acuity level and then relate it to staffing needs. Patient classification software is available from vendors. These systems attempt to categorize the levels of nursing care required by patients and then project appropriate nursing and ancillary staff. Some of these may be expensive to purchase and then modified to meet the needs of a specific hospital; they may also be costly to install and maintain. Critics argue that such systems cannot capture the invisible knowledge work of nursing. The systems often inadequately adjust for the experience level and varied expertise of RNs, such as a new graduate versus an experienced senior nurse.

In general, too little effort has been devoted to isolating actual nursing costs and determining the costs of nursing and the provision of care. With actual data, nurses are in a better position to demonstrate the economic value of their service, and nurse managers will have appropriate information with which to accurately manage nursing services.

PRODUCTIVITY

Understanding the concept of productivity and relating it to the management of professional nursing is a leadership skill that will serve nursing in an era of accelerating health care expenditures. Based on this understanding, the nurse manager will be able to determine the costs associated with providing nursing care. Productivity is defined as the relationship between output and the goods and services used to produce them.

Measures of Productivity

Various measures of productivity exist, but all involve relationships between volume of inputs and cost. Nurses' time is the critical input in the production of nursing care. Home health agencies measure their productivity in patient home visits and hours of care, hospitals measure patient days, and clinics measure the number of patient visits. The cost measure is the cost of the nursing time required to produce this care. Table 22.5 displays some productivity measures that track and benchmark unit performance and assist the unit manager in presenting unit-related fiscal outcomes to nurse executives and hospital leadership.

The oldest method of measuring nursing productivity is the analysis of HPPD. The input is the nursing hours worked. The number of hospitalized patient days is the output. This index is imprecise because of the wide variation in patient acuity, with the result that the measure of patient days is not equivalent across cases. Patient "churn" further complicates this calculation. The number of heads in a bed at midnight (midnight census) is often less than what is seen at noon or 4 pm. Table 22.6 shows staffing variance calculations, measuring actual staffing against budgeted staffing based on actual census.

A variety of data sources and productivity indices can also be considered. In nursing, productivity has been tightly linked to staffing numbers. For example, staffing—calculated as the total number of hours of a given staff for a given time period—can be compared with patient volume or census. Using this method, if the output (patient days) increased while staffing remained the same, then strictly speaking the productivity would be increased. This typically happens in hospitals, for example, when the influenza season is severe and a large number of geriatric patients are admitted to the hospital. In this short-term staffing crisis, the same numbers of staff are available to care for the high census, and productivity temporarily increases. However, the gains may be short lived in that the short-staffing situation may result in nurse burnout, overtime, and resignations. To this end, during the budget process, it is important that the

nurse executive advocate for expenses to fund a flexible workforce (as needed, float pool, overtime, and contract staff). Some organizations track productivity and quickly adjust for when it is both too high and too low.

No one measure of productivity adequately captures the knowledge-based work of nursing. Productivity measurement is complex for several reasons. The causal linkages between nursing interventions and patient outcomes are not always well established. There is little research that addresses economic efficiency—that is, what is the least cost combination of inputs required to produce an outcome.

Enhancing the productivity of nurses while protecting the quality of patient care will continue to be a major challenge for nurse leaders. As outcomes research continues, the nurse executive needs to share this information with hospital leadership to support increased nursing expenses.

CURRENT ISSUES AND TRENDS

Evaluation of Budget Expenditures

The public is becoming increasingly knowledgeable regarding the quality and safety of health care. Health care consumers and payers expect that money for new initiatives will be well invested and that a significant return on investment will be realized in terms of improved quality or safety of care. Business plans must include specific metrics that will be used to measure the impact of expenditures on clinical outcomes, quality, safety, and cost. Metrics should specify the impact on nurse-sensitive indicators when feasible to further validate the significant role that nurses play in improving the health status of patients.

TABLE 22.6	**Staffing Variance**				
Bud HPPD	**Act Census**	**Target Hrs/Day**	**Target RNs/Day**	**Act RNs/Day**	**Staffing Variance**
11.86	29	343.9	14.3	26	−81%
11.86	34	403.2	16.8	36	−114%
9.1	49	445.9	18.6	39	−110%
9.1	54	491.4	20.5	38	−86%

HPPD, hour per patient day; *RN*, registered nurse.

Nurse Workforce Participation

The continuing nurse shortage and related nurse workforce participation issues carry ramifications for budgeting and financial management. Two trends to watch are nurses nearing retirement and the educational capacity available for the nurse workforce. The concern is with the number of projected nurses retiring, although to date the projections have not been realized, possibly due to economic pressures. However, it appears to be a matter of time.

For replacement prospects, the job of an RN is attractive for its employment potential. The Bureau of Labor Statistics (2015) noted the positive job outlook for RNs: "Employment of registered nurses is projected to grow 16% from 2014 to 2024, much faster than the average for all occupations. Growth will occur for a number of reasons, including an increased emphasis on preventive care; growing rates of chronic conditions, such as diabetes and obesity; and demand for health care services from the baby-boom population, as they live longer and more active lives."

Educational capacity is a concern due to the finite number of slots in schools and colleges of nursing plus an even more severe nurse faculty shortage, which limits student capacity. The age of nursing faculty is an acute issue due to impending retirements. Strategies are needed to address the nurse faculty shortage.

It is possible that increased use of technology will be a partial solution to increasing nursing productivity. Computerized documentation and medication administration systems are widespread applications of technology that have resulted in time savings and subsequent increased productivity for nurses. Information technology is another enhancement to nurses' productivity. Medical records are easily accessed from multiple sites, results of diagnostics tests are communicated instantly, and monitoring devices detect deviations from normal limits and communicate these to the nurse as they occur. However, as the EHR captures key nursing data related to quality, safety, staffing, patient engagement, and satisfaction, it must do so in concert with the nursing process in order to avoid stress burnout and "death by data entry" (O'Brien et al., 2015).

Another responsibility of nurse leaders related to productivity is ensuring a future workforce by participating in the recruitment of future nurses. One conference speaker reported that as a colleague leaves her home for work each day, she tells her young children, "Mom is going to go to the hospital to save lives today." Although nursing does not *always* offer that level of drama, it certainly speaks of the importance of the work that nurses do. That importance needs to be communicated to the pool of potential nurses.

Integration of Economics in Clinical Practice

The incorporation of economic evaluation in clinical practice is important to productivity because health care resources are limited and choices must—and will—be made. In the years preceding managed care, health care providers acted as if health care resources were infinite, with the result that health care costs spun out of control. Today, providers are faced with difficult decisions about "who gets what." Although rationing health care is inherently unacceptable to most of the US population, it is true that rationing is occurring. Currently, rationing is done based on the ability to pay for health care, with the uninsured receiving less health care. Well-educated nurse leaders who understand economics and finance are in a unique position to bring the values of nursing to decision making about the allocation of health care resources.

Nurses are able to tap into their full skill set to assess, educate, intervene, and evaluate the care they provide to increasing numbers of patients. Care providers are evaluated in their ability to provide efficient and quality care, and their reimbursements are directly related to their ability to demonstrate best practices. Their results are compared with others, and performance that varies from agreed-on outcomes will not be reimbursed. This means nurses are encountering more patients than ever before, but the reimbursement for these services is negotiated and often times less than in the past.

Simply put, nurses need to commit to continued learning and professional development over the course of their careers, seek collaborative and productive partnerships with all members of the provider team and beyond with members of the community at large, and become increasingly comfortable using data to measure outcomes, demonstrate achievements, and drive improvements across the continuum.

▲ RESEARCH NOTE

Source

DiMattio, M. J. K., & Spegman, A. M. (2019, April 30). Educational preparation and nurse turnover intention from the hospital bedside. *OJIN: The Online Journal of Issues in Nursing, 24*(2). https://doi.org/DOI:10.3912/OJIN.Vol-24No02PPT22.

Purpose

Although there is a lot of evidence about why nurses leave their jobs, there has been little clear understanding about turnover from the hospital bedside as a specific setting for practice. The purpose of this article was to examine the relationship between educational preparation and turnover intent, defined as intention to leave the hospital bedside as a practice setting, and gain a better understanding of the relationship between registered nurse (RN) educational preparation and turnover intentions.

Method

Data were obtained from a larger study of career trajectories of nurses at an integrated health system in Pennsylvania focusing only on direct patient care nurses. A cross-sectional, comparative design using a non-probability sample of 424 RNs who identified their primary work setting to be at the point of care was used. Study measures included turnover intent, educational preparation, clinical expertise, years of experience, and practice environment. Results showed that having a baccalaureate degree or more and current enrollment in school independently predicted turnover intention from the hospital bedside as a practice setting. Hospitals with a higher percentage of Bachelor of Science in Nursing prepared nurses might unwittingly set themselves up for turnover.

Discussion

Turnover of baccalaureate nurses negatively impacts both safe patient care and hospital costs. Staff churn, inadequate staffing, decreased continuity of care, and adverse events are attributed to RN turnover. Documented nurse satisfaction scores among this group of highly educated direct patient care nurses trends higher as a reflection of "hard" work and exhaustion experienced. The need for nurses in expanded roles provides an incentive for career advancement, and it has been reported that nurses seek to advance their education as a means to leave or "escape" the hospital bedside. In light of career mobility available to the higher educated staff nurses and the associated costs of nurse turnover, researchers have suggested that the employment of associate degree nurses may produce a more consistent and less expensive RN workforce. Current patterns indicate that hospitals are training newly graduated baccalaureate nurses who have the intention of leaving that organization once they master certain bedside skills. The authors advocated for deliberate and intentional re-envisioning of the acute care hospital setting as one specialty among others with commensurate hiring practices, recognition, and advancement opportunities that include salary adjustments as a way to retain these nurses. It is suggested that future research focus on the impact of turnover when more advancement and educational opportunities are available, thus allowing the nurse to become a specialist.

Application to Practice

To support safe patient care through decreasing baccalaureate RN turnover, nurse leaders need to creatively re-envision bedside direct care nursing as a specialty. This includes recognizing nurses as human capital needing advanced education to meet the complexity and critical thinking needed in clinical care.

CASE STUDY

Medical Center A has a 47-bed intensive care unit (ICU) budgeted for an average daily census (ADC) of 35.2, with nursing hours per patient day (HPPD) of 21.5. Based on historical experience, budgeted patient days were spread in a bell shaped curve with "high census" months, November through February (fiscal year months 5 through 8), budgeted at an ADC of 45. The budgeted ADC for non-peak months averaged 22 to 35. Three months into the fiscal year, the ICU was experiencing a consistently strong ADC of 35, with many days reaching peak ADC levels of 40 and above.

As the unit's variable workforce is budgeted to meet average budgeted volumes, it is expected and planned that premium pay staff will be used during budgeted high census months. Unfortunately, those early months in the fiscal year, not budgeted at peak volumes, used up increasing amounts of premium pay labor to meet the experienced census levels of 40 and above.

CASE STUDY—cont'd

Since early in the fiscal year, unit and nursing leaders have been managing the increasing workforce needs in the ICU through multiple measures, such as floating nurses from other critical care units, deploying large numbers of float pool nurses to the intensive care unit, using contract nursing assignments, use of an extra shift bonus, and use of overtime pay. Unfortunately, the income from operations for the ICU has been marginalized at the per-unit of service level. During the early months of the fiscal year, the levels of premium pay required to meet patient care needs were not placed in the budget based on the lower patient day volumes. Although the ICU is aggressively hiring and onboarding new nurses, the time required for these activities coupled with normal attrition cannot fully solve staffing needs. At present, the unit is limited to hiring at budgeted levels only.

1. How many additional nurses above budget are required to meet actual patient levels experienced during the first 4 months of the fiscal year? How many additional nurses above budget are required to meet budgeted patient levels during the time period of November through March?
2. As Chief Nursing Officer, what information and metrics would you share with finance to support the need for increased nurses in the intensive care unit? If you were granted an "ask," how many nurses would you ask to hire outside of the budget?
3. To onboard additional nurses, what plans, programs, and strategies do you need to develop and implement in order to achieve your workforce goals?

■ CRITICAL THINKING EXERCISE

As manager of the Surgical Care Unit (SCU), Ms. Dawson has identified a trending increase in unit-related RN patient care staffing challenges, which are correlating with changing patterns in patient case mix. To this end, Ms. Dawson has shared with the nursing leadership team that several new surgical care attending physicians have joined the organization over the past nine months. These surgeons, national experts in colorectal and pelvic reconstruction and orthopedic specialties, such as spinal infusions, are adding new and expanded service lines to the organization.

Although the SCU has not experienced an RN shortage in over 3 years, Ms. Dawson is preparing a review of the SCU's budgeted hours per patient day, with the goal of demonstrating a need for an increase in budgeted nursing hours during the next budget cycle.

1. What guiding principles should frame the review?
2. What are the key components and metrics Ms. Dawson should address in her review?
3. What external benchmarks would help support Ms. Dawson's position? Please explain.
4. What financial outcomes/measures would interest the chief finance officer?
5. Should the SCU not receive increased nursing hours in the next budget year, what would be Ms. Dawson's next steps?

REFERENCES

Bannow, T. (2019). More hospitals calculating actual cost of care. *Modern healthcare.* May 18. https://www.modernhealthcare.com/finance/more-hospitals-calculating-actual-cost-care.

Bureau of Labor Statistics. (2015). *Occupational outlook handbook: Registered nurses.* https://www.bls.gov/ooh/healthcare/registered-nurses.htm.

Centers for Medicare & Medicaid Services (CMS). (2019). *National Health Expenditure Fact Sheet 2018–2027.* Centers for Medicare & Medicaid Services (CMS.Gov). cms.gov/Research-Statistics-Data-and-Systems/Statistics-Trends-and-Reports/NationalHealthExpendData/NHE-Fact-Sheet.

Gander, K. (2018, December 27). Hospital prices: Full cost lists must be published from January 1, new federal rule says. *Newsweek.* https://www.newsweek.com/cnd-hidden-costs-january-1st-all-us-hospitals-must-publish-price-lists-all-1272328.

Jones, C., Finkler, S. A., Kovner, C. T., & Mose, J. (2019). *Financial management for nurse managers and executives.* Amsterdam, NL: Elsevier, Inc. E-Book on Vital Source.

Nurses First Solutions. (2018, January 20). https://nursesfirstsolutions.com/patient-and-staff-satisfaction-on-a-budget/.

O'Brien, A., Weaver, C., Settergren, T., Hook, M., & Ivory, C. (2015). EHR documentation: The hype and the hope for improving nursing satisfaction and quality outcomes. *Nursing Administration Quarterly, 39*(4), 333–339.

Rundio, A. (2016). *The nurse managers guide to budgeting & finance*. Indianapolis, IN: Sigma Theta Tau International.

Salmond, S., & Echevarria, M. (2017). Healthcare transformation and changing roles for nursing. *Orthopedic Nursing, 36*(1), 12–25.

Viviano, J. (2019, January 7). Hospitals post prices online to meet federal requirement. *The Columbus Dispatch*. https://www.dispatch.com/news/20190107/hospitals-post-prices-online-to-meet-federal-requirement.

23

Performance Appraisal

Barbara Seifert

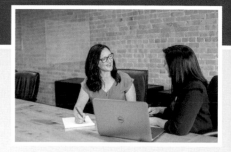

(e) http://evolve.elsevier.com/Huber/leadership

Insight into one's job performance is a critical component of not only keeping that job, but also for job satisfaction and promotional opportunities. The way to ensure that a nurse's performance is meeting, or exceeding, organizational standards, is through performance appraisal, which is a function of human resource management (HRM) systems. Appraisals guide managerial and administrative decisions that affect staffing and ensure competency for patient care standards, which are tied to organizational goals.

The purpose of an appraisal is to evaluate and improve the employee's performance, which in turn will enhance organizational effectiveness. Nursing leadership is in charge of guiding this process. In this chapter, the appraisal process, approaches to performance appraisals, developmental approaches to drive performance, and organizational goals will be discussed.

DEFINITIONS

In order to understand the concept of performance management, it is necessary to know the various meanings that underlie it.

360 review: A formal process whereby employees receive feedback on their behavior or outcomes from various individuals they regularly interact with. It is useful to assess individual, department, or team performance (360pev.com, 2013).

Coaching: A means of "partnering with clients in a thought-provoking and creative process that inspires them to maximize their personal and professional potential" (International Coach Federation, n.d.).

Feedback: "Information about reactions to a product or a person's performance of a task, which is used as a basis for improvement" (Lexico Dictionary, n.d.).

Peer-review: "The process by which practicing registered nurses systematically access, monitor, and make judgments about the quality of nursing care provided by peers as measured against professional standards of practice.... Peer review implies that the nursing care delivered by a group of nurses or an individual nurse is evaluated by individuals of the same rank or standing according to established standards of practice" (Haag-Heitman & George, 2011).

Performance: The accomplishment of a specific action; it is getting people to do the things we ask them to in a way that contributes to the goals of the business (Benedictine University, n.d.).

Performance appraisals: The process through which supervisors assess, after the fact, the job-related performance of their supervisees and allocate rewards to the supervisees based on that assessment (Capelli & Conyon, 2018); "the systematic evaluation of the performance of employees and to understand the abilities of a person for further growth and development" (Juneja, 2020).

Performance improvement plan (PIP): A formal performance action plan that is used as a tool to facilitate conversation in the form of constructive discussion between staff members and their managers or supervisors in order to clarify work performance and needed improvements (Heathfield, 2016). A PIP outlines specific goals to work towards, specific improvement steps to take, and specific time frames for improvements to be made.

Performance management: "A wide variety of activities, policies, procedures, and interventions designed to help employees to improve their performance. These programs begin with performance appraisals but also include feedback, goal setting, and training, as well as reward systems" (DeNisi & Murphy, 2017, p. 421).

Performance management systems/human resource information systems (HRIS): A software or online solution that is used for data entry, data tracking, and data management of all human resources (HR) operations of an organization, which aids in effective HRM and planning (Ghosh, 2019).

Self-evaluation: The aspect of performance appraisal whereby employees are asked to do their own evaluation of their job performance, which includes "evaluating progress towards pre-defined annual objectives and performance standards" (Performance-appraisals.org, 2018).

PURPOSE OF PERFORMANCE APPRAISALS

Administrative

Performance appraisals serve several administrative functions to meet compliance standards and organizational goals. These functions include helping to strengthen the appraisal process, improving employee performance, meeting compliance standards, and assisting with HR workforce planning, such as recruiting, compensation, and succession planning (Iqbal, 2017). HR can work in conjunction with administration to develop competencies and standards that lead to fair and effective evaluation with compensation tied to them. Appraisals help the nurse manager in updating personnel records and making decisions on staffing, including hiring, scheduling, promotions, or terminations. Another function is to assist with the culture, or "positive organizational climate, in which problems and grievances can be easily detected and handled" which leads to fairness and employee satisfaction" (Iqbal, 2017, p. 49).

Another administrative function of performance appraisal is that they function as psychological contracts, which is an unwritten agreement between employees and the organization (Geise & Thiel, 2015). This contract sets expectations for what the employer will provide, such as fair treatment, acceptable working conditions, and feedback on their job performance. As a result, employee expectations are to "demonstrate a good attitude, follow directions, and show loyalty to the organization" (Robbins & Judge, 2018, p. 140). Performance appraisals are a way to ensure that these unwritten expectations are carried out by the manager and employee.

Measurement

A second purpose for performance appraisals is to evaluate an employee's performance, which is done through various types of measurement standards. This helps the manager to determine if performance goals are met or if further development of the employee needs to be implemented. Performance measures should be tied to job duties and roles as well as to departmental and organizational goals. For example, a hospital that is working to win a Joint Commission Certification for Disease Management in Orthopedics, which sets standards and expectations for providing reliable care (The Joint Commission, n.d.), would have measurements that address pre-and post-operative care and how the nurse meets those standards to provide excellent, quality patient care. Processes such as these can determine if the measures are valid and reliable and actually measuring what they were intended to do.

Development

Employee development is a necessity from both the employee and employer. A worker can become complacent in their skills and duties, which can affect patient care and liability; the organization is able to identify and plan for developmental needs, such as training, certifications, or other resources to aid in employee development.

An appraisal allows for an employee to see their work from an external perspective, which they may not often see. An appraisal is a first step in ensuring legal compliance. Through observational feedback, the manager can make recommendations to advance the employee, such as by sending them to classes or for certifications that would build on their skills and lead to higher performance. It also allows for identification of potential leadership opportunities. However, when deficits are identified, it gives both the manager and the employee the ability to come up with a plan for improving either skills, behaviors, and/or attitudes. It also provides the manager with the opportunity to ensure formal documentation for employee improvements or hard decisions, such as by termination.

Relationships

Performance appraisal involves providing feedback to the employee (i.e., nursing staff) about their performance, with the intent of recognizing achievements and offer developmental opportunities. Therefore, the appraisal should not do harm to the relationship between the nurse manager and nursing staff. Research has shown that trust is an essential factor to moderate a positive relationship when providing feedback and leads to a positive interaction and feedback acceptance, with the belief that performance was accurately characterized. When specific feedback is provided, it moderates a positive relationship with trust and feedback acceptance which, in turn, leads to greater job satisfaction and involvement (Moon, 2019). The appraisal process should be conveyed as an open, positive experience by the manager. "Managers who take time outside of the formal performance appraisal process to seek common ground, practice reciprocity, understand their employees and provide informal feedback will develop trust and support that will enhance workforce productivity" (Teckchandani & Pichler, 2015, p. 16).

ISSUES IN PERFORMANCE MANAGEMENT

A long-held focus, by both researchers and HR practitioners, is the accuracy and measurements used in performance appraisals. Are they valid? Do they reflect actual performance? These questions will be addressed in this section.

What Is Being Measured in the Performance Appraisal?
Traits

Traits are characteristics that one possesses, such as initiative or work ethic. The Big Five Model is a highly recognized tool to identify five basic dimensions of one's personality. They are a predictor for how one behaves in a variety of situations and the stability of those behaviors. The five dimensions include: conscientiousness, emotional stability, extraversion, openness to experiences, and agreeableness (Robbins & Judge, 2018, p. 67). This rating

scale has positive relationships with both empathy and ethical decision-making. Other traits that may be rated include decision-making, ability to resolve conflict, or time management. Trait resilience is the ability to handle high levels of stress; individuals who possess this type of resiliency have been shown to handle higher workloads to either exceed standards and are aware of monetary and promotional results, as well as to avoid any negative consequences, such as discipline or termination.

Critics of trait models are against the use of these types of assessments as they may not be reflective of the worker as it puts them in a category that may not necessarily be accurate. Trait studies have been inconclusive in demonstrating whether trait results are actually indicative of performance. For instance, extroverts are often seen as leaders, due to their outgoing nature, but this does not always translate to effectiveness in a leader role, as some studies show that introverts are just as capable because they tend to think before reacting (Farrell, 2017).

Another issue with using a trait model is the rater's interpretation of the meanings of them, making them subjective in nature. One nurse might rate Agreeableness as a 2 if they had a conflict with that nurse, while another might give a rating of 5 if their interactions were positive. Although raters can be trained in trait assessments as to its meaning, there still can be misunderstanding and confusion as to how traits translate to performance.

Behaviors

Behaviors are more easily tied to performance appraisals when they are observable, thus reducing the subjectivity found in trait models. Employees are rated either by the frequency or the quantity of specific work actions. Examples include exhibits positive interactions with coworkers or patient's family members, willingness to stay to help the team, and responds to patient concerns in a timely manner. There are several means to formulate a behavioral rating; these can vary from a simple checklist or rating scale, based on 1–5 scale for each behavior, to structured assessments, such as the Behavioral Observation Scale (BOS) (Latham & Wexley, 1977) or the Behavioral Expectation Scale, also known as the Behaviorally Anchored Rating Scale (BARS) (Smith & Kendall, 1963).

Although researchers show that behavior models hold more validity than using traits, there are still some problems that can occur in their use. Behaviors are observable, yet the rater may not see every behavior an employee has, thus it can skew their assessment. It can lead the rater to rely on specific observations or from opinions of others. Another issue with this type of rating is that behaviors can change over time, thus requiring the evaluations to change and increase in their frequency. This can be confusing, costly, and time consuming for managers and staff.

Competencies

Competency-based models are commonly used in appraisals today. Schub (2014) defined competencies as the ability to perform a task based on clinical skills, knowledge, education, and experience. Competencies relate to demonstrating skills, knowledge, and abilities that enable and improve the efficiency of job performance. The focus is on behaviors and how they relate to a job task. Competencies should be evaluated regularly to assess and maintain the nurse's skills to achieve the best patient outcomes and within their scope of practice. Some examples of competencies are conducting a patient assessment, medication management, or proper hygiene procedures.

Competency assessments should relate back to specific behaviors of the job and be tied to goals of the department and the organization. There are nursing bodies that have developed competency-based assessments, such as the American Nurses Association (ANA), Association for Rehab Nurses (ARN), and National League for Nurses (NLN). States can independently develop their own nursing competences, such as the Massachusetts Nurse of the Future Core Competencies. Massachusetts core competencies is behaviorally based. It relies on individual perception by the rater, which can leave room for interpretation and bias.

Results

Results-based measures can be used to reduce any bias that may occur during the performance evaluation. The focus is on what is to be accomplished on the job versus observing traits or on-the-job behaviors. The focus is recognizing both quantitative and qualitative outcomes as it relates to the nurse's performance. These outcomes may result in compensation based on goal attainment. Robbins and Judge (2018) based this type of evaluation on the work of Peter Drucker (1954) and his Management by Objectives (MBO), which bases performance on set goals that are "tangible, verifiable, and measurable" (Drucker, 1954, as cited in Robbins & Judge,

2018, p. 107). Since results-based measures have clear objectives and outcomes, the nurse can work to fulfill these goals.

This method has its flaws. Due to its focus on goals, it can miss many other performance indicators or leave an employee only focusing on reaching the goals of results-based measures. This may cause employees to neglect other parts of their work, sometimes causing them to seem ineffective. This focus may lead to unrealistic expectations on all sides as to what can actually be accomplished. In addition, there may be circumstances that can occur outside of the scope of the nurse that may have an impact on their actual performance, such as if the pharmacy is taking too long to deliver a patient's medication (Weirks, 2007).

Which Performance Measurement Should be Used?

There is no uniform measure for performance appraisals. Each is developed based on an organization's needs. A tiered rating standard is utilized, either by a Likert scale of 1–5, or ratings of Meets Standards, Exceeds Standards, or Does Not Meet Standards. The intent is two-fold: (1) to review past employee performance, and (2) set a direction for future performance and development. Usually, a past appraisal is used to determine the progress on goals and improvements.

Rating Accuracy: Can We Measure It Accurately?

The question arises whether performance reviews are accurate in assessing performance and a person's abilities and effectiveness in their job role. There has been much research done to perfect the system, but problems still exist.

Rater Bias

Rater bias is an error in judgment when the rater uses their predetermined judgments and biases to affect their evaluation and decisions related to an employee. This is a big factor in ensuring accurate measurements. Bernardin et al. (2016, p. 325-325) found that: "a managers attributes may affect the importance attached to the various goals that can be pursued in the context of performance appraisal activities and that the relative importance raters assign to these various goals may in

TABLE 23.1   Definitions of Rater Bias Types
Rater Bias Term Definition
• **Central tendency:** The rater does not want to give too high a score, believe anyone merits the highest score, or want to be too strict and give a low score, so everyone is rated in the middle, or "average."
• **Contrast effect:** The rater bases their score on comparison with another employee, either overvaluing or undervaluing.
• **Halo effect:** The rater focuses only on a positive experience and rates all areas based on that measure.
• **Horns effect:** The rater focuses on a negative experience and rates on that measure
• **Leniency:** Ratings are higher than the employee deserves.
• **Recency of events error:** The rater considers only more recent events, rather than what occurred since the last evaluation period.
• **Severity, or strictness:** Awarding lower ratings than the employee deserves.
• **Similar to me:** The rater scores more highly those who are like them, such as gender, age, race, personality.

Reiken, J. (2018). *8 Rater biases that are affecting your performance management.* Trakstar https://www.trakstar.com/blog-post/8-rater-biases-impacting-performance-management/.

turn affect the levels of performance appraisal competencies manages develop and sustain".

This affirms that rater bias does occur, which is subjective to each rater. Some common types of rater bias are presented in Table 23.1.

The performance appraisal system should include rater training. This will help to mitigate and/or avoid biases, provide oversight by managers, and give accountability to the rater to ensure they are using fair practices in the evaluation. Rater training has been shown to increase a rater's understanding of the evaluation process, including potential biases, leading to more accurate performance assessments (Sanchez et al., 2019).

Political Motivations

Political motivations or influencing occurs with particular individuals or groups and does exist in the performance evaluation process (Dello Russo et al., 2017). This can include envy of another's occupational status or accomplishments (Henniger, 2016), personal feelings of affection for a favorite employee, or affinity bias (Include-empower.com, 2018). The opposite is also true, namely, to "punish" a difficult employee, or for financial compensation.

Larsen (2019) found that political motivations are intentional to favor one person or group, either positively or negatively, which leads to inaccuracies that may or may not be reflective of the nurse's performance. Rater training enhances the knowledge

and understanding of performance measures and lessens the risk of any adverse motivations that may affect a fair evaluation. More research must be done in this area to examine raters' use of political motivation.

Who Should Do the Rating?

The manager is responsible for evaluation and providing feedback on results. There have been improvements in recent years to involve others in the process. As the possibility for bias exists with a manager's rating, having the input from others is now becoming more the norm. Peer review and 360-degree feedback are two common techniques.

Peer-Reviewed

Many health care systems use a peer-review system to evaluate their staff. This can take the form of one-to-one review or with a panel. A peer review may involve observations or a skills test. The format involves feedback from peers regarding skills, performance, attitude, and competencies. The benefits of this format are that it can give the manager a more well-rounded view of the employee's strengths and challenges. The feedback will be used toward employee development such as training, competency acquisition, or building on their strengths.

A peer-review system can help provide feedback to individuals with high potential who do not seek recognition. However, these systems may have a negative effect. Peers may provide biased ratings, depending on their relationships with each other.

If employees receive negative feedback or strong criticism from the appraiser, an employee's relationship with their employer is more likely to be impacted. Employees might become reluctant to forge new working relationships, collaborate with colleagues, and might feel the pressure to provide feedback based on a group's consensus (Steele, n.d.). Negative reviews can also lead an employee to "adjust their roles to be around people who will give them more-positive reviews" (Berinato, 2018, p. 1). Worrying about potential feedback can increase stress levels of staff and have a detrimental result on performance, productivity, and team cohesion.

360-Degree Feedback

The 360-Degree Feedback is a tool that more organizations are beginning to use in the performance appraisal process. It has long been used for leadership development but is now becoming more popular as a tool for all employee levels in recent years. This appraisal involves multiple individuals who interact with the employee, specifically, the supervisor, peers, patients, families, staff from other departments, and outside vendors. The employee also completes a self-assessment (Chopra, 2017). The results are then discussed, and feedback is provided to compare and contrast results. This type of feedback provides a more rounded view of the employee, which does reduce bias to some extent.

There are both benefits and limitations to the 360-degree appraisal. Some limitations include expenses, timeliness, and the involvement of multiple people. Other issues may include raters having other duties, raters rushing through the evaluation to get it done quickly, raters able to over-or underinflate their results. When employees get to choose who is involved in the evaluation, bias can occur. Benefits of a 360 are that they give a more-rounded view of the employee because data are from multiple sources. In addition, (1) it gives the employee more recognition and validation of their duties, which can raise their confidence in their role; (2) it increases accountability to raise performance; (3) it promotes continuous improvement; and (4) it can change the culture through openness, accountability, and empowerment for role responsibility and professional development (Chopra, 2017).

DEVELOPING EMPLOYEES THROUGH THE PERFORMANCE APPRAISAL AND REVIEW

The Manager as Coach

The use of coaching by organizations is becoming more common, with the manager taking the role of the coach, where managers "give support and guidance rather than instructions, and employees learn how to adapt to constantly changing environments in ways that unleash fresh energy, innovation, and commitment" (Ibarra & Scoular, 2019, para 3). Managerial coaching can be described as empowering employees to exceed their performance and providing the tools and resources that allows them to do so (Ladyshewsky & Taplin, 2018).

Coaching has been found to raise self-awareness, self-confidence, and self-leadership while positively facilitating relationships with others. According to the International Coach Federation (ICF), 80% of those who received coaching reported an increase in self-confidence with 70% reported improved work performance and more effective communication skills. Organizations would benefit from training managers on the use of coaching as a leadership strategy (Institute of Coaching, n.d.).

Performance Improvement Plans

What happens if a nurse is not performing up to standards or has a critical incident that is averse to patient care or the team? A PIP is the first step to take before any major consequences occur, such as termination. The PIP gives the manager the opportunity to correct any actions in a formalized manner, as it is a tool that provides the opportunity for the nurse to make performance corrections. It should be used to help the employee improve and is not to be used as a punitive measure. It does not always mean that a termination is imminent, but it is the first step if it does occur (Society for Human Resource Management [SHRM], n.d.).

The PIP needs to be very detailed, with specific examples of identified problems, to avoid any confusion by the employee; it should also include specific and measurable goals and outcomes with a time frame for improvements to be made. The manager then meets with the employee to discuss reasons for the plan, improvements to be made, support needed, and if any resources, such as training or tools to accomplish job expectations. According to Kirkpatrick (2005), any adverse actions by the manager should also be identified in the root-cause of the problem, such as not keeping the employee updated on information or not clarifying what is needed for the job.

PIPs should be tied to job duties in the performance appraisal and should focus on employee strengths and overcoming challenge areas. Once signed by the employee, frequent check-ins should be made to see how the employee is performing and meeting their goals and if any revisions need to be made. A PIP can be extended if improvements are being observed to allow the employee the time to develop. If no improvements are observed, then moving to termination is the last step.

LEADERSHIP AND MANAGEMENT IMPLICATIONS

Elements of a Successful Performance Review

Managers drive the performance appraisal process, although they may bring in supervisors or others with whom the nurse has interacted. The manager will gather relevant data related to the employee, which can include notes, previous evaluations, and interviews with staff. This data should be collected on a continuous basis, lessening the chance of any bias. The manager then develops a written plan and writes an assessment according to the organization's appraisal format. The manager would include any observations on performance, recommendations that would continue to develop the nurse in skills, classes or certifications to take, or suggestions for behavioral change (such as improvement in documentation). Finally, an overall rating is tallied.

Now the manager can meet with the nurse to discuss the outcomes and recommendations and any compensation attached to the rating. The tone of this meeting is set by the manager so the more positive and open it is, the more positive the review process is looked at from both sides.

If the nurse was involved in the evaluation (self-rating), this is brought into the meeting and compared against the manager's evaluation. It is in this conversation that the nurse is allowed the opportunity to express views and concerns and any desired goals to attain over the next evaluation period, such as a desire to move into a new role.

Stress and Burnout

The effect of performance appraisals on the work effort of employees to meet performance standards can lead to performance pressure, or the urgency to achieve performance levels with rewards and consequences attached. This often leaves employees feeling the need to work harder and longer. This can compound the stress level of a nurse, who may already be under pressure to provide the highest level of care in dealing with staff and families and encountering pressure to meet regulatory compliance. Nurses must also regulate their own emotions in their work to calm patients and families and in carrying out their duties. Kim (2020) distinguished between deep acting and surface acting. Deep acting is changing one's emotions to meet demands of the job, and surface acting refers to hiding one's emotions. Both types of acing can lead to more stress and, eventually, burnout.

Job stress "results when the requirements of the job do not meet the capabilities, resources, or needs of workers" (National Institute for Occupational Safety and Health (NIOSH), 2009, p. 6). The American Institute of Stress (2019) reported that 40% of workers experience job stress, although that number continues to climb higher. Adverse effects of stress include physical problems and can lead to aggressive behavior (https://www.stress.org). This topic has many layers and implications, outside the scope of this chapter, but it is critical for health care organizations to be more aware of the emotional health of workers and for managers to have "check-ins" with staff to determine how they are doing, as well as providing tools and resources to address staff emotional reaction or level. Nurse managers who are aware of the signs and symptoms of stress are better able to assess the emotional needs of staff and mitigate adverse effects, such as absenteeism or inadequate patient care.

CURRENT ISSUES AND TRENDS

There is a growing trend to eliminate the current use of performance appraisals and move to a performance management system. According to a Gallup report (Wigert & Harter, 2017) about 14% or only 2 in 10 employees feel that performance appraisals motivate them to make improvements. As a subsequent, Sutton and Wigert (2019) concluded that the current system is ineffective.

Performance management systems benchmark employees to set standards that one either meets, exceeds, or needs improvement on. The set-up includes the use of a technology-based platform, or Human Resource Information Systems (HRIS). In this platform or system, job roles are entered, benchmarks for each of those roles, and thresholds to meet national standards. Goals are set to meet those thresholds, and feedback is done through an ongoing process. This process benefits both the manager and employee, as feedback is done in real time so problems can be immediately addressed, and corrective action taken. This benefits the nurse and the organization overall.

Along with benchmarks, many organizations are adding coaching, either from an internal coach or external coach. Coaching has been shown to help an employee to meet their goals faster by setting expectations, increasing communication skills, and attaining goals through accountability (Sherpa Coaching, 2019). Once benchmarks are set, the coach then works with the employee to meet required standards, and coaching has been shown to get them there faster (Sherpa Coaching, 2019). Training managers in coaching principles, as part of the HRIS system, would lead to faster development of employees in meeting work expectations.

Many major corporations have changed their performance appraisal system, or eliminated them entirely, and are setting the trend for other companies to follow. Netflix is a prime example. Netflix changed its performance management system in 2009 to a context environment, where the focus is less on goal setting and more on helping employees understand the context, specifically, "organizational goals, the priority of those goals, level of refinement required, key stakeholders, and the definition of success" (Cognology, n.d.). In this appraisal model, it is the responsibility of the manager to set the environment for employees to succeed. If an employee makes a mistake, the context and environment are first examined to determine whether they were conducive for goal attainment.

Netflix also moved to a continuous feedback system, as opposed to a yearly review, which led to better performance. Google uses a continuous feedback system as well, but it is based on a peer-review system: employees are not promoted if they do not get good reviews from their peers. Zappos is also based on feedback; however, half of their ratings focus on the relationship with the organization's culture and values (Cognology,

n.d.). These companies are discovering, through continuous feedback, that employees have higher performance and better alignment with core values, which leads to delivering high quality products, services, and customer service.

Agile Performance Management

Agile Management has been around for a long time, but it is mainly used in manufacturing and defense agencies. It is about efficiency, so services and resources are utilized in the most energetic and productive way. Due to that focus, health care organizations are now beginning to see the value and adopt this strategy. Agile Performance Management is a collaborative, continuous, and developmental strategy that is focused on processes that evaluate an employee over a period of time, such as 6-months to a year. "Agile Performance Management focuses on both the process and end goal. Continuous improvement is key" (Pawar, 2016). There are three processes in this model: (1) continuous feedback, (2) communication, and (3) coaching. Health care organizations are using this model to improve the quality of services and their competitive advantage: Mayo Clinic uses Agile with streamlining Information Technology (IT) functions to improve processes and systems without compromising patient care (Pool et al., 2019). Benefits of using the Agile model include: (1) increased accountability, (2) collaboration, and (3) communication through supportive leadership.

Deficit Versus Strengths Model

The new paradigm focuses on the strengths of an employee versus their deficits. Current feedback tends to focus on what an employee has done wrong and then sets the goals for improvement. However, this approach does not lead to improvement. This new paradigm is based on the model of Appreciative Inquiry, which is an organizational development process that has shifted from deficits to strengths, affirms past and present strengths, and acknowledges successes and the individual's potential (Cooperrider & Srivatsa, 1987). The employee (i.e., nurse) is then asked how they will apply their past behavior to current or future situations, thereby, bestowing accountability on them. By focusing on strengths and past successes, more awareness and accountability is given to the nurse who can override challenges they face. This is a much more positive experience in the feedback process for both the nurse and manager.

SUMMARY

The development of employee competencies leads to quality patient care or positive organizational outcomes based on the organizations mission. This is augmented through the performance appraisal system. This process allows managers to assess the knowledge, skills, and abilities of employees to aid in their development and future needs. Understanding various factors that make up the appraisal process will lead to a fair assessment and feedback that aligns the employee to individual, departmental, and organizational goals. Managers with an employee development mindset have the knowledge to drive the appraisal process to build relationships (i.e., with nurses and support staff) and have continuous feedback into their development. This allows the employee to be conscientious and take more responsibility in meeting set goals. Hospitals can meet organizational goals and standards of care through supporting a strong performance management system.

RESEARCH NOTE

Source
Setiawati, T., & Ariani, I. D. (2020). Influence of performance appraisal fairness and job satisfaction through commitment on performance. *Review of Integrative Business and Economics, 9*(3), 133–151.

Purpose
This quantitative study discussed the influence of performance appraisal fairness and job satisfaction through commitment on job performance among respondents working in a hospital in Indonesia.

Research

Purpose
The study aims were to determine the influence of performance appraisal fairness and job satisfaction through commitment on job performance. This study used a survey design with a questionnaire using a six-point Likert scale that was mailed to 187 people. Returned were 155 questionnaires. Participants were between the ages of 26 and 79 years old.

Discussion
Four key variables were used to operationalize the study. These include performance appraisal fairness, job satisfaction, commitment, and job performance. The authors tested nine hypotheses. Proven hypotheses included: (1) performance appraisal fairness has a positive effect on commitment, (2) job satisfaction has a positive effect on commitment, (3) commitment has a positive effect on job performance, (4) performance appraisal fairness has a positive effect on job performance, (5) job satisfaction has a positive effect on job performance, (6) performance appraisal fairness and job satisfaction have a positive effect on commitment, and (7) performance appraisal fairness and job satisfaction have a positive effect on job performance. Two unproven hypotheses were: (1) indirect influence of performance appraisal fairness on job performance with commitment as the intervening variable is greater than the direct influence, and (2) indirect influence of performance appraisal fairness on job performance with commitment as the intervening variable is greater than the direct influence.

Application to Practice
Similar studies have been done in other industries such as banking and hotels. These new findings are specific to health care. The authors have concluded that performance appraisal fairness and job satisfaction had positive effects on job performance. Therefore, these findings can inform health care in an era of nursing shortages and an increasing aging population.

With the increasing need to hire and develop staff, an effective way to do so is through an efficient performance management system. Fairness in the appraisal system will lead to equity and job satisfaction. Enhancing these can lead to higher performance, which this study proved. Although commitment was not supported, independently it can lead to higher levels of commitment to the job and ensure quality patient care.

CASE STUDY

Stephanie is a nurse manager in a large hospital system, where she is in charge of several departments, including two medical-surgical units that serve general medicine and orthopedics, with over 40 staff. Stephanie has been in nursing leadership for over 10 years and considers herself a caring manager. As she works to develop relationships with her employees to ensure their satisfaction, she knows that will result in high quality care.

Through the "grapevine," Stephanie heard that several of her nurses are unhappy, and unit level metrics indicate that there has been a higher rate of turnover in the last 6 months. Performance appraisals are done in the short-term, and Stephanie worries how the feedback will further affect her staff, considering that several of the nurses have been under-performing. She worries that there will be more staff dissatisfaction and, worse, more turnover.

Stephanie is a caring and involved leader. She reads about the latest trends, not just in nursing, but also in other fields.

During her research to assess problems and identify solutions, she discovered information about how some companies are implementing newer, best practices that focus on an employee's strengths, rather than on problems, and use benchmarks to develop employees, one of which is providing continuous feedback. Stephanie decides to work on implementing this practice by having regular meetings with each staff member to let them know how they are performing, to share information on events in the hospital, and to also get their feedback on how she is doing and for any ideas/or recommendations for improvements.

By collaborating with Human Resources (HR), Stephanie restructured the performance management program in her department. This made the process more fulfilling both for her employees and for her as the leader. The new program was well received by staff. She now intends to present the new program to her leadership for consideration to adopt enterprise-wide.

CRITICAL THINKING EXERCISE

Maxine has been in nursing for 30 years. She started as a floor nurse then expanded her skills in several specialties. For the last 5 years she worked in a nursing home and decided to return to a hospital setting, where she functions in the role of nurse manager for a medical-surgical unit.

Maxine is enjoying her new role but tends to be critical of newer nurses who she feels are not as dedicated as she is and tend to circumvent many practices in day-to-day events. She gets along with tenured nurses, and has difficulty relating to younger nurses. Maxine has upcoming performance appraisals in the next month and is feeling a bit awkward.

This "disconnect" is causing Maxine stress as she attempts to write fair appraisals. For the past month, she has been diligently working on them, despite feeling uneasy. HR has given her the schedule to receive their reviews. To her dismay, Maxine finds one of the young nurses is the first for a performance review, which includes not just writing the review, but meeting with them in person. Maxine now finds herself procrastinating and finding excuses to not write the appraisal. She realizes she needs to proceed with the meeting but has delayed it twice and now has heard from both HR and her immediate manager that the appraisal is past due.

1. What is the problem?
2. What is the cause, or causes, which could be leading to Maxine's behavior?
3. If you were Maxine's supervisor, what interventions would you take to address her delay in getting the appraisals completed?
4. What recommendations would you make to Maxine to get through the appraisals successfully?

REFERENCES

360pev.com. (2013). *Here you will find all you need to know about a 360 feedback.* http://360performanceevaluation.com/.

American Institute of Stress. (2019). *Workplace stress.* http://www.stress.org/workplace-stress/.

Benedictine University. (n.d.). *What is performance and how does it relate to culture?* https://online.ben.edu/programs/msmob/resources/what-is-performance.

Berinato, S. (2018). Negative feedback rarely leads to improvement: Mr. Green, defend your Research. *Harvard Business Review, 96*(1), 32–33.

Bernardin, J., Thomason, S., Buckley, M. R., & Kane, J. S. (2016). Rater rater-level bias and accuracy in performance appraisals: The impact of rater personality, performance management competence, and rater accountability. *Human Resource Management, 55*(2), 321–340.

Capelli, P., & Conyon, M. J. (2018). What do performance appraisals do. *ILR Review, 71*(1), 88–116.

Chopra, R. (2017). 360 degree performance assessments: An overview. *Global Journal of Enterprise Information System, 9*(3), 102–105.

Cognology. (n.d.). *What can Netflix, Hubspot, Zappos and Google teach you about the future of performance management.* https://www.cognology.com.au/can-netflix-hubspot-zappos-google-teach-future-performance-management/.

Cooperrider, D. L., & Srivasta, S. (1987). Appreciative inquiry in organizational life. *Research in Organizational Change and Development, 1*, 129–169.

Dello Russo, S., Miraglia, M., & Borgogni, L. (2017). Reducing organizational politics in performance appraisal: The role of coaching leaders for age-diverse employees. *Human Resource Management, 56*(5), 769–783. https://doi.org/10.1002/hrm.21799.

DeNisi, A. S., & Murphy, K. R. (2017). Performance appraisals and performance management. *Journal of Applied Psychology, 102*(3), 421–433.

Drucker, P. F. (1954). *The practice of management,* New York, NY: Harper & Row.

Farrell, S. (2017). Leadership reflections: Extrovert and introvert leaders. *Journal of Library Administration, 57*(4), 436–443.

Geise, K., & Theil, A. (2015). The psychological contract Chinese-African informal labor relations. *International Journal of Human Resource Management, 26*(14), 1807–1826.

Ghosh, P. (2019). What is HRIS? System, model, and application. *HR Technologist.* https://www.hrtechnologist.com/articles/performance-management-hcm/what-is-hris/.

Haag-Heitman, B., & George, V. (2011). Nursing peer-review: Principles and practice. *American Nurse Today, 6*(9), 48–52. https://www.mghpcs.org/eed_portal/Documents/ProfDev/Nursing-Peer-Review-Article.pdf.

Heathfield, S. M. (2016). *Performance improvement plan: Contents and sample form.* https://www.thebalance.com/performance-improvement-plan-contents-and-sample-form-1918850.

Henniger, N. (2016). *Appraisals and envy: The influence of situational factors on envious feelings and motivation.* (Doctoral dissertation). University of San Diego. California. https://escholarship.org/uc/item/823902nj.

Ibarra, H., & Scoular, A. (2019). The leader as coach. *Harvard Business Review, 97*(6), 110–119. https://hbr.org/2019/11/the-leader-as-coach.

Include-empower.com. (2018). *Explaining affinity bias: Preferring people like us.* https://cultureplusconsulting.com/2015/06/19/explaining-affinity-bias/.

Institute of Coaching. (n.d.). *Benefits of coaching.* https://instituteofcoaching.org/coaching-overview/coaching-benefits.

International Coach Federation (ICF). (n.d.). *Current competency model.* https://coachfederation.org/core-competencies.

Iqbal, M. Z. (2017). Expanded dimensions of the purposes and uses of performance appraisals. *Asian Academy of Management Journal, 17*(1), 41–63.

Juneja, P. (2020). *Performance appraisal.* Management Study Guide. https://www.managementstudyguide.com/performance-appraisal.htm.

Kim, J.- S. (2020). Emotional labor strategies, stress, and burnout among nurse: A path analysis. *Journal of Nursing Scholarship, 52*(1), 105–112.

Kirkpatrick, D. L. (2005). *The performance improvement plan. Improving employee performance through appraisal and coaching* (2nd ed.). New York, NY: American Management Association (pp. 66–78).

Ladyshewsky, R. K., & Taplin, R. (2018). The interplay between organizational learning culture, the manager as coach, self-efficacy and workload on employee work engagement. *International Journal of Evidence Based Coaching and Mentoring, 16*(2), 3–19.

Larsen, D. A. (2019). Using the elaborate likelihood model to explain performance appraisal inaccuracies. *Journal of Practice and Policy Management, 20*(4), 65–77.

Latham, G. P., & Wexley, K. N. (1977). Behavioral observation scales for performance appraisal purposes. *Personnel Psychology, 30*, 255–268.

Lexico Dictionary (n.d.). *Feedback.* https://www.lexico.com/definition/feedback.

Moon, K. (2019). Specificity of performance appraisal feedback, trust in manager, and job attitudes: A serial mediation model. *International Journal of Social Behavior and Personality, 47*(6), 2–12.

National Institute for Occupational Safety and Health (NIOSH). (2009). *Stress…at work*: DHHS (NIOSH) Publication No. 99–101. https://www.cdc.gov/niosh/docs/99-101/default.html.

Pawar, Y. (2016). Traditional versus agile performance management. *Uprise Together.* https://upraise.io/blog/traditional-vs-agile-performance-management/.

Performance-appraisals.org. (2018). *What is employee self-appraisal?* http://performance-appraisals.org/faq/selfappraisals.htm.

Pool, E. T., Poole, K., Upjohn, D. P., & Fernandez, J. S. (2019). Agile project management proves effective, efficient for Mayo Clinic. *American Association for Physician Leadership*. https://www.physicianleaders.org/news/agile-project-management-proves-effective-efficient-mayo-clinic.

Reiken, J. (2018). *8 Rater biases that are affecting your performance management*. Trakstar. https://www.trakstar.com/blog-post/8-rater-biases-impacting-performance-management/.

Robbins, S. P., & Judge, T. A. (2018). *Essentials of organizational behavior* (14th ed.). Upper Saddle River, NJ: Pearson.

Sanchez, C. R., Diaz-Cabrera, D., & Hernandez-Fernaud, E. (2019). Does effectiveness in performance appraisal improve with rater training? *PLoS One*, *14*(9), 1–20. https://doi.org/10.1371/journal.pone.0222694.

Schub, E. (2014). *Clinical competencies assessment*. Cinahl Information Systems. https://www.ebscohost.com/images-nursing/assets/ClinicalCompetenceAssessment.pdf.

Sherpa Coaching. (2019). *Executive Coaching Survey Report 2019*: Sasha Corporation. https://www.sherpacoaching.com/pdf_files/2019_Executive_Coaching_Survey_Summary_Report.pdf.

Smith, P. C., & Kendall, L. M. (1963). Retranslation of expectations: An approach to the construction of unambiguous anchors for rating scales. *Journal of Applied Psychology*, *47*, 149–155.

Society for Human Resource Management (SHRM). (n.d.). *How to establish a performance improvement plan*. https://www.shrm.org/resourcesandtools/tools-and-samples/how-to-guides/pages/performanceimprovementplan.aspx.

Steele, D. (n.d.). Pros and cons of peer-review in the workplace. Council for Adult and Experiential Learning. https://www.cael.org/blog/pros-and-cons-of-peer-review-in-the-workplace.

Sutton, R., & Wigert, B. (2019). *More harm than good: The truth about performance reviews*: Gallup Organization. https://www.gallup.com/workplace/249332/harm-good-truth-performance-reviews.aspx.

Teckchandani, A., & Pichler, S. (2015). Quality results in performance management. *Industrial Management*, *57*(4), 16–20.

The Joint Commission. (n.d.). *Orthopedic certification: Pathways to excellence in patient care*. https://www.jointcommission.org/-/media/enterprise/tjc/imported-page-assets/tjc-ortho-cert-brochure-v4pdf.pdf?db=web&hash=189A318A66F917F27AA76B3C901DAF36.

Weirks, T. G. D. (2007). *Behavior and result-based performance management and the performance of business management: An examination of the mediating relationships between proactive behavior between performance management and performance*. Tillburg, Netherlands: Tillburg University Master's thesis.

Wigert, B., & Harter, J. (2017). *Re-engineering performance management*: Gallup Organization. https://www.gallup.com/workplace/238064/re-engineering-performance-management.aspx.

24

Emergency Management and Preparedness

Kimberly K. Hatchel, Melinda Hirshouer

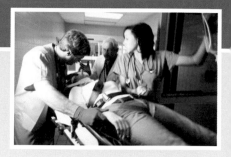

http://evolve.elsevier.com/Huber/leadership

Editors' note: In early February 2020, when this chapter was prepared and submitted, we all were unaware of what was about to happen: a severe worldwide coronavirus pandemic. Although COVID-19 was a new virus, it had been some 17 years since the last severe coronavirus outbreak (SARS). As this book goes into production, we are watching the responses by governments and organizations in real time. The need for emergency management and preparedness has been brought into sharp focus in the pressing urgency of what is now unfolding.

TRANSITIONING THEORY INTO PRACTICE FOR ALL-HAZARDS PREPAREDNESS

The events of September 11, 2001, a tragic day in history, changed Americans' perception of a "safe" world. In the years that followed the world has experienced numerous catastrophic events with causes across a continuum. A new disaster preparedness narrative has emerged as a result of the diversity, magnitude, and frequency of these events. People of all backgrounds have been forced to consider preparation in their homes, at their church, schools, and work environments for the eventuality of a disaster. It was once assumed that people were knowledgeable about how to prepare for potential natural disasters within their local regions. As disasters have impacted larger groups of people and events are impacting the same geographical areas including large rural and isolated areas in shorter periods of time, preparation has changed. Appropriate planning has become more crucial than ever. A list of man-made possibilities is endless: biological exposures, chemical spills, gun violence,

radiological exposures, nuclear blasts, conventional bombings, agricultural contamination, cyber viruses, and other unforeseen cataclysmic nature events may also occur. Thus developing a contingency plan for most types of disasters, including bioterrorism, is most appropriately termed **all-hazards disaster preparedness.**

Since the occurrence of major disasters such as the attack on the World Trade Center, Hurricane Sandy in 2012, and the devastating tornado in Joplin, Missouri in 2011, key community stakeholders such as local governments, fire and rescue workers, and hospitals have been focused on sharing information from a variety of resources, developing collaborative response plans, and preparing for a probable disaster. However, there are still gaps in the possession and execution of emergency preparedness knowledge. In a 2008 study, Niska and Shimizu (2011) found that while greater than 95% of hospitals had emergency preparedness plans for chemical, biological, or natural disasters, considerably fewer facilities were prepared for radiological-nuclear or explosive-incendiary incidents. Additionally, only 73% of facilities were prepared for loss of utilities. The American College of Emergency Physicians (ACEP) has recommended that hospitals use their Emergency Operations Plan (EOP) to develop their training plan and that they execute situational drills to ensure that the staff has retained knowledge and that the training remains a valuable tool for the hospitals. Of the 88% of facilities that had prepared plans to continue operations during an emergency, 15% of these hospitals had to enact these plans for an actual incident in 2007. Additionally, only 47% of hospitals were prepared to manage and shelter mobility or cognitively impaired patients (Niska & Shimizu, 2011). In 2014, there were 84 federally declared disasters in the United States and that is only a small portion of the emergency events that a hospital may encounter (Federal Emergency Management Agency, 2016).

In order to close some of these gaps, The Joint Commission (TJC) has advanced hospital efforts through the development of six crucial areas for emergency preparedness: communication, safety and security, resources and assets, staff responsibilities, utilities management, and patient clinical and support activities (TJC Resources, 2008, 2020). These crucial areas create a framework for all-hazards disaster preparedness planning. Hospitals must prepare for a variety of internal or external events that cause enough disruption that the normal operations are forced into crisis mode. If the employees chosen to lead the hospital in its response to casualties, property damage, or suspending patient care are unprepared or make ineffective decisions, the crisis will quickly escalate to a disaster (Sternberg, 2003). TJC requires hospitals to have a written EOP (TJC, 2020). The EOP must include how the hospital trains, prepares, and responds to potential events. What is certain is that patients and their family members will expect the hospital to continue to provide normal operations regardless of internal or external circumstances.

Health care executives across the country understand the need to dedicate resources to support effective all-hazards preparedness. The Health Insurance Portability and Accountability Act (HIPAA) and TJC require all health care facilities to have detailed all-hazard preparedness plans. Nursing leaders are an integral part of the planning process and should have knowledge of the national Emergency Response Plan promulgated by the Federal Emergency Management Agency (FEMA) (https://www.ready.gov/business/implementation/emergency), as well as state and local disaster response plans. Effective planning and evaluation skills for all-hazards preparedness is an essential management competency for nursing leaders. The ability to receive federal response grants must be compliant with the National Incident Management System (NIMS) (US Department of Homeland Security [DHS], 2020). Additionally, TJC requires hospitals to practice elements of their EOP and evaluate areas of success and opportunity (2016).

This chapter describes how to orchestrate a multilevel plan for a health care facility. A comprehensive all-hazards preparedness plan will assist in establishing (1) an organized hospital-based plan for both internal and external disasters at the department/unit level, (2) an interhospital plan for effectively collaborating with other hospitals within a health care system and within the vicinity, (3) a community plan that will integrate the hospital plan with other external community plans, and (4) a national plan that will guide nurse leaders in accessing financial assistance from federal and state all-hazards preparedness resources.

DEFINITIONS

From a health care perspective, a **disaster** is "a type of emergency that, due to its complexity, scope, or duration, threatens a health care center's capabilities … and requires outside assistance to sustain patient care, safety, or security functions" (TJC, 2008, p. 2). There are a wide variety of types and causes of disasters, including sudden onset (severe weather events or chemical spills) and slow-onset events (progressive disease outbreaks) (World Health Organization [WHO], 2013). Although often triggered by nature, disasters can be caused by human acts, including chemical, biological, radiological, nuclear, or explosives (CBRNE). Wars and civil disturbances that destroy homelands and displace people are included among man-made disasters. Causes of natural disasters include severe weather events such as blizzards, wildfires, floods, tsunamis, volcanic eruptions, earthquakes, tornadoes, hurricanes, and the devastation caused by Hurricane Sandy in 2012 or the earthquake and resulting tsunami in Japan in 2011. Disasters can be *internal*, such as a catastrophic event that occurs within a facility, such as a loss of utilities or an unplanned extended downtime of the electronic health record, making it difficult to maintain operations (TJC, 2012); or *external*, such as a catastrophic event that affects the community that may or may not affect the facility, such as the 2020 coronavirus 2019 (COVID-19) worldwide viral pandemic.

Other disaster-related definitions are:

- *All-hazards*: A general term that is descriptive of all types of natural and/or human terrorist events.
- *All-hazards disaster preparedness*: An effective and consistent response to any disaster or emergency regardless of the cause (Wright State University, 2016).
- *Crisis standards of care*: "Substantial change in the usual healthcare operations and the level of care it is possible to deliver … in a public health emergency, justified by specific circumstances, declared by a state government in recognition that crisis operations will be in effect for a sustained period" (Institute of Medicine [IOM], 2012).

- *CBRNE*: Chemical, biological, radiological, nuclear, explosives (US Department of Defense, 2015).
- *Biological disaster*: Disease epidemics and insect/animal plagues or an incident occurring as a result of the deliberate or unintentional release of biological materials that may adversely affect the health of those exposed (International Federation of Red Cross and Red Crescent Societies [IFRC], 2016; US Department of Defense, 2015).
- *Chemical disaster*: The deliberate or unintentional release of poisonous vapors, liquids, or solids that have a toxic effect on people, plants, and animals (Ready. gov, 2016).
- *Radiological/nuclear disaster*: Radiological or nuclear emergencies may be intentional (caused by terrorists) or unintentional (accidents that may result from accidents within a facility, e.g., the departments of nuclear medicine and radiation oncology or from external sources involving vehicles transporting radioactive materials) (Centers for Disease Control and Prevention [CDC], 2014).
- *Explosives*: A catastrophic event caused by the use of weapons such as guns, bombs, missiles, or grenades.
- *Cyber disaster*: A catastrophic event that results from an attack initiated from one computer against another computer with the purpose of compromising the information stored on it (Arnand, 2014).
- *Hazard vulnerability analysis*: An exercise that is a systematic approach to recognizing hazards and identifying an organization's potential emergencies, the likelihood of the event occurring, and the impact it would have on the organization. The risks associated with each hazard are analyzed to prioritize planning, mitigation, response, and recovery activities (California Hospital Association, 2011).
- *Mass casualty incident*: A natural or manmade event generating large numbers of patients requiring medical care and that overwhelms a health care facility and prevents it from delivering medical services that are consistent with accepted standards (Agency for Healthcare Research and Quality [AHRQ], 2012).

BACKGROUND

GETTING STARTED: FIRST STEPS

Starting any systems project can be complex and difficult. Beginning the work of establishing a comprehensive all-hazards preparedness plan is no exception.

Historically, most hospitals have had some type of disaster plan in place. Evaluating the hospital's existing EOP while focusing on maintaining a state of constant readiness can be a complicated process. One of the first steps to gaining participation from appropriate stakeholders and moving the evaluation process forward is the creation of an emergency management oversight committee, or an all-hazards preparedness task force. Based on the American Organization of Nurse Executive's (AONE, 2016) *Role of the Nurse Leader in Crisis Management,* the nurse executive—often called the *chief nursing officer (CNO)*—will play a pivotal role in facilitating the initial committee. The AONE guiding principles include:

- Nurse leaders are trained in media relations and understand the tenets of good communication.
- Leaders are skilled critical thinkers, collaborative, and able to manage ambiguity.
- Nurse leaders project calm, confidence, and authority in all situations. They also are empathetic to how people react to loss, challenges, and uncertainty.
- Nurse leaders are prepared to review and practice the organization's crisis readiness plan with nursing staff.
- The CNO is a member of the senior leadership team, whose role is clearly defined and sought by colleagues, particularly during a crisis.

Creating an Emergency Management Committee

As many nurses understand, effective projects start with the basic nursing process: assessment, planning, implementation, evaluation, and, if necessary, modification. The emergency management committee will follow a similar process when developing an emergency management plan, which will incorporate mitigation of potential hazards (assessment), developing a plan of what to do should the event occur (planning), responding to the actual event (implementation), and assisting the hospital and the community in the short- and long-term recovery that will follow (evaluation). Developing an original plan is best accomplished by establishing a high-level administrative committee whose purpose will be oversight of the multilevel emergency management plan development. Whether the hospital is part of a larger health care system or is a freestanding, independent hospital, the committee will function similarly.

Health care systems with multiple facilities are very familiar with the complexity and intricacies of trying to establish a standardized system-wide approach to care needs. In organizations such as these, system-wide executive administrators need to be part of the committee. Having a senior executive administrator of the health care system serve as the chairperson of the committee will provide the leadership needed to communicate the importance of emergency preparedness as a system priority. A representative CNO and emergency medicine physician, serving as co-chairs with the senior executive administrator, can create a dynamic team that is uniquely prepared to tackle any issues that arise. A project facilitator is helpful in getting the committee started and operational. The project facilitator can also serve in a pivotal maintenance role, keeping the emergency management plan current and in the forefront of the administration's strategic planning over time.

Establishing the committee requires that all departments be committed to the tasks at hand and cognizant of the need for consensus building and standardization of processes. Multidirectional communication is imperative. The standing membership should be composed of stakeholders representing all areas of the organization, both clinical and non-clinical. Because not all departments can logistically be on the committee, the members will have large areas of oversight and communication. Committee membership might typically look like that outlined in Table 24.1.

TABLE 24.1   Emergency Management Committee Membership Responsibilities

Responsibility Area(s)	Position Title	Detail of Area Covered
Executive owner (chair)	Executive administrator	Leads the emergency management committee as chair. If the hospital is part of a health care system, this person will be a system-wide senior administrator. If the hospital is a freestanding, independent facility, this person will be the hospital's chief operating officer.
Clinical operations (co-chair)	Chief nurse officer	Represents all nursing and clinical departments; co-chairs the emergency management committee.
Chemical, biological, radiological, nuclear, or explosives (CBRNE) threats (co-chair)	Emergency department/ medical director	Represents all aspects of emergency medicine and physician needs related to all-hazards preparedness. This person also will co-chair the committee.
Physician liaison(s)	Department chiefs	Serve as spokespersons for physician needs with regard to disaster preparedness. Facilitate communication of timely information should an event occur. Have oversight for physician credentialing in times of a disaster. Assist in approval of medical standards established for various types of disasters.
Chief operating officers (COOs) from health care system facilities	Chief operating officer(s)	Represent the needs of their facilities in establishing an effective all-hazards preparedness plan. Facilitate system-wide collaboration in standardizing practices and communicate essential information to employees.
Security	Safety and security director	Serves as liaison for system-wide safety and security departments in the system. Coordinates and synchronizes efforts of all departments as related to all-hazards preparedness. Responsible for rapid "lockdown" of all entrances and flow of people in the event of a disaster.
Communications	Chief information technology officer	Oversees successful operation of the integrated information system, including telephones, radios, and computers and satellite technology, during times of instability. Creates and maintains redundant systems to ensure an ability to communicate within facilities, outside to other hospitals, and partners with community.

TABLE 24.1	Emergency Management Committee Membership Responsibilities—cont'd	
Responsibility Area(s)	**Position Title**	**Detail of Area Covered**
Messages/media	Marketing director/ information officer	Plays an active role in communicating the all-hazards preparedness message to all employees, patients, and community. Acts on behalf of the health care system or hospital in speaking with press about impending or actual disaster situations.
Human resources	Human resources director	Serves as the staff's voice in meeting the needs of employees during a disaster. Creates manuals to guide staff in preparing for and responding to a disaster. Manages the human resources pool when the incident command center is active.
Financial reimbursement	Chief financial officer	Leads efforts in monitoring financial expenses related to establishing an effective all-hazards preparedness plan. Seeks out state/federal reimbursement opportunities for planning.
Government funding	Government affairs director	Serves as a vital link to local, state, and federal boards representing the system financial and operational needs regarding all-hazards preparedness. Advocates for funding related to all-hazards preparedness.
Biological threats	Infectious disease medical director	Serves as the liaison for all infection control (IC) departments in the system.
Infection control	Infection prevention and control practitioner	Coordinates and synchronizes efforts of all IC departments as related to all-hazards preparedness. Responsible for development, dissemination, and understanding of procedures related to biological events.
Legal	Executive attorney	Advises all-hazards preparedness task force in legal matters related to establishing an effective all-hazards preparedness plan.
Education planning	Education director	Has oversight for planning and implementing educational efforts for staff and patients. As needed, coordinates "just in time" training for any arising incident and is an integral partner in planning and implementing internal and external disaster drills.
Logistics	Pharmacy director	Serves as the liaison for all system pharmacies. Has oversight for stockpiling medications for use in a disaster. Establishes par levels of drugs for use in "patient surge" situations. Establishes contracts with pharmaceutical vendors to ensure adequate supply of medications in the event of a disaster. Has oversight for any medical supply trucks ready for deployment in times of a disaster (e.g., stocking par level of drugs used in a chemical disaster).
Logistics	Materials management director	Serves as an active participant on the task force. This liaison is the system representative for all materials management departments. Is very involved in setting par levels for supplies and equipment on the units at the time of a disaster. Establishes contracts with materials management vendors to ensure adequate supply of medications in the event of a disaster (e.g., stocking a supplemental supply truck for use in a disaster).
Logistics	Engineering	Directs any operational building redesign needed to prepare hospital for handling a disaster (e.g., decontamination showers).

Note: This assessment tool was developed by Inova Health System based on a bioterrorism preparedness survey created by a committee consisting of representatives from Baylor University's Graduate Program in Healthcare Administration, the US Army Center for Healthcare Education and Studies, and the University of Texas Health Science Center at San Antonio. (For more information, see Drenkard et al., 2002.) Courtesy Inova Health System, Falls Church, VA.

As the team evolves in its work, ad hoc members can be added as needed. Internal ad hoc members might include radiology, facility engineering, telecommunications, volunteer support, chaplain services, physician chairs, social work, case management, and dietary, respiratory, and laboratory services. External ad hoc members might include representatives from the local public health department, government liaison, police, fire and rescue, public school system, representatives from the faith community, community physicians, and even vendor representatives who can be contracted to provide such things as oxygen, ice, food, cots, and linens in the event of a disaster.

During the start-up, the system-wide committee will need to meet frequently. To begin, the committee should perform a hazard vulnerability analysis (HVA). The HVA will be used as a starting point to create an EOP that identifies risks and prioritizes likely emergencies in order to mitigate them when possible and develop strategies for preparedness (TJC Resources, 2016). For specific details on the HVA process, there are several resources available, including the FEMA and TJC Resources websites.

Performing an Effective Gap Analysis

There are many ways to perform an all-hazards preparedness gap analysis, and a multitude of online reference websites exist, including these examples:
- FEMA: https://www.fema.gov/media-library/assets/documents/27403.

- Office of Emergency Management, US Department of Health and Human Services: https://www.phe.gov/about/oem/Pages/default.aspx; the American Hospital Association (AHA): https://www.aha.org/2006-05-10-emergency-readiness-1.
- CDC: https://www.cdc.gov/.
- Agency for Healthcare Research and Quality (AHRQ): https://www.ahrq.gov/.
- Clinics and Community Health Centers (CCHC) Emergency Preparedness Gap Analysis: https://docplayer.net/2969385-Cchc-emergency-preparedness-gap-analysis.html.

The guiding principle for creating a hospital-specific all-hazards gap analysis is to keep it simple. One example of a simple way to assess the current state is to create an emergency preparedness survey that is easy to read and requires the department directors to answer in simple checklists one of two ways: (1) "Yes, we have it," or (2) "No, we don't have it." Survey questions need to be concise and clear. The goal is to begin by identifying the areas where there are gaps in the facility's preparedness plans. Questions should be addressed to appropriate departments who then assess the items and determine the current state. A review of the literature and online searches will assist the team in identifying the areas of assessment (Federal Emergency Management Institute (FEMA), 2014; Joint Commission Resources, 2008, 2016). Examples of questions to ask in the survey might include those listed in Box 24.1.

BOX 24.1　Hospital Gap Analysis Survey: Sample Questions

General
- Has your organization conducted a thorough hazard vulnerability analysis (HVA)?
- Does your organization have an emergency operations plan (EOP) that specifically addresses the four disaster phases?
- Does your EOP identify how to activate an emergency response and who is in charge of the command center in a disaster?
- Does your facility have an operational command center to coordinate the hospital's response to a disaster?
- Does your department staff know the chain of command in an emergency?
- Does your department know their role in each type of disaster?

- Does your hospital know their role in the community in an emergency situation?
- Are there specific plans for chemical, biological, radiological, nuclear, or explosives (CBRNE) emergencies?
- Is there a bed and staffing plan for surge capacity for 50 patients? 100 patients? 250 patients? Do you have the necessary supplies and equipment for use in a surge situation?

Human Resources
- Does your department staff know how to prepare themselves, their significant others, and pets in the event of a disaster?
- Is there a credentialing plan for health care professionals who come to the nearest facility in a disaster to volunteer their services?

BOX 24.1 Hospital Gap Analysis Survey: Sample Questions—cont'd

Safety and Security
- Does your facility have the following during an emergency:
- A lockdown plan?
- A plan for facility traffic flow and staff entry?
- Multi-language signage to direct people where to go?

Communication
- Does your hospital have emergency-powered phones in case of a disaster?
- Does your facility have a backup radio system and volunteer staff to run it?
- Does your facility have a tiered paging system that can reach multiple staff simultaneously?
- Does your department know the central command center telephone number (if there is one)?
- Is there an on-call procedure for notifying the administrator on-call and opening the command center in the event of a disaster?
- Are there established linkages to the external community (e.g., other hospitals in the region, fire department, police, emergency medical system, public schools, public health)?
- Is there a procedure for how to link patients and families both in your facility and in the community should a disaster occur?

Logistics
- Does your facility have:
- Backup emergency supplies, pharmaceuticals, and equipment?
- The ability to release and send pharmaceuticals, medical supplies, and equipment such as respirators to the areas in need in the event of a chemical or biological emergency?
- Prearranged plans with physicians, ambulances, nearby churches, and nursing homes to clear beds in an emergency? (What sites can take patients?)
- Contracts with vendors to bring in food, ice, oxygen, and other needed supplies?
- Is there an established written psychosocial role for social work, chaplains, psychiatry, employee health, and case management in the event of a disaster?
- Are there contingency plans for 4 to 5 days of no power, no water, no computers, and/or no food?
- Are there contingency plans for staff to report to nearest facility to work?

- Are there contingency plans for childcare during an emergency so that parents can work?
- Is there common nomenclature used during an emergency so that everyone understands what is happening and who has what responsibility?

Clinical Operations
- Does your facility have:
  - Procedures established to maximize staff safety in the event of a disaster?
  - Procedures for respiratory mask fit testing and training for personal protective equipment for staff?
  - The ability to track patients until discharge, admission, or death using HIPAA guidelines?
  - Clear established policies and procedures to respond to CBRNE emergencies?
  - A decontamination area and detailed step-by-step procedures on how to work in this area?
  - A backup staff to assist with people/patients arriving to the hospital?
- Does your facility have procedures for how to:
  - Track available beds, arriving patients, and discharges?
  - Track regular and volunteer staff and direct them to a designated area?
  - Operate every department of the hospital during an emergency?
  - Handle surge capacity situations including an understanding of crisis standards of care?
  - Handle operating room cases in the event of an emergency?
  - Track biological, chemical, or nuclear events and report them to authorities?

Financial
- Is there an established plan for tracking costs and submitting them for reimbursement or claims during an emergency?

Messages/Media
- Is there an established communication plan in case of an emergency?
- Is there an established communication script in the event of an emergency?
- Is there an alternative communication plan if wi-fi, power, telephones, and radios are not working?

Courtesy Inova Health System. From Drenkard, K., & Rigotti, G. (2002, updated 2016). *Inova Health System survey*. Falls Church, VA: Inova Health System.

Once the survey is created, it should be distributed to all stakeholders. Directors should be challenged to complete and return it within an appropriate deadline so that work can be initiated to address outstanding issues. The committee should review the survey results and start an issues list to address deficiencies. Nursing leaders will play key roles in creating aggressive timelines for resolving issues identified. Most resolutions will be modified and enhanced over time as the committee gains more knowledge about all-hazards planning. For issues that require multiple steps to correct, commonly seen with widespread education efforts, the use of SMART (specific, measurable, actionable, realistic, and time-bound) goals should be used.

From the gap analysis, the committee needs to establish high-level, multifaceted standards of practice and system-wide goals for all-hazards preparedness. These standards and goals will be implemented at the facility level and department level as directed by the chief operating officer (COO), CNO, and emergency department (ED) medical director. At this point, there is latitude for departments to design and implement the standards and goals based on the unique needs of the populations served. Annual review and evaluation of goals is an effective project management activity, with new goals being created based on the HVA, changing regulatory requirements, new threats, and the results of gaps identified during drills. Sustaining attention and focus on disaster preparedness efforts becomes a key role of the nurse executive in ensuring a constant state of organizational readiness. The project facilitator assists the nurse executive in researching new and evolving initiatives in the discipline of all-hazards preparedness, determining the importance of new trends to the effective operations of the health care organization's all-hazard plan, and implementing relevant enhancements that support the strategic vision for preparedness within the organization.

Keeping the Momentum Going

Once the gap analysis is completed and the issues are identified, development of a comprehensive plan is a critical next step. The work can appear daunting, and it is hard to know where to start. It is at this point that nursing leadership has the opportunity to take charge of the process. Even though the gap analysis may show a multitude of areas for improvement, issues are solvable one step at a time. The CNO and nurse

leaders can help focus the committee and department directors. Efforts should be directed toward creating a streamlined, comprehensive internal emergency management plan that will set the foundation for later steps when the hospital begins to work externally with the community.

Action Items List

Over the next phase, the development of an action items list will become the working action plan used to prioritize and organize work to be done. Subgroups made up of members from the task force who are content experts can be assigned to lead efforts to resolve issues. Issues need to be constantly added and resolved as the facility refines the plan. Reports from subgroups on their progress should be regularly submitted to the committee. The committee needs to have oversight of the subgroups and should strive to clear the road for subgroup progress as needed. Hospitals may need to address common issues such as allocation of resources, including funds to educate staff. Although the immediate return on investment may not be seen or may have a negative effect on productivity numbers during the training, Arbon et al. (2013) found that disaster training did positively influence an employee's willingness to report to work following a disaster. Nurses, in particular, were four times more likely to report to work if they had any pre-existing disaster knowledge or skills, and they were also more likely to respond during a disaster if they perceived their peers and employers were prepared (Arbon et al., 2013). Educating the nursing workforce will be critical to promote an effective disaster response. Planning and education will reduce variability and increase reliability in times of uncertainty.

Establishing a Common Nomenclature, Structure, and Role Definition for Writing All-Hazards Preparedness Plans

When working with the community, using common language becomes especially important for promoting interagency communication in crisis situations. Therefore the NIMS was created by the US DHS (2020) Secretary in response to specific deadlines first identified in Homeland Security Presidential Directive 5 after the September 11 terrorist attacks to further standardize and integrate response practices nationally (Committee on Homeland Security of the House of Representatives, 2008).

The NIMS is a systematic, proactive approach to guide departments and agencies at all levels of government, nongovernmental organizations, and the private sector to work together seamlessly and manage incidents involving all threats and hazards— regardless of cause, size, location, or complexity—in order to reduce loss of life, property and harm to the environment. The NIMS is the essential foundation to the National Preparedness System (NPS) and provides the template for the management of incidents and operations in support of all five National Planning Frameworks. (FEMA, 2016)

In the past, the limited focus of the disaster plan on file at a hospital usually related specifically to safety and security preparedness. Today the primary responsibility for the safety and security department, in conjunction with nursing leadership, is to develop or refine the hospital's EOP for incidents based on the HVA. The safety and security department need to have assigned oversight for facility security, quick lockdown or controlled access, and management of people flowing into and out of the hospital. This not only includes the time the incident is occurring but also during the time that family members are seeking reunification.

Nursing leadership needs to ensure that all facility departments understand their role in a disaster situation. Nurse leaders are the coordinators in synchronizing department plans so that everything fits together to meet the essential needs of the staff, patients, hospital, and community. Once the comprehensive emergency management plans are complete, every department should understand its identified written role.

Creating Procedural Annexes to All-Hazards Preparedness Plans

In addition to overall all-hazards preparedness plans, the hospital will need to define procedures regarding what will be done in any CBRNE disaster and what the surge capacity needs will be related to any of these events. *Surge capacity* is a measurable representation of the ability to manage a sudden influx of patients (ACEP, 2011). These specific procedures are added separately to the plan and are called annexes. The committee can assign the creation of each of these procedures to a subgroup.

These teams are often led by nursing leadership and the emergency medicine director, with appropriate ad hoc participation. For example, the infection prevention and control department, in partnership with public health, can co-lead the biological planning efforts; the radiology department can co-lead the nuclear/radiological efforts partnering closely with local authorities; and nursing, pharmacy, and emergency medicine can co-lead the explosives, chemical, and surge capacity efforts, partnering closely with police, fire, and rescue. The goal with these procedural annexes is to create easy, step-by-step action plans, fact sheets, and algorithms for identifying, intervening, and notifying the appropriate authorities. As with most all-hazards preparedness literature, the most current references will be online. Some essential websites to assist in writing specific hospital procedures include the CDC, the DHS), and the US Department of Labor's Occupational Safety and Health Administration (OSHA).

In establishing procedural annexes and the overall all-hazards disaster preparedness plan, TJC's emergency management accreditation standards call for hospitals to sustain disaster operations for at least 96 hours should an external disaster occur that affects the local area or region (TJC, 2012). Lessons learned from Hurricane Katrina illustrate just how long it can take before assistance is available. This means surge capacity planning must go beyond the traditional areas of the ED and operating rooms. Hospital leadership needs to make sure every operating unit and department is prepared. The following are only a few examples of what hospitals will need:

- A conservative stockpile of essential antibiotics for biological threats
- Antidotes for chemical exposures
- Basic food and bottled water surpluses for environmental contamination events
- Preplanned contracts with local supply companies and businesses for ice, oxygen and other gases, and emergency power
- Alternative communication methods and plans, both internal and external, in case of power outage
- Staff and volunteer credentialing and identification procedures
- Established entrances for staff during lockdowns or controlled access situations
- Patient identification and tracking systems for families in search of loved ones

- Downtime procedures for cyber threats (with the ability to function up to 5 days)
- Accommodations for staff to bring in their children for care while they are working
- Mutual aid agreements to assist with levels of care not usually available (e.g., pediatrics) or to assist in accelerating discharges or post-acute placements.

Creating a Planning Subgroup

Even with comprehensive emergency management plans and annexes, the unexpected will happen, such as in threats and incidents involving anthrax, severe acute respiratory syndrome (SARS), smallpox, potentially harmful H1N1 influenza, and the Ebola and Zika viruses. Initially no one will know whether these are true terrorist threats or isolated spontaneous incidents. The hospital must be ready to respond at all times. An ongoing emergency management planning group needs to be formed at the local level and chaired by a nurse executive who sits on the system emergency management committee along with key stakeholder membership (including ED, employee health staff, and infection prevention and control). Based on the changing needs of the events, this planning group will enable the facility to respond quickly to the "just in time" educational needs of the staff, allow for rapid procedural planning for community needs, and ensure appropriate authority notification in the event of a disaster. For example, the staff will be expected to recognize the symptoms and presentation of Ebola and respond by critical thinking, as follows:

- Triaging and isolating the patient on admission to the ED and placing the patient in the hospital or facility's negative pressure room if available
- Obtaining and having the staff don and doff appropriate personal protective equipment (PPE)
- Controlling access to the ED and possibly the entire hospital
- Identifying (name, address, telephone number) all patient contacts, transport services (emergency medical services [EMS]), staff, and patients in the waiting room
- Notifying the infection prevention and control practitioner, hospital/facility infectious disease physician or epidemiologist, public health officials, and police

Biological and chemical terrorism are examples of unexpected severe events needing a strategic plan for preparedness and response. The CDC (2001) provided recommendations for biological and chemical terrorism. They noted that:

> Terrorist incidents in the United States and elsewhere involving bacterial pathogens (3), nerve gas (1), and a lethal plant toxin (e.g., ricin) (4), have demonstrated that the United States is vulnerable to biological and chemical threats as well as explosives. Recipes for preparing "homemade" agents are readily available (5), and reports of arsenals of military bioweapons (2) raise the possibility that terrorists might have access to highly dangerous agents, which have been engineered for mass dissemination as small-particle aerosols. Such agents as the variola virus, the causative agent of smallpox, are highly contagious and often fatal. Responding to large-scale outbreaks caused by these agents will require the rapid mobilization of public health workers, emergency responders, and private health-care providers. Large-scale outbreaks will also require rapid procurement and distribution of large quantities of drugs and vaccines, which must be available quickly.

There are numerous potential biological and chemical agents. Attacks with biological agents are more likely to be covert. There are three categories of biological agents, with the highest priority agents including emerging pathogens that could be engineered for mass dissemination in the future. Chemical agents that might be used by terrorists range from warfare agents to toxic chemicals commonly used in industry: nerve gas, blood agents, blister agents, heavy metals, volatile toxins, pulmonary agents, incapacitating agents, pesticides, polychlorinated biphenyls (PCBs), nitro compounds, flammable gasses and liquids, poisons, and corrosive acids and bases.

Managing causes of biological or chemical mass casualty or terrorism events includes strategies for preparedness and prevention, detection and surveillance, diagnosis and characterization of biological and chemical agents, and response and rapid deployment in the event of an overt attack. Hospitals and hospital systems will need to make sure they are aware of how to access national or system stockpiles should the need arise, because an organization can quickly become overwhelmed with a surge of patients. Effective communication is also an essential element. For example, educational materials need to be prepared to inform the public during and after an attack. The initial detection of a covert biological or chemical attack will probably occur at the local level. Thus disease surveillance systems at state and local health agencies need to be capable of detecting unusual patterns of disease or injury, including those caused by unusual or unknown threat agents (CDC, 2001). Early identification and notification of the threat to emergency medical services and hospitals must also be provided in order to maintain surveillance.

Despite the best PPE guidance by the CDC (https://www.cdc.gov/vhf/ebola/healthcare-us/ppe/index.html), the Ebola crisis highlighted serious issues in the health care delivery system, such as gaps in training, the cost of PPE, and a story reported by *60 Minutes* about a company accused of providing faulty surgical gowns to US hospitals and the US strategic national stockpile, although the company denied the allegations (CBS News, 2016). Because Ebola is so lethal, these gaps and the ways organizations responded to protect their employees came to the forefront. Nurses and other health care workers were directly affected. PPE availability quickly became a critical issue in the COVID-19 pandemic.

Developing a Command Center

In the event of a disaster, the hospital would need a dedicated centralized command center where all department directors can report for instructions. The four essential elements of a command center, explained in more detail in later sections, are as follows:

1. Setting up the room
2. Developing processes in the command center
3. Establishing the hospital's role in the community
4. Testing the all-hazards preparedness plans and command center functionality

Setting Up the Command Center Room

The location of the incident command center will depend on the organization's physical layout, but it often is located near the safety and security department. It is commanded by the on-call administrator along with the CNO, the ED medical director, and the safety and security director, although if the event occurs outside of normal business hours, the command center may be opened by personnel pre-designated by administration or by the employee with the best set of qualifications to handle the event. Not knowing when a disaster may occur makes it essential

for the emergency management oversight committee to involve leaders at all levels of the organization and determine what training each leadership level will require. TJC has determined a basic set of training requirements in order to work within the command center. The following equipment should be available in the room:

- Multiple telephones/telephone lines with speed dial for frequently called numbers
- Computer access (with both intranet and Internet capabilities)
- Printing capability
- Batch copying capabilities
- Alternative phone options (e.g., 800 MHz radio technology and/or Voice over Internet Protocol [VoIP] technology—a phone system that operates over Internet lines with functioning antenna) and people trained to use them
- Tiered paging capability
- Television access
- Office-related supplies such as paper, pens, easels, dry erase boards, worktables, phone books, and reference materials such as the all-hazards preparedness plans for each hospital area

The command center should be available at a moment's notice and fully functional within minutes. A common scenario is that the call comes into the ED, but many internal disasters, such as utility failures, may come from other sources. When an external disaster occurs, nursing leadership staff in the ED, along with medical staff, will determine the gravity of the situation and decide whether the incident can be handled in the ED or whether the hospital administrator needs to be contacted. Internal disasters function in a similar manner with the affected unit escalating concerns through the appropriate channels and contacting the hospital administrator if necessary. If it is deemed appropriate to contact the hospital administrator, there will be dialogue among nursing leadership, medical leadership, and the administrator to decide whether the command center should be opened. If the command center is to be opened, the hospital administrator will start the process and call in the additional staff necessary to assist with incident command operations. In the event that the disaster involves the area where the command center is located, the hospital will have to have a predetermined plan to establish a backup command center in another location. In the case of a multifacility system, the alternate command center could be at another hospital.

Developing Processes in the Command Center

Because one of the rotating on-call administrators may be called on to open the command center, the creation of a simple, step-by-step, short document (one to two pages) of how to open, operate, and close down the command center is important. A more extensive manual can also be created, but in times of a disaster, the short "How to Open the Command Center" document is crucial. If the facility does not have an on-call administrator list, one should be established, and staff must know how to reach the on-call person(s). A clear decision matrix should be in place outlining when to open the command center and who needs to be notified. It may be helpful to create a communication tree identifying the process for quickly notifying the administrative team and emergency management committee members. Using a group paging function can be helpful for rapid notification of the leadership team.

To facilitate the incident command structure during a disaster, many hospitals have adopted the Hospital Incident Command System (HICS) for their all-hazards preparedness plans, because it allows logical standardization with common nomenclature that is understood both in the hospital environment and in the community setting (US Department of Health & Human Services, 2012). In addition, the HICS organizational chart provides a comprehensive structure that is scalable to the size of the event and has standardized role descriptions. Techniques such as using vests to identify people in charge during a disaster, with a one-page job action sheet in each vest pocket, are essential in a crisis situation. Color-coded vests may also be useful in identifying the role of each leader based on the incident command structure utilized. All hospital and department all-hazards preparedness plans must be on hand and clearly labeled in the command center, along with in-house phone and pager directories.

Testing the Emergency Management Plans and Command Center

The benefits of conducting biannual emergency drills, both announced and unannounced, includes being able to test the EOP, the command center, and staff roles and responsibilities. Announced drills have the added benefit of teaching opportunities. Tabletop exercises test a group's ability to cooperate and their readiness to respond to a disaster situation (FEMA, 2015a). There are many types of drills, including:

- *Internal drills* to test specific department and/or hospital responses. Examples include setting up and operating the command center, recognizing a biological event both in the ED and on the units, locking down the hospital entrances, simulating decontamination processes, using downtime procedures during a communications or cyber disaster event, and handling various surge capacity situations.
- *External drills* in collaboration with community agencies and departments involving patients (police, fire, and rescue; public health); tabletop drills simulating an unknown biological, nuclear/radiological, or chemical scenario and prioritizing the response by departments; and surge capacity drills testing a community's ability to respond to overwhelming demand. Joint command centers and mutual aid agreements may also be tested.

All of these drills offer great insight into the merit of the all-hazards preparedness plan and allow facilities the opportunity to modify plans to improve processes. Regardless of the type of drill or who is involved, the drill should always be set up as a safe place where participants are encouraged to ask questions and be provided an opportunity to learn from any mistakes.

Establishing the Hospital's Role in the Community

The hospital will play an important role in the community in the case of a disaster. Knowing how the hospital fits in the all-hazards disaster response plan from the perspective of such entities as the police and fire departments, EMS, public health department, and the local school system will be important in coordinating efforts. The emergency management committee will be instrumental in defining the hospital's role locally in the community and nationally to meet federal government expectations and regulatory compliance. Additionally, the public expects the same level of competent care to be provided at all times regardless of the situation.

On a local level, the lead person of the committee (often this will be a designated hospital administrator) will partner with public health, local police, fire departments, EMS, community physicians, regional alliances with other health care facilities, and local emergency management agencies/councils. It will be important to define the hospital's and community's role in emergency situations. Testing of plans using local community disaster drills, often biannually, is essential to continually improve processes. The hospital should strive to test its internal all-hazards preparedness plans whenever there is a planned community drill in order to get a full picture of its ability to respond in a disaster in step with the community response.

Nationally, each hospital will play an important role in the political arena by helping local and federal government personnel understand that hospitals, like police and fire departments, are first responders in a disaster. The materials, equipment, and training required for hospitals to prepare adequately for their role in responding to disasters are very expensive. Capital expenditures will be required to create decontamination facilities; purchase PPE; train and educate staff on effective all-hazards preparedness; stockpile emergency equipment, supplies, and pharmaceuticals; ensure adequate isolation rooms; and outfit a hospital command center. Replacement of expired supplies and pharmaceuticals will also need to be considered. Hospitals need financial assistance to do this well, and the committee members can be advocates for federal and state funding. It is helpful to establish a financial subgroup whose mission will be to develop a set plan for capturing costs related to the event as the disaster unfolds. The financial subgroup can also partner with individual units to develop a business continuity plan that can be incorporated into the EOP. This will enable the hospital to submit immediately for any reimbursement funding that becomes available after the event. This may include business disruption insurance. In addition, the subgroup can identify potential federal grants or public funding that might be available to support costly financial expenditures.

Helping Staff Overcome Fear Associated With Disaster and All-Hazards Preparedness

It is important to know that the first rule of disaster preparedness is to keep staff safe. In a disaster, the paradigm of keeping the patient safe first must be modified to focus on helping staff members (and their families) feel as safe as possible. This may be a shift in thinking, but the reality is that if staff members do not feel comfortable coming to work, then the patients' needs cannot be met.

Nursing leadership, in partnership with human resources and the education department, will need to develop educational tools to assist staff in creating personal disaster preparedness plans for themselves and their

significant others. Many websites and mobile apps are available to assist in developing educational tools, such as the FEMA and America Red Cross websites. Tools such as personal disaster preparedness plans should be effectively communicated so that employees know that the organization's first priority in a disaster is to keep staff safe. Arrangements will need to be made for 24-hour childcare somewhere close to the hospital or on-site. Employee assistance programs need to be available at all times to help employees cope with fear related to a disaster. It is important that nurse leaders understand the psychological impact of a disaster on the victims as well as the staff (Tillman, 2011), so that staff can positively influence victims of a disaster. This requires educating nurses about how to provide care during extreme conditions.

CRISIS STANDARDS OF CARE

During times of crisis in health care delivery, it may become necessary to make decisions about allocating resources. When the number of patients exceeds the available supplies, equipment, and medications, health care organizations may have to change the way they use their resources in order to deliver the best care to the most people. In 2012 the Institute of Medicine (IOM, now called the National Academies of Science, Engineering, and Medicine, Health and Medicine Division) developed *Crisis Standards of Care* to help with this decision-making process with the understanding that these decisions are complex and must be made using fair and equitable principles (Hodge et al., 2013). The framework for these decisions works to inspire fairness and trust and includes heightened ethical sensitivity, understanding what is at stake ethically, adequate planning and policy-making, and flexibility (McLean, 2013). *Crisis Standards of Care* have specific applications based on changing situations. The decisions are often difficult for caregivers but are designed to be consistent in their execution across all disciplines. This type of framework allows for ethical decision-making based on caring for the community as a whole in a disaster situation (McLean, 2013).

LEADERSHIP AND MANAGEMENT IMPLICATIONS

Moving Into the Future With Confidence

Nursing leaders can effect change and ensure that a fully functional emergency management plan for the hospital is developed within 6 to 12 months. Nursing leadership competencies in disaster planning and crisis management are invaluable, and fortunately they have been developed by a collaborative group led by the Department of Veterans Affairs, Office of Nursing Services. These disaster competencies are categorized into four domains: assessment of the disaster scene, technical skills, risk communication, and critical thinking (Coyle et al., 2007).

Clearly, nurse executives are in a position to take a greater role in planning and implementing a disaster response for their organizations. Nursing leaders, from charge nurses through nursing executives are called on to take charge, make decisions, successfully implement protocols, and then modify their action plans based on routine evaluation. Expectations exist that nursing leaders at all levels will act in their patients' best interests and will follow appropriate procedures. In addition, being willing to take risks is an important attribute of the nursing leader. Nurse executives are in a unique position to forge new pathways in the arena of emergency management because of their combination of clinical skills, strong organizational ability, networking expertise, and training in clinical crises. If the emergency management committee is not diligent in its efforts to keep everyone continually focused on preparedness, a sense of complacency about refining the emergency management plan may result. With strong nursing leadership at the managerial and executive level, the oversight of disaster planning can be proactively addressed, and a constant state of readiness can be achieved. Engagement of staff nurses—often through shared governance committees or organization-wide all-hazards disaster preparedness planning—is essential for keeping readiness high. Participation in disaster drills is one example of action learning.

CURRENT ISSUES AND TRENDS

Current nursing and medical literature is focused on specific departments and how they are establishing their unique roles and responsibilities in a disaster. Nurse leaders can use these benchmark articles to motivate units and departments to move forward in fully assessing and defining their roles in all-hazards preparedness. For instance, making decisions about consolidating care sites may require closing clinics, emergency care centers, and community health programs during a disaster to free up clinical staff to assist in a hospital's surge

capacity planning in a disaster, provide staff for vaccination teams in a biological event, or help with decontamination in a chemical exposure event. Allocation of staff may be required to build capacity in outpatient and community arenas depending on the disaster threat. Decisions about alternate care sites should be considered well ahead of an event and often require regional collaboration across many disciplines and agencies. Clinical staff may need to flex up or assume roles not usual to their job assignment.

All-hazards preparedness has become a way of life, and knowledge about the level of alertness is an everyday expectation. Hospital staff and leadership have begun to settle in at a heightened state of preparedness. In April 2011, the federal government implemented a new alert system, the National Terrorism Advisory System (NTAS), which replaced the colored-coded system implemented by the DHS. The new two-level system will alert the American public about an "elevated threat" in the event of a credible terrorist threat or an "imminent threat," if a credible and specific terrorist threat is about to occur (US DHS, 2011).

One area of all-hazards preparedness that has not been fully developed, yet has great potential in disaster planning, is the role of various community resources such as outpatient centers, schools, and even churches. The nurse executive can facilitate the establishment of partnerships between the hospital and the community facilities. Once established, these partnerships can be used to set up communication centers where people can congregate to receive support and obtain information about the disaster situation or family and friends who may have been injured.

To effectively manage large-scale events, networking beyond the hospital will be critical to create partnerships with other facilities, hospitals, community agencies, and local, state, and federal departments. To assist in this process, it may be helpful to have a signed agreement or memorandum of understanding (MOU) with community organizations and businesses for assistance. A trend is underway, as evidenced by a growing alliance between regional hospitals and the community at large throughout the United States, to strategically plan for allocation and sharing of federal and state resources in the event of a disaster. As an example, in Virginia, a Regional Hospital Command Center (RHCC) has been established in which 14 northern Virginia hospitals have been networked to more effectively respond in a disaster. This is accomplished via radio communication and a shared web-based bed availability tracking system displaying each hospital's ability to take varying levels of patient acuities. These hospitals can directly link with hospitals in Washington, DC, to coordinate efforts during an event and communicate effectively with fire, police, EMS, public health, the emergency operating center (a local command center for overseeing the event), and the field incident commander in coordinating the disaster response. Similar to the Virginia RHCC just mentioned, cohorts of hospitals, firefighters, EMS, law enforcement, schools, public health, and businesses are joining together to form regional alliances and collaborations to leverage their capability to respond in a coordinated manner.

Under the direction of FEMA, incident management assistance teams (IMATs) were created to provide rapidly deployable (within 2 hours) supplemental assistance to the region affected by a disaster. These teams consist of trained personnel from different departments, organizations, agencies, and jurisdictions, activated to support incident management at major or complex emergency incidents. IMATS function as an initial interface with regional and state responders (FEMA, 2015b).

Building on the idea of partnering with the community to strengthen preparedness, in 2012 FEMA established a community-based assistance program called FEMA Corps. FEMA Corps is dedicated to disaster preparedness, response, and recovery. It is designed to help communities prepare for, respond to, and recover from disasters by supporting disaster recovery centers; assisting in logistics, community relations, and outreach; and performing other critical functions (Corporation for National & Community Service, n.d.). The FEMA Corps provides a pool of trained personnel and pays long-term dividends by adding depth to existing workforce reserves. Hospital executives need to stay abreast of these newly emerging resources and explore ways to partner with them. These types of programs will be pivotal in providing extra human resources and support services desperately needed for hospitals to function effectively in times of crisis.

One other emerging issue that challenges care during a disaster is allocation of scarce resources when the system is overwhelmed. This need was directly experienced in the United States during the Hurricane Katrina and Sandy events, was also witnessed with the Haiti earthquake, with devastating tornadoes in Joplin, Missouri, and with the COVID-19 pandemic. As a result of these catastrophic events, both state and national disaster preparedness leaders examined planning needs for response requirements when resources are scarce. These efforts include substantial planning efforts to address immediate needs, including ethical considerations and planning assumptions, as well as management issues regarding responder protection, with the health care workforce as a primary concern. In recommendations of the Ethics Subcommittee of the Advisory Committee to the Director, CDC, ethical guidelines were outlined for pandemic planning (CDC, 2007) and are a useful resource. To maximize the level of national and regional preparedness, these principles included the identification of clear overall goals, principles of transparency in decision-making, public engagement and involvement in the process, use of sound scientific evidence for decision-making, and thinking in a global context.

The guidelines recommended early planning efforts that balance utilitarian concepts with respect of persons, nonmaleficence, and justice. The recommendations gave examples of distribution criteria that will need to be considered well ahead of the time of an actual event. The development of triage criteria for allocation of scarce resources has been documented in several articles (Hick & O'Laughlin, 2006; Kraus et al., 2007). Further, adopting standards of care under altered conditions has been described and addressed in numerous documents from states and associations seeking to offer guidelines to care providers (American Nurses Association, 2008; New York State Department of Health Task Force on Life and the Law, 2007; Phillips & Knebel, 2007). Each nursing leader and team needs to understand these guidelines and begin the planning process at both the local and regional levels for developing protocols to allocate scarce resources and implementing triage criteria for care in overwhelming events. Implementing periodic tabletop discussions regarding how to allocate resources in a time of scarcity will prove to be a powerful tool in setting the stage for what to do if such an event occurs. Collaborative professional staff and hospital leadership discussions about scarce resource allocation will present ethical dilemmas that need to be thoughtfully considered in a planning time that is devoid of emotion. Questions to be discussed at the tabletop include the following: (1) Which hospital and/or clinical leader will make the final decision about ventilator allocation and other scarce resource distribution? (2) What are the criteria used to determine which patients receive aggressive treatment and which will receive palliative care, both imminently and long term, as other life-threatening complications ensue? (3) How are prophylactic pharmaceutical dissemination plans going to be activated to protect staff

and their families? Knowing the hospital's approach to handling these types of scenarios will be a critical precursor in implementing an effective plan in the event of a disaster that is compounded by a shortage of resources.

RESEARCH NOTE

Source
Arbon, P., Ranse, J., Cusack, L., Considine, J., Shaban, R. Z., Woodman, R. J., et al. (2013). Australasian emergency nurses' willingness to attend work in a disaster: A survey.
Australasian Emergency Nursing Journal: AENJ, 16(2), 52–57.

Purpose
All types of hospital staff would be required to show up for work during an internal or external disaster and many hospitals consider staffing shortages as a barrier to efficiently operationalize their response plans. Identifying factors that would encourage willingness of the staff to be present in times of disaster would mitigate some of the family and other external factors that place employees into conflict. The purpose of this research was to confirm if previously identified factors that influenced nurse absenteeism could be mitigated and to develop strategies for sufficient staffing for use during times of disaster.

Discussion
A 10-minute survey was designed and distributed to greater than 1000 emergency nurses in the country of Australia. Characteristics of the individuals in addition to their willingness to come to work under different types of circumstances were analyzed. Out of the 451 participants who submitted the survey, the majority were female with a mean age of 39.8 years. Although there was a general willingness to attend work during a disaster, participants were 23.9 times more likely to be willing to come to work for events such as earthquakes and fires versus pandemics and chemical events. Gender and level of nursing education/licensure did not influence willingness to be

present during time of disaster, but employment status measured by full time equivalents did. Nurses who had different types of disaster training or perceived that their peers and leaders were prepared for a disaster were also more likely to be willing to come to work. Although the participants who lived with children at home were the most likely to be unwilling to attend work during a disaster, those who had a personal disaster plan were almost eight times more likely to be willing to work.

Application to Practice
Health care facilities will need to consider individual, family, and workplace factors that may influence a nurse's willingness to come to work during a disaster. Proactive personal disaster planning and the ability to communicate with loved ones during these times appeared to have the biggest influence. Hospitals can develop mitigation strategies by encouraging nurses to develop personal plans using disaster preparedness checklists and having crucial conversations prior to any events with their support systems. Educating nurses to use these checklists to develop plans for their families or others that they care for outside of the work environment can also provide peace of mind and increase willingness to come to work if they feel their families are cared for. Hospitals can also work to provide disaster education at the workplace for nurses, allied health, and hospital leaders as the perception of peer and workplace readiness also increased willingness to work. Implementing strategies around these types of practices provide hospitals an opportunity to mitigate staffing shortages during times of crisis.

CASE STUDY

Shooting Incident

Day 1 (Sunday)
At approximately 10:05 pm on the final evening of a 3-day music festival held in a large metropolitan city and known for being a world-renowned tourist attraction, more than 1000 shots were fired over a 15 minute time-frame, with shooting occurring in the concert venue. The venue was outdoors, on a flat area of nearly 15 acres. Approximately

22,000 concert goers were in attendance over the course of the event. The hospitals servicing the area were a mix of for-profit and not-for profit facilities with Level 1 and Level 2 trauma centers within miles of the concert venue.
  The shooter was across the street from the venue and began shooting down from about 30 stories, and about 300 yards away. The crowd was initially disoriented by

CASE STUDY—cont'd

the sound and assumed it was part of the show. When people in the crowd began to fall from gun-shot wounds, the crowd began to run for their lives. All points of egress became quickly over-run, and some began jumping over temporary barriers, including fencing meant to outline the concert boundaries.

Utilizing all resources available to them, concert goers began to stabilize wounds, stop bleeding, and help as many of the injured as possible escape the area and seek shelter or emergency care. That night 31 people were killed before reaching a hospital, and an additional 800 were injured. Fleeing on foot the crowd expanded beyond the 15-acre site an additional 4 miles into the densely populated city.

Day 1–2 (Post Incident–After Midnight–Pre-Hospital)

There were about 800 injured patients. The injured eventually found their own transportation to surrounding hospitals. Many were routed to medical care through the use of smartphones or mapping applications. The Emergency Medical Personnel were responding to approximately 20 sites around the perimeter of the event to treat or transport the wounded who had fled on foot. It is reported that each site had as few as 3 patients and as many as 40 patients. To complicate communication there were multiple calls being placed to law enforcement regarding potential additional active shooters. The massive use of cell phones quickly overwhelmed already heavily utilized cell towers.

Day 1–2 (Post Incident–After Midnight–Hospital)

The occurrence of the event on a Sunday night and other events discussed above created unique circumstances around patient arrivals. Many hospitals reported not having supplies restocked or having already flexed off extra staff. It was at this time that the surge of patients started coming in. Carloads, truck loads, Uber drivers, and taxi drivers were arriving without prior notice. The closest hospitals to the concert began to receive the largest number of patients and began to manage the volume as a mass casualty. No prior field triage or formal pre-hospital care had occurred, and hospitals reported lines longer than a quarter of a mile. For example, one of the hospitals received 200 patients in need of treatment within 8 hours of the event.

Questions for Reflection

1. How do you plan for the following areas of potential impact on patients arriving via privately owned vehicles in large numbers with no forward notification?
2. How does EMS respond to more than 20 locations in a 15-acre area with some order and priority?
3. How should orchestrated communication occur when cell phone towers are overwhelmed?

Mass Casualty Disaster Plan Implementation

Communications

Day 1: Check and test redundant communications systems (telephone, VoIP, radio, satellite, Internet).
Communicate with hospital leadership and established community partners regarding the hospital's emergency plan.

Day 1: Open the incident command center and review action plans for the next 24 to 48 hours. Open the manpower pool to communicate with staff, including surgeons, to be prepared to stay at the hospital and work extra shifts if necessary. Notify community partners regarding the plan for the duration of the mass casualty event. Prepare spaces for staff to change clothes if soiled and be able to get back to work quickly.

Day 4: The incident command center should be fully staffed and operational. Review internal surge plan specific to bed capacity, discharges, and staff. Communicate the plans to physicians and leadership. The appointed media relations personnel will provide accommodations for media. Communicate with local, state, regional, and federal resources for support including supplies, personnel, and infrastructure. Provide frequent situational updates to staff and visitors. Receive frequent updates from department leadership for effective decision-making. Request support from state and/or local authorities to help transport personnel to the hospital to relieve on-duty staff if possible.

Day 5: Connect with local and regional partners to update your situation, request help if needed, and offer assistance if possible.

(continued)

CASE STUDY—cont'd

Safety and security	**Day 1:** Complete a facility safety survey regarding incoming patient surge and potential visitor surge. **Day 3:** Do frequent facility surveys inside and outside to check communication infrastructures. **Day 4:** Prepare for an influx of patients in the emergency department. Set up a space for the "worried well" (community members who are not ill but are distressed about the mass casualty). Monitor patients and visitors for stress-related behavioral problems. **Day 5:** Monitor the exterior building and grounds for any safety hazards. Including where you will set up extra morgue sites.
Resources and assets	**Day 1:** Inventory supplies including food, fuel, water, medical supplies, and staff. Order for any shortages from vendors. **Day 3:** Organize emergency supplies for rapid deployment to units. Food service changes to surge-level meal planning. **Day 4:** Consider allocating resources and medical supplies according to crisis standards of care. Request any needed supplies from the central warehouse if available. **Day 5**: Inventory supplies, food, water, linens, and pharmaceuticals. Begin restocking units with available supplies.
Staff responsibilities	**Day 1–2:** Remind staff to prepare to be able to respond to the hospital's needs as essential personnel. This includes arranging for child, elder, or pet care; securing their homes against damage; and having adequate supplies for their families. Be certain that you communicate with employees to be proactive for Day 2 and continue care. **Day 1–2:** Work to arrange timely discharge for appropriate patients and receive new admits from the emergency department. **Day 2:** Staff should be prepared for the possibility of working in an area other than their home unit. Prepare for "just in time" training. **Day 2:** Alter the nurse/patient ratio to accommodate surge levels and train personnel who will work in a different area. Coordinate patient tracking with EMS.
Utilities management	**Day 1:** Check and test redundant utilities systems including having a 96-hour supply of fuel. **Day 3:** Transfer all essential equipment to emergency outlets. Continue to check utility operations frequently including outside the facility for infrastructure problems. **Day 4:** Monitor fuel supply, equipment operations, and infrastructure. Respond to any internal or external damage. **Day 5:** Restore equipment to main power source. Arrange generator fuel delivery, and test that systems are functioning adequately including air handlers, water, and lighting.
Clinical and support activities	**Day 1:** Consider discharging appropriate patients and canceling elective surgeries to increase bed capacity. **Day 1–2:** Consider a discharge holding area for patients who are discharged but not able to go home. **Day 1–2:** Incident commander orders surge capacity plan in effect. Open surge beds. Incident commander and medical director review *Crisis Standards of Care* for possible implementation. Monitor blood supply and storage capability. Inventory pharmaceutical supplies and consider using the emergency supply if necessary. **Day 1–2:** Arrange for discharges to accommodate emergency department patients.

CASE STUDY—cont'd

After Action

An after-action meeting is necessary to evaluate the hospital's response to the emergency event. Leaders will discuss what went well and what did not, what could have been done better, and how to plan for the next event. It is also an opportunity to evaluate and make needed updates or changes to the emergency operations plan. Some common questions for this meeting may include:

1. Did your incident command team maintain planning using the six critical areas of preparedness (communications, resources and assets, safety and security, staff responsibilities, utilities management, and patient clinical and support activities)?
2. Did you document every action over the past 6 days, with time, date, and names?
3. Were communications effective?
4. Were you able to integrate your response with state, regional, and local authorities?
5. How could you have improved your response to the surge situation?
6. Were the crisis standards of care decisions consistent and decided using fair and equitable principles?

CRITICAL THINKING EXERCISE

It is a Friday evening in the middle of winter. Cold and influenza season continues. The Centers for Disease Control & Prevention has just confirmed a small outbreak, less than 10 patients, in your city of a novel virus that has symptoms listed as influenza-like illnesses. You have been working in health care for greater than 10 years and remember the outbreaks of H1N1 and different corona viruses that created surge capacity events in areas throughout North America and other parts of the world. The emergency department (ED) is staffed with nine registered nurses, three ED physician providers, and one emergency medical technician. Information continues to change rapidly, including the inclusion criteria for testing. Your infection prevention department has told you to isolate symptomatic patients and place them in droplet and contact precautions. On a normal day, the ED sees 150–200 patients, and you know that an increase in symptomatic patients or even the walking well will easily create a surge event. You have concerns about the ability to triage patients quickly while keeping staff and others from contracting the virus. The ED team has requested other areas of the hospital be available as secondary triage and the ability to fast track confirmed admissions.

Planning process: Epidemic planning process for a novel virus.

Purpose: To prepare and educate all staff on a surge capacity event and plan for staffing shortages resulting from community impact on social services including day cares and schools.

Background information: You are one of several nursing directors at a 400-bed hospital with a 30-bed emergency room in a large metropolitan city. There are multiple hospitals in the city who are also anticipating surge events. The staff at the hospital have done drills for emerging diseases after SARS and Ebola events, and have identified and trained a group of initial responders for positive cases. You are the administrator on duty and have been tasked with leading the effort to quickly develop a plan for surge capacity.

1. How and where can the ED screen the walking well while maintaining all of the elements of Emergency Medical Treatment and Labor Act (EMTALA)?
2. What triage and safety considerations need to be put in place for separating influenza like illness apart from other non-infectious chief complaints?
3. What considerations will need to be addressed for personal protective equipment (PPE)?
4. How will you manage staffing shortages that may occur from surge, fear, or employees that have to stay home to care for loved ones?
5. What education needs to be provided to staff? Is this different by discipline?
6. How do you manage additional foot traffic, including visitors and vendors?
7. What should be done to secure the campus and manage media requests?
8. Do you have enough respiratory equipment including ventilators? What is your process for securing more if needed?
9. Are positive patients appropriate to cohort? What is your first area for admission placements and where do you expand to if additional beds are needed?

10. Are there additional or potential disruptions in the supply chain? How will you manage scare resources or items affected by backorders?

11. Can non-essential staff be redeployed to assist in other areas?

12. How will you maintain your processes should the surge event last longer than 7 days?

REFERENCES

Agency for Healthcare Research and Quality (AHRQ). (2012). *Allocation of scarce resources during mass casualty events*. https://effectivehealthcare.ahrq.gov/products/mass-casualty-events-scarce-resources.

American Nurses Association (ANA). (2008). *Adapting standards of care under extreme conditions: Guidance for professionals during disasters, pandemics, and other extreme emergencies*. https://www.aft.org/sites/default/files/ept_sect2_ana-care-standards.pdf.

American Organization of Nurse Executives (AONE). (2016). *AONE guiding principles: Role of the nurse leader in crisis management*. https://www.aonl.org/sites/default/files/aone/role-of the-nurse-leader-in-crisis-management.pdf.

Arbon, P., Ranse, J., Cusack, L., Considine, J., Shaban, R. Z., Woodman R. J., et al. (2013). Australasian emergency nurses' willingness to attend work in a disaster: A survey. *Australasian Emergency Nursing Journal: AENJ, 16*(2), 52–57.

Arnand, K. (2014). *Cyber attacks—Definition, types, prevention*. Retrieved from http://www.thewindowsclub.com/cyber-attacks-definition-types-prevention.

California Hospital Association. (2011). *Emergency preparedness: Hazards vulnerability analysis*. http://www.calhospitalprepare.org/hazard-vulnerability-analysis.

CBS News. (2016). *60 Minutes investigates medical gear sold during Ebola crisis*. http://www.cbsnews.com/news/60-minutes-investigates-medical-gear-sold-during-ebola-crisis/.

Centers for Disease Control and Prevention (CDC). (2007). *Ethical guidelines in pandemic influenza*. https://www.cdc.gov/od/science/integrity/phethics/panFlu_Ethic_Guidelines.pdf.

Centers for Disease Control and Prevention (CDC). (2001). *Biological and chemical terrorism: Strategic plan for preparedness and response*. https://www.cdc.gov/mmwr/preview/mmwrhtml/rr4904a1.htm.

Committee on Homeland Security of the House of Representatives. (2008). *Compilation of homeland security presidential directives (HSPD) (updated through 39 December 31, 2007): Prepared for the use of the committee on homeland security of the House of Representatives*: US Government Printing Office.

Corporation for National & Community Service. (n.d.). *What is FEMA Corps?* https://www.nationalservice.gov/programs/americorps/americorps-programs/fema-corps/fema-corps-faqs#12439.

Coyle, G., Sapnas, K., & Ward-Presson, K. (2007). Dealing with disaster. *Nursing Management, 38*(7), 24–29.

Drenkard, K., & Rigotti, G. (2002, updated 2016). *Inova Health System survey*. Falls Church, VA: Inova Health System.

Drenkard, K., Rigotti, G., Hanfling, D., Fahlgren, T., & LaFrancois, G. (2002). Healthcare system disaster preparedness, part 1: Readiness planning. *Journal of Nursing Administration, 32*(9), 461–469.

Federal Emergency Management Agency. (2006). *NIMS Implementation Activities for Hospitals and Healthcare Systems* (pp. 1–26) (United States of America, Department of Homeland Security, Federal Emergency Management Agency). http://www.fema.gov/pdf/emergency/nims/06_training.pdf.

Federal Emergency Management Agency (FEMA). (2015a). *Emergency planning exercises*. https://www.fema.gov/emergency-planning-exercises.

Federal Emergency Management Agency (FEMA). (2015b). *Fact sheet: Incident management assistance teams*. http://www.fema.gov/media-library-data/1440617086827-f6489d2de59dddeba8bebc9b4d419009/IMAT_July_2015.pdf.

Federal Emergency Management Agency (FEMA). (2016). *National incident management system*. http://www.fema.gov/national-incident-management-system.

Federal Emergency Management Institute (FEMA). (2014). *Academic emergency management and related courses (AEMRC) for the higher education program: Comparative emergency management book*. https://training.fema.gov/hiedu/aemrc/booksdownload/compemmgmtbookproject/.

Hick, J. L., & O'Laughlin, D. T. (2006). Concept of operations for triage of mechanical ventilation in an epidemic. *Academic Emergency Medicine, 13*(2), 223–229. http://dx.doi:10.1197/j.aem.2005.07.037.

Hodge, J. G., Jr., Hanfling, D., & Powell, T. (2013). Practical, ethical, and legal challenges underlying crisis standards of care. *Journal of Law, Medicine, and Ethics, 41*, 50–55, 2012. Public Health Law Conference: Practical Approaches to Critical Challenges, Spring 2013.

Institute of Medicine (IOM). (2012). *Crisis standards of care—A systems framework for catastrophic disaster response*. National Academics Press. http://hmd.nationalacademies.org/hmd/Activities/PublicHealth/DisasterCareStandards.aspx.

International Federation of Red Cross and Red Crescent Societies (IFRC). (2016). *Biological hazards: Epidemics*. http://www.ifrc.org/en/what-we-do/disaster-management/about-disasters/definition-of-hazard/biological-hazards-epidemics.

Joint Commission Resources. (2008). *Emergency management in health care: An all-hazards approach*. Oakbrook Terrace, IL: Author.

Joint Commission Resources. (2016). *Emergency management in health care: An all-hazards approach* (2nd ed.). https://store.jointcommissioninternational.org/emergency-management-in-health-care-an-all-hazards-approach-4th-edition/.

Kraus, C. K., Levy, F., & Kelen, G. D. (2007). Lifeboat ethics: Considerations in the discharge of inpatients for the creation of hospital surge capacity. *Disaster Medicine and Public Health Preparedness, 1*(1), 51–56. http://dx.doi.org/10.1097/DMP.0b013e318065c4ca.

McLean, M. R. (2013). Allocating resources—A wicked problem. *Health Progress, 94*(6), 60–67.

New York State Department of Health Task Force on Life and the Law. (2007). *Allocation of ventilators in an influenza pandemic*. www.health.state.ny.us/diseases/communicable/influenza/pandemic/ventilators/.

Niska, R. W., & Shimizu, I. (2011). *Hospital preparedness for emergency response United States, 2008*. US Dept. of Health and Human Services, Centers for Disease Control & Prevention, National Center for Health Statistics.

Phillips, S. J., & Knebel, A.(Eds.). (2007). *Mass medical care with scarce resources: A community planning guide*. (Prepared by Health Systems Research, Inc., an Altarum company, under contract No. 290-04-0010. AHRQ Publication No. 07–0001). Agency for Healthcare Research and Quality. http://archive.ahrq.gov/research/mce/mceguide.pdf.

Ready.gov. (2016). *Chemical threats*. https://www.ready.gov/chemical.

Sternberg, E. (2003). Planning for resilience in hospital internal disaster. *Prehospital and Disaster Medicine, 18*(4), 291.

The Joint Commission (TJC). (2008). *Accreditation program: Hospital emergency management*. Author. https://store.jcrinc.com/2020-comprehensive-accreditation-manual-for-hospitals-pdf-manual-/ebcah20/.

The Joint Commission (TJC). (2012). *Comprehensive accreditation manual for hospitals 2012: Emergency management accreditation standards*. Author.

The Joint Commission. (2016). Joint Commission Resources Portal. Retrieved February 20, 2016 from https://e-dition.jcrinc.com/Frame.aspx.

The Joint Commission. (2020). *Joint Commission resources portal*. https://e-dition.jcrinc.com/Frame.aspx.

Tillman, P. (2011). Disaster preparedness for nurses: A teaching guide. *The Journal of Continuing Education in Nursing, 42*(9), 404–408. http://dx.doi:10.3928/00220124-20110502-02.

US Department of Defense. (2015). *DOD dictionary of military terms*. https://www.jcs.mil/Portals/36/Documents/Doctrine/pubs/dictionary.pdf.

US Department of Health & Human Services. (2012). *Emergency management and the incident command system*. https://www.phe.gov/preparedness/planning/mscc/handbook/chapter1/Pages/emergencymanagement.aspx.

US Department of Homeland Security. (2011). *NTAS public guide*. https://www.dhs.gov/xlibrary/assets/ntas/ntas-public-guide.pdf.

US Department of Homeland Security. (2020). *National incident management system (NIMS)*. https://www.fema.gov/national-incident-management-system.

World Health Organization (WHO). (2013). *Emergency response framework*. Geneva, Switzerland: WHO. http://apps.who.int/iris/bitstream/10665/89529/1/9789241504973_eng.pdf.

Wright State University. (2016). *Emergency preparedness*. https://www.wright.edu/police/emergency-preparedness.

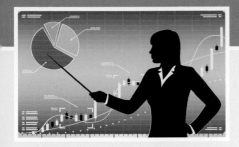

25

Nursing Informatics for Leaders in Clinical Nursing

Karen Dunn-Lopez, Lisa Janeway, Michele A. Berg

Nursing informatics is a subspecialty of nursing that applies computer, data, and information science to nursing science and practice, and emerged as a subspecialty in nursing in the mid-1970s. For those who did not understand the need for the subspecialty, in the early 1990s, Norma Lang articulated the importance saying, "If we cannot name it, we cannot control it, practice it, teach it, finance it or put it into public policy" (Clark & Lang, 1992, p. 128). Today, given the vast array of clinical care activities, data recorded, and rule-based prompts mediated by computers, software, and other technologies, informatics plays an increasingly prominent role in nursing. In fact, the American Association of Colleges of Nursing (AACN) requires that nurses at all levels outside the subspecialty of informatics, including nurse leaders, have basic competencies in nursing informatics (AACN, 2019).

The business of health care information technologies is evolving rapidly in all settings where people spend time, including schools, work settings, homes, and where they shop. Management of the health care industry and care delivery relies extensively on not only the device capture, collection, and analysis of data, but also on the workflow process for what, when, where, who, and how the data are captured. Data about the patient, provider, outcomes, and processes of care delivery are collected from many individuals practicing in different specialties and must be standardized, integrated, coordinated, and managed. Moreover, widespread demand to use these data for performance measurement and reporting to accountable care customers, regulators, and accrediting/certification bodies comes at a time when reimbursement and incentive payments to providers and health care institutions are linked with performance on selected patient outcome

measures. Whereas the imperative in nursing used to be that nurses needed their nursing-specific data, now a subspecialty of nursing informatics has become rooted and is growing in clinical care management as nurses migrate to using their data for care management. The purpose of this chapter is to delineate what clinical nursing informatics is and discuss informatics competencies, regulatory and policy issues, current trends, and the implications that all these areas have for clinical nursing leaders.

DEFINITIONS

What Is Nursing Informatics?

Informatics is a multidisciplinary field defined by the American Medical Informatics Association (AMIA) as applying principles of computer and informatics science to advance life science research, health professions education, patient care, and public health (AMIA, 2020). The application of informatics knowledge is applied by clinical informaticists who facilitate the delivery of health care.

The field of **nursing informatics** has been defined in multiple ways in the past decades, including technology-, conceptual-, and role-focused definitions. Staggers and Thompson (2002) articulated one of the most encompassing versions of the definition as follows:

Nursing informatics is a specialty that integrates nursing science, computer science, and information science to manage and communicate data, information, and knowledge in nursing practice. Nursing informatics facilitate the integration of data, information, and knowledge to support patients, nurses, and other providers in their decision-making in all roles and settings. This support is accomplished through the use of information structures, information processes, and information technology. (Staggers & Thompson, 2002, p. 260)

The language of data management and clinical informatics contains many acronyms and specific technical terminology. Selected terms are:

Clinical informatics: The area of informatics that is applied to facilitate the delivery of health care.

Clinical nursing informatics: The area of informatics that is applied to facilitate the delivery of nursing care.

Contingency plans: Preparations to continue the safe care of patients throughout the continuum in case electronic health records or technology systems are not available for use.

Data set: A collection of patient specific variables.

Electronic health records: A longitudinal record of patient information that is stored electronically that crosses encounters and the continuum of care.

Electronic medical records: An electronic version of a medical record that contains medical information from one provider or health care facility.

End users: Persons who are the intended and actual user of a product or technology.

Information blocking: Blocking of information by health care providers, organizations, or developers that interferes or prevents health information from being exchanged and is punishable by law.

Interoperability: The ability of an information system to accurately exchange information with another system.

Medical device integration: A method that allows medical devices to flow patient data from one system to another using software programs known as middleware or interface engines.

mHealth: Patient health care and wellness that is supported by mobile devices such as mobile phone, wearable monitors, and other wireless devices.

Ransomware: A threat where a malicious software causes system access issues and a monetary threat to organizations, holding patient data hostage.

Usability: The degree to which a technology is easy to learn and remember, and efficient and pleasant to use. In addition, technologies that are useable have limited errors that are easy to detect and recover from.

BACKGROUND

Nursing informatics can best be described, understood, and contextualized using the *Data, Information,* *Knowledge, and Wisdom (DIKW)* Framework (Nelson, 2019). The model (Fig. 25.1) includes four major constructs defined in Table 25.1. Although it may seem that nursing informatics focuses on health information technologies used by nurses, the DIKW framework demonstrates increasing levels of critical thinking or "knowledge work" at each level.

Although this framework provides an important lens to understand nursing informatics broadly, we propose a new informatics area, **Clinical Nursing Informatics**. In contrast to those nursing informatics scientists who focus on the creation of generalizable knowledge about nursing informatics using scientific methods, we believe that clinical nursing informatics focuses on optimizing quality and safety of patients using information and communication systems through the delivery of nursing care. Although it is necessary to have clinical informatics departments in health systems, this alone is not adequate to ensure that informatics solutions will be applied that optimize nursing's unique role in health care. Rather, organizations need to have a well-educated cadre of clinical nursing informaticist nurses who specialize in *nursing* informatics, along with nurse leaders and bedside nurses who have robust competencies in nursing informatics.

Nursing Informatics Competencies

Professional nursing organizations have developed, and regularly revise, competencies for the profession, including competencies in nursing informatics for all clinical roles. AACN develops competencies to guide faculty members to develop and integrate curricula that support these competencies at the prelicensure through graduate levels. Of interest, the AACN is currently in the process of re-envisioning its essentials (AACN, 2019). Early drafts suggest an increasing emphasis on informatics. The Quality and Safety Education for Nurses Institute (QSEN) focuses on preparing nurses to improve the quality and safety of the organizations they work in (QSEN, 2020). A core area for this initiative is informatics.

Other leading interdisciplinary organizations (e.g., Health Information Management Systems Society's TIGER Initiative and AMIA) have also developed competencies. Table 25.2 highlights some of the competencies that focus on informatics skills for nurses. This is an important distinction. We believe nurses who have nursing informatics competencies are likely to have a more focused impact on advancing the profession

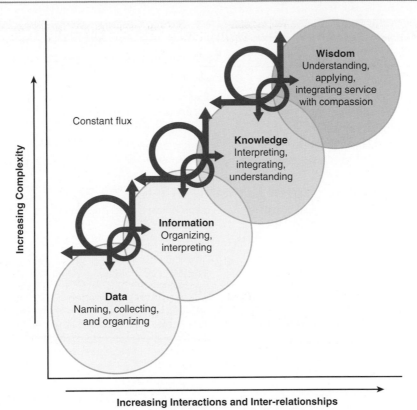

Fig. 25.1 Data, Information, Knowledge, Wisdom, Framework. Source: Nelson, R. (2019). Informatics: evolution of the nelson data, information, knowledge and wisdom model: part 1. *OJIN: The Online Journal of Issues in Nursing, 23*(3). https://ojin.nursingworld.org/MainMenuCategories/ANAMarketplace/ANAPeriodicals/OJIN/Columns/Informatics/Informatics-Evolution-of-Nelson-Model-Part-1.html.

TABLE 25.1	Data, Information, Knowledge, Wisdom Core Constructs	
Construct	**Definition**	**Example**
Data	Single uninterpreted variables	Weight, blood pressure, body temperature
Information	A group of variables that are organized in a manner that meaning can be interpreted	Body mass index is a measure of body size based on height, weight and gender
Knowledge	The formalization of relationship and rules between data and information	Knowledge that patients with cancer are often at risk for infection guides the action to check patients' body temperature when they exhibit chills
Wisdom	The application of data, information and knowledge to make decisions with compassion to meet the needs of the patients, families, and communities	Providing highly immunosuppressed cancer patient exhibiting signs of infection with rapid assessments, mobilization of the needed members of the health care team, while providing interventions to decrease their fever and ease their discomfort.

Source: Nelson, R. (2019). Informatics: evolution of the nelson data, information, knowledge and wisdom model: part 1. *OJIN: The Online Journal of Issues in Nursing, 23*(3). https://ojin.nursingworld.org/MainMenuCategories/ANAMarketplace/ANAPeriodicals/OJIN/Columns/Informatics/Informatics-Evolution-of-Nelson-Model-Part-1.html.

TABLE 25.2   Nursing Informatics Competencies Across Levels of Clinical Nurses

AACN Informatics Related Competencies[a-c]	QSEN Informatics Knowledge Competencies[d]
Bachelors Essential IV	**Prelicensure**
1. Demonstrate skills in using patient care technologies, information systems, and communication devices that support safe nursing practice.	1. Explain why information and technology skills are essential for safe patient care
2. Use telecommunication technologies to assist in effective communication in a variety of health care settings.	2. Identify essential information that must be available in a common database to support patient care
3. Apply safeguards and decision-making support tools embedded in patient care technologies and information systems to support a safe practice environment for both patients and health care workers.	3. Contrast benefits and limitations of different communication technologies and their impact on safety and quality
4. Understand the use of CIS systems to document interventions related to achieving nurse sensitive outcomes.	4. Describe examples of how technology and information management are related to the quality and safety of patient care
5. Use standardized terminology in a care environment that reflects nursing's unique contribution to patient outcomes.	5. Recognize the time, effort, and skill required for computers, databases and other technologies to become reliable and effective tools for patient care
6. Evaluate data from all relevant sources, including technology, to inform the delivery of care.	
7. Recognize the role of information technology in improving patient care outcomes and creating a safe care environment.	
8. Uphold ethical standards related to data security, regulatory requirements, confidentiality, and clients' right to privacy.	
9. Apply patient care technologies as appropriate to address the needs of a diverse patient population.	
10. Advocate for the use of new patient care technologies for safe, quality care.	
11. Recognize that redesign of workflow and care processes should precede implementation of care technology to facilitate nursing practice.	
12. Participate in evaluation of information systems in practice settings through policy and procedure development.	
Master's Essential V	**Graduate**
1. Analyze current and emerging technologies to support safe practice environments, and to optimize patient safety, cost-effectiveness, and health outcomes.	1. Contrast benefits and limitations of common information technology strategies used in the delivery of patient care. Evaluate the strengths and weaknesses of information systems used in patient care.
2. Evaluate outcome data using current communication technologies, information systems, and statistical principles to develop strategies to reduce risks and improve health outcomes.	2. Formulate essential information that must be available in a common database to support patient care in the practice specialty. Evaluate benefits and limitations of different communication technologies and their impact on safety and quality.

(Continued)

TABLE 25.2   Nursing Informatics Competencies across Levels of Clinical Nurses (cont'd)

3. Promote policies that incorporate ethical principles and standards for the use of health and information technologies.

3. Describe and critique taxonomic and terminology systems used in national efforts to enhance interoperability of information systems and knowledge management systems.

4. Provide oversight and guidance in the integration of technologies to document patient care and improve patient outcomes.

5. Use information and communication technologies, resources, and principles of learning to teach patients and others.

6. Use current and emerging technologies in the care environment to support lifelong learning for self and others.

Doctorate in Nursing Practice Essential V

1. Design, select, use, and evaluate programs that evaluate and monitor outcomes of care, care systems, and quality improvement including consumer use of health care information systems.

2. Analyze and communicate critical elements necessary to the selection, use, and evaluation of health care information systems and patient care technology.

3. Demonstrate the conceptual ability and technical skills to develop and execute an evaluation plan involving data extraction from practice information systems and databases.

4. Provide leadership in the evaluation and resolution of ethical and legal issues within health care systems relating to the use of information, information technology, communication networks, and patient care technology.

5. Evaluate consumer health information sources for accuracy, timeliness, and appropriateness.

[a] (American Association of Colleges of Nursing, 2008).
[b] (American Association of Colleges of Nursing, 2011).
[c] (American Association of Colleges of Nursing, 2006).
[d] (Quality and Safety Education for Nursing, 2020).
Source: Based on AACN's Essentials for Baccalaureate, Master's and Doctorate in Nursing practice Education and QSEN Informatics Competencies. https://qsen.org/competencies/pre-licensure-ksas/.

and practice of nursing as compared to nurses who are trained primarily in the interdisciplinary informatics context, because nurses who are primarily trained in interdisciplinary informatics are more likely to be pulled away from nursing to lead overarching informatics programs and projects, and may become disconnected from nursing care.

Regulatory and Policy Issues Related to Clinical Informatics

Recent federal policy initiatives have had a wide range and transformative impact on clinical informatics. In 2009 the United States government enacted the *Health Information Technology Act* (HITECH) as part of the

American Recovery and Reinvestment Act (ARRA). HITECH required organizations to adopt electronic health records, offering incentives for meaningful use (MU). MU focused on three key areas of clinical data: capture and storage, advancing clinical processes, and improving outcomes (Adler-Milstein & Jha, 2017). The overarching goal of the HITECH act was to use technology to arm providers with the tools to be able to manage care better in a safe and secure methodology, and improve the quality of care (O'Grady et al., 2016). Electronic health records (EHRs) have the technology to share information electronically across multiple organizations through health information exchanges and are equipped with interoperability, a method to communicate information between systems. However, systems must be secure, and patient information must be private. *The Health Insurance Portability and Accountability Act* (HIPAA) of 2009 was instituted to protect patients' privacy in electronic records (Cohen & Mello, 2018).

As the nation moved beyond meaningful use, there were new provisions following the Medicare Access and Children's Health Insurance Program (CHIP) that have had an impact on clinical informatics. *The Reauthorization Act* of 2015 (MACRA) changed the reimbursement landscape, adding a quality payment program (QPP) under the premise of value, quality, and better care (Kahn & Baum, 2020). The new payment model will impact organizations as metrics will drive reimbursement rates and create a potential need to modify electronic health records systems and report outcomes.

The 21st Century Cures Act (2015) amends the HITECH Act and became public law in 2016 (Lye et al., 2018). The Office of the National Coordinator for Health Information Technology (ONC, 2016) is responsible for implementing parts of the act through "delivery, advancing interoperability, prohibit information blocking and enhancing the usability, accessibility and privacy and security of HIT." Unintended consequences of health information technology (HIT) have led to new problems enfolding, including security threats in the form of ransomware, an increase in the burden of documentation, usability problems, and safety concerns. New regulatory policies, which often have implications for the delivery of nursing care, are in constant development to address these problems. It is imperative for clinical leaders in nursing to stay informed and be responsive to this changing landscape.

CURRENT ISSUES AND TRENDS

Nursing informatics is a current issue and trend. Nurses comprise the majority of the workforce in health care are the most abundant "end-users" of EHRs. Technological advances to improve patient care and safety during the delivery of care are continuing to develop at a fast pace. Several current issues and trends impacting the profession of nursing are described next.

Dashboards and Reports

There is now a vast amount of information stored from all of these systems and available to provide data analytics in the form or reports or dashboards to nurse leaders. Nurse leaders need to take part in the development of these reports to ensure data validity and be able to understand the output of the reports for monitoring and decision-making. Examples of analytical reports are bar code compliance, late medication administration, and missing or late documentation. Dashboards can be specific and group information together, such as capacity management, quality and safety metrics, and staffing information. Information can also be reused in the form of complex algorithms and decision trees to make predictions based upon a data set, for example, for sepsis, falls, and readmissions (Alexander et al., 2019).

Clinical Decision Support Systems

Clinical decision support systems (CDS) is a method embedded in electronic systems, providing actions and relevant information for clinicians to make decisions related to patient care (Lowry et al., 2012). Clinical decision support is represented in the form of active and passive alerts, banners, icons, or order entry. These interventions must be carefully designed and developed using best practices to increase adoption, reduce over-dependency, over-warning, and linked to measurable goals and monitored (Osheroff, 2012). Before implementing CDS, nurse leaders need to ensure that decisions are for the right reason, have clear measurable objectives, and a plan to monitor. Using a framework such as the Five Rights of clinical decision support (Osheroff, 2012), in collaboration with key stakeholders and governance, will lessen potential pitfalls.

The Five Rights consider:

1. **What:** The right information provides clear direction to the clinicians about the next steps to consider.
2. **Who:** The right person ensures that the CDS is aimed at the correct provider.

3. **How:** The right format is the type of tool used.
4. **Where:** The right channel describes the place information is delivered.
5. **When:** The right time ensures that the intervention occurs in the precise moment of the workflow.

Patient Education

Informatics tools are shaping the way patients engage in learning. These informatics tools have flipped the format of nurse-only led patient education to allow for asynchronous on-demand education for patients and their caregivers. Nurses play a pivotal role in ensuring that the education is evidence-based, culturally sensitive, and addresses health literacy for patients. Nurses should be involved in vetting the materials to ensure they are written at or below a fifth-grade reading level (Stossel et al., 2012). Usability is also a high priority action (Dunn Lopez & Fahey, 2018) that nurses can engage in to ensure patients can easily log in to these applications and navigate through learning materials.

In addition to the reading level and usability, ensuring the patient understands the material presented remains a critical role of nurses. Nurses need to follow up with the patient using teach-back and/or validation methods via verbal understanding. Nurse leaders and clinical nurse educators need to evaluate which tools best fit their IT infrastructure and the long-term costs associated with maintaining such systems. For example, patients may prefer watching videos compared to reading from a handout, and can review the content multiple times.

Clinical Documentation Burden

In February 2020 the ONC finalized the report on reducing regulatory and administrative burden relating to the use of health IT and the EHR (United States Department of Health and Human Services, 2020). There are three primary goals:

1. Reduce the effort and time required to record information in the EHR
2. Reduce the effort and time needed to meet regulatory reporting requirement for clinicians, hospital and health care organizations
3. Improve the functionality and intuitiveness.

The ONC has put forth three major strategies (Table 25.3) to reduce documentation burden that has important implications for nurses. Nursing leaders should be familiar with the strategies and collaborate with informatics and operations personnel to implement local level strategies and processes to reduce the burden of documentation.

Mobile Health

Mobile health applications (known as mHealth) are on the rise in the health care industry as more patients have access to smartphones, tablets, and wearable sensor technologies (e.g., smart watches, etc.). mHealth apps contain multimodal interventions such as diaries, patient-entered data, education, reminders, symptom and activity trackers, and text messages, and can be connected to wearables or other external devices such as scales, glucometers, or blood pressure devices (Alexander et al., 2019). Less common, but expected to rise, are feedback loops to providers that can be interfaced to electronic health records and can inform providers of patients' changes real time, to modify treatment plans or intervene without an office visit. Like technologies to support patient education, nurses need to be aware of the quality of mHealth their patients may be using. Assessment of quality should include how readable and useable the app is, the degree to which the information is guided by high quality evidence, and whether the mHealth secures patient privacy.

Mobile Devices in Clinical Settings

Mobile devices are also used by clinicians at the point-of-care to enter information, place orders, and review patient records. Electronic health record vendors are developing applications to supplement computer-based charting and increasing functionality. Examples include bar code scanning of medication, blood, and infusion pumps. The advantage of this technology is to reduce the burden on nursing of having a toolkit of hardware to perform safe and quality care. Mobile devices also allow nurses to look up reference information. As organizations deploy these types of devices, there are cost and security implications. Middleware software must be deployed to form a bridge between the devices to other systems and still be secure.

Bring Your Own Device and Medical Device Management (MDM)

Due to the cost of commercial mobile devices, some organizations are allowing nurses to bring their own device (BYOD). The convenience of performing such activities on devices, however, requires strict mobile device management to ensure HIPAA compliance and security.

TABLE 25.3 Clinical Documentation Burden: Strategies and Recommendations for Nurse Leaders

ONC Strategy[a]	Recommendations for Nurse Leaders
Reduce regulatory burden around documentation requirements for patient visits	Recognize that this policy is a major driver of nursing documentation. Identify ways to align documentation practice with documentation policies. Engage nurse users in analysis for streamlining documentation processes. Identify and remove redundant nursing documentation. Develop best practice for copy and paste or copy forward. Use nursing governance structures to manage these changes.
Continue to partner with clinical stakeholders to encourage adoption of best practices related to documentation requirements	Implement training programs that focus on both on both quality and efficiency of documentation. Identify potential outside resources via professional organizations for documentation best practices for nurses. Engage with vendors to improve the usability of vendors' documentation in the EHR. Partner with vendors and clinical implementation teams to address documentation redundancies. Build cross-institutional interdisciplinary teams who meet on a regular basis to evaluate performance metrics after large changes. Advocate at the federal level for high quality nursing documentation for outcomes related to patient safety and care quality.
Leverage health IT to standardize data and processes around ordering services or equipment and related prior authorization processes	Integrate supply chains and order sets for equipment used by nursing. Evaluate other workflow factors related to the burden of nurse ordered equipment.

[a] (United States Department of Health and Human Services, 2020).

There are implications for nursing leadership when nurses are using mobile devices to deliver care and should include policies to ensure the data and information are secure. Whether the device is issued by the organization or brought by the staff, hospitals may decide to manage the device encryption and applications on the phones in-house, or via a third-party MDM provider. Devices must be encrypted, and employees are required to "opt in" or consent to organizational security policies when using personal phones. Employees will sign a consent to the security and enrollment policies set forth by the IT department. For example, if a phone is lost or stolen, the applications associated with patient data can be removed using a remote "wipe" function. Adding to the complexity, all devices need to run the same operating system defined by the organization. This ensures each device can support the applications and resources. Organizations may find that supplying company owned devices is less cumbersome than managing applications and security on personal phones. An example of how to ensure this security includes disabling the phone from taking screenshots of patient information and limiting what is stored on the mobile device within the application.

Nurse Communication Systems, Middleware, and Alarm Management

Nurse call and communications systems are now integrated into mobile devices, which push physiologic alarms and calls from patient rooms to nurses' phones. Alarms can originate from the patient monitor, their ventilator, intravenous pump, or any connected device. This decentralization of monitoring from the nursing station to the phone allows the nurse to manage multiple patients and their physiological alarms on the go.

Middleware serves as a bridge that connects the patient monitor and call light to the phone. Nurse leaders should plan for future applications and select middleware that will connect any other device they anticipate using. For example, middleware used for inpatient systems may need to integrate or work with the outpatient middleware if they serve similar functionality. Extreme caution and care must be followed to ensure any system is programmed with safety in mind and that nurses are educated on the policies and procedures used to mitigate risk. These include and are not limited to defining time limits for answering alarms, defining alarm priority (critical versus warning alarms), standardizing default alarm settings and sounds, planning for backup if systems fail, and ensuring alarms for the patient population are appropriate. For example, when making staff assignments, nurse managers should have a method of communicating which patients are at the most risk for deterioration based on their alarm frequency and clinical history. Nursing leaders should lean on the shoulders of others and understand what has worked in their clinical setting based on the existing and progressing literature from patient safety organizations such as ECRI (https://www.ecri.org/) and the Association for the Advancement of Medical Instrumentation (https://www.aami.org/).

Usability

As organizations have adopted electronic health records and emerging technologies are on the rise, a new problem has arisen that impacts nursing. Technologies that are not easy to use can cause unintended consequences such as documentation mistakes, workarounds, interpretation errors, missing information, decrease in productivity, delay in patient care, increased cognitive load, patient safety concerns, and dissatisfied users (Coiera et al., 2016).

Nursing informaticists play a vital role in assessing the usability of technologies. Along with nursing informaticists, nurse leaders need to ensure that the voices of frontline nursing staff, who are the primary users of systems, are heard (Dunn Lopez & Fahey, 2018), that systems are highly useable, and avoid unintended consequences that compromise patient safety.

Patient Acuity and Staffing Systems

Patient acuity and staffing systems assist management in determining patient acuity levels, workload intensity, and the type of care needed by nurses through electronic systems. Organizations have the ability to track and monitor expenses and resources to promote patient care with patient acuity systems. These systems can also assist with forecasting future trends and strategize on changing market trends (Hawkins et al., 2019). One of the advantages of having systems for patient acuity and staffing is to monitor and improve nurse patient staffing levels and provide documentation for regulatory agencies. On the other hand, some external staffing systems require manual intervention to update, are not real time, and increase organizational costs to maintain. Also, the information is typically entered by resources not in the direct care of the patient, which can lead to subjective information that does not account for patient complexity. More forward-thinking tools can predict nurse staffing needs based on existing nursing documentation of the nurses' assessment of patient outcomes (Garcia & Lovett, 2018).

Nursing Documentation

For many EHRs have moved from adoption to optimization. Nurses are interested in leveraging the EHR to make nursing work more efficient, data driven, transferable, shareable, and measurable, to improve quality and outcomes. Others want to be able to conduct queries to understand what nursing interventions will lead to the highest quality outcomes in a given patient population. However, in order to leverage nursing documentation, it must be based on the use of valid, reliable, interoperable nursing terminologies.

There are five standardized nursing terminology sets endorsed by the American Nurses Association that represent the nursing process, three of which are comprehensive and can be used across patient care populations. This include: (1) NANDA-I, Nursing Outcome Classification (NOC) and Nursing Intervention Classification (NIC) that include linkages to each other for nursing diagnosis, interventions, and outcomes; (2) The International Classification of Nursing Practice (ICNP), and (3) Clinical Care Classification (Macieira et al., 2019). Of note, all of these comprehensive terminology sets can be integrated into EHRs for interoperable flow of nursing information, but there is greater evidence supporting the successful integration of NANDA-I, NIC, and NOC (Macieira et al., 2019).

Electronic Health Record Downtime

With the implementation of the EHR system, downtime presents challenges to organizations and especially nurses who are accustomed to having systems available. Downtime is used to describe the inability to access information systems and can be scheduled or unplanned. There are multiple reasons that outages occur with EHR, including system maintenance, upgrades, hardware failure, software problems, loss of power, security threats, and natural disasters. Nursing workflow can be disrupted by not having patient-level data information easily accessible, the ability to document electronically, and the operation of clinical decision support systems (CDS) results, medication information, and provider order entry.

System downtime, either planned or unplanned, can lead to unintended consequences causing a decrease in productivity, medication errors, delays in patient care, and safety and quality issues resulting in adverse effects. Nurse and other organizational leaders need to be prepared for downtime by having policies and procedures in place, contingency plans, and operational readiness. System outages can last one hour or up to days. It is essential that information systems (IS) work in partnership with Nursing Departments to ensure the plan encompasses all aspects of patient care and workflow. Downtime documentation forms are important to accreditors (e.g., The Joint Commission and Centers for Medicare & Medicaid Services) and should be readily available in designated areas so patient care and documentation are not interrupted. Some departments chose to create "safety stations" with binders of documentation forms and emergency preparedness workflows.

According to the ONC, a recommended practice is to have downtime and reactivation policies that are complete, available, and reviewed regularly. The policies should describe when a downtime should be called, who will be in charge, notifications, and how orders will be executed (ONC, 2016). Not only are downtime procedures important but equally imperative is the reactivation procedures. According to the Safer Guides, Safety Assurance Factors for EHR Resilience (ONC, 2016), organizations should regularly conduct downtime simulations or drills.

Nursing leaders need to consider incorporating downtime training for new hires and annual competencies for nursing staff. Formal training related to downtime procedures and policy will allow nurses to be more efficient, potentially decrease workflow or patient safety concerns, and negative feelings during downtime.

Materials, including procedures and downtime forms, must be accessible in the departments and on a schedule to be regularly reviewed.

LEADERSHIP AND MANAGEMENT IMPLICATIONS

Widespread adoption of meaningful EHRs in the US has been ongoing for over a decade. EHRs provide an opportunity for clinicians and leaders to learn about the care delivered in their organization in order to support real time decision-making and improve care outcomes. This is sometimes referred to as "Practice Based Evidence" (Linder et al., 2017) and "Learning Health Systems" (Friedman et al., 2015).

Data generated by nurses about their clinical decisions for patients, including identification of appropriate nursing diagnosis, selection of nursing interventions, and assessment of patients progress towards outcomes need to be an important part of learning health systems. Unfortunately, many organizations do not have systems for capturing nursing documentation data in a standardized manner. Fortunately, forward-thinking nurse leaders can advocate for the inclusion of standardized nursing terminologies as part of routine nursing documentation in order to capture important data about nursing care.

Standardized terminologies representing nursing diagnoses, interventions, and outcomes were developed by teams of nurse scientists with input from practicing nurses using rigorous research methods over four decades ago. For example, NIC (interventions) (Butcher et al., 2018) and NOC (outcomes) (Moorhead et al., 2018) were funded by the National Institute of Nursing Research. Standardized nursing terminologies have successfully been integrated into many EHRs and used by researchers to understand the impact of nursing care and predictive models (Macieira et al., 2019). Moorhead described ten ways to use NIC and NOC for practice-based evidence. These range from working with the EHR vendor to develop reports based on nursing documentation data and improving quality of care based on NIC and NOC data.

The constantly changing landscape of health information technologies' increasing use and regulatory issues have many implications for clinical nursing operations. In order to manage these changes, clinical nurse leaders need to leverage and sometimes improve their governance and organizational structures. Nurse leaders are also responsible for managing large- and small-scale implementation of technology.

Governance and Organizational Structure

Informatics processes touch every aspect of the health care system, from medication administration to mandatory health screening. It is essential to have not only interdisciplinary teams, but also ensure nursing leaders support informatics as project sponsors and operationalize the vision of the informatics team. Shared governance structures supported by nurse leaders and the prioritization of informatics work are imperative for new HIT initiatives and optimizing existing information systems. Nursing leaders and clinical informaticians collaborate on parallel committees with stakeholders such as IS, nursing councils, risk management, and accreditation departments to support a structured and sustainable clinical operation. Although there are many organizational structures for clinical informaticians, the role of the bedside nurse informs leadership of nursing work, where formalized informaticists positions serve to bridge the gap between IS and nurse end-users.

Some have found that EHR and other health information technology implementation is successful when (1) clinicians can define technology needs, (2) informatics goals are aligned with organizational strategy, (3) defined principles for EHR decision-making are aligned with strategy, (4) escalation protocols are well defined, (5) clinical informatics models are representative of shared governance models, and (6) clinical informatics are devoted full time to informatics positions with no patient care (Collins et al., 2015).

Managing Implementation of New Health Information Technologies

Not only must hospitals meet business objectives, but also external regulatory policy changes require leadership to work with interdisciplinary stakeholders to stay ahead and comply with new policies. Clinical nursing informaticians are in a unique position to create a structure of connectivity between top-level leadership, IS, and bedside nurses.

Organizational readiness projects should be assessed early to anticipate barriers to adoption and opportunities for engaging motivated stakeholders. Technology will not solve ineffective workflows, and failure to clearly implement a technology around the task needs of the nurse may potentially increase work/inefficiencies. Projects involving technology implementations are not technology projects, but people projects. Therefore prior assessments of culture, a clear understanding of the problem to be solved, analysis of the current state, and proposed future state must be defined. Creating effective teams and training, measuring key performance metrics, and sharing information with stakeholders early increases the chance of success.

Communications Plans

After assessing readiness to change, a communications plan and effective training strategy needs to be developed. New HIT changes come in many forms, from quarterly updates, to entire work processes that change how nurses perform daily tasks. Change is expected, and developing a standard communications plan will help users anticipate how to adjust smoothly. For example, quarterly updates should be in a standard template format and come from a leader who is invested in that change. A Vice President of Nursing Operations may send the message to the entire organization or the message may come directly from IS. Regardless of the sender, the communication needs to allow the user to reference current state with future state, and how the change will affect their work. Most importantly, how is the new state going to make the job easier and more efficient? Nurses need to know: what's in it for them?

Vetting the message with clinical nursing staff prior to delivery ensures it is congruent with the language nurses use to interpret the message's meaning. Nursing and IS may team up for traveling "road shows" and communicate changes in person or present at town hall meetings. Shift change reports and staff meetings are time-honored traditions for sharing new content. Whatever method, it is important to file the communications in a shared file where it may be referenced later.

Education Planning

Nurses expect change, whether it is a new piece of equipment or entire clinical process change and responsibilities. Any new HIT implementation should be coordinated with nursing leadership, frontline staff, and patients. The same holds true for education. Education should be done well before implementation, and the materials should relate to nursing work and contain expectations for what to do in case of failure. In-person education with protected time away from patients allows for focus and no interruptions. Asking a nurse to learn during patient care is distracting and unsafe. Training modules may be developed with nurses and subject matter experts to ensure alignment with clinical context and the environment of care.

Boilerplate education from IT vendors needs to be reviewed carefully or edited to match what is happening at the organization. Materials need to be available both electronically and via paper form during implementation. Relating any new technology or processes back to the previous one will help reinforce the existing mental model. What are the differences and similarities about how this process was done? What are the new tools needed, and how does the nurse get there? Nurses should know how to use any new tools and allow "hands on" testing before roll out. Technology documents from the manufacturer must be readily available and reviewed with nurses before implementations. When technical documents are not written in plain language or are cumbersome, shortened "quick tips" sheets written by nursing educators help the user when problems arise.

Creating Stakeholder Teams

Effective interdisciplinary teams ensure that the transition to a new technology is effective and efficient. The diffusion of new information technology innovations is dependent upon many factors, especially those most likely to be early adopters (Rogers, 2003). Nurses who welcome change and risk will be the "cheerleaders" for new HIT. Early adopters are respected leaders who communicate the message through social channels and influence others to do the same.

Frontline nurses should be part of the interdisciplinary team and inform leadership what happens at the bedside during new HIT implementations to eliminate unintended consequences like bottlenecks to workflow and nursing productivity at the bedside. If patients are part of the new change, they need to be part of the plan before it starts. For example, patients should be part of patient portal development and can guide usability and the way information is presented on the home screen. Nursing and patients can participate in usability testing months prior to roll out to ensure the right information is presented in a comprehensive, concise format.

CONCLUSION

In today's health care world of increasing reliance on technologies, all nurses need to have basic competencies in nursing informatics to provide safe and high-quality care. Nurse leaders can play a particularly important role in ensuring that the voice of nursing, as it relates to clinical technology use, is well represented in nursing governance structures and throughout every level of the organization. Clinical nursing informaticists play a key role in technology implementations, assessment, daily use, as well as the inclusion of nursing data in EHRs that fully represent nursing care. Their combined expertise in health care technologies and nursing work and workflow can save organizations money, prevent unintended consequences, and promote the success of technology implementations.

RESEARCH NOTE

Source

Mosier, S., Roberts, W.D., & Englebright, J. (2019). A systems-level method for developing nursing informatics solutions: The role of executive leadership. *Journal of Nursing Administration, 49*(11), 543–548.

Purpose

The challenge for nurse executive and nurse informaticists is how best to coordinate the efforts of experts from diverse fields to design, develop, and deploy solutions to complex systems problems. The purpose of this study was to describe the systems-level method and two successful applications of creating nursing informatics solutions to enhance patient care.

Discussion

The project was conducted within a large network of hospitals and facilities in the US and the UK. The Chief Nurse Executive developed a method to harmonize the work efforts of disparate groups of both clinical and informatics experts. The three guiding principles of the framework were clear lines of responsibility and authority, respect for each type of expertise needed, and clear commitment to the aims of the project. A visual model was displayed. Two large-scale nursing informatics solutions were discussed: one clinically focused (evidence-based clinical documentation for the flow of information in a patient-centric record), and one leadership focused (development of a nursing data portal with a common platform for sharing nursing performance data).

(Continued)

Application to Practice

Nurse executives advance the use of nursing knowledge by creating a data culture, developing data competencies, and establishing a data infrastructure. It takes specific leadership to guide a group of experts through idea development, design, development, data mapping, visualization, and subsequent application of the products that are developed. All of this goes through a technology and informatics life cycle. Clarity of roles was crucial. Leadership engagement stimulated ultimate adoption of the resulting solutions in two examples.

CASE STUDY

Clinical Decision Support System for Neonatal Hypoglycemia

Hypoglycemia is a very treatable condition with early intervention. A serious safety event was reported at a hospital where a neonate was not treated for hypoglycemia twelve hours after birth. Hypoglycemia is defined as low blood glucose concentration, is found in 5% to 15% of newborns, and is increasing in frequency. Hypoglycemia can lead to neurologic damage and abnormalities, such as seizures, and can result in learning disabilities (Wight et al., 2014).

A root cause analysis was completed by a team of clinicians, informatics nurses, and Information Technology Professionals (IT). It was determined there was a nursing educational gap, policies and procedures needed revision, hypoglycemia assessments were absent, and the system lacked alerts, reminders, or protocols. After the root cause analysis was performed, a project team was formed.

Stakeholders

Stakeholders for the project included Labor and Delivery and Special Care Nursery nurses, the Director and Manager of Women's and Children's Services, Quality Manager, Patient Safety Liaison, Project Manager, Informatics Nurse, Systems Analyst, Interface Engineer, analytics, and trainer.

Objectives

The objectives of the intervention were to improve adherence in testing neonates who are at risk for hypoglycemia or have signs and symptoms by obtaining blood glucose levels within the first hour of birth, to increase adherence to following hypoglycemic protocols in neonates who have abnormal glucose levels, and for an increase in staff satisfaction with the ERH related to functionality in the electronic health record to support clinical decision-making for the right patient at the right time in the workflow.

Interventions

The leadership team reviewed and updated the Hypoglycemia Policy and Procedure. Also, necessary documentation assessment points that were missing were added to the system. Finally, a hypoglycemic protocol was designed. There would be three Clinical Decision Support (CDS) interventions.

A clinical alert was designed by the project team and is based on the **Five Rights of CDS**. Table 25.4 summarizes each right and provides examples. The **Right information** will appear for the nurse when a newborn is at risk for hypoglycemia. The **Right person** is elicited from documented maternal risk factors during labor and delivery and neonatal assessment. The alert will appear for nurses who are caring for the mother and/or the neonate. The **Right format** is an active alert that requires input. The **Right channel** will be the Nursing Documentation System within the EHR. The format will contain a pop-up box with text suggesting the neonate is at risk for hypoglycemia and a link to hypoglycemia protocol. The **Right point in the workflow** is while the mother is in labor, during the newborn assessment, and when a point-of-care test result is entered into the system. The Five Rights of clinical decision support are mapped to an example in Table 25.4.

Workflow

Labor and Delivery

The first CDS intervention will occur while the mother is in labor. The patient must be admitted, be in labor, and have associated risk factors on the problem list or history. Upon opening up the record of a patient who meets the criteria, an active alert will appear. The nurse will be presented with the following information "this patient's newborn is at risk for hypoglycemia." The nurse is required to acknowledge the alert and has the option to review the policy and procedure: "select not applicable or remind me later." If the policy and procedure is not selected, the alert will continue to pop up every two hours. The purpose is to alert the nurse that the neonate may be at risk for hypoglycemia.

Neonatal

The second CDS intervention will occur after the neonate is born and will be directed toward the nurse who is

CASE STUDY cont'd

TABLE 25.4   Five Rights of Clinical Decision Support Mapped to Case Study

5 Rights[a]	Example
(What) Right information	A pop up alert for the nurse when a newborn is at risk for hypoglycemia: "This patient's newborn is at risk hypoglycemia." A pop-up alert for the nurse when the neonate is exhibiting signs and symptoms of hypoglycemia with a link to a suggested protocol to place orders.
(Who) Right person	The alert will appear for nurses caring for moms who are at risk for an infant with hypoglycemia or the infant that is exhibiting signs and symptoms. Based upon patient history and assessments documented in the EHR
(How) Right format	The alert will be active and display on the screen with the right information and will be required to acknowledge.
(Where) Right channel	The electronic health record
(When) Right point in the workflow	The alert will appear upon opening the laboring mom, newborns record, or when the point-of-care test is entered with an abnormal result.

[a] Adapted from Osheroff, J. A. (Ed.) (2012). *Improving outcomes with clinical decision support: an implementer's guide* (2nd ed.). Chicago, IL: HIMSS.

caring for the patient. The alert is based upon new documentation question selections added to the newborn admission history. The assessment will include maternal risk factors and signs and symptoms of hypoglycemia. When any of the choices are selected, the following information will appear in a pop-up box, "this patient is at risk for hypoglycemia, order the hypoglycemia protocol." The protocol will be based orders based and will require a response. After the order is placed a banner will appear in the electronic health record indicating the patient is at risk for hypoglycemia, nursing tasks will be added to the worklist related to feeding schedules and blood glucose levels. Nursing problems and goals will appear in the care plan.

Point-of-Care Testing
The third CDS intervention will be presented during the point-of-care testing. Blood glucose levels are interfaced from the point-of-care testing system. When the blood glucose is not within the parameters, the nurse is presented with the same alert in Intervention two. Also, graphical reports will display the glucose levels. Once the orders are placed, the active alert will cease.

Evaluation
Analytical reports were created for Nurse Managers to monitor patients who are at risk for neonates with hypoglycemia and neonates who have low blood glucose levels.

Staff Training
The project will include a training program that provides for baseline measurement of nurse's knowledge of hypoglycemia risk factors and interventions with a post quiz. Nurses needed to be trained on the new assessments, alerts, tasks, reports, and reminders.

The implementation of clinical decision support to alert nurses of mothers who may deliver a baby who is at risk or develop hypoglycemia will result in a higher quality of care and lead to improved outcomes. To achieve success multiple interventions at different points in the workflow needed to be implemented. Analytics were available to ensure clinical accuracy. The key to success in solving serious patient safety issues is to involve appropriate team members and engaging stakeholders. This will result in the right solution for the right person at the right time with the right information, at the right point in the workflow using the right channel.

CRITICAL THINKING EXERCISE

Nurses in all units of a large medical center are required to print and label patient point-of-care lab specimens that are automatically generated by physician orders in the EHR. Once an order is written and electronically "signed off" by the nurse, the label prints on a local printer designated for labs only.

Leaders from several nursing units have noticed an uptick in mislabeled specimens, and they need a way to improve compliance. Mislabeled specimens not only impede timely care, but can also potentially lead to the wrong care when specimens are labeled for the wrong patient. The nursing leadership team asked the Nursing Informatics department and Information Systems (IS) to help develop a solution to the problem by investigating the process by which labels are generated and applied to specimens.

The IS team decided to create a verification process where once the label is generated, a separate "task" of scanning the patient's ID band would need to be completed in the patient's room, whereby the label is linked to the patient. This "task" also shows up as a nursing task in a list in the EHR. After the band is scanned, the task will show as "completed" in the EHR and disappear from the list. Any labels that are not verified in the patient room showed up as unfinished tasks in the EHR. Leaders would then be able to monitor adherence via an unfinished task window in the EHR.

Prior to implementation, communications were sent out by IS to the nursing units on the process. There was no in-person training and during the implementation day, scanning tasks did not complete the nursing "task" in the list, and some patient labels did not scan. Nurses went back to the traditional method to print labels and send specimens. In some cases, nurses had to ask physicians to reorder labs just to generate lab labels. It was found later that during integration of the lab information system to the EHR, orders that were generated before the new process were not included in the new workflow. In addition, nurses had questions about how to scan multiple labels in one task, and how that would be captured in the EHR. IS could not answer whether that workflow was possible. Of note, IS was the only stakeholder to validate the process before go-live, and all testing occurred outside of the production environment.

1. Which stakeholders were missing in the development of this new process?
2. Where should the new process have been tested prior to implementation?
3. How should the process have been better tested?
4. What type of training would have been beneficial prior to the implementation?
5. What key performance metric would have been more effective in measuring outcomes besides task list completion? (Hint: number of mislabeled specimens after implementation)
6. What role do nursing leaders have in ensuring the success of any new HIT project?
7. How could education about the new process have been communicated better?
8. What types of communication channels are needed in HIT implementations such as this one?
9. What other unintended consequences and extra work came out of this new process?
10. What would you have done differently and why?

REFERENCES

Adler-Milstein, J., & Jha, A. K. (2017). HITECH Act drove large gains in hospital electronic health record adoption. *Health Affairs, 36*(8), 1416–1422.

Alexander, S., Frith, K. A., & Hoy, H. (2019). *Applied clinical informatics for nurses* (2nd ed.). Burlington, Mass: Jones and Bartlett Learning.

American Association of Colleges of Nursing (AACN). (2006). *DNP essentials*. https://www.aacnnursing.org/dnp/dnp-essentials.

American Association of Colleges of Nursing (AACN). (2008). *The essentials of baccalaureate education for professional nursing practice*. http://www.aacnnursing.org/portals/42/publications/baccessentials08.pdf.

American Association of Colleges of Nursing (AACN). (2011). *The essentials of master's education in nursing*. http://www.aacnnursing.org/portals/42/publications/mastersessentials11.pdf.

American Association of Colleges of Nursing. (2019). *AACN Essentials, DRAFT Domains and descriptors*. https://www.aacnnursing.org/Portals/42/Downloads/Essentials/Essentials-Revision-Domains-Descriptors.pdf.

American Medical Informatics Association. (2020). *What is informatics?* https://www.amia.org/fact-sheets/what-informatics.

Butcher, H. K., Bulechek, G. M., Dochterman, J. M. M., & Wagner, C. M. (2018). *Nursing interventions classification*

510 PART 5 Business Skills

(NIC)-E-Book. Amsterdam, NL: Elsevier Health Sciences.

Clark, J., & Lang, N. (1992). Nursing's next advance: an internal classification for nursing practice. *International Nursing Review, 39*(4), 109–111 128.

Cohen, I. G., & Mello, M. M. (2018). HIPAA and protecting health information in the 21st century. *Journal of the American Medical Association, 320*(3), 231–232.

Coiera, E., Ash, J., & Berg, M. (2016). The unintended consequences of health information technology revisited. *Yearbook of Medical Informatics, 25*(01), 163–169.

Collins, S. A., Alexander, D., & Moss, J. (2015). Nursing domain of CI governance: recommendations for health IT adoption and optimization. *Journal of the American Medical Informatics Association, 22*(3), 697–706.

Dunn Lopez, K., & Fahey, L. (2018). Advocating for greater usability in clinical technologies: The role of the practicing nurse. *Critical Care Nursing Clinics, 30*(2), 247–257.

Friedman C., Rubin J., Brown J., Buntin M., Corn M., Etheredge L., et al. (2015). Toward a science of learning systems: a research agenda for the high-functioning Learning Health System. *Journal of the American Medical Informatics Association, 22*(1), 43–50.

Garcia, A., & Lovett, R. (2018). Use of nursing outcomes classification to measure patient acuity and optimize nurse staffing. In S. Moorhead, E. Swanson, M. Johnson, & M. Maas (Eds.), *Nursing Outcomes Classification.* Amsterdam, NL: Elsevier.

Hawkins, M., Messier, A., Myers, K., Nihsen, A., & Kniewel, M. (2019). Using an acuity tool that interfaces with the electronic health record to balance nursing workload. *Manager's Journal on Nursing, 9*(2), 36.

Kahn, M. J., & Baum, N. (2020). MIPS MACRA and Payment Models. In N. Baum, & M. J. Kahn (Eds.), *The Business Basics of Building and Managing a Health Care Practice* (pp. 75–79). New York, NY: Springer.

Linder, L. A., Gerdy, C., Abouzelof, R., & Wilson, A. (2017). Using practice-based evidence to improve supportive care practices to reduce central line–associated bloodstream infections in a pediatric oncology unit. *Journal of Pediatric Oncology Nursing, 34*(3), 185–195.

Lowry S., Quinn M., Ramaiah M., Schumacher R., Patterson E., North R., et al. (2012). *Technical evaluation, testing, and validation of the usability of electronic health records.* Gaithersburg, MD: National Institute of Standards and Technology. *NISTIR*(780).

Lye, C. T., Forman, H. P., Daniel, J. G., & Krumholz, H. M. (2018). The 21st Century Cures Act and electronic health records one year later: will patients see the benefits? *Journal of the American Medical Informatics Association, 25*(9), 1218–1220.

Macieira, T. G., Chianca, T. C., Smith, M. B., Yao, Y., Bian, J., Wilkie, D. J., et al. (2019). Secondary use of standardized nursing care data for advancing nursing science and practice: a systematic review. *Journal of the American Medical Informatics Association, 26*(11), 1401–1411.

Moorhead, S., Johnson, M., Maas, M. L., & Swanson, E. (2018). *Nursing Outcomes Classification (NOC)-E-Book: Measurement of Health Outcomes.* Elsevier Health Sciences.

Mosier, S., Roberts, W. D., & Englebright, J. (2019). A systems-level method for developing nursing informatics solutions: The role of executive leadership. *Journal of Nursing Administration, 49*(11), 543–548.

Nelson, R. (2019). Informatics: evolution of the nelson data, information, knowledge and wisdom model: part 1. *OJIN: The Online Journal of Issues in Nursing, 23*(3). https://ojin.nursingworld.org/MainMenuCategories/ ANAMarketplace/ANAPeriodicals/OJIN/Columns/ Informatics/Informatics-Evolution-of-Nelson-Model-Part-1.html.

O'Grady, E., Mason, D., Hopkins Outlaw, F., & Gardner, D. (2016). Frameworks for action in policy and politics. In D. Mason, D. Gardner, F. Hopkins Outlaw, & E. O'Grady (Eds.), *Policy politics in nursing in health care* (7th ed.). Philadelphia, PA: Saunders.

Osheroff, J. A. (2012). *Improving outcomes with clinical decision support: an implementer's guide* (2nd ed.). Chicago, IL: HIMSS.

Quality and Safety Education for Nursing (QSEN). (2020). *About QSEN.* https://qsen.org/about-qsen/.

Rogers, E. M. (2003). *Diffusion of innovations* (5th ed.). New York, NY: Free Press.

Staggers, N., & Thompson, C. B. (2002). The evolution of definitions for nursing informatics: A critical analysis and revised definition. *Journal of the American Medical Informatics Association, 9*(3), 255–261. https://doi-org. proxy.lib.uiowa.edu/10.1197/jamia.M0946.

Stossel, L. M., Segar, N., Gliatto, P., Fallar, R., & Karani, R. (2012). Readability of patient education materials available at the point of care. *Journal of General Internal Medicine, 27*(9), 1165–1170.

The Office of the National Coordinator for Health Information Technology. (2016). *Safety assurance factors for EHR resilience.* https://www.healthit.gov/ sites/default/files/safer/guides/safer_high_priority_ practices.pdf.

United States Department of Health and Human Services (USDHHS). (2020). *Strategy on reducing regulatory and administrative burden relating to the use of Health IT and EHRs.* https://www.healthit.gov/topic/usability-and-provider-burden/strategy-reducing-burden-relating-use-health-it-and-ehrs.

Wight, N., & Marinelli, K. A. (2014). ABM clinical protocol# 1: Guidelines for blood glucose monitoring and treatment of hypoglycemia in term and late-preterm neonates, Revised 2014. *Breastfeeding Medicine, 9*(4), 173–179.

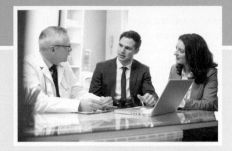

26

Marketing

Lyn Stankiewicz Losty

http://evolve.elsevier.com/Huber/leadership

Marketing is as old as civilization itself. In ancient Greece, the agora was the center of all aspects of economic life. Market stalls were set up and traders actively engaged in persuasive communications (Fig. 26.1). Marketing is also mentioned in the Bible, with references to marketplaces and the exchange of goods and services in both the Old and New Testament. Marketing is essential for any business to thrive as it helps to build and maintain an organization's goods and services while building the brand equity of the organization. Marketing also assists in building a relationship of trust and understanding with customers. Marketing also creates revenue opportunities for an organization. Since health care systems are businesses, they rely on promotion and advertising to attract patients; thus, marketing is paramount to health care.

Traditionally, nurses are educated to care for patients and their families. Nurse leaders and nurse managers are challenged to care not only for patients and families but also for organizations, especially in today's turbulent

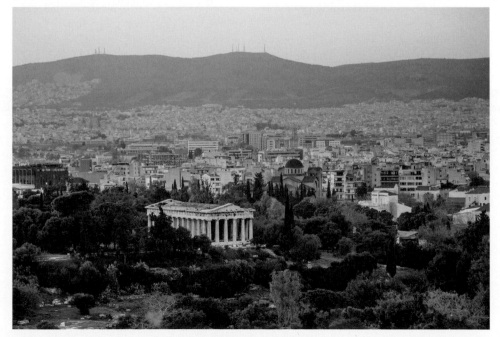

Fig. 26.1 Greece agora.

(Copyright iStock Photo; Credit: MarioGuti.)

times. Nurse leaders and managers have a responsibility to foster collaborative relationships among all individuals within our health care organization in order to implement the mission and vision of the organization. They are responsible for recruiting, hiring, orienting new providers, evaluating performances, budgeting, setting policies and procedures, and most importantly, delivering safe and effective care to the patients served. All of these activities are included in the discipline of marketing. The purpose of this chapter is to present key marketing concepts and definitions, identify key current issues and trends of marketing in health care, and discuss implications for nurse leaders and nurse managers.

DEFINITIONS

Defining the Discipline of Marketing

Marketing seems relatively simple because it is about identifying and meeting human and social needs. However, similar to nursing, marketing is both an art and a science as it is achieved by careful planning and execution using state-of-the-art tools and techniques. To understand marketing, some definitions of the discipline of marketing are presented:

- **Armstrong and Kotler** (2017, p. 5) defined marketing as "engaging customers and managing profitable customer relationships."
- **Kotler and Keller** (2016, p. 5) articulated marketing as "the art and science of choosing target markets and

getting, keeping, and growing customers through creating, delivering, and communicating superior customer value."

- The **American Marketing Association** (AMA, 2020) described marketing as "the activity, set of institutions, and processes for creating, communicating, delivering, and exchanging offerings that have value for customers, clients, partners, and society at large."
- **Peter Drucker**, a famous management theorist, described "the aim of marketing is to know and understand the customer so well that the product or service fits him and sells itself. Ideally, marketing should result in a customer who is ready to buy. All that should be needed then is to make the product or service available" (Kotler & Keller, 2016, p. 5).

From these definitions, it is apparent that much of what the average person understands about marketing focuses on the words such as "relationships," "customers," and "needs." Simply put, marketing is about meeting a need. **Marketing** is the art and science of identifying a private or social need and turning it into a profitable business opportunity. For example, when Google recognized that people needed to more effectively and efficiently access information on the internet, they created a powerful search engine that organized and prioritized information. When Apple saw that people wanted to carry one device that was a phone, music player, and organizer, they created the iPhone. Overall, there are ten different categories of entities that are marketed by organizations all over the world (Table 26.1).

TABLE 26.1	**Types of Marketed Entities**
Goods	Physical goods constitute the bulk of most countries' marketing efforts. Examples include furniture, cars, machines, sports equipment, etc.
Services	Services include the work of airlines, hotels, car rental firms, barbers and beauticians, maintenance and repair people, and accountants, bankers, lawyers, engineers, doctors, software programmers, and management consultants. Many market offerings mix goods and services, such as a fast-food meal.
Events	Marketers promote time-based events, such as major trade shows, artistic performances, and company anniversaries. Global sporting events such as the Olympics and the World Cup are promoted aggressively to companies and fans. Local events include craft fairs, bookstore readings, and farmer's markets.
Experiences	By orchestrating several services and goods, an organization can create, stage, and market experiences. Walt Disney World's Magic Kingdom lets customers visit a fairy kingdom, a pirate ship, or a haunted house.
Persons	Artists, musicians, CEOs, physicians, high-profile lawyers and professional athletes are examples of people who are marketed. For example, NFL quarterback Peyton Manning, talk show veteran Oprah Winfrey and rock-and-roll legend, Tom Petty are branded.

Continued

TABLE 26.1	**Types of Marketed Entities—cont'd**
Places	Cities, states, regions, and whole nations compete to attract tourists, residents, factories, and company headquarters. For example, Atlanta is the "hub" for Delta Airlines.
Properties	Property are intangible rights of ownership to either real property, real estate, or financial property such as stocks and bonds.
Organizations	Museums, art studios, corporations, and non-profits all use marketing to boost their public image and compete for audiences and funds.
Information	Information is essentially what books, schools, and universities produce, market, and distribute "this information" to consumers.
Ideas	Most products and services are platforms for some idea or benefit. Such ideas include "Friends Don't Let Friends Drive Drunk," "Just Say No," or "A Mind Is a Terrible Thing to Waste."

BACKGROUND

Marketing is not much different in health care, where the literature is replete with examples of the need for marketing. First, health care revenues were approximately $3.6 trillion in 2018, making it the single largest industry in the United States at 17.7% of GDP (Centers for Medicare & Medicaid Services [CMS], 2019a). Second, the industry faces many challenges, ranging from financial, regulatory, technological, and environmental that often create the need for radical, complex change. Continued consolidation among health care organizations has created a multi-faceted, convoluted, competitive environment. Overlying these challenges, health care leaders and managers need to balance concerns of quality of life and quality of care with "bottom line profits in a way that no other industry is challenged to do" (Kennett et al., 2005, p. 5). Thus, marketing skills are and will continue to be one of the key tools for nurse leaders and managers in the health care field.

Here is a scenario. A working mother with a family of four and an aging father to care for, may wonder if her father's unstable gait should be a concern or if it is part of the normal aging process. She commits to exploring possible solutions and Googles terms like "unstable walking" or "unstable gait in the elderly." She finds the webpage for the local hospital, which provides information about "change in gait for older adults" and sees that the hospital offers an evening program geared towards assisting adult children of aging parents. She calls the program and plans to attend as she has determined that her father's unstable gait is of concern and is committed to seeking a suitable solution. She attends the meeting, meets a geriatric nurse practitioner, and schedules an appointment for her father.

In this brief scenario, the individual becomes aware of an issue (an identified need), considers possible solutions, decides on the type of solution that works best, and commits to the solution. Before any of these events occurred, the marketing team at the local hospital recognized that assisting adult children of aging parents was a need for the community, thus became a priority for their organization. By understanding the customers' needs prior to "actual occurrence of the need," organizations are able to anticipate and meet the customer's need by marketing the solution prior to the need being identified. Thus, when a customer is ready to receive the information that he or she is looking for, an organization is "one step ahead" by advertising and marketing that good or service.

In health care, marketing is focused on establishing customer relationships and satisfying customer identified needs and wants. It is here that nurse leaders and managers are crucial members of the hospital marketing team. Nurse leaders and managers may provide input regarding the organization's marketing strategy; but more importantly, nurse leaders and managers also supervise the team that most directly affects the value that a customer (the patient and family) receives and, ultimately, may report in terms of outcomes. Every interaction between a patient and a nurse creates and communicates value—the very definition of marketing. Therefore, it is imperative that a health care environment which is to be built on patient satisfaction, is created and enhanced through the discipline of marketing.

Marketing Activities

Marketing activities within health care organizations occur at the organizational, departmental, and unit levels. Such activities are also classified as **internal or**

external, with each targeting a different audience or market. Target audiences can be patients and families, physicians, payers, and employees. Marketing departments within health care agencies take the lead in organizational-level, departmental-level, and unit-level activities to ensure that customer-driven marketing strategies and programs are in alignment with the organization's mission, vision, and strategic plan. The primary product that is offered and marketed by health care organizations is care delivery (a service), which includes the nurses who deliver most care in health care organizations. Patient satisfaction is a common and accepted indicator of the service, and a high level of satisfaction is imperative to viability in today's competitive marketplace (Kennedy et al., 2013). This is an example of an internal marketing strategy: marketing the quality of care to patients. For example, the nurse communication section of the Hospital Consumer Assessment of Healthcare Providers and Systems (HCAHPS) survey, which is a standardized survey of patients' perspectives about hospital care, has an important impact on patients' satisfaction with hospitalization. Thus, nurses and nurse leaders are important members of the marketing team because of their primary focus on providing patient care and managing patients' health care needs.

Not only are nurses at the center of health care delivery, but nurse leaders are also accountable for the workforce that provides this service. Marketing initiatives that focus on care delivery, customer satisfaction, and recruitment and retention of the nursing workforce are essential in hospitals. Nurse leaders who possess marketing acumen within their business skill set are invaluable to the development of more sensitive customer/patient service programs delivered by a competent, experienced nursing workforce. These initiatives may be internal (retention) or external (recruitment) or a blend of both.

Previous chapters in this text have addressed the challenges faced by top-level and frontline nurse leaders. These challenges include delivery of high-quality patient-centered care; recruitment and retention of a culturally diverse, competent workforce; promotion of a positive and inspiring image of nursing; design of a healthy work environment; and development of practices to satisfy patients and improve outcomes. Marketing initiatives can be designed and implemented to assist the nurse leader and nurse manager to successfully identify and meet these challenges.

KEY MARKETING CONCEPTS

The Market

Traditionally, a "market" was a physical place where buyers and sellers came together to buy and sell tangible goods. However, in today's environment, markets operate a bit differently. A market is a collection of buyers and sellers who interact over a particular product, product class or service, such as the housing market or the grain market. Manufacturers go to resource markets (raw material markets, labor markets, money markets), buy resources, turn them into goods and services, and sell finished products to intermediaries, who sell them to consumers. Consumers sell their labor and receive money with which they pay for goods and services. The government collects tax revenues to buy goods from resource, manufacturer, and intermediary markets and uses these goods and services to provide public services.

Each nation's economy consists of interacting sets of markets linked through exchange processes. Marketers view sellers as the industry and use the term "market" to describe customer groups. There are a variety of market types, such as need markets (the diet-seeking market), product markets (the shoe market), demographic markets (the "millennium" youth market), geographic markets (the Chinese market), voter markets, labor markets, and donor markets (Fig. 26.2). Sellers communicate to the market through ads and direct mail in the hope that the "market" or customer will purchase their goods and services, and, in return, the sellers receive money for the goods and services and information such as customer attitudes and sales data from the interaction. The inner loop shows an exchange of money for goods and services; the outer loop shows an exchange of information (Fig. 26.3).

Market Brand

A brand is a name, term, design, symbol, or any other feature that identifies a seller's good or service as distinct from those of other sellers. Brands are used in business, marketing, and advertising for recognition. Name brands are sometimes distinguished from generic or store brands. Interestingly, the practice of branding begun with the ancient Egyptians, who were known to have engaged in livestock branding as early as 2700 BCE. Branding was used to differentiate one person's cattle from another's by means of a distinctive symbol burned into the animal's skin with a hot branding

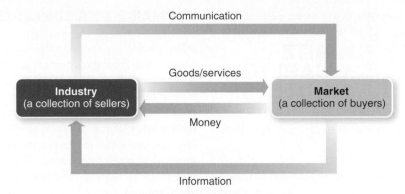

Fig. 26.2 A simple marketing system.

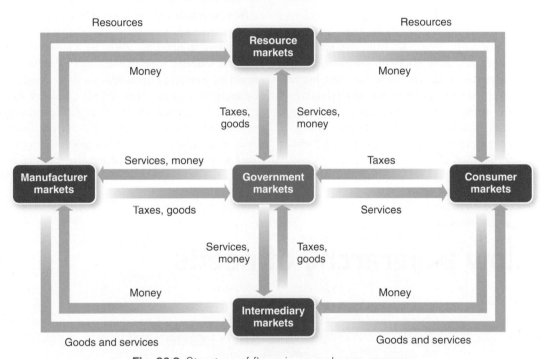

Fig. 26.3 Structure of flows in an exchange economy.

iron. If a person stole any of the cattle, anyone else who saw the symbol could deduce the actual owner. The term has been extended to mean a strategic personality for a product or company, so that "brand" now suggests the values and promises that a consumer may perceive and buy into. Over time the practice of branding objects extended to a broader range of packaging and goods offered for sale including oil, wine, cosmetics, and fish sauce. Branding in terms of painting a cow with symbols or colors at flea markets was considered to be one of the oldest forms of the practice.

In the modern era, the concept of branding has expanded to include the marketing and communication techniques that help to distinguish a company or products from competitors, aiming to create a lasting impression in the minds of customers. The key components that form a brand's toolbox include a brand's identity, brand communication (such as by logos and trademarks), brand awareness, brand loyalty, and various branding (brand management) strategies. Many companies believe that there is often little to differentiate between several types of products in the 21st century,

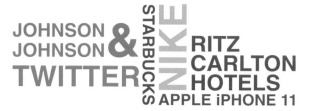

Fig. 26.4 Can you identify these popular brands by their logo?

hence branding is among a few remaining forms of product differentiation (Fig. 26.4).

Product Differentiation

Product differentiation is a marketing strategy that businesses use to distinguish a product from similar offerings on the market. The difference could be something concrete, like speed, power, performance, and better service. Or, it could be a more ephemeral quality, such as just being cooler or more stylish than your competitors. For small businesses, a product differentiation strategy may provide a competitive advantage in a market dominated by larger companies.

When an organization uses a differentiation strategy that focuses on the cost value of the product versus other similar products on the market, it creates a perceived value among consumers and potential customers. A strategy that focuses on value highlights the cost savings or durability of a product in comparison to other products. The cost savings can revolve around the initial selling price of the product, or focus on longer-term, life cycle costs. An energy-saving product, for example, might save consumers money in the long run, even if they pay a bit more at the front end.

Needs, Wants, and Demands

Needs. Needs are considered to be the basic human requirements such as for air, food, water, and shelter. The core of marketing starts with understanding the customer's needs. One of the most effective ways that nurses have accessed patients' needs is using Maslow's Hierarchy of Needs (Fig. 26.5). Maslow's Hierarchy of Needs is a motivational theory in psychology that depicts a classification system that reflects the universal needs of society as its base, then proceeds upward in the shape of a pyramid. Interestingly, marketing also uses

Maslow's hierarchy of needs

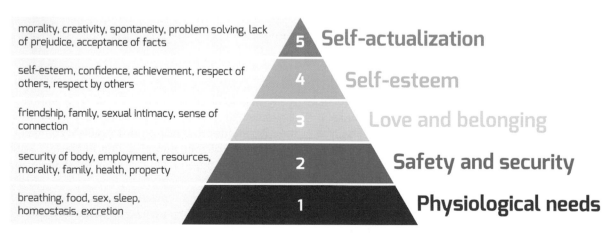

Fig. 26.5 Maslow's hierarchy of needs. *(©iStock.com (Credit:PytyCzech))*

Maslow's Hierarchy of Needs. The levels of the pyramid include:

- **Physiological:** Food, clothing, shelter, money, sleep, and homeostasis.
- **Safety:** Financial security, personal safety, health and wellness, and stability.
- **Love and Belonging:** Close bonds, recognition, compassion for others and affection.
- **Self-Esteem:** Respect, status, recognition, praise, confidence, and independence.
- **Self-Actualization:** Desire to become the most that one can be; full use and exploitation of talents, capabilities, and potentials.

Although the theory is generally portrayed as a fairly rigid hierarchy, Maslow noted that the order in which these needs are fulfilled does not always follow this standard progression. For example, he noted that for some individuals, the need for self-esteem is more important than the need for love. For others, the need for creative fulfillment may supersede even the most basic needs. Interestingly, some people consider health care to be a need while others see health care as a luxury, thus representing different levels on the hierarchy. When the Affordable Health Care Act (ACA) was passed in 2010, the law had three primary goals:

1. To make affordable health insurance available to more people with incomes between 100% and 400% of the federal poverty level,
2. Expand the Medicaid program to cover all adults with incomes below 138% of the federal poverty level, and
3. Support innovative medical care delivery methods designed to lower the costs of health care generally.

As a result of the ACA, individuals faced rigid fines for being without coverage. Despite this federal mandate, millions of working Americans remain uninsured because they are unable to afford the premiums, thus, unable to meet their need for health care.

Wants. Wants are a type of need when an individual is directed to a specific object that may satisfy a specific need. When deciding whether something is a need or a want, start with the basic definitions outlined in economics. A need is something necessary to survive. Without meeting a need, one would be in grave danger or even die as one's safety and health depend on it. If one can survive without something, then it's not a need. On the other hand, a want is simply something one desires but can live without.

Interestingly, research has determined that patients want safety more than savings when differentiating

between various providers for necessary health care. In fact, 97% of the time, consumers will choose hospitals that are rated safer, regardless of cost (Byrnes, 2015). However, wants are not fixed. Wants change because both related factors and priorities can shift. For example, private insurance mitigates the impact of cost on patient choices. If the insurance environment changes, cost may become a more important factor in the choices patients make to meet their health care needs.

Demands. Demands are the "wants" for specific products backed by an ability to pay. In other words, demand refers to a buyer's desire to purchase goods and services at given price. For example, a person may want a diamond necklace; however, only a few individuals can actually buy one. We may want health care, but health care comes at a cost. Marketers spend a considerable amount of money to determine the amount of demand the public has for a good or a service. How much of their goods will they actually be able to sell at any given price? Incorrect estimations either result in money left on the table if demand is underestimated or losses if demand is overestimated. Demand is what helps fuel the economy, and without it, businesses would not produce anything.

Demand is closely related to supply. Consumers try to pay the lowest prices they can for goods and services, suppliers try to maximize profits. If suppliers charge too much, the quantity demanded drops and suppliers do not sell enough product to earn sufficient profits. If suppliers charge too little, the quantity demanded increases, but lower prices may not cover suppliers' costs or allow for profits. Some factors affecting demand include the appeal of a good or service, the availability of competing goods, the availability of financing, and the perceived availability of a good or service.

Supply and Demand

Supply and demand are perhaps one of the most fundamental concepts of economics, and it is the backbone of a market economy. Demand refers to how much (quantity) of a product or service is desired by buyers. The quantity demanded is the amount of a product people are willing to buy at a certain price; the relationship between price and quantity demanded is known as the demand relationship. Supply represents how much the market can offer. The quantity supplied refers to the amount of a certain good producers are willing to supply when receiving a certain price. The correlation between price and how much of a good or service is supplied to the market is known as the supply relationship. Price, therefore, reflects supply and demand.

Interestingly enough, there are only four basic laws that govern supply and demand. They include:
- If demand increases and supply remains unchanged, it leads to a higher price and higher quantities.
- If demand decreases and supply remains unchanged, it leads to a lower price and lower quantities.
- If supply increases and demand remains unchanged, it leads to a lower price and a higher quantity.
- If supply decreases and demand remains unchanged, it leads to a higher price and lower quantity.

So, exactly how does this work? Think about demand and the "want" for something. A new Apple watch or a reservation at the newest restaurant in New York are in high demand. As a result of the high demand, suppliers can charge a higher price, because there is a demand and the quantity of the goods will slowly increase to meet that demand. In health care there is a demand for services, however, the quantity is limited. For example, a hospital may have 350 available beds and 357 patients that need a bed (the demand is greater than the supply). An outpatient clinic may have five providers that can see 10 patients per day (50 appointments), but there are only 46 appointments (the supply is greater than the demand). This principle was in sharp focus during the 2020 COVID-19 pandemic.

Market Equilibrium

The point at which supply and demand meet represents the market clearing or market equilibrium price. An increase in demand shifts the demand curve to the right. The curves intersect at a higher price, and consumers pay more for the product. Equilibrium prices typically remain in a state of flux for most goods and services because factors affecting supply and demand are always changing. Free, competitive markets tend to push prices toward market equilibrium (Fig. 26.6).

Market Demand Versus Aggregate Demand

The market for each good in an economy faces a different set of circumstances, which vary in type and degree. Aggregate demand in an economy is examined by macroeconomics. Aggregate demand refers to the total demand by all consumers for all good and services in an economy across all the markets for individual goods. Because aggregate includes all goods in an economy, it is not sensitive to competition or substitution between different goods or changes in consumer preferences

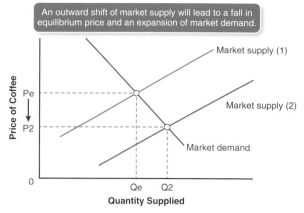

Fig. 26.6 Market equilibrium.

between various goods in the same way that demand in individual good markets can be.

Utility

Utility is an abstract concept rather than a concrete, observable quantity. The units to which we assign an "amount" of utility, therefore, are arbitrary, representing a relative value. Total utility is the aggregate sum of satisfaction or benefit that an individual gain from consuming a given amount of goods or services in an economy. The amount of a person's total utility corresponds to the person's level of consumption. Usually, the more the person consumes, the larger their total utility will be. Marginal utility is the additional satisfaction, or amount of utility, gained from each extra unit of consumption.

Although total utility usually increases as more of a good is consumed, marginal utility usually decreases with each additional increase in the consumption of a good. This decrease demonstrates the law of diminishing marginal utility. Because there is a certain threshold of satisfaction, the consumer will no longer receive the same pleasure from consumption once that threshold is crossed. In other words, total utility will increase at a slower pace as an individual increases the quantity consumed.

Take, for example, a chocolate bar. Let us say that after eating one chocolate bar your sweet tooth has been satisfied. Your marginal utility (and total utility) after eating one chocolate bar will be quite high. But if you eat more chocolate bars, the pleasure of each additional chocolate bar will be less than the pleasure you received from eating the one before - probably because you are starting to feel full or you have had too many sweets for one day (Table 26.2).

TABLE 26.2	Chocolate Bars and Utility	
Chocolate Bars Eaten	Marginal Utility	Total Chocolate Utility
0	0	0
1	70	70
2	10	80
3	5	85
4	3	88

The Four Ps of Marketing

The four Ps of marketing are the four essential factors that come into play when a good or service are being marketed to the public (Fig. 26.7). Neil Borden popularized the idea of the Four Ps in the 1950s and E. Jerome McCarthy (1964) updated the Ps in 1960. The Four Ps include:

Product. Product refers to a good or service that a company offers to customers. Ideally, a product should fulfill a certain consumer demand or be so compelling that consumers believe they need to have it. To be successful, marketers need to understand the life cycle of a product, and business executives need to have a plan for dealing with products at every stage of their life cycles. The type of product also partially dictates how much businesses can charge for it, where they should place it, and how they should promote it in the marketplace.

Price. Price is what the consumer pays. Some industries garner only a small markup on price, while others have huge profit margins, because they are highly sought after. Price is affected by sales cycles, product life cycles, supply and demand. Business strategies might consider a cost leadership strategy by trying to beat the market with the lowest price, or a business strategy might choose to inflate the price, based on a luxury component or brand image.

Place. As a strategy, place has become a more significant component of marketing success. Place involves where the product is stored, perhaps even where it is manufactured. The internet has created a dramatic evolution of where products are sold and distributed, from small, local companies to global. This strategy also considers where the product is advertised and in which format, including radio, infomercials, magazines, online ads, and even in film product placements.

Promotion. This strategy component is tied directly to the other three Ps. The promotional strategy aims to show consumers why they need to buy this specific product over others. Timing heavily influences the amount of promotional marketing, and when. It may also adjust the location, such as commercials during football season games that target pizza delivery deals. It may try to entice consumers to try a product with an irresistible promotional or introductory offer. In today's digital age, the "place" and "promotion" factors are as much online as offline. Online considerations include where a product appears on a company's web page or social media, as well as which types of search functions trigger corresponding, targeted ads for the product.

An Important Fifth "P": PEOPLE

One of the most important Ps is the fifth P: people. Interestingly, a leader could have the best strategy in the world, but if the people are unable to execute the strategy

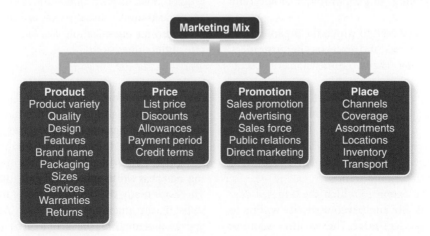

Fig. 26.7 Four Ps of marketing.

or closing sale, then there will not be a successful marketing campaign. For people to be positive factors in executing the strategy, the leader needs to take the time to properly hire, onboard, train, and monitor the team. Finding talent is one of the most difficult things any business leader must do. There is a great deal of competition for people who are looking for work, but there is a smaller pool of people who are a great fit for a company. Spend the time needed to review team positions and the team's exact needs. Understand what is required to make someone successful on the team.

When new hires are brought on board ("onboarding"), the leader needs to share their vision and the strategy for success. Having new employees buy into the company vision from day one sets the tone for success. Properly train people in the process of sales or service, whichever division they will be responsible for. Every person is a promotional face for the company, whether they know it or not. If your employee is leaving work and speaking negatively about their job, it is a reflection on the company.

The Four As of Marketing

In reviewing the Four Ps, it is evident that the Four Ps are completely company driven. The organization decides on the price, builds the product, decides where to distribute it and how to promote it. The missing piece is that it does not consider the customer. Sheth and Sisodai (2006) made the case that customer knowledge is more reliable. Thus, their framework emphasizes consumer value in terms of the Four As. This approach is organized around the values that matter most to the customers as it focuses on the four distinct roles that customers play in the market: acceptability, affordability, accessibility, and awareness.

Acceptability. The extent to which the organization's product or service meets and exceeds the customers' needs and expectations. The two dimensions of acceptability include:

Functional Acceptability: Indicated by the functionality of the product, performance attributes, ease of use, and reliability.

Psychological Acceptability: includes brand image, social and emotional value. Psychological acceptability is often associated with "luxury brands".

Affordability. The extent to which the targeted customers are economically and psychologically willing to pay the product or service's price. The two dimensions of affordability include:

Economic Affordability: The ability to pay for the product or service as determined by factors such as income, assets, financing, and fit within a budget. In other words, does the customer have sufficient economic resources to pay a product or service's price?

Psychological Affordability: The willingness to pay for a product or service determined by the perceived value for money, perceived price fairness, and price relative to other options.

Accessibility. The extent to which a customer is able to readily acquire and use the product or service. Accessibility has two dimensions:

Availability: As determined by factors such as supply and demand; the degree to which a product is kept in-stock and readily available to customers.

Convenience: Determined by the time and effort in acquiring the product, the ease in which the product can be found and accessed.

Awareness. The extent to which customers are informed regarding a product's characteristics and are in the process of making a decision that demonstrates they are "on board" with the product, ranging from the most obvious, a purchasing decision, to a surrogate, such as clicking on a coupon to print out. Awareness has two dimensions:

Product Knowledge – as demonstrated by interest or understanding

Brand Awareness – as demonstrated by brand recall or brand association.

In order for an organization to benefit from the four A's, Sheth and Sisodai (2006) posit that an organization be measured on each "A" on a 0 to 100 percent scale for a target market as each element is important. To succeed, an organization must do well on all four dimensions. However, an organization can fail simply by failing in one of the dimensions.

Marketing Mix

Previous sections of this chapter have focused on marketing at the organizational level to external markets. Familiarity with the marketing terminology and concepts that have been presented are imperative to building business skills and to applying the marketing mix. There are many complex marketing models that depict steps in the marketing process. Most begin with an appraisal and understanding of the environment and potential customers, include the design and delivery of a customer-driven marketing strategy, and end with customer loyalty and equity. A more in-depth understanding of such models is required as nurses advance in their career. At this point, understanding basic aspects of the marketing process is more meaningful. The marketing mix is the set of tactical tools used in the marketing process. The marketing mix was introduced almost 50 years ago (McCarthy, 1964) but remains a useful organizing framework for successful marketing programs. Nurse leaders at all levels can apply this framework in programs and initiatives designed to meet everyday challenges.

Although the Four Ps framework has been in existence for more than five decades, both frameworks are helpful in understanding how nurses can deliver health care effectively. The Four Ps framework is particularly well suited to a manufacturing and industrial economy and reflects a business-centric perspective. As the US economy has become more service-oriented, an alternative framework that assumes a customer-centric perspective might be more helpful in conceptualizing the ways in which a hospital's products are priced, placed, and promoted.

The Four As, therefore, describe a business environment in which the patient has far more influence over the marketing mix. This has been facilitated by the development of a digital marketplace, where services can be delivered without the more traditional boundaries established by brick and mortar buildings and regular business hours. The health care market is increasingly located in digital environments like electronic medical health records, computers and smartphones. In fact, Deloitte (2014) predicted that 75 million physician visits in North America annually would occur via some form of electronic technology.

Marketing Orientation

Organizations develop distinctive orientations or viewpoints that define their organizational culture. Hospital organizational cultures also have distinctive orientations. Orientation is usually presented in one of four ways:
- **Product orientation:** An organizational culture that assumes what the customer wants is the very best quality, regardless of cost.
- **Selling orientation:** An organizational culture that assumes the customers must be persuaded to buy the firm's products.
- **Marketing orientation:** An organizational culture that assumes the customer's needs and wants should determine the quality, price, and availability of the product.

- **Holistic orientation:** An organizational culture that focuses on the customer's needs and wants, as well as the societal impact of products that meet those needs and wants. Communication and promotion of the products involve both employees and potential customers.

Institutions that are committed to sustaining a relationship with their customers strive for a culture that can be labeled as a **marketing** or **holistic orientation**. Nurses can reflect on and evaluate these four orientations (product orientation, selling orientation, marketing orientation, and holistic orientation) and describe which of these most closely resembles their current workplace (or a prior workplace). What practices can be identified as evidence of the company's orientation? How does this company orientation affect the nurses' work? How are nurses' relationships with patients and colleagues affected by the culture that this orientation describes?

Segmentation → Targeting → Positioning
Segmentation. Segmentation is the process of dividing a market into distinct groups of buyers by identifying demographic, psychographic, and behavioral differences between them (Kotler & Keller, 2016). Segmentation has become particularly crucial as hospitals work to refine ways of predicting which patients are more or less likely to be hospitalized initially or readmitted after discharge. Identifying such segments of the population and creating relevant, effective interventions can save significant health care costs. Given this, there are many different approaches an organization can take when segmenting the target market. Generally speaking, there are four different types of market segmentation. These segmentation helps an organization to define a population into smaller "segments" so that each segment can be targeted. For example, in a health care organization, segmenting by lifestyle stage (infants, toddlers, adults, and geriatrics) can assist in identifying the specific needs of the group (Fig. 26.8).

Targeting. Targeting is the process through which an organization identifies users that they would like to reach and then advertises to them through various channels. For example, an organization may divide their population into segments by age and gender and then target specific groups, such as child-bearing women for their new maternity wing. By identifying which segment is most relevant presents the greatest opportunity for a given business (Kotler & Keller, 2016).

Market Segmentation

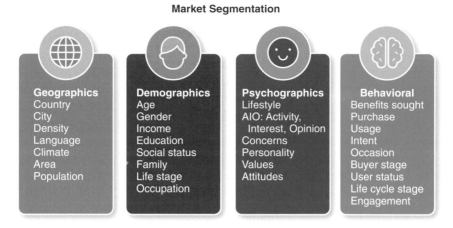

Fig. 26.8 Market segmentation.

Positioning. Positioning focuses on how the customer ultimately views the product or service in comparison to the competition. In other words, it is what a business should do to market its products and services. The more intense a positioning strategy, the more effective the market strategy is for an organization. In positioning, the marketing department creates an image for the product based on its intended audience. This is created through the use of promotion, price, place, and product.

Nurses are essential providers of the health care product and are engaged in marketing when delivering care. This is in part because interpersonal relationships are an important part of the therapeutic "product" of care. A health care organization dedicated to achieving excellence realizes this and works hard to inform all care providers and support staff about meeting customer needs. In excellence-driven organizations, particularly those with a holistic company orientation, marketing is more than a department; it is at the core of the organizational business framework. The American Organization for Nursing Leadership (AONL) has noted the identification of marketing opportunities and the development of marketing strategies as key business skills for nurse leaders in executive practice and for those with a career goal of leadership (AONL, 2015). Nurse leaders and aspiring nurse leaders who operate within a business framework benefit from understanding marketing concepts that underlie programs and initiatives in health care organizations.

Marketing Strategy

Strategic planning, a process discussed in Chapter 14, sets the overall direction for an organization. Defining the business, determining the mission, and developing long-term objectives form the basis of an organization's strategic plan. Marketing strategies and programs need to be aligned and guided by the organization-wide strategic plan (Kotler & Keller, 2016). This cannot be done effectively without investing adequate time and resources in evaluating the organization's competitive environment.

A market research approach is used for environmental scanning and is a critical step in both the strategic and marketing planning processes. During the environmental scanning, marketing departments explore and evaluate the internal and external environments to gain an understanding of demographic and societal trends, competition, and potential customers. Also, internal business performance indicators such as profits (or losses), customer and staff satisfaction, and quality indicators are evaluated. To be most effective, compilation, review, and analysis of environmental data should involve every functional area in an organization, including the nursing department. The results of the market research need to be shared across business units, and all key stakeholders need to participate in the subsequent planning process.

Marketing strategy is based on how target markets are defined. Markets are both broad and narrow. Mass marketing, which is broad, offers a product to an entire external market. Niche marketing represents a narrower view and focuses on capturing a small but important part of the market. Consider the difference between a full-service community hospital and a children's hospital. The former serves a broad market; the latter targets very specific customers: children and their families. Understanding the application of four critical concepts of segmentation, targeting, product differentiation, and positioning is essential to becoming fluent in the language of marketing.

By analyzing information about the competitive market, a hospital can determine key strategies to meet the unmet needs in its service area. A small rural community hospital in a market 200 miles from any other hospital will adopt strategies for defining and serving its market that are very different from the strategies of a large suburban hospital in a market with four other hospitals within a 25-mile radius. The rural hospital would likely position itself as a full-service facility capable of meeting the most frequently occurring needs of their target audience or the local community. For example, its profile of services is likely to include women's services, emergency care, diagnostic care, and general surgery. On the other hand, the large suburban hospital in a highly competitive market might seek to differentiate itself from competitors by creating a specialty center for heart disease or cancer. However, product or service lines are not the only way to differentiate.

In today's health care environment, differentiation is often based on quality measures and other distinctions that are prevalent today. Measures used to assess and compare the quality of health care organizations are classified one of three ways: structure, process, or outcome measures. This is known as the Donabedian model (1966).

Structure. Structure includes all of the factors that affect the context in which care is delivered. This includes the physical facility, equipment, and human resources, as well as organizational characteristics such as staff training and payment methods. These factors control how providers and patients in a health care system act and are measures of the average quality of care within a facility or system. Structure is often easy to observe and measure, and it may be the upstream cause of problems identified in process.

Process. Process is the sum of all actions that make up health care. These commonly include diagnosis, treatment, preventive care, and patient education but may be expanded to include actions taken by the patients or their families. Processes can be further classified as technical processes, how care is delivered, or interpersonal processes, which all encompass the manner in which care is delivered. According to Donabedian (1966), the measurement of process is nearly equivalent to the measurement of quality of care because process contains all acts of health care delivery. Information about process can be obtained from medical records, interviews with patients and practitioners, or direct observations of health care visits.

Outcome. Outcome contains all the effects of health care on patients or populations, including changes to health status, behavior, or knowledge as well as patient satisfaction and health-related quality of life. Outcomes are sometimes seen as the most important indicators of quality because improving patient health status is the primary goal of health care. However, accurately measuring outcomes that can be attributed exclusively to health care is very difficult. Drawing connections between process and outcomes often requires large sample populations, adjustments by case mix, and long-term follow ups as outcomes may take considerable time to become observable.

Although it is widely recognized and applied in many health care related fields, the Donabedian (1966) Model was developed to assess quality of care in clinical practice. The model does not have an implicit definition of quality care so that it can be applied to problems of broad or narrow scope. Donabedian noted that each of the three domains has advantages and disadvantages that necessitate researchers draw connections between them in order to create a chain of causation that is conceptually useful for understanding systems as well as designing experiments and interventions.

A handful of analytic frameworks for quality assessment have guided measure development initiatives in the public and private sectors. One of the most influential is the framework put forth by the Institute of Medicine (IOM, 2001), which includes the following six aims for the health care system:

Safe: Avoiding harm to patients from the care that is intended to help them.

Effective: Providing services based on scientific knowledge to all who could benefit and refraining from providing services to those not likely to benefit (avoiding underuse and misuse, respectively).

Patient-centered: Providing care that is respectful of and responsive to individual patient preferences, needs, and values and ensuring that patient values guide all clinical decisions.

Timely: Reducing waits and sometimes harmful delays for both those who receive and those who give care.

Efficient: Avoiding waste, including waste of equipment, supplies, ideas, and energy.

Equitable: Providing care that does not vary in quality because of personal characteristics such as gender, ethnicity, geographic location, and socioeconomic status.

Frameworks like the (IOM 2001) make it easier for consumers to grasp the meaning and relevance of quality measures. Studies have shown that providing consumers with a framework for understanding quality helps them value a broader range of quality indicators. For example, when consumers are given a brief, understandable explanation of safe, effective, and patient-centered care, they view all three categories as important. Further, when measures are grouped into user-friendly versions of those three IOM domains, consumers can see the meaning of the measures more clearly and understand how they relate to their own concerns about their care.

Setting marketing strategy is a shared responsibility within a health care organization. This critical activity needs to be guided by the strategic plan with input from every key stakeholder group, especially nursing, that is engaged in meeting customer needs during many and varied exchanges. Likewise, the organization's marketing team is engaged at the start when new services are planned. With multiple perspectives represented at the planning table, an organization will respond more effectively to the needs and challenges of its markets.

LEADERSHIP AND MANAGEMENT IMPLICATIONS

At a glance, nurses may consider that marketing is outside of the realm of nursing and care delivery. However, nurses (and nursing) are critical components to health care marketing. This is because marketing is about building relationships with customers so that needs and wants are satisfied and value is created. Marketing goals are incorporated in the organizational strategic plan. These goals focus on satisfying and creating value with respect to customers. They also may be focused on attracting new customers or increasing volume to enhance financial viability. Nursing is affected by such strategies and also can have an impact on goal achievement.

Health care marketing can be challenging in today's environment as health care marketing refers to marketing strategies that targets providers, insurers, suppliers, advocacy groups, patients, and families in order to increase awareness of their business and attract new patients. An understanding of the marketing framework as well as basic marketing concepts allows nurse leaders and managers to be knowledgeable contributors at the table where high-level goals are established and decisions about meeting goals are made. Nursing executive leadership generally would be involved in corporate strategic planning. Nurse leaders and managers then implement corporate strategies at the marketing management level by promoting the value nursing brings to the organization and managing the implementation of the marketing mix. Financial viability comes through the delivery of high-quality care product across varied settings and in a timely and efficient manner and price. Nurse leaders can challenge themselves and their colleagues to ask and answer questions such as:

- How do I create value for my organization?
- How do I help my organization become more patient centric?
- How do I help my organization recognize the centrality of nursing care in affecting the organization's reputation and brand?

The nurse's interactions with patients and their families are critical to patent satisfaction and good clinical outcomes. Nursing relationship management is a major component of the product/service element of the marketing mix. All employees need to focus on establishing and maintaining satisfactory customer relationships. In hospitals and other health care organizations, frontline nurses are critical in creating value for customers.

Advertising messages and promotion about nurses and nursing care can reinforce a positive image of nursing to internal and external markets. One opportunity for promotion of nursing to all markets is to have a nursing focus on the hospital's website. Nurse leaders can ensure the promotion of nursing and nursing roles in as many venues as possible to communicate the importance of nursing, nursing practice, or nursing care to potential target markets (Hoeve et al., 2013; Walker, 2014). This can be done by capturing stories of nurses who have been exemplars of compassionate and skilled care and featuring them on the hospital's intranet. These stories help define the profession and strengthen the organization's self-image as a place where branding tag lines such as "the skill to heal" and "the spirit to care" intersect with and exemplify the commitment to health and healing.

Kotler and Keller (2016) believed the future of marketing will be horizontal: consumer-to-consumer. They say that the economic downturn has not fostered trust in the marketplace and that customers now increasingly turn to one another for credible advice and information when selecting products (Kotler & Keller, 2016). In their book *Social Media for Nurses: Educating Practitioners and Patients in a Networked World,* Nelson and colleagues (2013, p. 2) noted that "Over the last several decades, the role of the patient has been evolving from passive recipients of health care to informed, empowered, and engaged patient/consumer." Digital marketplaces have empowered consumers to improve their own health literacy, research providers, and write reviews of health care services (Hotopf, 2013). Nurse managers can work with their colleagues to creatively imagine how social media (promotion) can be used to leverage this technology as well as this growing cultural trend of patient-to-patient trust to build patient loyalty and brand strength. Nurse leaders and managers are responsible for promoting the merits of nursing service internally and externally.

Finally, another marketing application for nurse leaders and managers relates to workforce characteristics. Nurses who are employed make up an internal market, and the pool of nurses who are potential new hires makes up an external market. In these instances, nurses are the customers. Nurse leaders can use marketing to increase "customer" retention and attraction. When considering nurse retention and recruitment, leaders consider what value proposition (product) the nursing department or unit offers to nurses. Highlighting department or unit characteristics deemed important, such as shared governance and professional development opportunities, provides details about the product. Leaders can give attention to the unit (place) where nurses provide service. Consideration of the physical layout and whether the unit design is conducive to an efficient and effective workflow is important. Nurse leaders can ensure that nurses' salaries are competitive and that nurses do not feel underpaid and undervalued (Evans, 2013). Market research in collaboration with the human resources department can analyze salaries (price) in the external market and adjust accordingly.

CURRENT ISSUES AND TRENDS

The hospital industry continues to evolve, streamlining and improving patient care, integrating big data and moving from a fee-for-service to a fee-for-outcome payment model. The hospitals of yesterday were quite different from the sprawling health care centers that are common in the United States today. Although the previous focus was on payment and legal changes that would be required to move health care forward, more recently the focus has been more about how the private sector has responded and shifted to answer new challenges. A brief environmental analysis of marketing in health care reveals an emphasis on issues of social media, cost and transparency, patient-centered care, the nursing shortage, geriatric workforce shortage, work–life balance, and data analytics.

A Dramatically Changed Marketplace

Overall, the first half of the 20th century began with childbirth, influenza, and everyday trauma inflicting high casualties. Medical education improved such that in 1911, the average patient seeing an average doctor for an average problem had better than a fifty-fifty chance of benefiting from the transaction. By the mid 1950s, progress in sanitation, immunizations, and antibiotics led to the eradication of polio and smallpox, the expectation of living to old age, and new wonder drugs. Knowledge, technologies, and entrepreneurism accelerated ever faster. Acute diseases have been replaced by new illnesses of body and psyche such as coronary heart disease, chronic fatigue syndrome, pain syndromes, arthritis, cancers, teenage suicide, and addictions of all varieties. Gauging the quality of health care systems is often difficult and restricted by the availability of data. One method for measuring quality is to look at mortality rates, which, though influenced by a myriad of factors, are in part affected by the quality of the health care system in addressing diseases for which mortality is amenable to health care.

Social Media

In this era of information and communication technology, every sector is taking advantage of social media, and the health care industry is no exception. In particular, social media can help engage patients, providers, and the public with relevant and timely information as well as communicate the value and credibility of health care organization. Research has demonstrated that posts with *links to more information* are the most preferred type of content on social media. In addition, 30% of consumers posited that social media is the primary way to receive information. Thus, any organization that desires to be in the public domain has to use social media.

Health care has now become patient-centered which makes patient engagement and satisfaction a top priority, hence the need to implement a social media strategy. Hospitals need social media experts, a new emerging opportunity, as well as a public relations department. Employing a social media expert has become one of the necessities for many health care organizations. For example, organizations can facilitate patient empowerment and patient education by enabling and engaging in patient forums and research networks online. For example, many organizations allow patients to manage their own health conditions by discussing treatment options with other patients who have similar conditions through social media. Moreover, organizations can use social media to physician alignment and collaboration.

Another example is *The Medical Directors Forum,* a social networking site for medical directors that provides a verified, secure, closed-loop environment for peer-to-peer interaction. The resources on this site include a comprehensive library, discussion groups, calendar postings, and alerts. The site also provides dedicated group pages for medical directors working in a wide range of sectors, including hospital, veterans' affairs, Medicare, group practice, employer, behavioral health, managed care, correctional facility, and long-term care.

It is important to understand that social media has the potential to be both beneficial and challenging to an organization. Health Insurance Portability and Accountability Act (HIPAA) compliance is one the biggest challenges of social media-facing organizations today.

Health care professionals are leery of entering into the social media fray for fear that they will compromise patient privacy, either through what they post or by exposing their networks to viruses or hacking. Although HIPAA offers specific guidelines on how to safely post information, comments, photos, or videos online without violating patient privacy laws, organizations must be diligent in their online security. Some of the guidelines include "de-identification" of patients by removing or omitting names, insurance or Social Security numbers, date of birth, photos, and eliminating specific details of rare medical issues, including the dates they occur. Health care providers can also obtain consent from patients to post their photos on social media sites.

When nurses post on social media sites such as Facebook, HIPAA and privacy violations may occur. A robust social media policy needs to exist and be enforced. Health care professionals worry that their presence on social media may label them as unprofessional with potential patients. Thus, it is important to consider the extent and reach of posts as a medical professional. Every post does offer more detail into you as a person, much less as a health care professional and care should be taken to post only content that is appropriate. The American College of Physicians and the Federation of State Medical Boards have been working on guidelines for health care professionals that can help physicians and providers make better choices regarding what is posted on social media. Overall, health care organizations have a duty to protect patients and providers by ensuring that the best possible information is made public to its customers through social media.

Cost and Transparency

Price transparency in health care is an important issue to watch for in health care. Prior to January 1, 2019, California was the only state that required hospitals to post their prices online for consumers to view. As of January 1, 2019, the CMS required all hospitals to post prices online (CMS, 2019b). However, prices don't provide the whole story as a patient's costs remain non-specific. For example, if a patient has a hip replacement surgery at an outpatient center versus in a hospital as an inpatient, the costs are going to vary considerably and include a wide range of variables. To aid consumers in understanding the billing process, the state of Maryland hosts a website where total cost is available for some procedures. The site shows the hospital costs and a potential total cost per condition, along with some quality metrics related to that condition for individual hospitals. This is a good example of how states can help improve transparency for consumers, enabling them to make informed choices about their health care.

An important consideration for nurses related to cost and value is that current payment models do not unbundle nursing care from room and board, thus making adjustments for nursing intensity in billing mechanisms impossible. Recommendations for incorporating a nursing intensity adjustment to existing inpatient billing could lead to determination of the economic value of nursing care. The marketing mix could more closely reflect the "price" of nursing care, which would contribute to the establishment of a value-based purchasing system for hospitals (Kavanagh et al., 2012).

There will be continued efforts and initiatives to address the costs of nursing care and subsequent reimbursement decisions in order to deliver and market cost-effective and efficient care. Nurses also need to stay informed about, and engaged in, evolving accountable payment models in order to create care delivery systems that prevent negative outcomes for which reimbursement will be withheld and/or to capture payment as an Advance Practice Provider. The shift away from fee-for-service models places an increasing emphasis on customer relationships and increasing pressure on nurses to manage such relationships and build value for the customer and the system (Healthcare Financial Management Association, 2015).

Patient-Centered Care

The focus on patient-centered care began in the 1970s, but implementation remains an issue for many health care organizations. Varied patient-centered models and frameworks exist. Attributes in patient-centeredness include patient satisfaction, the patient experience of care, patient engagement, and shared decision-making. Evidence supports the view that patient-centered care improves patient outcomes and is one approach to addressing racial, ethnic, and socioeconomic disparities in health care and health care outcomes (Long, 2012; Radwin et al., 2013).

Planetree is a designation that differentiates a hospital on the basis of excellence in patient- and person-centered care. The Planetree philosophy reveals a simple view of what it means to be patient-centered (Planetree, 2018). Components of the Planetree model that move an organization toward a culture of patient-centeredness can be found on their website. It is easy to determine the importance of patient-centeredness to marketing goals and ultimately to patient satisfaction, therefore models for delivery of patient-centered care will continue to evolve (Millenson & Macri, 2012).

Nursing Shortage

The US is projected to experience a shortage of registered nurses (RNs) that is expected to intensify as Baby Boomers age and the need for health care grows (American Association of Colleges of Nursing [AACN], 2020). According to the Bureau of Labor Statistics (BLS, 2015), RNs are listed among the top occupations in terms of job growth through 2026. Moreover, the Bureau projects the need for an additional 203,700 new RNs though 2026 to fill newly created positions and to replace retiring nurses. Buerhaus et al, (2017) estimated that one million RNs will retire by 2030 because according to a 2018 survey, nearly 51% of the RN workforce is aged 50 or older. Compounding this concern is that by 2050, the number of US residents aged 65 and over will almost double to 83.7 million. With this larger number of older adults, there will be an increased need for geriatric care, including care for individuals with chronic diseases and comorbidities.

Despite these needs, US nursing schools have turned away more than 75,000 qualified applicants from baccalaureate and graduate nursing programs in 2018 due to insufficient number of faculty, clinical sites, classroom space, and clinical preceptors, and budget constraints. The AACN (2020) projected a shortage of 260,000 nurses nationally by 2024 (Irish, 2014). This trend calls for internal marketing initiatives that address nurse turnover, job satisfaction, and occupational and organizational commitment. External marketing challenges will be encountered by hospitals seeking a more qualified nurse workforce (i.e., those with baccalaureate [BSN] degrees). This is supported by the American Nurses Credentialing Center's (ANCC) Magnet Recognition Program® (ANCC, 2016) as well as studies finding that higher percentages of RNs with BSN degrees in hospitals are linked to lower patient mortality rates (Aiken et al., 2014; Blegen et al., 2013; Kutney-Lee et al., 2013). This calls for competitive marketing strategies to recruit successfully from the target market of BSN-prepared nurses.

Geriatric Workforce Shortage

The baby boomer population as a whole will increase the demand for health care services over the next several decades (Irish, 2014). The combination of the aging of the baby boom population, increases in life expectancy, and decreases in the number of younger persons will mean that older adults make up a much larger percentage of the US population than ever before. As a result, the scarcity of workers specializing in the care of older adults, the eldercare workforce, will be even more pronounced (Bureau of Labor Statistics, 2015). This is an external marketing opportunity to recruit young people into nursing.

Work–Life Balance

About two-thirds of the close to 3 million nurses who live in the United States work in hospitals. Generally speaking, hospitals are high-stress environments. In one study, only 23% of female participants who worked in health care indicated that they were able to balance their personal and professional lives well (Delina & Raya, 2013). Research shows the importance of caring for oneself in order to provide outstanding patient care. Fatigue can lead to dangerous or costly mistakes, thereby affecting one's professional reputation and mental well-being (Steege & Pinekenstein, 2016). Nurse leaders need to advocate for policies that promote work–life balance in health care organizations and use this in internal marketing in order to improve retention of qualified nurses and increase the value of care provided to their customers.

Data and Analytics

The health care industry is at a point where core, foundational technology for the end user is almost fully digitized and automated. Structured data captured in data warehouse-centric models and electronic health records (EHRs) provides information that can be executed on in real time to improve patient care. Reducing the prevalence of hospital-acquired conditions (HACs) continues to be an output of new technology and tools combining with data and analytics. Early warning systems for sepsis that utilize continually updated EHR data, and subsequent treatment protocols, are helping organizations successfully lower sepsis rates nationwide. Algorithms for fall risk management, catheter-associated urinary tract infection (CAUTI) prevention, and diabetes management are now commonplace.

Avoiding costly and preventable readmissions is one area where health care has seen the valuable application of data and machine learning. Conservative estimates put the cost of readmissions at more than $41 billion annually for hospitals, and 30-day readmissions continue to be a quality measure for health care organizations. As hospital outcome data become more transparent, hospitals with excellent outcomes have a marketing advantage.

CONCLUSION

In a marketplace where patient needs and wants are the primary drivers of value, nurses are crucial participants in the marketing efforts of the health care organizations where they work. An understanding of the concepts and tools that are the foundation of modern marketing will enable nurses and nurse managers to advocate for their profession within health care organizations, recruit and retain high-quality peers, and build relationships with patients that facilitate meaningful exchange.

RESEARCH NOTE

Source: Elrod, J.K., & Fortenberry, J.L. (2018). Formulating productive marketing communications strategy: A major health system's experience. *BMC Health Services Research, 18*(1), 1–5.

Purpose

Health care organizations traditionally have selected marketing strategies from a standard marketing communications mix, including advertising (i.e., the paid use of mass media to deliver messages), personal selling (i.e., the use of sales agents to personally deliver messages), sales promotion (i.e., the use of incentives, such as contests and free giveaways, to encourage patronage), direct marketing (i.e., the delivery of messages via mail, the Internet, and similar routes directly to customers), and public relations (i.e., the use of publicity and other unpaid promotional methods to deliver messages). The purpose of this article is to describe one health system's expansion of marketing strategies.

Discussion

Willis-Knighton Health System decided to forge a new and different communications pathway, with this innovative course fostering its expansion initiatives and providing insights that influence its communications approach. The Willis-Knighton Health System was a small system desirous of growth. However, despite having a skill at identifying innovations emerging outside of the health care industry for use within that led to numerous product-related advancements that were driving growth, it also had to communicate effectively with target audiences. Submitting press releases to news media organizations and requesting these be placed with associated stories was not an effective strategy, so they experimented with and embraced advertising at a time when this was not common. Advertising required payment. They pursued two media types: newspaper advertising and billboard advertising. For example, the initial billboard advertisement provided a public service message promoting childhood immunizations. Advertising was well received by stakeholders. This evolved into a full communications strategy and formal marketing operation.

Application to Practice

Without effective communications as a centerpiece of the marketing strategy, current and prospective patients will remain unaware of available offerings. Health care organizations are a key community resource for improving health and wellness, yet this needs to be effectively communicated. Forging a new pathway created expertise in provider-patient engagement initiatives and leading to an enduring marketing communications approach. Being a trailblazer gave the organization an advantage over other competitors. As a result there was the opportunity to innovate, leading to communications prowess, informed audiences, and lasting mutual benefits resulting in growth.

CASE STUDY

Health System A is the only children's hospital in Soufriere for the last 75 years. This system has the entire market share for pediatric hospitalizations and many pediatric services. For the past five years, Health System B has conducted market research. This research required environmental scanning. Some actions included exploring and evaluating the internal and external environments, examining demographic and societal trends, examining competitors, and searching for potential customers. Findings revealed a need for children's services both inpatient and outpatient.

The results of the market research were shared across business units, and all key stakeholders had the opportunities to participate in the evaluation of the data and the planning process. Therefore, after 5 long years, the C-suite leadership in Health System B decided that it was time to build a children's hospital.

Mid-level leadership thought that continuing to provide supportive services for teenagers was sufficient and were not motivated with the future goal to penetrate the Children's space. Many thought that since Health System A was Magnet, it would be very difficult to penetrate.

You are a Nursing Director and the liaison for marketing. You noticed that one of the reasons Health System A is increasing their market share is because customers prefer to go to one system for all services. You communicate to marketing that ensuring customer knowledge will be the key in gaining market share. You started to brainstorm ways to build the new children's brand. Using the framework below how will you develop value for both current customers and new ones. Below here are the updated 4As with their prompts:

Acceptability: How will you ensure that this new service meets and exceeds the customers needs?

Affordability: Will old and new clientele have the resources to pay for an improved service within the community?

Accessibility: Will old and new clientele see this service as convenient?

Awareness: How will you ensure awareness in a market where Health Care System A, has had the market share for 75 years? What type of content will you need to differentiate your system?

CRITICAL THINKING EXERCISE

1. Review your organization's mission, vision, and values statement. How are these components marketed to individuals such as:
   a. The organization's employees?
   b. The organization's customers?
   c. The organization's stakeholders?
   d. The community at large?
2. Identify two to four service lines of your organization.
   a. What methods are used to market these service lines?
   b. Are these methods effective? What measures are used?
   c. How could the marketing efforts be enhanced?
3. Identify your organization's brand.
   a. What does your brand represent?
   b. How is your brand related to your organization?
   c. Does your organization's brand need to be updated? Why or why not?
4. In their book *Marketing Management,* Kotler and Keller (2016) suggested that marketing communications allow companies to link their brands to other people, places, events, experiences, feelings, and things.
   a. Identify three major organizations, their brand, and the target audience for their brand.
   b. Have these organizations changed their brand over time? If so, how?
   c. What factors may influence an organization to change its brand?
5. Often, such communications are understood in terms of advertisements or social media campaigns designed to promote a company's brand. In health care, however, the most important link between brands and experiences or feelings depends largely on communication between one patient and one nurse. Using your organization's website, how does your organization brand and market its nursing services? What strategies would you use to enhance the marketing of nursing services in your organization to:
   a. New nurses
   b. Current patients
   c. Potential patients
   d. Stakeholders

6. In 2015, Johnson & Johnson (J&J) pulled advertising from ABC's "The View" after controversial comments were made about nurses by the show's host. The company decided to "put some of the money we saved" by donating a dollar for every photo shared through the company's website to National Nurses Association.
   a. What potential harm, if any, did J&J avoid by pulling its ads?
   b. What does this say about the importance of marketing?
   c. What implications does this have for nursing as a profession?
7. Simon Sinek (2009), author of the national bestseller, *Start With Why,* posits that good marketing and good leadership begins with purpose, not product. View the TED talk: How Great Leaders Inspire Action found at https://www.ted.com/talks/simon_sinek_how_great_leaders_inspire_action?language=en
   a. What is your personal "why, how, and what"?
   b. What is your organization's ""why, how, and what"?
   c. What is the relationship between your own "why" and the "why" of your organization?
   d. As a nurse manager, how can you identify or screen for an individual's "why" in your recruitment and retention process?
8. At Good Hope Hospital, the HCAHPS scores for physician communication are consistently lower than those for nurses. Research has demonstrated that patients are more likely to accept the instructions of their physicians without question, despite having concerns about the instructions (Kennedy et al., 2013). Using this research as a basis, create a list of possible marketing campaigns to increase the physicians' HCAHPS scores at Good Hope Hospital.
9. Between Memorial Day and Labor Day, research has demonstrated that the risk of death and injury increasing significantly among teens aged 13 to 18. To raise awareness of these risks, the Arkansas Children's Hospital developed and marketed the "#100DeadliestDays" campaign. Search the web for examples of other marketing campaigns that are health related.
   a. How are these campaigns used?
   b. Are these campaigns successful?
   c. What strategies would you use to improve these campaigns?

10. Nurses must often manage patient care circumstances that require a complex balance between respecting individual autonomy, maintaining a high standard of care, and providing excellent customer service that is the basis for marketing. An indigenous patient is nearing the end of his life. As you discuss palliative care with the patient, who is now unable to leave his hospital bed, he makes a request. Because he subscribes to a deeply held set of religious beliefs, the patient asks that you facilitate adherence to end-of-life rituals involving ceremonies performed around an open fire.

a. How would you respond to this request?
b. What information and/or guidelines would you investigate and use to assist you in your response.
c. What elements of this request would you be able to honor and in what way?
d. How would this patient experience reflect your organization's mission and vision?
e. How would this patient experience reflect your organization's marketing plan?

REFERENCES

Aiken, L. H., Sloane, D. M., Bruyneel L., Van den Heede, K., Griffiths, P., Busse, R., et al. (2014). Nurse staffing and education and hospital mortality in nine European countries: A retrospective observational study. *Lancet, 383*, 1824–1830.

American Association of Colleges of Nursing (AACN). (2020). *Nursing shortage.* https://www.aacnnursing.org/news-information/fact-sheets/nursing-shortage.

Americ Marketing Association. (2020). *Definition of marketing.* https://www.ama.org/the-definition-of-marketing-what-is-marketing/.

American Nurses Credentialing Center (2016). *Magnet Recognition Program®: Testimonials and case studies.* https://www.nursingworld.org/organizational-programs/pathway/overview/testimonials-and-case-studies/.

American Organization for Nursing Leadership (AONL). (2015). *Nurse executive competencies.* http://www.aone.org/resources/nurse-executive-competencies.pdf.

Armstrong, G., & Kotler, P. (2017). *Marketing: An introduction* (13th ed.). New York, NY: Pearson Education, Inc.

Blegen, M. A., Goode, C. J., & Park, S. H. (2013). Baccalaureate education in nursing and patient outcomes. *Journal of Nursing Administration, 43*(2), 89–94.

Buerhaus, P. I., Skinner, L. E., Auerbach, D. I., & Staiger, D. O. (2017). State of the registered nurse workforce as a new era of health reform emerges. *Nursing Economic, 35*(5), 229–237.

Bureau of Labor Statistics. (2015). *Employment projections – 2014-24* (BLS Publication No. USDL-15-2327). http://www.bls.gov/news.release/pdf/ecopro.pdf.

Byrnes, J. (2015). The value proposition in action. *Healthcare Financial Management, 69*(5), 106–107.

Centers for Medicare & Medicaid Services (CMS). (2019a). *Historical.* https://www.cms.gov/Research-Statistics-Data-and-Systems/Statistics-Trends-and-Reports/NationalHealthExpendData/NationalHealthAccountsHistorical.

Centers for Medicare & Medicaid Services (CMS). (2019b). *Trump administration announces historic price transparency requirements to increase competition and lower healthcare costs for all Americans.* https://www.cms.gov/newsroom/press-releases/trump-administration-announces-historic-price-transparency-requirements-increase-competition-and.

Delina, G., & Raya, R. P. (2013). A study on work-life balance in working women. *International Journal of Commerce, Business and Management, 2*(5), 274–282.

Deloitte. *eVisits: The 21st century housecall.* (2014). https://www2.deloitte.com/content/dam/Deloitte/au/Documents/technology-media-telecommunications/deloitte-au-tmt-evisits-011014.pdf.

Donabedian, A. (1966). Evaluating the quality of medical care. *Milbank Memorial Fund Quarterly, 44*(3), 166–206.

Elrod, J. K., & Fortenberry, J. L. (2018). Formulating productive marketing communications strategy: A major health system's experience. *BMC Health Services Research, 18*(1), 1–5.

Evans, J. D. (2013). Factors influencing recruitment and retention of nurse educators reported by current nurse faculty. *Journal of Professional Nursing, 29*(1), 11–20.

Healthcare Financial Management Association. (2015). Developing a blueprint for accountable care. *Healthcare Financial Management, 69*(11), 1–8.

Hoeve, Y., Jansen, G., & Roodbol, P. (2013). The nursing profession: Public image, self-concept, and professional identify. *Journal of Advanced Nursing, 70*(2), 295–309.

Hotopf, M. (2013). How patients' review sites will change health care. *Journal of Health Services Research and Policy, 18*(4), 251–254.

Institute of Medicine (IOM). (2001). *Crossing the quality chasm: A new health care system for the 21st century*: Washington, DC: National Academies Press.

Irish, K. (2014). Trends affecting the future of home healthcare. *Home Healthcare Nurse, 32*(9), 567–568.

Kavanagh, K. T., Cimiotti, J. P., Abusalem, S., & Coty, M. (2012). Moving healthcare quality forward with nursing-sensitive value-based purchasing. *Journal of Nursing Scholarship, 44*(4), 385–395.

Kennedy, B., Craig, J. B., Wetsel, M., Reimels, E., & Wright, J. (2013). Three nursing interventions' impact on HCAHPS scores. *Journal of Nursing Care Quality, 28*(4), 327–334.

Kennett, P. A., Henson, S. W., Crow, S. M., & Hartman, S. J. (2005). Key tasks in healthcare marketing: Assessing importance and current level of knowledge. *Journal of Health & Human Services Administration, 27*(4), 414–427.

Kotler, P., & Keller, K. L. (2016). *Marketing management* (15th ed.). New York, NY: Pearson.

Kutney-Lee, A., Sloane, D. M., & Aiken, L. H. (2013). An increase in the number of nurses with baccalaureate degrees is linked to lower rates of post-surgery mortality. *Health Affairs, 32*(3), 579–586.

Long, L. (2012). Impressing patients while improving HCAHPS. *Nursing Management, 43*(12), 32–37.

McCarthy, E. J. (1964). *Basic marketing: A managerial approach* (rev. ed.). New York, NY: McGraw-Hill.

Millenson, M. L., & Macri, J. (2012, March). Will the Affordable Care Act move patient-centeredness to center stage? Timely analysis of immediate health policy issues. *Urban Quick Strike Series*, 1–10. http://www.rwjf.org/en/library/research/2012/03/will-the-affordable-care-act-move-patient-centeredness-to-center.html?cid=XEM_A5765.

Nelson, R., Joos, I., & Wolf, D. M. (2013). *Social media for nurses: Educating practitioners and patients in a networked world.* New York, NY: Springer Publishing Company.

Planetree. (2018). *Person-centered care.* https://www.planetree.org/.

Radwin, L. E., Cabral, H. J., & Woodworth, T. S. (2013). Effects of race and language on patient-centered cancer nursing care and patient outcomes. *Journal of Health Care for the Poor and Underserved, 24,* 619–632.

Sheth, J. N., & Sisodia, R. (2006). *The 4 A's of marketing: Creating value for customer, company and society.* Milton Park, UK: Routledge.

Sinek, S. (2009). *Start with why: How great leaders inspire everyone to take action.* Westminster, MD:Penguin Group.

Steege, L. M., & Pinekenstein, B. (2016). Addressing occupational fatigue in nurses. *Journal of Nursing Administration, 46*(4), 193–200.

Walker, L. (2014). Promoting nursing's professionalism. *Nursing New Zealand, 20*(3), 2.

Answers for Next-Generation NCLEX ® Case Studies and Item Types

CHAPTER 1: LEADERSHIP AND MANAGEMENT PRINCIPLES

Case Study

The medical/surgical units at St. Helens Community Hospital are busy with a complex mix of patient diagnoses and conditions and have a staff of 88 employees, with a few nurses of long tenure, but mostly new graduates and nurses with less than 2 years of experience. They have four very different leaders:

1. Nurse Manager Dan has 3 years of experience as a nurse manager. He prefers to tell the followers what to do and how to do it in order to get tasks done.
2. Nurse Manager Maria has 3 years of experience as a nurse manager. She prefers to use her outgoing personality and likability to achieve success, using positive motivation and team morale.
3. Nurse Manager Jorge has 3 years of experience as a nurse manager. He prefers to have a hands-off approach and let his employees assume responsibility in the decision-making process.
4. Nurse Manager Olivia has 3 years of experience as a nurse manager. Her unit is busy with a complex mix of patient diagnoses and conditions. She prefers to use her inspiring energy and personality to create a magnetic workplace by engaging with others, centering on followers' needs and goals, and thus raising each other to higher levels of motivation.

SLO/Objective: Analyze leadership styles for effectiveness
NGN Item Type: Matrix
Cognitive Skill: Analyze cues

Question

Use the numbered scenarios above, to indicate the best approach and priority area to lead the unit.

Nursing Situation	Best Approach
The entire facility has a power outage in a storm. Backup generators do not come on in the ICU.	#1
Nurses complain about being understaffed for Christmas vacation.	#4
Nurses have organized a shared governance committee.	#2
The bariatric unit does not have an adequate number of Hoyer lifts, and the NM is concerned about future back injuries.	#3

Answers/Rationales

1. The primary priority approach is #1. This situation will require an all-hands-on-deck approach, and a leader who does not operate in isolation, but one who requires cooperation and collaboration: specifically, one who will guide and motivate nurses to achieve the goal of patient safety during a power outage supported by effective followers.
2. The second priority approach is #2. In this situation the leader has empowered the nursing staff using a shared governance committee. In this case, she is acting as a servant leader. The leader is ensuring that other people's highest priorities are being addressed so that she promotes personal growth and helps others become freer and more autonomous.
3. The third priority approach is #3. In this situation, the leader is recognizing that the bariatric unit has increasing admissions and that there are not adequate resources to manage their care. This is a great example of clinical leadership using interpersonal understanding.

4. The fourth priority approach is #4. In this situation nurses are voicing a potential issue. This scenario is future-oriented and provides the leader with the opportunity to model an authentic leader approach. She can use self-awareness: How would I feel in this situation? She would use an internal moral perspective, determine what is relevant, and be open about the situation with subordinates.

Reference: Huber & Joseph (2021). Chapter 1.

CHAPTER 5: MANAGING TIME AND STRESS

Case Study

Caitlin has been working on 2 North for 6 months since graduating from nursing school. Every day seems stressful, and every new situation makes her feel like she does not have what it takes to be a nurse. She often feels overwhelmed. There are very few senior experienced nurses on the unit, and they are burned out from constantly orienting new nurses. Productivity and effectiveness are low. Caitlin is concerned about her own coping yet also wants to build a higher-functioning and more resilient team. There are lots of recommended stress reduction techniques. Key to success is choosing techniques that are practical and able to be accomplished by a busy nurse daily.

SLO/Objective: Determine highest priority actions
NGN Item Type: Cloze
Cognitive Skill: Take action

Choose the most likely options for the information missing from the question below by selecting from the list of options provided.

Question

Caitlin spent 2 days observing the employees on the unit and noticed that they were always busy, skipped breaks and lunch, drank lots of coffee, and never had down time, confirming her personal perceptions. The top three strategies an employee may use while at work to relieve stress are:

1. _____ (Drink 8 glasses of water a day),
2. _____ (Use your getaway place),
3. _____ (Take scheduled lunches).

Options for Strategies
Getting a massage at the massage parlor 10 min from work
Eat French fries
Drink 8 glasses of water a day
Taking scheduled lunches
Taking a long walk in nature
Taking yoga classes in your neighborhood
Eat at your desk
Use your getaway place

Answers/Rationales
The only three correct anti-stress strategies that are feasible while at work include drinking water for hydration, taking scheduled breaks, and going to your getaway spot. The other choices will require that you leave work (massage parlor 10 min away, walk in nature, and yoga class in your neighborhood) and engage in activities that are not healthy (eat at desk and eat French fries).

Reference: Huber & Joseph (2021). Chapter 5.

CHAPTER 8: COMMUNICATION LEADERSHIP

Case study: Nurse Manager

Tyler has been in his job for 9 months in a busy academic medical center and is just beginning to settle in. He has noticed a spike in medication errors on the unit. It is difficult to manage health care providers' incoming orders as well as the confusion and complexity of multiple provider teams (e.g., neuro, cardiovascular, oncology) rounding independently and making medication and treatment changes that sometimes conflict. Tyler just got the latest data on his unit's quality and safety measures. The medication error rate has increased. He calls the Chair of the unit's Shared Governance Council (SGC) to help evaluate ideas to address communication breakdowns.

SLO/Objective: Apply knowledge of communication theory to determine effective actions
NGN Item Type: Extended multiple response
Cognitive Skill: Analyze cues

Question

Which communication strategies will Tyler, the nurse manager, use to support effective communication interventions? **Select all that apply.**

_____ A. Confrontive communication style

__X___ B. AHRQ's CUS assertive statements.

_____ C. Incident reporting

__X___ D. Crucial conversations

_____ E. Formal referral to immediate supervisor

__X__ F. TeamSTEPPS SBAR

Answers/Rationales

The correct responses (AHRQ's CUS assertive statements, crucial conversations, and TeamSTEPPS SBAR) are proactive communication tools or strategies to enable a constructive outcome. However, the incorrect responses (confrontive communication style, incident reporting, and referral to immediate supervisor) are all disciplinary in nature.

Reference: Huber & Joseph (2021). Chapter 8.

CHAPTER 13: DECENTRALIZATION AND GOVERNANCE

Case study

After 1 year of employment on 3 South, nurse Maria was invited to join the unit's Shared Governance Council Committee (SGCC). Maria has listened to her fellow nurses complain about not being listened to or valued, and the unit's nurse turnover rate is climbing. Morale is low. She is thrilled that this will be a venue to communicate ways to mitigate the increasing turnover and to communicate her peer's perceptions of being powerless and not having a voice. However, it is important that the SGCC operate as an effective structure. At the first meeting, Maria decided to observe and gain trust with the group versus voicing her concerns. After the meeting, Maria made an appointment with the chairperson (Elyssa) to discuss her observations about how the SGCC operates. Elyssa was open to her feedback.

SLO/Objective: Utilize competencies of shared governance
NGN Item Type: Extended multiple response
Cognitive Skill: Take action

Choose the most likely options to complete the question below.

Question

Which actions, observed while on the committee, indicate that the Shared Governance Council is demonstrating effectiveness? **Select all that apply.**

1. The council meetings are skillful.
2. The council enables leadership.
3. The information discussed is useful.
4. The committee goals are supported by management.
5. The council members are empowered to act.
6. The council is improving patient safety.
7. The council is improving nursing practice.

Answers/Rationales

All responses apply and define council effectiveness.

Reference: Huber & Joseph (2021). Chapter 13.

According to the General Effective Multilevel Theory for Shared Governance (GEMS), there are seven competencies that demonstrate council effectiveness, and these are all provided as the correct responses.

CHAPTER 21: NURSING WORKFORCE STAFFING AND MANAGEMENT

Case Study

Nurse Manager Dan's budget has been cut and is projected to have increasing cuts over the next 2 years due to COVID-19 implications. He made the decision to not hire new employees and use the existing employees to cover staffing needs. Employees on his unit are feeling overworked. Many employees are being asked to do mandatory overtime without adequate compensation. Dan's director was told by human resources that employees are feeling overwhelmed with the increasing staffing demands without adequate compensation. The director pulls Dan's non-salary YTD expense report to examine where opportunities may exist to reallocate funds toward staffing.

SLO/Objective: Evaluate solutions to reallocate funding for staffing management
NGN Item Type: Extended multiple response
Cognitive Skill: Take action

Question

Utilizing the non-salary expense report, the director makes the recommendation for Dan to redirect dollars from some itemized items in the budget. Dan decides to redirect budgetary dollars. Which options indicate an effective strategy to fund staffing?

Select all that apply.

1. Redirect dollars from food service to staffing.
2. Redirect dollars from equipment rental to staffing.
3. Redirect dollars from departmental supplies to staffing.
4. Redirect dollars from travel to staffing.
5. Redirect dollars from other expenses to staffing.

YTD Non-Salary Expense Report

Non-salary expense	Actual	Budget	Var %	Prior
Purchase professional	350	0	0.0%	0
Patient non-chargeable (e.g., Kleenex, bath wipes, deodorant)	100,655	60,656	(65.0%)	59,999
Drugs	0	178	100.0%	0
Food service	6,252	4,200	(48.0)%	4,736
Medical supplies	0	449	100.0%	0
Department supplies	8,668	8,546	(1.4)%	5, 429
Forms and access to databases	1,025	1,255	18.3%	1,204
Minor equipment (e.g., vital signs machine, IV vein finder)	0	1,080	100%	0
Equipment rental (e.g., wound VAC, low bed, bariatric bed)	6,148	6,800	9.5%	1,529
Publications	350	50	(600)%	44
Dues and Memberships	0	8	100%	0
Travel	567	1,058	46.4%	1,325
Other expenses (e.g., outside catering, holiday parties, recognition trophies)	0	8000	100%	3,000
Total non-salary expenses	124,015	92,280	34.3%	77,266

Answers/Rationales

- #4 Redirect dollars from travel for staffing and
- #5 Redirect dollars from Other Expenses

Answer #4: The itemized budget line for "travel" is $1,058, but only $540 has been utilized. Therefore, these funds may be redirected toward staffing and traveling can be put on hold.

Answer #5: The itemize budget line for "other expenses" is $8,000, and $0 has been utilized. Therefore, the $8,000 may be redirected to staffing fully or partially. To consider the redirection of partial budgeted funds, the manager must look at historical spending in that category. They may keep the same or reduce the amount previously allocated.

Reference: Huber & Joseph (2021). Chapter 21 and Chapter 22.

Page numbers followed by *b*, *t*, and *f* indicate boxes, tables, and figures, respectively